Primary Immunodeficiency Diseases: Diagnosis and Management

Primary Immunodeficiency Diseases: Diagnosis and Management

Editor: Ocean Garfield

hayle medical

New York

Hayle Medical,
750 Third Avenue, 9th Floor,
New York, NY 10017, USA

Visit us on the World Wide Web at:
www.haylemedical.com

ISBN 978-1-64647-573-5 (Hardback)

Cataloging-in-Publication Data

Primary immunodeficiency diseases : diagnosis and management / edited by Ocean Garfield.
p. cm.
Includes bibliographical references and index.
ISBN 978-1-64647-573-5
1. Immunological deficiency syndromes. 2. Immunological deficiency syndromes--Diagnosis.
3. Immunological deficiency syndromes--Treatment. 4. Immunodeficiency. 5. Immunologic diseases.
I. Garfield, Ocean.
RC606 .P75 2023
616.979--dc23

Contents

Preface

This book aims to highlight the current researches and provides a platform to further the scope of innovations in this area. This book is a product of the combined efforts of many researchers and scientists, after going through thorough studies and analysis from different parts of the world. The objective of this book is to provide the readers with the latest information of the field.

Immunodeficiency refers to a condition in which the immune system's ability to fight infections is weakened or missing. The majority of cases occur because of extrinsic factors, which impact the patient's immune system, such as nutrition and HIV infection. Primary immunodeficiency (PID) is a disease in which a portion of the body's immune system is absent, or is not able to function properly. A condition will be considered PID if the cause of immune deficiency is not secondary in nature, such as a condition caused due to drug treatment or other disease. The diagnosis of PID includes evaluation of immunoglobulin levels and a full blood cell count. The treatment of these diseases relies on the severity of the abnormality. Majority of the treatments are palliative and passive, which can be categorized into two modalities, which include boosting the immune system and managing infections. This book contains a detailed explanation of the various diagnostic and management techniques associated with primary immunodeficiency diseases. Those in search of information to further their knowledge will be greatly assisted by it.

I would like to express my sincere thanks to the authors for their dedicated efforts in the completion of this book. I acknowledge the efforts of the publisher for providing constant support. Lastly, I would like to thank my family for their support in all academic endeavors.

Editor

1

Evaluating STAT5 Phosphorylation as a Mean to Assess T Cell Proliferation

Michael Bitar [1†], Andreas Boldt [1†], Marie-Theres Freitag [1], Bernd Gruhn [2], Ulrike Köhl [1,3,4] and Ulrich Sack [1]*

[1] Medical Faculty, Institute of Clinical Immunology, University of Leipzig, Leipzig, Germany, [2] Department of Pediatrics, Jena University Hospital, Jena, Germany, [3] Hannover Medical School, Institute of Cellular Therapeutics, Hannover, Germany, [4] Fraunhofer Institute for Immunology and Cell Therapy (IZI), Leipzig, Germany

Correspondence:
Michael Bitar
michael.bitar@medizin.uni-leipzig.de

† These authors have contributed equally to this work

Here we present a simple and sensitive flow cytometric—based assay to assess T cell proliferation. Given the critical role STAT5A phosphorylation in T cell proliferation, we decided to evaluate phosphorylation of STAT5A as an indicator of T cell proliferation. We determined pSTAT5A in T cell treated with either CD3/CD28 or PHA. After stimulation, T cells from adult healthy donors displayed a strong long-lasting phosphorylation of STAT5A, reaching a peak value after 24 h. The median fluorescence intensity (MFI) of pSTAT5A increased from 112 ± 17 to 512 ± 278 (CD3/CD28) (24 h) and to 413 ± 123 (PHA) (24 h), the IL-2 receptor-α (CD25) expression was greatly enhanced and after 72 h T cell proliferation amounted to 52.3 ± 10.3% (CD3/CD28) and to 48.4 ± 9.7% (PHA). Treatment with specific JAK3 and STAT5 inhibitors resulted in a complete blockage of phosphorylation of STAT5A, CD25 expression, and suppression of T cell proliferation. Compared with currently available methods, STAT5A phosphorylation is well-suited to predict T cell proliferation. Moreover, the method presented here is not very time consuming (several hours) and delivers functional information from which conclusions about T cell proliferation can be drawn.

Keywords: STAT5 activation, T cell proliferation, T cell activation, flow cytometry, CD25

INTRODUCTION

The decision of T cells to start an appropriate activation- proliferation program upon encountering an antigen presented by an antigen presenting cell is a critical step of the adaptive immune reaction (1, 2).

Following engagement of the T cell receptor (TCR), three transcription factors, namely nuclear factor of activated T cells (NFAT), nuclear factor kappa-light-chain-enhancer of activated B cells (NF-κB), and activator protein 1 (AP-1) will be activated (3, 4). The interaction between these molecules leads to the synthesis of important cytokines such as Interleukin−2 (IL-2) and Interferon gamma (IFN-γ) (5), as well as the up-regulation of Janus kinase 3 (Jak3) expression (**Figure 1**) (4, 6–8).

TCR stimulated production of IL-2 and other cytokines starts the cascade of signaling events, leading to the activation of Jak3, which in turn phosphorylates signal transducer and activator of transcription 5 (STAT5) (**Figure 1**) (8). STAT5 consists of two highly related proteins, STAT5A and STAT5B, which share over 90% identity and differ in their carboxyl (C)—terminus (9, 10). Both STAT5A and STAT5B regulated genes are involved in cell proliferation, survival, differentiation and apoptosis (10, 11).

Phosphorylated STAT5 (pSTAT5) translocates into the nucleus to regulate transcription of the target genes including the IL-2 receptor α (IL-2Rα) (CD25) (**Figure 1**) (5, 12–14), a prerequisite for the formation of the high affinity IL-2Rαβγ (12, 15, 16). The induction of the functional system composed of IL-2 and the high affinity IL-2R is critical for G1 progression and for mounting an effective immune response (**Figure 1**) (12, 17).

One standard procedure to quantify cellular immune responses to antigens is based on the measurement of cell proliferation (1, 2). Today, the assays are mainly carried out by the use of flow cytometry (FCM). One of the methods consists of serial halving of the fluorescence intensity of the vital dye (18). The current assays have many drawbacks including the need of bulk cultures and long incubation times (3–5 days). This is especially inconvenient when rapid diagnosis is desirable. Therefore, a fast and simple flow cytometric method enabling the early and reliable detection of lymphocyte entry into an activation program would be of great interest.

In this work, we asked whether phosphorylation of STAT5A is an appropriate candidate to predict the behavior of T cells upon activation. We established and validated a rapid, sensitive, flow cytometric based pSTAT5A assay to detect T cell proliferation. We showed that there was a strong correlation between the early CD3/CD28 or polyclonal mitogen phytohemagglutinin (PHA) induced STAT5A phosphorylation and T cells proliferation. Moreover, due to its simplicity and robustness, the flow cytometric based pSTAT5 assay is especially appropriate to rapidly assess primary immune deficiencies (PIDs) associated with STAT5 defects including autoimmune diseases, CD25 deficiency and T cells proliferation defects (11, 19–22).

METHODS AND MATERIAL

Collection of Blood Samples

Heparinized peripheral blood samples (7 ml) were taken from 19 adult healthy donors (median of age = 31), at the Institute of Clinical Immunology at the University of Leipzig. Additionally, we analyzed a blood from a patient selected by their clinical representations: anemia, clubfeet, and pancytopenia. Written informed consent was obtained from all included individuals. Sample collection and processing were completed according to the Medical Faculty, University of Leipzig standard operating guidelines and regulations.

Isolation of PBMCs and Staining With Violet Proliferation Dye 450

Peripheral blood mononuclear cells (PBMCs) were isolated from fresh peripheral blood samples by density gradient centrifugation over Ficoll-Hypaque (Pan Biotech, Germany), as described previously (23, 24). PBMCs ($1 * 10^7$ cells/ml) were diluted with phosphate-buffered saline (PBS, pH 7.2) (Gibco life Technologies, USA) and stained with Violet Proliferation Dye 450 (VPD450) (3 μM) (BD Biosciences) for 15 min at 37°C. Subsequently, PBMCs were washed and re-suspended in RPMI 1,640 containing 10% fetal bovine serum, penicillin ($1 * 10^5$ mg/ml) and streptomycin ($1 * 10^5$ mg/ml) (Gibco life Technologies, USA) and finally adjusted to $1 * 10^6$ cells/ml.

Stimulation of PBMCs and Treatment With Specific Inhibitors

PBMCs ($1 * 10^6$ cells/ml) were seeded into 48 well cell culture plates ($5 * 10^5$ cells/well) at 37°C. After 2 h, PBMCs were stimulated with either CD3/CD28 (eBioscience, clones OKT3, CD28.2) (100 ng/ml) or with PHA (Sigma) (10 μg/ml).

Following pharmacological inhibitors: JAK3 inhibitor [JAK3i, 4-(4′-Hydroxyphenyl) amino-6, 7-dimethoxyquinazoline] (12 μM), STAT5 inhibitor [STAT5i, N′-((4-Oxo-4H-chromen-3-yl) methylene) nicotinohydrazide] (35 μM), Cyclosporin A (CsA) (500 nM) (Calbiochem, USA) or DMSO (0.07%) were added 2 h before stimulating the cells.

In parallel, cells were either cultured for 24 h to determine pSTAT5A and CD25 in T cells or for 72 h to determine T cell proliferation in a humidified atmosphere of 5% CO_2 at 37°C.

Determination of pSTAT5A and CD25 Expression in T Cells by Flow Cytometry

Cultured PBMCs were harvested after 24 h, pelleted by centrifugation, lysed and fixed by using "lyse and fix" buffer (BD Biosciences) and incubated at 37°C in a water bath for 12 min. The cells were centrifuged, the supernatant was discarded and the pellet was washed with 4 mL PBS.

The samples were permeabilized by using cold perm buffer III (1 ml) (BD Biosciences) and left on ice for 30 min. The pellet was washed three times with a fetal bovine serum stain buffer (FBS) (2 ml) (BD Biosciences) and finally re-suspended in 200 μl FBS. For flow cytometric analysis, the T cells were stained with PerCP-Cy™ 5.5 mouse anti-human CD3 (2.5 μL, clone UCHT1, BD Biosciences), PE mouse anti-human CD25 (5 μL, clone 2A3, BD Biosciences) Alexa Fluor 647 mouse anti human -STAT5A (10 μL, PY694, Clone 47/Stat5, BD Biosciences) and Alexa Fluor 647 mouse anti human FoxP3 (10 μl, clone 259D, c7, BD Biosciences). Mouse IgG1-k- Alexa Fluor 647 isotype control (10 μl, clone MOPC-21, BD Biosciences) was used for assessing the background staining of cells. After 1 h of incubation in the dark at room temperature, the cells were washed with 2 mL stain buffer, centrifuged and were suspended in 300 μL of stain buffer. To analyze STAT5A phosphorylation: based on the following gating strategy (1) forward scatter (FSC) vs. side scatter (SSC) and (2) CD3 vs. SSC, the T cells ($CD3^+$) were separated (**Supplementary Figure 1**). Now, after clear separation of T cells from the non-T cells, 30,000 $CD3^+$ T cells per sample were detected. The phosphorylation of STAT5A was calculated as median fluorescence intensity (MFI) in $CD3^+$ T cells.

Abbreviations: TCR, T cell receptor; NFAT, nuclear factor of activated T cells; IL-2, Interleukin−2; Jak3, Janus kinase 3; pSTAT5, phosphorylated signal transducer and activator of transcription 5; CD25, IL-2 receptor α; FCM, flow cytometry; PHA, phytohemagglutinin; PBMCs, Peripheral blood mononuclear cells; Jak3i, Janus kinase 3 inhibitor; STAT5i, signal transducer and activator of transcription 5 inhibitor; CsA, Cyclosporin A; MFI, median fluorescence intensity.

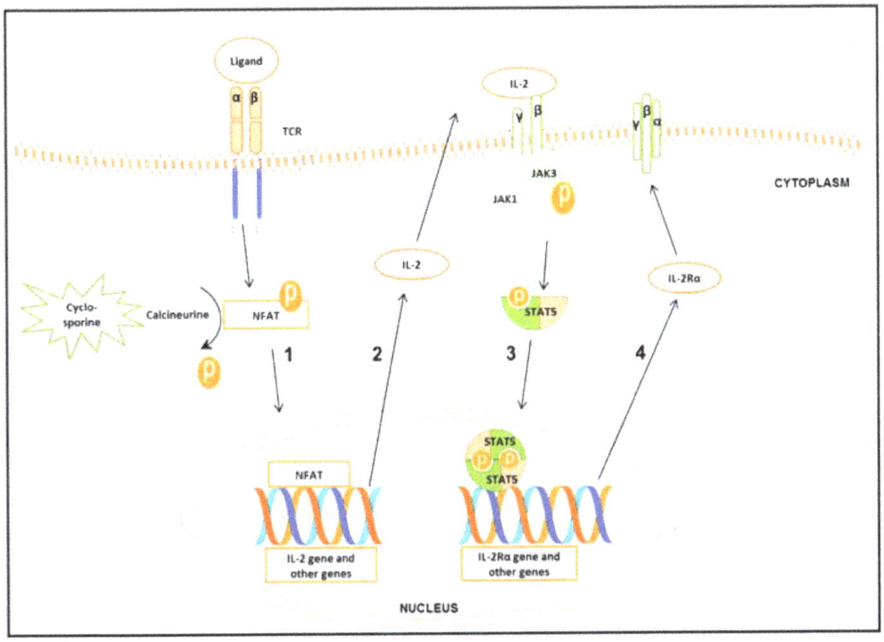

FIGURE 1 | Schematic presentation of the signal cascade following T cells stimulation **(1)** Binding of the ligand to the T cell receptor (TCR) leads to the activation of nuclear factor of activated T cell (NFAT). Cyclosporine by inhibiting calcineurine prevents activation of NFAT. Activated NFAT translocates to the nucleus where it activates target genes including IL-2. **(2-3)** Binding of IL-2 to IL-2 receptorβγ (IL-2Rβγ) leads to the activation of Janus kinase 3 (Jak3) which in turn phosphorylates signal transducer and activator of transcription 5 (STAT5). Phosphorylated STAT5 forms homo- and heterodimers that translocate to the nucleus, leading to the transcription of target genes including the IL-2Rα gene. **(4)** IL-2Rα together with IL-2Rβγ forms the high affinity IL-2Rβγα.

Determination of T Cell Proliferation by Flow Cytometry

Cultured PBMCs were harvested after 72 h and washed with 2 mM EDTA PBS. The pellet was re-suspended in 200 μl PBS and stained with APC–H7 mouse anti-human CD45 (2.5 μl, clone 2D1, BD Biosciences) and FITC mouse anti-human CD3 (5 μl, clone SK7, BD Biosciences) at 37°C. After 15 min, cells were washed with 2 mL 2 mM EDTA PBS, centrifuged and suspended in 300 μL PBS.

To analyze T cell proliferation: based on two lymphocyte collection gates (1) FSC vs. SSC and (2) CD45 vs. SSC (mathematical connected by AND-operation) the T cells ($CD3^+$) were separated in a third dot plot (CD3 vs. SSC). Now, the decrease of VPD450 dye intensity in proliferated $CD3^+$ cells was measured, 50,000 $CD3^+$ cells per sample were detected (**Supplementary Figure 2**). Data analysis was done using FlowJo.7.6.5 software (Ashland, OR, USA) (25).

Cell Viability

7-Amino-Actinomycin D (7-AAD) staining was used to determine cell viability. 7-AAD is excluded by viable cells but can penetrate cell membranes of dead cells. 7-AAD (10 μl) (BD Biosciences) was added to pre-stained T cells (as described above) for 10 min, before cells were analyzed by flow cytometry.

Flow Cytometric Analysis

FACSCanto II based flow cytometry was conducted to measure the samples as previously described (26, 27). Briefly, the system was set up with three lasers: a violet laser 405 nm, a blue laser 488 nm, and a red laser 647 nm. Prior to running samples, the instrument was calibrated using calibration beads (BD Biosciences). BD FACSDiva software was used for acquisition of events.

Determination of IL-2 Production in PBMCs

PBMCs ($1 * 10^6$ cells/ml) were cultured with PHA (Sigma) (10 μg/ml) for different times (12, 24, 48, 72 h). The cell supernatants were then collected and assayed for IL-2 by enzyme immunoassay (EIA; R&D system, Minneapolis, USA).

Adaptation of Methods to DIN EN ISO 15189 Requirements

To exclude or diminish false positive or false negative results, the international standard DIN EN ISO 15189 recommended proceedings to fulfill highest requirements for the quality and competency of medical laboratories. This includes the validation of all data by performing intra-assay and inter-assay precision (28).

Note: in case of using two or more different FACS Canto, differences in technical adjustments among different devices leading to various results in the mean fluorescence and should be considered. Therefore, a transfer of the instrument setting among the devices has to be performed. Especially the voltage power in each channel in all devices should be equilibrated by the use of calibrate beads to get comparable MFI signals.

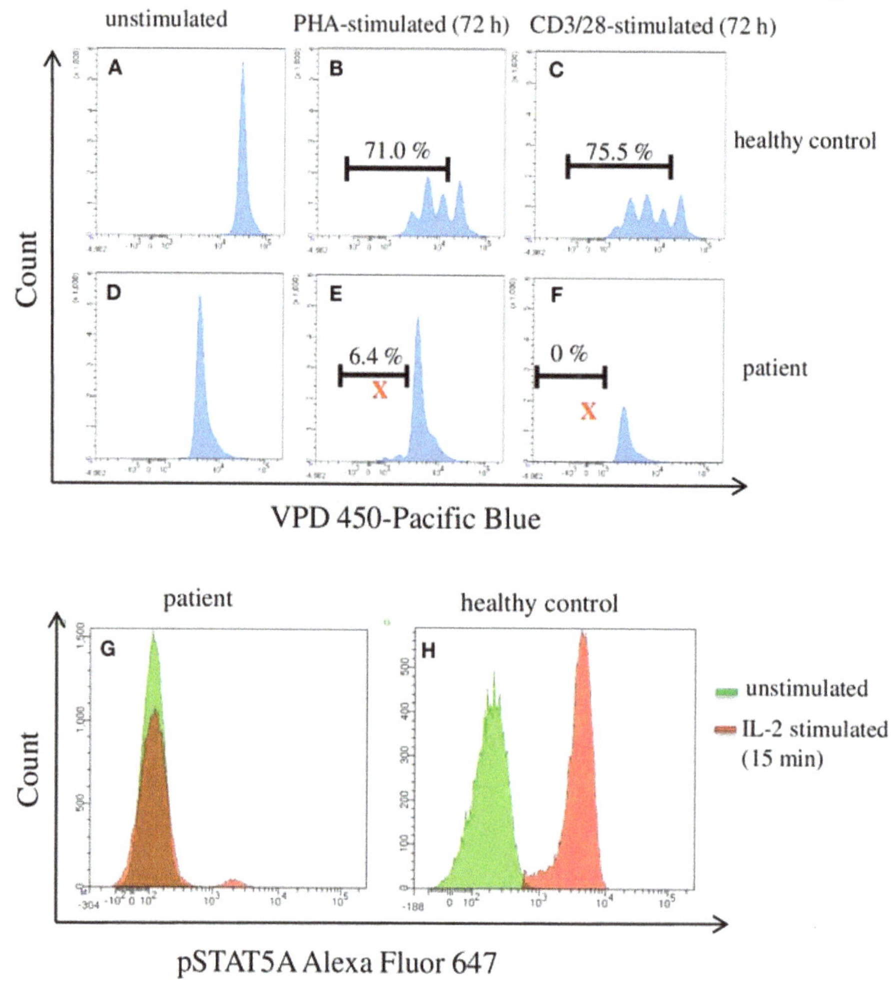

FIGURE 2 | Flow cytometric analysis of pSTAT5A and T cell proliferation in PBMCs from a patient suffering from a congenital pancytopenia. PBMCs (1 * 10^6 cells/ml) were treated with PHA (10 µg/ml) **(B,E)**, CD3/CD28 (100 ng/ml) **(C,F)**, or with IL-2 (100 ng/ml) **(G,H)**. After 15 min and 72 h, IL-2 stimulated pSTAT5A **(G,H)** and T cells proliferation **(A–F)** were determined, respectively.

Statistical Analysis

The statistical analysis was performed using the Graph Pad Prism 5 software (Graph Pad Prism software, Inc., San Diego, CA, USA). Curves were evaluated by the non-parametric Friedman test. The adjusted *P*-values were deemed by Wilcoxon's test (ns not significant, $^{*}P \leq 0.05$; $^{**}P \leq 0.01$; $^{***}P \leq 0.001$). Correlations were calculated with Spearman's correlation coefficient.

RESULTS

Immunodeficiency Is Accompanied by a Diminished Proliferation of T Cells and Down Regulation of pSTAT5A

An infant (female, 2 months old) of healthy, non-consanguine parents exhibited clinical symptoms such as umbilical hernia and clubfeet. Laboratory examinations revealed congenital pancytopenia: 0% neutrophils, 0% thrombocytes, and 100% naïve T cells. Nor B- or NK-cells could not be detected. For analyzing the function/proliferation of the T cells, we stimulated with CD3/CD28 or PHA (72 h) to investigate proliferation and with IL-2 (15 min) to measure pSTAT5A. As shown in **Figure 2**, the phosphorylation of STAT5A was completely deficient in patient T cells accompanied by severely limited T cell proliferation. Trio-exome sequencing did not reveal any abnormalities and excluded genetic defects in: IKZF1, GATA2, SAMD9, and SAMD9L. Finally, 14 month after successful unrelated bone marrow transplantation, the patient is in a very good clinical condition. Based on these data, we investigated in how far phosphorylation of STAT5A is a valid parameter to predict proliferation of T cells.

Concentration and Time Dependent STAT5 Phosphorylation and Proliferation

First, we tested the influence of different CD3/CD28 and PHA concentrations on STAT5A phosphorylation and T cell proliferation (**Figure 3**). We found that CD3/CD28 at a very low concentration of 0.25 ng/ml was sufficient to induce maximal

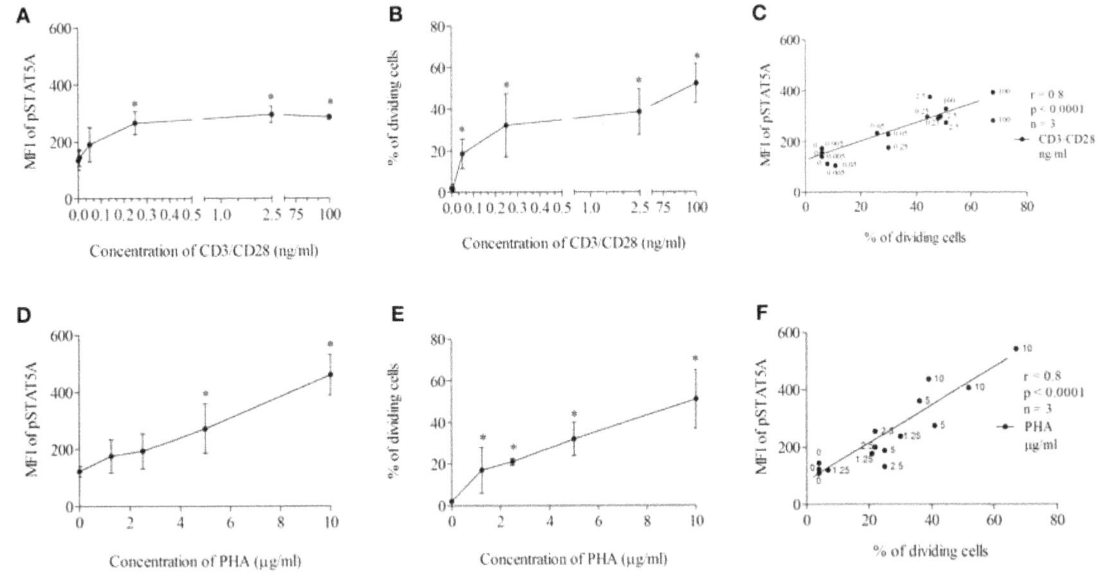

FIGURE 3 | Concentration dependent correlation between the percentage of dividing cells and STAT5A phosphorylation. PBMCs (1 * 10^6 cells/ml) were treated with CD3/CD28 (0, 0.005, 0.05, 0.25, 2.5, and 100 ng/ml) or PHA (0, 1.25, 2.5, 5, and 10 µg/ml). After 24 and 72 h, pSTAT5 **(A,D)** and proliferation **(B,E)** were determined, respectively. Correlation between the percentage of dividing cells (72 h) and STAT5A phosphorylation (24 h) dependent on the concentration of the stimulus **(C)** CD3/CD28, **(F)** PHA.*$p < 0.05$; r, Spearman's correlation coefficient; $n = 3$ independent experiments, MFI, median fluorescence intensity.

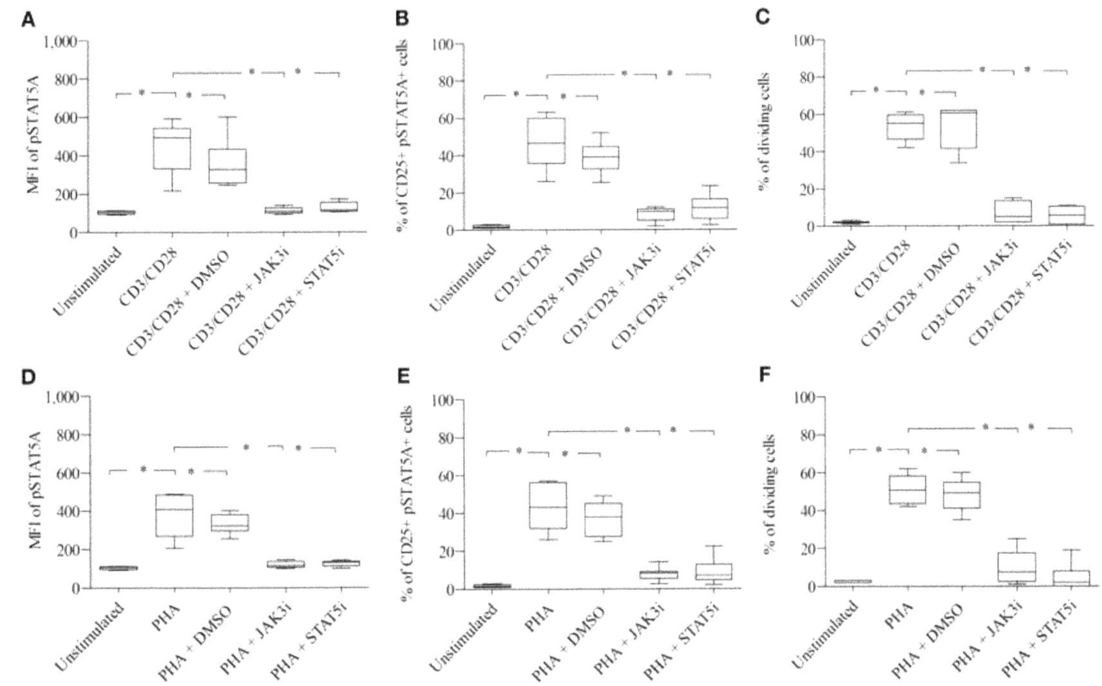

FIGURE 4 | Role of pSTAT5A in T cell proliferation. CD3/CD28 or PHA stimulated T cells were treated either with DMSO (solvent control, 0.07 %), JAK3i (12 µM) or STAT5i (35 µM). After 24 h the MFI of pSTAT5 **(A,D)** the percentage of $CD25^{+}pSTAT5A^{+}$ cells **(B,E)** and after 72 h proliferation **(C,F)** were determined, The bold line inside each box plot shows the median, upper and lower lines indicate the maximum and minimum values, respectively (Curves were evaluated by the non-parametric Friedman test). *$p < 0.05$ (Wilcoxon's test); $n = 6$ independent experiments; MFI, median fluorescence intensity; Jak3i, Janus kinase 3 inhibitor; STAT5i, signal transducer and activator of transcription 5 inhibitor.

TABLE 1 | Summary of MFI of pSTAT5A, % of CD25$^+$ pSTAT5A$^+$cells and % of dividing cells, before and after treatment with JAK3 and STAT5 inhibitors in CD3/CD28 stimulated cells ($n = 6$).

Control group	Unstimulated	CD3/CD28 (100 ng/ml)	CD3/CD28 (100 ng/ml) + DMSO (0.07 %)	CD3/CD28 (100 ng/ml) + JAK3i (12 μM)	CD3/CD28 (100 ng/ml) + STAT5i (35 μM)
MFI of pSTAT5A[a]	103 ± 8	449 ± 134	358 ± 131	112 ± 17	127 ± 27
% of CD25$^+$pSTAT5A$^+$[b]	1.75 ± 0.7	46.6 ± 13.5	38.7 ± 8.7	8.3 ± 3.7	11.6 ± 7.2
% of dividing Cells[c]	2 ± 0.6	53.3 ± 7.3	53.8 ± 12	7 ± 5.7	5.5 ± 4.5

[a]*Median fluorescence intensity (MFI) of STAT5A after 24 h, calculated as mean ± SD.*
[b]*Percent of CD25$^+$ pSTAT5A$^+$ cells after 24 h, calculated as mean ± SD.*
[c]*Percent of dividing cells after 72 h, calculated as mean ± SD.*

TABLE 2 | Summary of MFI of pSTAT5A, % of CD25$^+$ pSTAT5A$^+$cells and % of dividing cells, before and after treatment with JAK3 and STAT5 inhibitors in PHA stimulated cells ($n = 6$).

Control group	Unstimulated	PHA (10 μg/ml)	PHA (10 μg/ml) + DMSO (0.07 %)	PHA (10 μg/ml) + JAK3i (12 μM)	PHA (10 μg/ml) + STAT5i (35μM)
MFI of pSTAT5A[a]	103 ± 8	380 ± 111	331 ± 51	119 ± 15	125 ± 15
% CD25$^+$pSTAT5A$^+$[b]	1.75 ± 0.7	42.8 ± 11.4	36.5 ± 8.7	8.1 ± 3.6	8.9 ± 6.7
% of dividing cells[c]	2 ± 0.6	51 ± 7.6	48.2 ± 8.5	9.8 ± 9	4.5 ± 7

[a]*Median fluorescence intensity (MFI) of STAT5A after 24 h, calculated as mean ± SD.*
[b]*Percent of CD25$^+$ pSTAT5A$^+$ cells after 24 h, calculated as mean ± SD.*
[c]*Percent of dividing cells after 72 h, calculated as mean ± SD.*

phosphorylation of STAT5A (plateau phase) (**Figure 3A**) and that the percentage of dividing cells was highest at 100 ng/ml (**Figure 3B**). When stimulating the cells with PHA both pSTAT5A (**Figure 3D**) and the percentage of dividing cells (**Figure 3E**) steadily rose with increasing concentration of PHA up to 10 μg/ml. Thus in further experiments, we used CD3/CD28 at 100 ng/ml and PHA at 10 μg/ml.

As demonstrated in **Figures 3C,F** independent of the stimulus used a strong correlation [Spearman's correlation coefficient (r) = 0.8, $p < 0.0001$] could be observed between STAT5A phosphorylation and the percentage of dividing cells.

To determine the optimal time to analyze STAT5A phosphorylation, we performed a series of kinetics. We found that the CD3/CD28—induced phosphorylation of STAT5A reached a peak value after 24 h and that it declined thereafter (**Supplementary Figure 3A**). Peak values after the stimulation with PHA were reached between 12 and 24 h (**Supplementary Figure 3B**). Clearly, production of IL-2 was highest at 24 h (**Supplementary Figure 3C**). Thus, in further experiments, we analyzed pSTAT5A at 24 h.

Inhibition of the JAK3/STAT5 Signal Cascade Leads to an Inhibition of pSTAT5A Signaling and T Cell Proliferation

As seen in **Figures 4A,B**; **Table 1**, CD3/CD28 stimulated T cells showed a significant increase in both the MFI of pSTAT5A (from 103 ± 8 to 449 ± 134) and the percentage of CD25$^+$ pSTAT5A$^+$ cells (from 1.75 ± 0.7 to 46.6 ± 13.5 %) after 24 h.

Furthermore, after 72 h as determined by VPD450 dye staining 53.3 ± 7.3% of the T cells treated with CD3/CD28 proliferated (**Figure 4C**). Similar results were obtained upon activation with PHA (**Figures 4D–F**; **Table 2**)

When CD3/CD28 or PHA stimulated T cells were pre-incubated with STAT5i, the MFI of pSTAT5A was substantially abrogated or barely detectable [127 ± 27 (CD3/CD28), 125 ± 15 (PHA)] (**Figures 4A,D**; **Tables 1, 2**) and the percentage of CD25$^+$ pSTAT5A$^+$ cells was extremely low [11.6 ± 7.2% (CD3/CD28), 8.9 ± 6.7% (PHA)] (**Figures 4B,E**; **Tables 1, 2**). Importantly, inhibition of phosphorylation of STAT5A was associated with a suppression of dividing T cells [5.5 ± 4.5% (CD3/CD28), 4.5 ± 7 % (PHA)] (**Figures 4C,F**; **Tables 1, 2**) after 72 h.

Similar results were obtained upon inhibition with JAK3i (**Figures 4A–F**; **Tables 1, 2**)

The inhibitory effect of JAK3i or STAT5i on proliferation was not due to an increased cytotoxicity, the percentage of dead cells hardly changed after 72 h of treatment (**Figures 5A,B**). To test whether the CD25$^+$ cell population contained any regulatory T cells, we stimulated the cells with PHA or CD3/CD28 and measured the expression of the transcription factor FOXP3. Almost all CD25$^+$ cells were FOXP3$^-$ cells, the percentage of CD25$^+$ FOXP3$^+$ cells was low not exceeding 5–8% (data not shown).

Inhibition of IL-2 Gene Transcription Leads to a Decrease of pSTAT5A Signaling and T Cell Proliferation

To examine the role of IL-2 in STAT5A phosphorylation, we used CsA an inhibitor of calcineurine, which blocks the NFAT activity (3). After antigen recognition by the TCR, NFAT binds to the promoter region of the IL-2 gene leading to its transcription.

As shown in **Figure 6**; **Table 3** treatment with CsA led to a substantial decrease of MFI values of pSTAT5 (from 398 ± 123 to 249 ± 74) in CD3/CD28 and (from 435 ± 143 to 325 ±144) in PHA stimulated cells (**Figures 6A,D**; **Table 3**). This decrease

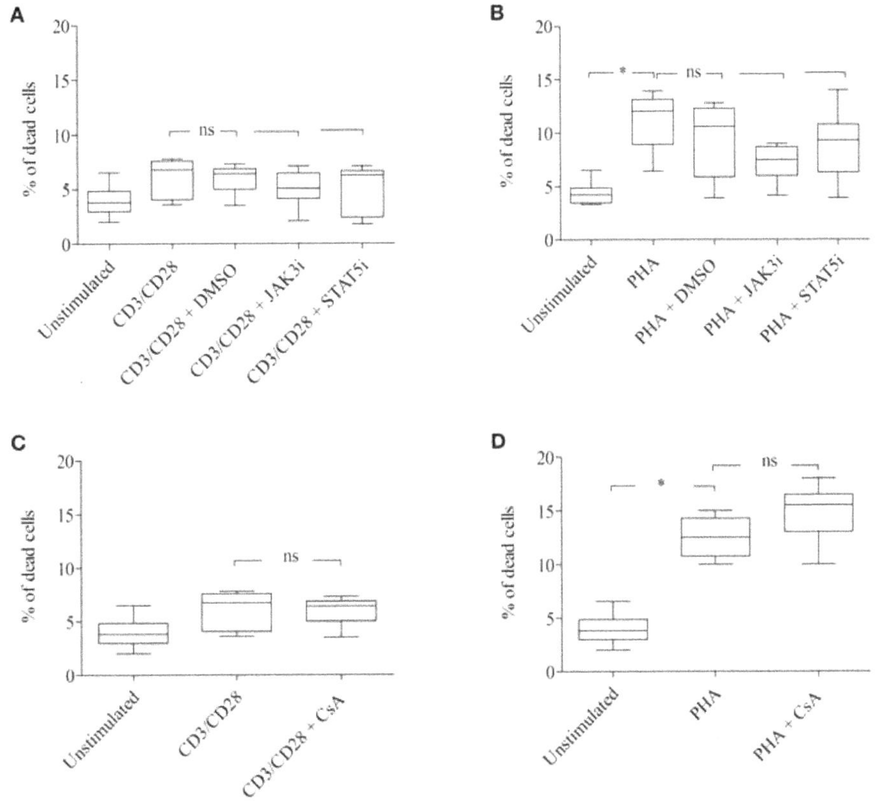

FIGURE 5 | Effect of JAK3, STAT5 inhibitors and cyclosporine (CsA) on cell viability. CD3/CD28 or PHA stimulated T cells were treated with DMSO (0.07 %), JAK3i (12 μM), STAT5i (35 μM) **(A,B)** or CsA (500 nM) **(C,D)** for 72 h. The percentage of dead cells was calculated after 7-AAD staining. The bold line inside each box plot shows the median, upper, and lower lines indicate the maximum and minimum values, respectively (Curves were evaluated by the non-parametric Friedman test). Ns, no significant; $^{*}p < 0.05$ (Wilcoxon's test); $n = 6$ independent experiments; Jak3i, Janus kinase 3 inhibitor; STAT5i, signal transducer and activator of transcription 5 inhibitor.

was associated with a low percentage of $CD25^{+}$ $pSTAT5A^{+}$ cells stimulated with CD3/CD28 (from 41.5 ± 9.9 to 21.3 ± 10.9%) or with PHA (from 36.6 ± 11.9 to 24 ± 10%) (**Figures 6B,E; Table 3**). The number of proliferating T cells was reduced [from 50.9 ± 5.7 to 26.5 ± 5.8% (CD3/CD28), from 51.6 ± 11.1 to 31.8 ± 12.6% (PHA)] (**Figures 6C,F; Table 3**).

Importantly, the phosphorylation of STAT5A and the percentage of $CD25^{+}$ $pSTAT5A^{+}$ of CsA—treated T cells (**Figures 6A–E**), but not the proliferation (**Figures 6C,F; Table 3**) was rescued by adding exogenous IL-2 (100 ng/ml). We could exclude that the inhibitory effect of CsA on T cell proliferation was due to a loss of cell viability as assessed 72 h after treatment (**Figures 5C,D**).

Validation of STAT5A Phosphorylation in Healthy Donors to DIN EN ISO 15189 Requirements and for Use in Diagnostic Application

To establish a rapid flow cytometric assay to evaluate STAT5A phosphorylation and to provide reference values for healthy adult controls, we analyzed the MFI of pSTAT5A and proliferation of T cells simultaneously ($n = 19$). In both, CD3/CD28 or PHA treated cells, the MFI of pSTAT5A was strongly increased [from 112 ± 17 to 512 ± 278 (CD3/CD28), 413 ± 123 (PHA)] (**Figure 7A; Table 4**). The percentage of $CD25^{+}$ $pSTAT5A^{+}$ cells was significantly up-regulated and the amount of $CD25^{+}$ $pPSTAT5A^{+}$ cells (24 h) correlated with the amount of dividing cells (72 h) (**Figures 7D,E**).

Flow cytometric analysis revealed that the percentage of $CD25^{+}$ $pSTAT5A^{+}$ cells (47.1 ± 13.2% [CD3/CD28), 42.6 ± 9% (PHA)] after 24 h nearly mirrored the percentage of dividing cells after 72 h [52.3 ± 10.3% (CD3/CD28), 48.4 ± 9.7% (PHA)] (**Figures 7B–E; Table 4**).

Subsequently, to ensure that our analytical method is accurate, reproducible and precise, validation of our data included the definition of intra- and interassay precision values (28). A coefficient of variation up to 25 percent was considered tolerable and fulfilled the criteria of the International Standard EN ISO 15189.

DISCUSSION

Lymphocyte proliferation is commonly accepted as a reliable measurement of lymphocyte activation (1). The current assays

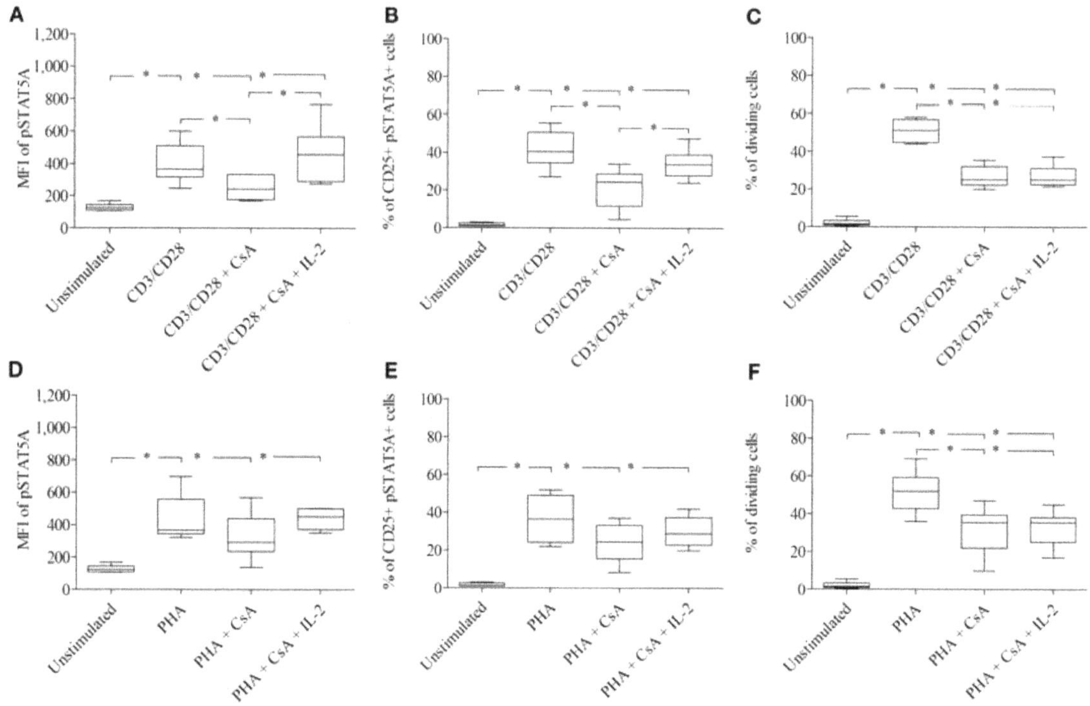

FIGURE 6 | Inhibition of IL-2 transcription by Cyclosporine (CsA) correlates with an inhibition of JAK3/STAT5 mediated signal transduction and proliferation. CD3/CD28 **(A–C)** or PHA **(D–F)**—stimulated T cells were either treated with CsA (500 nM) or with CsA (500 nM) + IL-2 (100 ng/ml). After 24 h the MFI of pSTAT5 A **(A,D)**, the percentage of $CD25^+$ $pSTAT5A^+$ cells **(B,E)** and after 72 h proliferation were determined **(C,F)**. The bold line inside each box plot shows the median, upper and lower lines indicate the maximum and minimum values, respectively (Curves were evaluated by the non-parametric Friedman test). $^*p < 0.05$ (Wilcoxon's test); $n = 6$ independent experiments; MFI, median fluorescence intensity.

TABLE 3 | Summary of MFI of pSTAT5A, % of $CD25^+$ $pSTAT5A^+$cells and % of dividing cells before and after treatment with Cyclosporine (CsA) in CD3/CD28 and PHA stimulated cells ($n = 6$).

Control group	Unstimulated	CD3/CD28 (100 ng/ml)	CD3/CD28 (100 ng/ml) + CsA (500 nM)	CD3/CD28 (100 ng/ml) + CsA (500 nM) + IL- 2 (100 ng/ml)	PHA (10µg/ml)	PHA (10µg/ml) + CsA (500 nM)	PHA (10 µg/ml) + CsA (500 nM) + IL- 2 (100 ng/ml)
MFI of pSTAT5A[a]	128 ± 22	398 ± 123	249 ± 74	458 ± 176	435 ± 143	325 ± 144	438 ± 64
% $CD25^+pSTAT5A^+$[b]	1.6 ± 0.8	41.5 ± 9.9	21.3 ± 10.9	33.9 ± 7.9	36.6 ± 11.9	24 ± 10	30 ± 8.3
% of dividing cells[c]	2 ± 1.8	50.9 ± 5.7	26.5 ± 5.8	26.8 ± 5.7	51.6 ± 11.1	31.8 ± 12.6	32.8 ± 9.4

[a]*Median fluorescence intensity (MFI) of STAT5A after 24 h, calculated as mean ± SD.*
[b]*Percent of $CD25^+$ $pSTAT5A^+$ cells after 24 h, calculated as mean ± SD.*
[c]*Percent of dividing cells after 72 h, calculated as mean ± SD.*

have many drawbacks including the need of bulk cultures and long incubation times (3–5 days), which is inconvenient when rapid diagnosis is desirable. Therefore, we tried to establish a rapid, reliable method that can be used as an indicator of proliferation. We asked whether the phosphorylation of STAT5A is a trustworthy marker for predicting T cell proliferation.

We analyzed the effect CD3/CD28 or PHA on signaling pathways that are essential for T cell proliferation. Our results revealed that a moderate expression of pSTAT5A starts after a few hours of stimulation (6 h) by CD3/CD28 and PHA. It leads to an increased expression of CD25, a prerequisite to form the high affinity IL-2 receptor. Hence, IL-2 can achieve its biological effects such as inducing a sustained IL-2 dependent JAK3/STAT5 signal cascade, which leads to high phosphorylation of STAT5 (after 24 h) and cell proliferation (after 72 h). Our data displayed a strong correlation between these two events.

Interestingly, loss of phosphorylation of STAT5A by the specific inhibitors, that target the activity of STAT5 directly like STAT5i or indirectly like JAK3i led to down-regulation of the percentage of $CD25^+$ $pSTAT5A^+$ cells, accompanied by a diminished PHA or CD3/CD28—driven T cell proliferation.

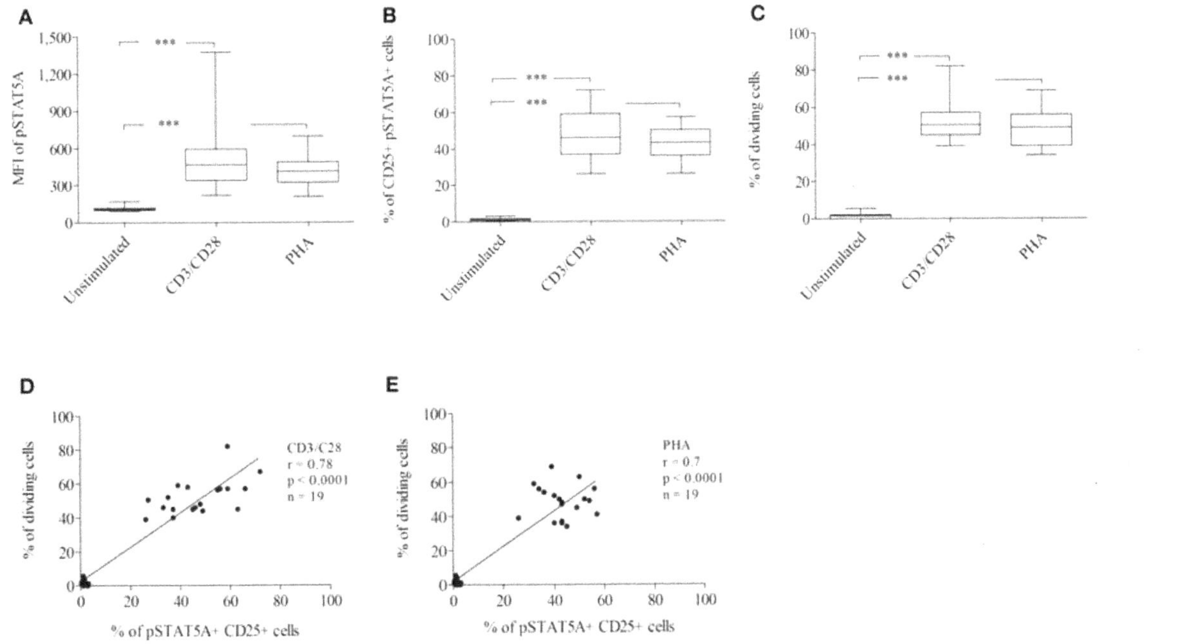

FIGURE 7 | Analysis of STAT5A phosphorylation and percentage of $CD25^+$ $pSTAT5A^+$ cells and dividing cells by flow cytometry ($n = 19$). T cells were stimulated with CD3/CD28 or PHA. After 24 h the MFI of STAT5A **(A)** the percentage of $CD25^+$ $pSTAT5^+$ cells **(B)** and after 72 h proliferations **(C)** were determined. The correlation between the percentage of dividing cells (72 h) and percentage of $CD25^+$ $pSTAT5A^+$ cells (24 h) **(D)** CD3/CD28, **(E)** PHA. The bold line inside each box plot shows the median, upper and lower lines indicate the maximum and minimum values, respectively. ***$p < 0.001$ (Wilcoxon's test); r, Spearman's correlation coefficient; MFI, median fluorescence intensity.

TABLE 4 | Summary of MFI of pSTAT5A, % of $CD25^+$ $pSTAT5A^+$ cells and % of dividing cells in CD3/CD28 or PHA stimulated cells for healthy adult controls ($n = 19$).

Control group	Unstimulated	CD3/CD28 (100 ng/ml)	PHA (10 µg/ml)
MFI of pSTAT5A[a]	112 ± 17	512 ± 278	413 ± 123
% of $CD25^+pSTAT5A^+$[b]	1.3 ± 0.8	47.1 ± 13.2	42.6 ± 9
% of dividing cells[c]	1.5 ± 1.4	52.3 ± 10.3	48.4 ± 9.7

[a]*Median fluorescence intensity (MFI) of STAT5A after 24 h, calculated as mean ± SD.*
[b]*Percent of $CD25^+$ $pSTAT5A^+$ cells after 24 h, calculated as mean ± SD.*
[c]*Percent of dividing cells after 72 h, calculated as mean ± SD.*

In agreement with other studies (9, 12), these observations confirm that STAT5A activation, downstream of TCR signaling, plays an important role in inducing the transcription of the CD25 gene. This in turn leads to the formation of the high affinity IL-2R, which results in sustained prolonged JAK3/STAT5 activity and long-term CD25 up-regulation (9, 12).

We could not distinguish between STAT5A and STAT5B being involved in CD25 expression, because both proteins were affected by the inhibitors. Previously, Ivashkiv LB and Hu X 2004 (29) reported that T cells from STAT5A deficient mice displayed reduced proliferation rates secondary to a diminished expression of the IL-2Rα chain. Likewise, Kanai et al. (10) reported that STAT5B deficient patients have reduced numbers of natural killer cells, T cells and impaired IL-2 signaling. They showed that in humans the anti-apoptotic factor BCL2L1 is regulated by STAT5A, whereas FOXP3, and CD25 expression are regulated by STAT5B. Moreover, Lin and Leonard (14) described the importance of the functional cooperation of STAT5 with other transcription factors in regulating CD25 expression (14).

In order to clarify the role of IL-2 in the activation of the JAK3/STAT5 signal cascade, expression of CD25 and cell proliferation, we used CsA which is known to inhibit the nuclear entry of the transcription factor NFAT that is required for IL-2 gene transcription (30). The treatment with CsA substantially decreased the phosphorylation of STAT5A, the percentage of $CD25^+$ $pSTAT5A^+$ cells and the percentage of dividing cells.

Importantly, the phosphorylation of STAT5A and the percentage of $CD25^+$ $pSTAT5A^+$ in CsA treated cells was rescued by adding exogenous IL-2, but the percentage of dividing cells was not (after 72 h incubation). It is very well possible that CsA by inhibiting the phosphatase calcineurine displays effects that are not restricted to NFAT and thus interferes with mechanisms that are IL-2 independent.

Taken together, our data underline the general perception on TCR mediated proliferation. Signaling basically involves two steps, the first leading to the transcription of the IL-2 gene, the second starting with the activation of JAK3/STAT5 signaling which results in generating the high affinity IL2R. Thereafter, the irreversible decision to replicate DNA and proliferate is made.

In the current study, we showed a strong correlation between the STAT5A phosphorylation and percentage of dividing cells. According to our results including the data derived from the T cells of an immunodeficient patient, we suggest pSTAT5A as a new and rapid diagnostic flow cytometric marker. Additionally, we analyzed T cells from 19 healthy donors to identify a threshold for pSTAT5A values after stimulation with CD3/CD28 or PHA. However, each laboratory should determine and validate its own threshold value following appropriate validation procedures.

In conclusion, we introduced a rapid und straightforward flow cytometric—assay for the assessment of T cell proliferation, based on the staining of phosphorylated STAT5A. Our assay is unique because it identifies T cell proliferation by detecting immediate phosphorylation of STAT5A after stimulation. Because this method is rapid, robust and adaptable, it could be implemented for the measurement of T cells in patient's samples in a variety of clinical settings.

AUTHOR CONTRIBUTIONS

MB: generation and analysis of data, writing of the manuscript. AB: analysis and interpretation of data. M-TF: analysis of IL 2 production. BG: supervision of the patient. UK: validation of data. US: study supervision, design of the experiments.

ACKNOWLEDGMENTS

We thank Heike Knaack, Katrin Bauer, and Bettina Glatte for excellent technical assistance and Anja Grahnert, Ronald Weiß, Erik Schilling, Danni Issa for support and advice. We thank Sauna Hauschildt for discussing the data and for critically reading the manuscript. MB is very grateful for grant support from Cusanuswerk, Germany. The authors acknowledge support from the German Research Foundation (DFG) and Leipzig University within the program of Open Access Publishing.

REFERENCES

1. Cretel E, Touchard D, Bongrand P, Pierres A. A new method for rapid detection of T lymphocyte decision to proliferate after encountering activating surfaces. *J Immunol Methods.* (2011) 364:33–9. doi: 10.1016/j.jim.2010.10.007
2. Caruso A, Licenziati S, Corulli M, Canaris AD, Francesco MA de, Fiorentini S, et al. Flow cytometric analysis of activation markers on stimulated T cells and their correlation with cell proliferation. *Cytometry.* (1997) 27:71–6. doi: 10.1002/(SICI)1097-0320(19970101)27:1<71::AID-CYTO9>3.0.CO;2-O
3. Frischbutter S, Schultheis K, Patzel M, Radbruch A, Baumgrass R. Evaluation of calcineurin/NFAT inhibitor selectivity in primary human Th cells using bar-coding and phospho-flow cytometry. *Cytometry A.* (2012) 81:1005–11. doi: 10.1002/cyto.a.22204
4. Jutz S, Leitner J, Schmetterer K, Doel-Perez I, Majdic O, Grabmeier-Pfistershammer K, et al. Assessment of costimulation and coinhibition in a triple parameter T cell reporter line: simultaneous measurement of NF-kappaB, NFAT and AP-1. *J Immunol Methods.* (2016) 430:10–20. doi: 10.1016/j.jim.2016.01.007
5. Podtschaske M, Benary U, Zwinger S, Hofer T, Radbruch A, Baumgrass R. Digital NFATc2 activation per cell transforms graded T cell receptor activation into an all-or-none IL-2 expression. *PLoS ONE.* (2007) 2:e935. doi: 10.1371/journal.pone.0000935
6. Macian F. NFAT proteins: key regulators of T-cell development and function. *Nat Rev Immunol.* (2005) 5:472–84. doi: 10.1038/nri1632
7. Barten MJ, Gummert JF, van Gelder T, Shorthouse R, Morris RE. Flow cytometric quantitation of calcium-dependent and -independent mitogen-stimulation of T cell functions in whole blood: inhibition by immunosuppressive drugs *in vitro*. *J Immunol Methods.* (2001) 253:95–112. doi: 10.1016/S0022-1759(01)00369-6
8. Ellery JM, Nicholls PJ. Possible mechanism for the alpha subunit of the interleukin-2 receptor (CD25) to influence interleukin-2 receptor signal transduction. *Immunol Cell Biol.* (2002) 80:351–7. doi: 10.1046/j.1440-1711.2002.01097.x
9. Paukku K, Silvennoinen O. STATs as critical mediators of signal transduction and transcription: lessons learned from STAT5. *Cytokine Growth Factor Rev.* (2004) 15:435–55. doi: 10.1016/j.cytogfr.2004.09.001
10. Kanai T, Seki S, Jenks JA, Kohli A, Kawli T, Martin DP, et al. Identification of STAT5A and STAT5B target genes in human T cells. *PLoS ONE.* (2014) 9:e86790. doi: 10.1371/journal.pone.0086790
11. Rani A, Murphy JJ. STAT5 in cancer and immunity. *J Interferon Cytokine Res.* (2016) 36:226–37. doi: 10.1089/jir.2015.0054
12. Shatrova AN, Mityushova EV, Vassilieva IO, Aksenov ND, Zenin VV, Nikolsky NN, et al. Time-dependent regulation of IL-2R alpha-Chain (CD25) expression by TCR signal strength and IL-2-induced STAT5 signaling in activated human blood T lymphocytes. *PLoS ONE.* (2016) 11:e0167215. doi: 10.1371/journal.pone.0167215
13. Serfling E, Berberich-Siebelt F, Chuvpilo S, Jankevics E, Klein-Hessling S, Twardzik T, et al. The role of NF-AT transcription factors in T cell activation and differentiation. *Biochim Biophys Acta.* (2000) 1498:1–18. doi: 10.1016/S0167-4889(00)00082-3
14. Lin JX, Leonard WJ. The role of Stat5a and Stat5b in signaling by IL-2 family cytokines. *Oncogene.* (2000) 19:2566–76. doi: 10.1038/sj.onc.1203523
15. Wang X, Rickert M, Garcia KC. Structure of the quaternary complex of interleukin-2 with its alpha, beta, and gammac receptors. *Science.* (2005) 310:1159–63. doi: 10.1126/science.1117893
16. Lockyer HM, Tran E, Nelson BH. STAT5 is essential for Akt/p70S6 kinase activity during IL-2-induced lymphocyte proliferation. *J Immunol.* (2007) 179:5301–8. doi: 10.4049/jimmunol.179.8.5301
17. Smith KA, Griffin JD. Following the cytokine signaling pathway to leukemogenesis: a chronology. *J Clin Invest.* (2008) 118:3564–73. doi: 10.1172/JCI35819
18. Lyons AB. Analysing cell division *in vivo* and *in vitro* using flow cytometric measurement of CFSE dye dilution. *J Immunol Methods.* (2000) 243:147–54. doi: 10.1016/S0022-1759(00)00231-3
19. O'Shea JJ, Holland SM, Staudt LM. JAKs and STATs in immunity, immunodeficiency, and cancer. *N Engl J Med.* (2013) 368:161–70. doi: 10.1056/NEJMra1202117
20. Atkinson TP. Immune deficiency and autoimmunity. *Curr Opin Rheumatol.* (2012) 24:515–21. doi: 10.1097/BOR.0b013e32835680c6
21. Pertovaara M, Silvennoinen O, Isomaki P. STAT-5 is activated constitutively in T cells, B cells and monocytes from patients with primary Sjogren's syndrome. *Clin Exp Immunol.* (2015) 181:29–38. doi: 10.1111/cei.12614
22. Owen DL, Farrar MA. STAT5 and CD4 (+) T Cell Immunity. *F1000Res.* (2017) 6:32. doi: 10.12688/f1000research.9838.1
23. Tsai W-J, Yang S-C, Huang Y-L, Chen C-C, Chuang K-A, Kuo Y-C. 4-Hydroxy-17-methylincisterol from agaricus blazei decreased cytokine production and cell proliferation in human peripheral blood mononuclear cells via inhibition of NF-AT and NF-kappaB activation. *Evid Based Complement Alternat Med.* (2013) 2013:435916. doi: 10.1155/2013/435916
24. Kuo YC, Yang NS, Chou CJ, Lin LC, Tsai WJ. Regulation of cell proliferation,

gene expression, production of cytokines, and cell cycle progression in primary human T lymphocytes by piperlactam S isolated from Piper kadsura. *Mol Pharmacol.* (2000) 58:1057–66. doi: 10.1124/mol.58.5.1057

25. Roederer M. Interpretation of cellular proliferation data: avoid the panglossian. *Cytometry A.* (2011) 79:95–101. doi: 10.1002/cyto.a.21010
26. Bitar M, Boldt A, Binder S, Borte M, Kentouche K, Borte S, et al. Flow cytometric measurement of STAT1 and STAT3 phosphorylation in CD4(+) and CD8(+) T cells-clinical applications in primary immunodeficiency diagnostics. *J Allergy Clin Immunol.* (2017) 140:1439–41.e9. doi: 10.1016/j.jaci.2017.05.017
27. Boldt A, Borte S, Fricke S, Kentouche K, Emmrich F, Borte M, et al. Eight-color immunophenotyping of T-, B-, and NK-cell subpopulations for characterization of chronic immunodeficiencies. *Cytometry B Clin Cytom.* (2014) 86:191–206. doi: 10.1002/cytob.21162
28. Sack U, Barnett D, Demirel GY, Fossat C, Fricke S, Kafassi N, et al. Accreditation of flow cytometry in Europe. *Cytometry B Clin Cytom.* (2013) 84:135–42. doi: 10.1002/cyto.b.21079
29. Ivashkiv LB, Hu X. Signaling by STATs. *Arthritis Res Ther.* (2004) 6:159–68. doi: 10.1186/ar1197
30. Brandt C, Liman P, Bendfeldt H, Mueller K, Reinke P, Radbruch A, et al. Whole blood flow cytometric measurement of NFATc1 and IL-2 expression to analyze cyclosporine A-mediated effects in T cells. *Cytometry A.* (2010) 77:607–13. doi: 10.1002/cyto.a.20928

2

Functional Analysis of Anti-cytokine Autoantibodies Using Flow Cytometry

Patricia A. Merkel[1], *Terri Lebo*[2] *and Vijaya Knight*[1*]

[1] *Section of Allergy and Immunology, Department of Pediatrics, University of Colorado School of Medicine, Denver, CO, United States,* [2] *Advanced Diagnostic Laboratories, National Jewish Health, Denver, CO, United States*

***Correspondence:**
Vijaya Knight
vijaya.knight@childrenscolorado.org*

Autoantibodies to cytokines are increasingly being detected in association with immunodeficient, autoimmune and immune dysregulated states. Presence of these autoantibodies in an otherwise healthy individual may result in a unique phenotype characterized by predisposition to infection with specific organisms. The ability to detect these autoantibodies is of importance as it may direct treatment toward a combination of anti-microbial agents and immunomodulatory therapies that decrease autoantibody levels, thereby releasing the immune system from autoantibody-mediated inhibition. Ligand binding assays such as ELISA or bead multiplex assays have been used to detect these antibodies. However, not all anti-cytokine autoantibodies have demonstrable function *in vitro* and therefore their clinical significance is unclear. Assays that evaluate the functionality of anti-cytokine autoantibodies can supplement such ligand binding assays and add valuable functional information that, when viewed in the context of the clinical phenotype, may guide the use of adjunctive immunomodulatory therapy. This mini review provides an overview of anti-cytokine autoantibodies identified to date and their clinical associations. It also describes the use of flow cytometry for the functional analysis of anti-IFNγ and anti-GM-CSF autoantibodies.

Keywords: autoantibodies, cytokines, interferon gamma, GM-CSF, non-tuberculous mycobacteria, flow cytometry, phosphorylation

INTRODUCTION

The association of anti-cytokine autoantibodies (AAbs) with primary or acquired immunodeficiency, immune dysregulation and autoimmunity has been increasingly documented in literature (1–3). In fact, immunodeficiency or immune dysregulation due to autoantibodies that target specific cytokines or cytokine pathways now form a unique category in the latest International Union of Immunological Societies (IUIS) PID expert committee (EC)'s classification of immunodeficiencies (4). This category, termed "phenocopies of primary immunodeficiencies (PIDs)," includes acquired immunodeficiency due to certain anti-cytokine AAbs, notably to interferon gamma (IFNγ), interleukin-6 (IL-6), interleukin-17 (IL-17), interleukin-22 (IL-22), and Granulocyte Macrophage Colony Stimulating Factor (GM-CSF) that result in phenotypes similar to those that occur due to pathogenic variants in genes encoding either these specific cytokines, their receptors or molecules mediating cytokine signal transduction.

Anti-cytokine AAbs can be found in circulation and may mediate diverse infectious and/or immunological manifestations depending on the cytokine that they specifically target. Anticytokine

AAbs may decrease bioavailability of cytokines by inhibiting binding to their cognate receptors or by sequestering the cytokine in high molecular weight complexes that subsequently undergo Fc-dependent degradation (5). Alternatively, these AAbs may prolong the action of the cytokine by forming immune complexes that promote increased cytokine activity through interaction with stimulatory receptors, FcγRII and FcγRIII. For example, IL8:IL8 AAb complexes have been shown to interact with FcγRIIa and increase IL-8 mediated neutrophil activity in acute respiratory distress syndrome (ARDS) (6).

The ability of anti-cytokine AAbs to mediate disease manifestations may depend on their ability to neutralize or potentiate cytokine function which in turn, may be dependent on the concentration of the AAb in circulation or in tissue, the avidity of the AAb, or the epitopes recognized by the AAb (5). In an analysis of anti-GM-CSF AAbs isolated from patients with Pulmonary Alveolar Proteinosis (PAP), Piccoli and colleagues showed that while monoclonal anti-Granulocyte Macrophage Colony Stimulating Factor (GM-CSF) AAbs showed diminished capacity to neutralize the cytokine in a bioassay, combinations of three non-competing anti-GM-CSF AAbs were effective in neutralizing the biological activity of GM-CSF. Additionally, healthy individuals were shown to have anti-GM-CSF AAbs at concentrations or in combinations that were non-neutralizing, whereas PAP patients generally had polyclonal antibodies at concentrations and titers that were capable of neutralizing the cytokine (5).

Anti-cytokine AAbs are generally polyclonal IgG in nature, however, low titer, non-neutralizing IgA AAbs to interleukin-10 (IL-10) have been detected in the serum of patients with inflammatory bowel disease (IBD) (7). Because the majority of IgA is secreted and only 15% of circulating immunoglobulins are of the IgA isotype, it is possible that these AAbs accumulate in inflamed tissue or at mucosal surfaces rather than in serum, suggesting that investigation of IgA AAbs should be perhaps be performed in relevant tissues or mucosal secretions.

Anti-cytokine AAbs can also be detected in a majority of healthy individuals and in therapeutic human immunoglobulin preparations (8). In fact, a study of over 8,000 healthy blood donors revealed that AAbs to IL-1α, IL-6, IL-10, and GM-CSF were not uncommon in healthy individuals and were noted to reach potentially neutralizing concentrations, chiefly in the case of anti-IL-6 AAbs (9). Although the significance of anti-cytokine AAbs in healthy individuals has not been definitively established, analysis of their functional activity, whether antagonistic to or agonistic with the biological activity of the cytokine is helpful to determine their significance in a disease setting (7, 10).

Under physiological conditions, anti-cytokine AAbs may potentially play a role in the regulation of biological activities of cytokines either by neutralizing excessive cytokine production or by prolonging the half-life of cytokines in circulation by forming cytokine-antibody immune complexes (6). This potential regulatory function is evidenced by the increase in levels of anti-cytokine AAbs with increasing amounts of cytokines (11). Under certain pathological conditions such as in rheumatoid arthritis (RA) or systemic lupus erythematosus (SLE), these AAbs have been observed to rise with decrease in clinical symptoms, suggesting that anti-cytokine AAbs may be used as tools to monitor severity or resolution of disease (12, 13).

There is growing evidence that suggests certain anti-cytokine AAbs play a direct pathogenic role in increasing susceptibility to infection or development of immune dysregulated states. For example, AAbs to interferon gamma (IFNγ), a cytokine responsible for protective immune responses against intracellular organisms, are associated with chronic, disseminated, treatment refractory infections with intracellular organisms such as mycobacteria (14) and AAbs to Granulocyte Macrophage Colony Stimulating Factor (GM-CSF), the principal orchestrator of maturation and function of pulmonary alveolar macrophages, are associated with autoimmune Pulmonary Alveolar Proteinosis (PAP) as well as with increased susceptibility to infection with Nocardia, Cryptococcus and Aspergillus species (5, 15).

In other clinical conditions, the presence of anti-cytokine AAbs might correlate with disease resolution; for example, an increase in anti-IL-1 AAbs correlates with milder disease course in rheumatoid arthritis (12), anti-interferon alpha (IFNα) AAbs have been noted to have an inverse correlation with disease severity in SLE (13), and high levels of anti-IFNγ AAbs correlate with resolution of Guillain-Barre Syndrome (16). The presence of the AAbs may also merely be an association rather than causative of disease (e.g., anti-Granulocyte Colony Stimulating Factor (G-CSF) AAbs in Felty's syndrome) (17).

The genetic and/or environmental factors that influence the development and potential pathogenicity of these anti-cytokine AAbs in an individual remain poorly defined. Understanding the true prevalence, titer and biological significance of anti-cytokine AAbs in healthy individuals or in specific disease cohorts is confounded by the diversity of techniques used to detect them. Therefore, it is important to measure not only the titer of the AAbs, but to also use functional assays, that may help to determine if the AAbs are functional and therefore more likely to be pathogenic. Appropriate recognition of these AAbs in the context of disease is also important because it may direct treatment toward a combination of adjunctive immunotherapy to modulate the AAb titer while continuing appropriate anti-microbial or other suitable therapy.

Table 1 lists anti-cytokine AAbs associated with various disease states identified to date and the assays, both binding and functional, that have been used to characterize these AAbs. Several of these AAbs may be associated with multiple disease states and may either lead to increased susceptibility to certain pathogens or may be immunoregulatory and dampen autoimmune-mediated disease symptoms. Therefore, the biological significance of anti-cytokine AAbs must be evaluated in the context of disease.

Abbreviations: AAbs, Autoantibodies; ELISA, Enzyme Linked Immunosorbent Assay; PID, Primary Immunodeficiency; PAP, Pulmonary Alveolar Proteinosis; NTM, Non-tuberculous Mycobacteria; IFNγ, Interferon gamma; GM-CSF, Granulocyte Macrophage Colony Stimulating Factor; STAT, Signal Transducer and Activator of Transcription.

TABLE 1 | Disease-associations of anti-cytokine AAbs and *in vitro* detection methods.

Cytokine	Clinical Phenotype	Possible biological role	Assay	References
PRIMARILY INFECTIOUS MANIFESTATIONS				
Interferon gamma (IFNγ)	Disseminated extra-pulmonary, NTM infections, infections with *Salmonella typhi*, Toxoplasma, CMV, reactivation of VZV. Likely immunomodulatory in Guillain-Barre Syndrome	Neutralizing, abrogates the IFNγ response, leading to compromised cellular immune responses. Neutralizes IFNγ thereby decreasing inflammation in GBS	Ligand-binding assay (ELISA) Functional, abrogation of p-STAT1 in human monocytes.	(1, 18, 19) (16)
Interleukin-17 (IL-17A, IL-17F)	APS-1, CMC	Neutralizing, abrogates IL-17 responses essential for anti-fungal immunity	ELISA Inhibition of IL-6 production by IL-17 responsive fibroblasts	(20, 21)
Interleukin-22 (IL-22)	APS-1, CMC	Found in association with anti-IL17 AAbs and may play a role in anti-fungal immunity. Not conclusively established.	Particle based ligand binding assay	(22, 23)
Granulocyte Macrophage Colony Stimulating Factor (GM-CSF)	Autoimmune PAP, intracellular infections with *Mycobacterium avium* and Cryptococcus, Nocardia, and Aspergillus species	Neutralizing, impaired alveolar macrophage development leading to compromised surfactant clearance, impaired macrophage, and neutrophil function	ELISA, proliferation of TF-1 cells in response to recombinant GM-CSF, Inhibition of p-STAT5 detection by flow cytometry	(5, 15, 24, 25)
Interleukin-12 (IL-12)	APS-1, thymoma associated autoimmune disease. Burkholdaria lymphadenitis (one documented case)	Neutralizing capability may increase susceptibility to intracellular organisms, however, biological role not conclusively established	Particle based ligand binding assay Inhibition of p-STAT4 in PHA-induced T cell blasts	(23, 26, 27)
INFECTIOUS OR AUTOIMMUNE MANIFESTATIONS				
Interleukin-6 (IL-6)	Documented association with systemic sclerosis, recurrent staphylococcal infections with low CRP levels.	Neutralizing, leads to decreased CRP levels, increased susceptibility to infection. May form stable complexes with IL-6 and contribute to disease progression in systemic sclerosis.	Luciferase immunoprecipitation (LIPS) ELISA, Western blot, inhibition of TF-1 cell growth Radioimmunoprecipitation	(28–30)
Interferon-alpha (IFN-α)	SLE, APS-1, Thymoma, immune deficiency associated with hypomorphic RAG mutations, NFKB2 mutations (one patient), IPEX syndrome	Neutralizing activity may increase susceptibility to infections. Neutralizing activity associated with reduction in disease severity in SLE, Sjogren's syndrome, and RA.	ELISA Viral growth inhibition Multiplex bead assay Inhibition of p-STAT1	(27, 31–33)
Granulocyte Colony Stimulating Factor (G-CSF)	Neutropenia, Felty's syndrome	May contribute to neutropenia through neutralization of G-CSF, however, robust evidence not available.	ELISA Western blotting Inhibition of proliferation of G-CSF receptor expressing 32D cell line.	(17)
Interleukin-1 (IL-1)	Pemphigus, psoriasis, rheumatoid arthritis, Sjogren's syndrome (non-destructive form of polyarthritis)	Shown to be neutralizing, negatively correlated with disease severity and may modulate disease.	Radioimmunoprecipitation, ELISA	(12, 34, 35)
B Cell Activating Factor (Baff)	Systemic Lupus Erythematosus, associated with CVID	Associated with decreased disease activity in SLE, but role unclear. Associated with CVID but does not correlate with pathogenesis of disease	ELISA	(36, 37)
PRIMARILY AUTOIMMUNE OR IMMUNE DYSREGULATION				
Tumor Necrosis Factor-alpha (TNF-α)	SLE, Multiple Sclerosis, psoriasis, RA	May play a role in disease modulation in SLE, RA, and Psoriasis. Role unclear in MS.	ELISA TNF-α induced apoptosis in U937 cells	(38)
Interleukin-8 (IL-8)	Acute Respiratory Distress Syndrome	Complexes with IL-8 thereby extending its proinflammatory activity including recruitment of neutrophils	ELISA to detect IL-8-anti-IL-8 complexes Ability to trigger neutrophil degranulation and release of superoxide	(10, 39)

(Continued)

TABLE 1 | Continued

Cytokine	Clinical Phenotype	Possible biological role	Assay	References
Erythropoietin (EPO)	Acquired pure red cell aplasia (PRCA)	Neutralizing AAbs to exogenous recombinant EPO cross react with endogenous EPO, inhibiting growth of erythroid progenitor cells.	Radioimmunoprecipitation. Ability of serum from EPO-treated patients to inhibit the proliferation of erythroid progenitor cells from healthy donor bone marrow.	(40)
Osteopontin (OPN)	Rheumatoid arthritis, hepatocellular carcinoma, prostate cancer.	Unclear, may have a role in modulating disease activity in RA, Potential early serum biomarker for prostate cancer. Diagnostic and prognostic biomarker for hepatocellular carcinoma	ELISA Western blotting,	(41, 42) (41, 42)
Osteoprotegerin	Osteoporosis, celiac disease, increased bone resorption in rheumatoid arthritis	Biological role unclear.	Direct and Competitive ELISA	(43, 44)

AAbs, Autoantibodies; NTM, Non-tuberculous mycobacteria; CMV, Cytomegalovirus; VZV, Varicella Zoster Virus; APS-1, Autoimmune Polyglandular Syndrome-1; CMC, Chronic Mucocutaneous Candidiasis; PAP, Pulmonary Alveolar Proteinosis; CRP, C-reactive protein; RAG, Recombination Activating Gene; NFKB2, Nuclear Factor Kappa B Subunit 2; IPEX, Immune dysregulation, polyendocrinopathy, enteropathy, X-linked; SLE, Systemic Lupus Erythematosus; RA, Rheumatoid Arthritis; CVID, Common Variable Immunodeficiency; PRCA, Pure Red Cell Aplasia; EPO, Erythropoietin.

ANALYSIS OF ANTI-CYTOKINE AUTOANTIBODIES

Although the association of anti-cytokine AAbs with immunodeficiency, dysregulation and autoimmunity is well-recognized, diagnostic testing for these AAbs is limited. Apart from validated diagnostic testing in a few clinical laboratories for the detection anti-GM-CSF AAbs in suspected or confirmed autoimmune PAP, anti-cytokine AAb testing is generally not routinely performed by most clinical laboratories. Analysis of anti-cytokine AAbs can be performed by laboratory-developed ELISA, radioimmunoassay, multiplex bead arrays or other ligand binding assays, and offers the ability to report an antibody titer and/or concentration. Ligand binding assays are, in general, high throughput, cost effective and automatable, and the methods can be fairly easily adapted by most clinical laboratories. Functional assessment of autoantibodies provides further information regarding their biological significance in the context of disease and requires demonstration of their neutralizing or potentiating capacity. These assays, while providing important functional information, are generally performed in laboratories that specialize in high complexity testing. Functional assessment of either the antagonistic or agonistic action of these AAbs has been performed in a variety of ways including demonstration of inhibition of proliferation of cytokine-responsive cell lines, inhibition of the ability of certain cytokines to restrict viral growth in permissive cell lines, inhibition of cytokine-driven differentiation of responsive cell lines, inhibition of cytokine-specific phosphorylation signals or potentiation of cellular function.

Flow cytometry is becoming more widely available in clinical laboratories and can be utilized to demonstrate inhibition of cytokine signaling pathways by neutralizing AAbs, and by inference, an indication of their ability to neutralize cytokine function *in vivo*. Although currently not widely available, flow cytometry based assays have been established for IFNγ and GM-CSF AAbs by exploiting knowledge of their signaling pathways. These assays and their relevance in diagnosis or monitoring disease states will be discussed below.

INTERFERON GAMMA AABS

The key role of IFNγ in generation of protective immunity to mycobacterial infections and other intracellular infections is underscored by the fact that mutations of genes encoding *IFNGR1* and *IFNGR2*, (the ligand-binding and intracellular, signaling subunits, respectively, of the IFNγ receptor), and *STAT1* (Signal Transducer and Activator of Transcription 1), that is downstream of the IFNγ receptor, often lead to severe infections with intracellular organisms of low pathogenicity such as the *Bacille Calmette Guerin* (BCG) vaccine or non-tuberculous mycobacterial (NTM) species (45). Such infectious manifestations tend to occur in childhood. In adults, such infections are generally rare and if they occur, are generally associated with an acquired immune deficient state, such as HIV infection or immunosuppression following solid organ or hematopoietic stem cell (HSCT) transplant (46–50).

The initial identification of an acquired immune defect that disrupted the IFNγ pathway was published in 2004 and described an adult Filipino patient with high titer, neutralizing AAbs to IFNγ and associated extra-pulmonary NTM infection (51). Following this report, several cases of intracellular infections associated with AAbs to IFNγ have been documented in otherwise healthy individuals (14, 18, 52). The general clinical manifestation in these patients is extra-pulmonary, disseminated, treatment refractory infections with NTM, although *Salmonella typhi*, cytomegalovirus, cerebral toxoplasmosis and reactivation of varicella zoster virus (VZV) have been reported as well (53). The common features of this autoimmune phenomenon that contribute to an immune deficient state are that patients are, in general, otherwise healthy adults, predominantly Southeast Asian, female, and not obviously immunocompromised. IFNγ AAbs in these patients are neutralizing in nature and tend to be of a very high titer.

While the reason behind development of anti-IFNγ AAbs in certain individuals is not clear, recent data suggest that molecular mimicry and specific HLA types may play a role, therefore indicating that both environment and genetics may be responsible for this phenomenon. In 2013, Chih-Yu Chi et al. published studies showing a strong correlation between two HLA alleles, DRB1*16:02 and HLA-DQB1*05:02 and the occurrence of anti-IFNγ AAbs, suggesting a potential genetic basis for the development of these antibodies (54). Additionally, the group showed that the IFNγ epitope targeted by the anti-IFNγ AAbs was highly homologous to a stretch of amino acids in the Noc2 protein of Aspergillus spp (55). Together, these findings raise the possibility of molecular mimicry leading to development of a cross reactive antibody response to a self-antigen in the context of certain HLA types, leading to an acquired form of immunodeficiency.

GM-CSF AABS

PAP is a rare disease in humans and may be congenital, secondary or acquired (56). The acquired form of PAP has been shown to be due to AAbs to GM-CSF that neutralize the cytokine *in vivo*, compromising alveolar macrophage function and leading to accumulation of pulmonary surfactant in the lungs (5). Impairment of alveolar macrophage adhesion, chemotaxis, phagocytosis, and killing as well as neutrophil phagocytosis, adhesion, oxidative burst and bactericidal activity have been demonstrated in patients with acquired PAP, suggesting that neutralization of GM-CSF *in vivo* compromises critical functions in these cell types (57, 58). These observations also provide an explanation for the increased frequency of infections with opportunistic pathogens including *Mycobacterium avium* complex, Cryptococcus, Nocardia, Histoplasma and Aspergillus species in patients with PAP (59, 60). Anti-GM-CSF AAbs have also been described in otherwise immunocompetent patients with disseminated, extrapulmonary Nocardia infection and invasive aspergillosis, none of whom had an accompanying diagnosis of autoimmune PAP prior to presenting with these infections (15). In at least one of these patients, the presence of anti-GM-CSF AAbs predated clinical presentation, suggesting that these AAbs are likely to be causative of disease rather than a reaction to disease (15). It is currently unclear why certain individuals progress to PAP and others to increased susceptibility to infections with intracellular, opportunistic pathogens. These descriptions have added to the spectrum of clinical presentations in which the presence of anti-GM-CSF AAbs should be investigated (24).

FLOW CYTOMETRY ANALYSIS; EXPLOITING CYTOKINE SIGNALING PATHWAYS

Interferon gamma, a type II interferon secreted chiefly by T lymphocytes and Natural Killer cells, plays a critical role in host defense against intracellular pathogens such as mycobacteria and salmonella. The IFNγ receptor is highly expressed on antigen presenting cells (monocytes, macrophages and dendritic cells) and to a lesser extent on lymphocytes (61). Binding of IFNγ to its cognate receptor leads to activation of Janus kinases 1 and 2 (Jak 1 and 2) followed by phosphorylation of STAT1 on a single tyrosine residue (Y701). Phosphorylated STAT1 dimerizes and is translocated to the nucleus where it initiates transcription of IFNγ regulated genes (**Figure 1A**) (61).

GM-CSF mediates its functions through binding to its receptor, a heterodimer that is comprised of a specific a subunit (GMRα) and a dimeric b subunit (βc) that is shared with other cytokines of the βc family. Following binding of GM-CSF to its receptor, the βc subunit associates with Jak2 that then leads to phosphorylation of STAT5, leading to intranuclear translocation and transcription of GM-CSF regulated genes (**Figure 1A**) (62). Compromised GM-CSF signaling leads to functional deficits in multiple cell types including macrophages and neutrophils.

The IFNγ and GM-CSF signaling pathways have been used to develop flow cytometry based strategies for the functional detection of autoantibodies to these cytokines. The basis of this assay is a short stimulation of isolated peripheral blood mononuclear cells (PBMC) from a healthy donor with either recombinant human IFNγ or GM-CSF to induce phosphorylation of STAT1 or STAT5, respectively. Isolated PBMCs are first stained with fluorophore-conjugated anti-CD14 to identify monocytes. Stained PBMCs are then incubated at 37°C with an optimized concentration of either recombinant IFNγ or GM-CSF for 10–15 min. PBMCs are fixed immediately at the end of the stimulation period with 4% paraformaldehyde to preserve their phosphorylation status and permeabilized using methanol to allow staining for intracellular proteins. Intracellular phosphorylated STAT1 (p-STAT1) or STAT5 (p-STAT5) is detected in monocytes by staining PBMCs with fluorophore conjugated monoclonal antibodies to p-STAT1

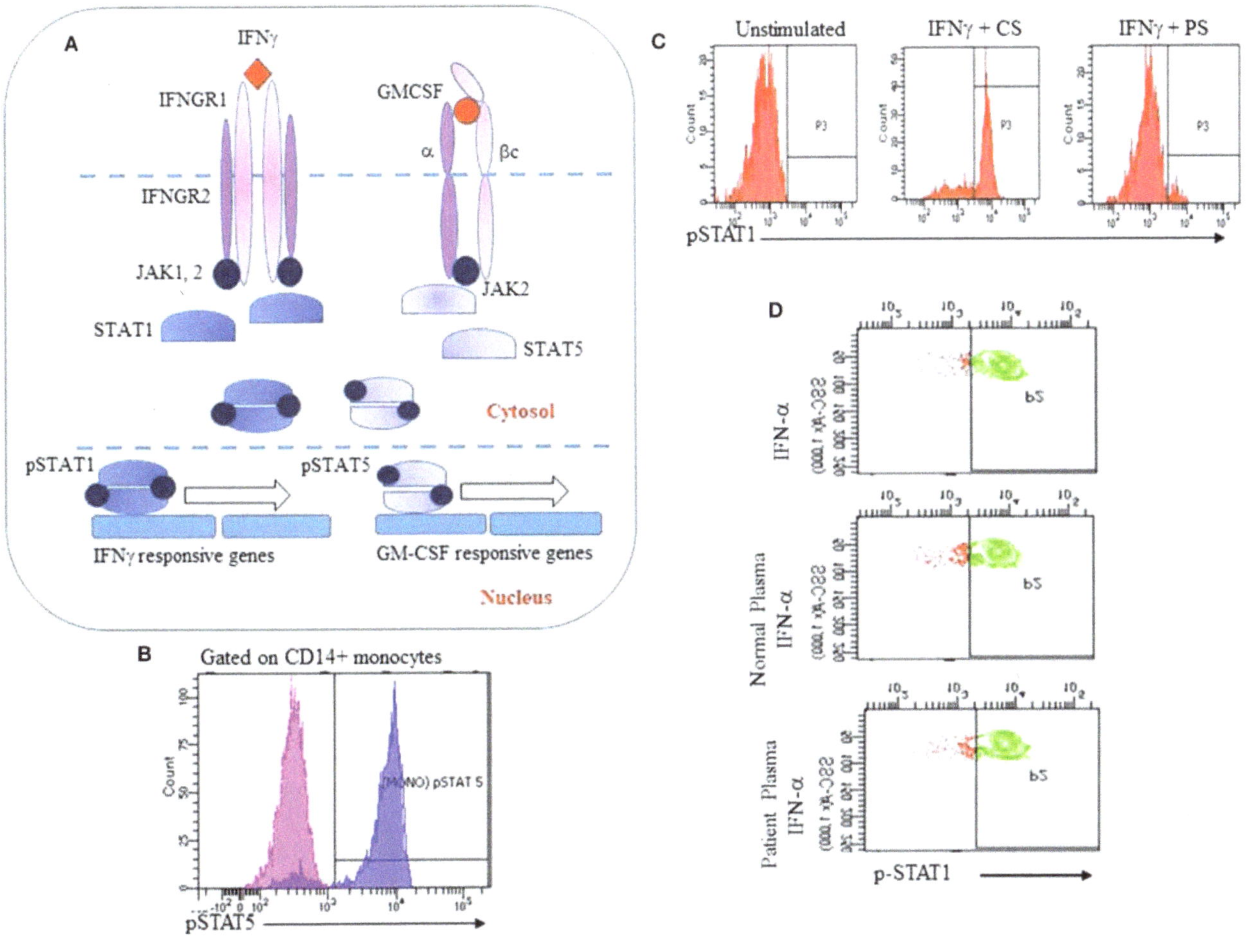

FIGURE 1 | Utility of the IFNγ and GM-CSF signaling pathways for analysis of anti-IFNγ or anti-GM-CSF AAbs. **(A)** IFNγ or GM-CSF bind to their cognate receptors causing Jak1 or 2 to be phosphorylated, leading to phosphorylation and dimerization of STAT1 or STAT5, respectively. Phosphorylated STAT1 and STAT5 dimers translocate to the nucleus and initiate transcription of IFNγ or GM-CSF responsive genes respectively; **(B)** Recombinant GM-CSF induces phosphorylation of STAT5 in human monocytes (pink: unstimulated cells; blue: stimulated cells); **(C)** Human PBMCs were incubated with recombinant IFNγ and control serum (CS) or serum from a patient with disseminated NTM (PS). PS strongly inhibited IFNγ-induced phosphorylation of STAT1; **(D)** Specificity of the flow cytometry assay for detection of anti-IFNγ AAbs. Human PBMC were stimulated with IFNα alone, or with IFNα and control serum or patient serum. Patient serum did not inhibit IFNα-induced phosphorylation of STAT-1 indicating that p-STAT1 inhibition was specific to IFNγ AAbs.

(Tyr701) or p-STAT5 (Tyr694) (**Figure 1B**). Addition of serum or plasma suspected to contain AAbs to IFNγ or GM-CSF to this system is expected to result in decreased fluorescence for p-STAT1 (**Figure 1C**) or p-STAT5. Because IFN-α also utilizes p-STAT1 for signal transduction, PBMC stimulation with IFN-α is performed to demonstrate specificity of the assay for anti-IFNγ AAbs (**Figure 1D**).

FLOW CYTOMETRY ANALYSIS: LIMITATION AND CHALLENGES

As with most functional assays, flow cytometry analysis of p-STAT1 and p-STAT4 may be affected by factors other than specific AAbs in patient serum that might interfere with these pathways. Functional assays do not directly detect an AAb and only infer its activity through the effect observed on specific biological activity attributed to the cytokine. Thus, it is important to address the specificity of the assay by combining it with a ligand binding assay in order to demonstrate the presence of an AAb, and to utilize a control cytokine that uses the same signaling molecules in order to demonstrate neutralization of a specific cytokine. For instance, the assay for IFNγ AAbs makes use of IFNα as a control for specificity because both cytokines signal through STAT-1. In clinical practice, ligand binding assays may be used as a high throughput screen for anti-cytokine AAbs followed by a functional assay as confirmation.

As these assays make use of PBMCs, it is necessary to develop a pool of previously screened donors for the assay. Donor PBMCs for these assays are initially evaluated for their response to IFNγ and GM-CSF and the ability of previous characterized inhibitory serum to effectively neutralize the IFNγ or GM-CSF response to these cytokines. In our laboratory practice, freshly isolated PBMC from acceptable donors are utilized for clinical testing. It may also be possible to utilize cryopreserved PBMC from acceptable donors, however, we have not tested the performance of cryopreserved PBMC for phosphorylation assays extensively. An alternative strategy may be to utilize cell lines that are responsive to these cytokines.

DIAGNOSTIC UTILITY

These functional assays enable the detection of functional, neutralizing AAbs to IFNγ or GM-CSF and have been validated for clinical use in a few clinical laboratories. As illustrated in **Figure 1C**, serum from a patient with extra-pulmonary, treatment-refractory NTM infection inhibited IFNγ-mediated phosphorylation of STAT1 while IFNα responses were unaffected (**Figure 1D**), indicating specificity for the IFNγ pathway. Using protein A purification for immunoglobulins, we demonstrated that the inhibitory component resides in the immunoglobulin fraction of patient's serum (63). In our experience, ELISA analysis of serum samples with known neutralizing activity demonstrated the presence of anti-IFNγ IgG AAbs, therefore proving that inhibition of the IFNγ pathway is IgG mediated. We have additionally shown that these autoantibodies are biologically significant because they abrogate the ability of *Listeria monocytogenes*-infected human monocytes to clear infection when activated by IFNγ (63). Similar to the flow cytometry assay for anti-IFNγ AAbs, inhibition of phosphorylation of STAT5 by serum from patients with clinically proven PAP following GM-CSF stimulation of PBMCs has been established as a clinical assay for functional evaluation of anti-GM-CSF AAbs. In our experience, as with anti-IFNγ AAbs, serum samples that had significant neutralizing activity for GM-CSF mediated phosphorylation of STAT5 also showed increased binding to GM-CSF in an ELISA, confirming that p-STAT5 inhibition by serum samples from these patients was antibody mediated.

CLINICAL AND THERAPEUTIC MONITORING

These flow cytometry-based assays can not only be used to demonstrate the presence of anti-cytokine AAbs in serum samples, but can also be used to monitor the success of immune modulation. Encouraging evidence is emerging for the efficacy of rituximab, an anti-CD20- monoclonal antibody that leads to depletion of B lymphocytes, in IFNγ AAb-mediated acquired immunodeficiency (19, 63, 64). The efficacy of rituximab in inducing and maintaining disease remission has been described in several case reports of patients with anti-IFNγ autoantibodies and treatment-refractory NTM infection (19, 63, 65). Monitoring p-STAT1 expression in conjunction with B cell numbers and percentages is of utility in such patients in order to assess the efficacy of immune modulation. We and others have shown a correlation between the decrease in peripheral blood B cells and improvement in IFNγ-induced phosphorylation of STAT1 as an indication of the release of the IFNγ signaling pathway from anti-IFNγ AAb mediated inhibition (63).

Recombinant GM-CSF (subcutaneous or inhaled) and B cell depleting agents such as rituximab have been used to treat autoimmune PAP due to anti-GM-CSF autoantibodies (66–68). Monitoring anti-GM-CSF AAb levels and their neutralizing capability may be of utility along with the assessment of clinical parameters for determining the efficacy of treatment.

CONCLUSIONS

Anti-cytokine AAbs causing immunodeficiency or dysregulation now form a distinct group of PIDs that share phenotypic characteristics with PIDs that occur due to pathogenic variants in genes encoding proteins involved in cytokine signaling pathways. As the management of patients with anti-cytokine AAbs differs from those with genetically disrupted cytokine signaling pathways, laboratory analysis for these AAbs is essential to enable not just improved phenotyping of these patients, but also to provide diagnostic and immune monitoring tools.

The neutralizing capability of anti-cytokine AAbs can be assessed by the analysis of the phosphorylation status of signaling molecules downstream of the relevant cytokine receptor. Such assays should be combined with ligand binding assays such as ELISA to demonstrate the presence of an antibody that correlates with neutralizing activity. Since signaling molecules such as STAT1 and STAT5 are phosphorylated by several cytokines, it is necessary to demonstrate specificity of these assays by utilizing alternate recombinant cytokine controls where possible. These assays that demonstrate the neutralizing capability of anti-cytokine AAbs are of utility in immune monitoring, particularly to demonstrate recovery of these cytokine pathways if immune depletion of B cells or plasmapheresis is employed to remove the source of the autoantibody or the autoantibody itself.

AUTHOR CONTRIBUTIONS

VK conceptualized and developed content for the manuscript. PM contributed to writing the manuscript. TL performed flow cytometry analysis of the AAb assays.

ACKNOWLEDGMENTS

The authors thank Andrew Gibula for performing the anti-GM-CSF autoantibody analysis.

REFERENCES

1. Browne SK. Anticytokine autoantibody-associated immunodeficiency. *Annu Rev Immunol.* (2014) 32:635–57. doi: 10.1146/annurev-immunol-032713-12 0222
2. Browne SK, Holland SM. Immunodeficiency secondary to anticytokine autoantibodies. *Curr Opin Allergy Clin Immunol.* (2010) 10:534–41. doi: 10.1097/ACI.0b013e328340 2b41
3. Browne SK, Holland SM. Anti-cytokine autoantibodies explain some chronic mucocutaneous candidiasis. *Immunol Cell Biol.* (2010) 88:614–5. doi: 10.1038/icb.2010.72
4. Bousfiha A, Jeddane L, Picard C, Ailal F, Bobby Gaspar H, Al-Herz W, et al. The 2017 IUIS phenotypic classification for primary immunodeficiencies. *J Clin Immunol.* (2018) 38:129–143. doi: 10.1007/s10875-017-0465-8
5. Piccoli L, Campo I, Fregni CS, Rodriguez BM, Minola A, Sallusto F, et al. Neutralization and clearance of GM-CSF by autoantibodies in pulmonary alveolar proteinosis. *Nat Commun.* (2015) 6:7375. doi: 10.1038/ncomms8375
6. Allen TC, Fudala R, Nash SE, Kurdowska A. Anti-interleukin 8 autoantibody:interleukin 8 immune complexes visualized by laser confocal microscopy in injured lung. *Arch Pathol Lab Med.* (2007) 131:452–6.doi: 10.1043/1543-2165(2007)131[452:AAICVB]2.0.CO;2
7. Frede N, Glocker EO, Wanders J, Engelhardt KR, Kreisel W, Ruemmele FM, et al. Evidence for non-neutralizing autoantibodies against IL-10 signalling components in patients with inflammatory bowel disease. *BMC Immunol.* (2014) 15:10. doi: 10.1186/1471-2172-15-10
8. Watanabe M, Uchida K, Nakagaki K, Kanazawa H, Trapnell BC, Hoshino Y, et al. Anti-cytokine autoantibodies are ubiquitous in healthy individuals. *FEBS Lett.* (2007) 581:2017–21. doi: 10.1016/j.febslet.2007.04.029
9. von Stemann JH, Rigas AS, Thorner LW, D.Rasmussen GK, Pedersen OB, Rostgaard K, et al. Prevalence and correlation of cytokine-specific autoantibodies with epidemiological factors and C-reactive protein in 8,972 healthy individuals: results from the Danish blood donor study. *PLoS ONE.* (2017) 12:e0179981. doi: 10.1371/journal.pone.0179981
10. Kurdowska A, Noble JM, Steinberg KP, Ruzinski J, Hudson LD, Martin TR. Anti-IL-8 autoantibodies in alveolar fluid from patients at risk for ARDS and with well-defined ARDS. *Chest.* (1999). 116(1Suppl.):9S. doi: 10.1378/chest.116.suppl_1.9S
11. Cappellano G, Orilieri E, Woldetsadik AD, Boggio E, Soluri MF, Comi C, et al. Anti-cytokine autoantibodies in autoimmune diseases. *Am J Clin Exp Immunol.* (2012) 1:136–46.
12. Graudal NA, Svenson M, Tarp U, Garred P, Jurik AG, Bendtzen K. Autoantibodies against interleukin 1alpha in rheumatoid arthritis: association with long term radiographic outcome. *Ann Rheum Dis.* (2002) 61:598–602. doi: 10.1136/ard.61.7.598
13. Gupta S, Tatouli IP, Rosen LB, Hasni S, Alevizos I, Manna ZG, et al. Distinct functions of autoantibodies against interferon in systemic lupus erythematosus: a comprehensive analysis of anticytokine autoantibodies in common rheumatic diseases. *Arthritis Rheumatol.* (2016) 68:1677–87. doi: 10.1002/art.39607
14. Asakura T, Namkoong H, Sakagami T, Hasegawa N, Ohkusu K, Nakamura A. Disseminated *Mycobacterium genavense* Infection in patient with adult-onset immunodeficiency. *Emerg Infect Dis.* (2017) 23:1208–1210. doi: 10.3201/eid2307.161677
15. Rosen LB, Rocha Pereira N, Figueiredo C, Fiske LC, Ressner RA, Hong JC, et al. Nocardia-induced granulocyte macrophage colony-stimulating factor is neutralized by autoantibodies in disseminated/extrapulmonary nocardiosis. *Clin Infect Dis.* (2015) 60:1017–25. doi: 10.1093/cid/ciu968
16. Elkarim RA, Dahle C, Mustafa M, Press R, Zou LP, Ekerfelt C, et al. Recovery from Guillain-Barre syndrome is associated with increased levels of neutralizing autoantibodies to interferon-gamma. *Clin Immunol Immunopathol.* (1998) 88:241–8. doi: 10.1006/clin.1998.4573
17. Hellmich B, Csernok E, Schatz H, Gross WL, Schnabel A. Autoantibodies against granulocyte colony-stimulating factor in Felty's syndrome and neutropenic systemic lupus erythematosus. *Arthritis Rheum.* (2002) 46:2384–91. doi: 10.1002/art.10497
18. Koya T, Tsubata C, Kagamu H, Koyama K, Hayashi M, Kuwabara K, et al. Anti-interferon-gamma autoantibody in a patient with disseminated *Mycobacterium avium* complex. *J Infect Chemother.* (2009) 15:118–22. doi: 10.1007/s10156-008-0662-8
19. Koizumi Y, Sakagami T, Nishiyama N, Hirai J, Hayashi Y, Asai N, et al. Rituximab restores IFN-gamma-STAT1 function and ameliorates disseminated *mycobacterium avium* infection in a patient with anti-interferon-gamma autoantibody. *J Clin Immunol.* (2017) 37:644–649. doi: 10.1007/s10875-017-0425-3
20. Sarkadi AK, Tasko S, Csorba G, Toth B, Erdos M, Marodi L. Autoantibodies to IL-17A may be correlated with the severity of mucocutaneous candidiasis in APECED patients. *J Clin Immunol.* (2014) 34:181–93. doi: 10.1007/s10875-014-9987-5
21. Puel A, Doffinger R, Natividad A, Chrabieh M, Barcenas-Morales G, Picard C, et al. Autoantibodies against IL-17A, IL-17F, and IL-22 in patients with chronic mucocutaneous candidiasis and autoimmune polyendocrine syndrome type I. *J Exp Med.* (2010) 207:291–7. doi: 10.1084/jem.20091983
22. Humbert L, Cornu M, Proust-Lemoine E, Bayry J, Wemeau JL, Vantyghem MC, et al. Chronic mucocutaneous candidiasis in autoimmune polyendocrine syndrome type 1. *Front Immunol.* (2018) 9:2570. doi: 10.3389/fimmu.2018.02570
23. Ding L, Mo A, Jutivorakool K, Pancholi M, Holland SM, Browne SK. Determination of human anticytokine autoantibody profiles using a particle-based approach. *J Clin Immunol.* (2012) 32:238–45. doi: 10.1007/s10875-011-9621-8
24. Applen Clancey S, Ciccone EJ, Coelho MA, Davis J, Ding L, Betancourt R, et al. Cryptococcus deuterogattii VGIIa infection associated with travel to the pacific northwest outbreak region in an anti-granulocyte-macrophage colony-stimulating factor autoantibody-positive patient in the United States. *MBio.* (2019). 10:e02733-18. doi: 10.1128/mBio.02733-18
25. Kuo CY, Wang SY, Shih HP, Tu KH, Huang WC, Ding JY, et al. Disseminated cryptococcosis due to anti-granulocyte-macrophage colony-stimulating factor autoantibodies in the absence of pulmonary alveolar proteinosis. *J Clin Immunol.* (2017) 37:143–152. doi: 10.1007/s10875-016-0364-4
26. Sim BT, Browne SK, Vigliani M, Zachary D, Rosen L, Holland SM, et al. Recurrent Burkholderia gladioli suppurative lymphadenitis associated with neutralizing anti-IL-12p70 autoantibodies. *J Clin Immunol.* (2013) 33:1057–61. doi: 10.1007/s10875-013-9908-z
27. Shiono H, Wong YL, Matthews I, Liu JL, Zhang W, Sims G, et al. Spontaneous production of anti-IFN-alpha and anti-IL-12 autoantibodies by thymoma cells from myasthenia gravis patients suggests autoimmunization in the tumor. *Int Immunol.* (2003) 15:903–13. doi: 10.1093/intimm/dxg088
28. Karner J, Pihlap M, Ranki A, Krohn K, Trebusak Podkrajsek K, Bratanic N, et al. IL-6-specific autoantibodies among APECED and thymoma patients. *Immun Inflamm Dis.* (2016) 4:235–43. doi: 10.1002/iid3.109
29. Nanki T, Onoue I, Nagasaka K, Takayasu A, Ebisawa M, Hosoya T, et al. Suppression of elevations in serum C reactive protein levels by anti-IL-6 autoantibodies in two patients with severe bacterial infections. *Ann Rheum Dis.* (2013) 72:1100–2. doi: 10.1136/annrheumdis-2012-202768
30. Takemura H, Suzuki H, Yoshizaki K, Ogata A, Yuhara T, Akama T, et al. Anti-interleukin-6 autoantibodies in rheumatic diseases. Increased frequency in the sera of patients with systemic sclerosis. *Arthritis Rheum.* (1992) 35:940–3. doi: 10.1002/art.1780350814
31. Meager A, Visvalingam K, Peterson P, Moll K, Murumagi A, Krohn K, et al. Anti-interferon autoantibodies in autoimmune polyendocrinopathy syndrome type 1. *PLoS Med.* (2006) 3:e289. doi: 10.1371/journal.pmed.0030289
32. Walter JE, Rosen LB, Csomos K, Rosenberg JM, Mathew D, Keszei M, et al. Broad-spectrum antibodies against self-antigens and cytokines in RAG deficiency. *J Clin Invest.* (2016) 126:4389. doi: 10.1172/JCI91162
33. Rosenberg JM, Maccari ME, Barzaghi F, Allenspach EJ, Pignata C, Weber G, et al. Neutralizing anti-cytokine autoantibodies against interferon-alpha in immunodysregulation polyendocrinopathy enteropathy X-linked. *Front Immunol.* (2018) 9:544. doi: 10.3389/fimmu.2018.00544
34. Forslind K, Svensson B, Svenson M, Bendtzen K. Anti-IL-1alpha autoantibodies in early rheumatoid arthritis. *Scand J Rheumatol.* (2001) 30:167–8. doi: 10.1080/030097401300162950
35. Lindqvist E, Eberhardt K, Bendtzen K, Heinegard D, Saxne T. Prognostic laboratory markers of joint damage in rheumatoid arthritis. *Ann Rheum Dis.* (2005) 64:196–201. doi: 10.1136/ard.2003.019992

36. Howe HS, B.Thong YH, Kong KO, Chng HH, Lian TY, Chia FL, et al. Associations of B cell-activating factor (BAFF) and anti-BAFF autoantibodies with disease activity in multi-ethnic Asian systemic lupus erythematosus patients in Singapore. *Clin Exp Immunol.* (2017) 189:298–303. doi: 10.1111/cei.12975
37. Pott MC, Frede N, Wanders J, Hammarstrom L, Glocker EO, Glocker C, et al. Autoantibodies against BAFF, APRIL or IL21 - an alternative pathogenesis for antibody-deficiencies? *BMC Immunol.* (2017) 18:34. doi: 10.1186/s12865-017-0217-9
38. Bergman R, Ramon M, Wildbaum G, Avitan-Hersh E, Mayer E, Shemer A, et al. Psoriasis patients generate increased serum levels of autoantibodies to tumor necrosis factor-alpha and interferon-alpha. *J Dermatol Sci.* (2009) 56:163–7. doi: 10.1016/j.jdermsci.2009.08.006
39. Krupa A, Kato H, Matthay MA, Kurdowska AK. Proinflammatory activity of anti-IL-8 autoantibody:IL-8 complexes in alveolar edema fluid from patients with acute lung injury. *Am J Physiol Lung Cell Mol Physiol.* (2004) 286:L1105–13. doi: 10.1152/ajplung.00277.2003
40. Casadevall N, Nataf J, Viron B, Kolta A, Kiladjian JJ, Martin-Dupont P, et al. Pure red-cell aplasia and antierythropoietin antibodies in patients treated with recombinant erythropoietin. *N Engl J Med.* (2002) 346:469–75. doi: 10.1056/NEJMoa011931
41. Sakata M, Tsuruha JI, Masuko-Hongo K, Nakamura H, Matsui T, Sudo A, et al. Autoantibodies to osteopontin in patients with osteoarthritis and rheumatoid arthritis. *J Rheumatol.* (2001) 28:1492–5.
42. Ying X, Zhao Y, Wang JL, Zhou X, Zhao J, He CC, et al. Serum anti-osteopontin autoantibody as a novel diagnostic and prognostic biomarker in patients with hepatocellular carcinoma. *Oncol Rep.* (2014) 32:1550–6. doi: 10.3892/or.2014.3367
43. Hauser B, Zhao S, Visconti MR, Riches PL, Fraser WD, Piec I, et al. Autoantibodies to osteoprotegerin are associated with low hip bone mineral density and history of fractures in axial spondyloarthritis: a cross-sectional observational study. *Calcif Tissue Int.* (2017) 101:375–383. doi: 10.1007/s00223-017-0291-2
44. Real A, Gilbert N, Hauser B, Kennedy N, Shand A, Gillett H, et al. Characterisation of osteoprotegerin autoantibodies in coeliac disease. *Calcif Tissue Int.* (2015) 97:125–33. doi: 10.1007/s00223-015-0023-4
45. Boisson-Dupuis S, Bustamante J, El-Baghdadi J, Camcioglu Y, Parvaneh N, El Azbaoui S, et al. Inherited and acquired immunodeficiencies underlying tuberculosis in childhood. *Immunol Rev.* (2015) 264:103–20. doi: 10.1111/imr.12272
46. McCarthy KD, Cain KP, Winthrop KL, Udomsantisuk N, Lan NT, Sar B, et al. Nontuberculous mycobacterial disease in patients with HIV in Southeast Asia. *Am J Respir Crit Care Med.* (2012) 185:981–8. doi: 10.1164/rccm.201107-1327OC
47. Varley CD, Ku JH, Henkle E, Schafer SD, Winthrop KL. Disseminated nontuberculous mycobacteria in HIV-infected patients, Oregon, USA, 2007-2012. *Emerg Infect Dis.* (2017) 23:533–535. doi: 10.3201/eid2303.161708
48. Dorman S, Subramanian A, AST Infectious Diseases Community of Practice. Nontuberculous mycobacteria in solid organ transplant recipients. *Am J Transplant.* (2009). 9(Suppl. 4): S63–9. doi: 10.1111/j.1600-6143.2009.02895.x
49. Longworth SA, Blumberg EA, Barton TD, Vinnard C. Non-tuberculous mycobacterial infections after solid organ transplantation: a survival analysis. *Clin Microbiol Infect.* (2015) 21:43–7. doi: 10.1016/j.cmi.2014.07.001
50. Al-Anazi KA, Al-Jasser AM, Al-Anazi WK. Infections caused by non-tuberculous mycobacteria in recipients of hematopoietic stem cell transplantation. *Front Oncol.* (2014) 4:311. doi: 10.3389/fonc.2014.00311
51. Doffinger R, Helbert MR, Barcenas-Morales G, Yang K, Dupuis S, Ceron-Gutierrez L, et al. Autoantibodies to interferon-gamma in a patient with selective susceptibility to mycobacterial infection and organ-specific autoimmunity. *Clin Infect Dis.* (2004) 38:e10–4. doi: 10.1086/380453
52. O'Connell E, Rosen LB, LaRue RW, Fabre V, Melia MT, Auwaerter PG, et al. The first US domestic report of disseminated *Mycobacterium avium* complex and anti-interferon-gamma autoantibodies. *J Clin Immunol.* (2014) 34:928–32. doi: 10.1007/s10875-014-0073-9
53. Hanitsch LG, Lobel M, Muller-Redetzky H, Schurmann M, Suttorp N, Unterwalder N, et al. Late-onset disseminated *mycobacterium avium* intracellulare complex infection (MAC), cerebral toxoplasmosis and salmonella sepsis in a german caucasian patient with unusual anti-interferon-gamma IgG1 autoantibodies. *J Clin Immunol.* (2015) 35:361–5. doi: 10.1007/s10875-015-0161-5
54. Chi CY, Chu CC, Liu JP, Lin CH, Ho MW, Lo WJ, et al. Anti-IFN-gamma autoantibodies in adults with disseminated nontuberculous mycobacterial infections are associated with HLA-DRB1*16:02 and HLA-DQB1*05:02 and the reactivation of latent varicella-zoster virus infection. *Blood.* (2013) 121:1357–66. doi: 10.1182/blood-2012-08-452482
55. Lin CH, Chi CY, Shih HP, Ding JY, Lo CC, Wang SY, et al. Identification of a major epitope by anti-interferon-gamma autoantibodies in patients with mycobacterial disease. *Nat Med.* (2016) 22:994–1001. doi: 10.1038/nm.4158
56. Trapnell BC, Whitsett JA, Nakata K. Pulmonary alveolar proteinosis. *N Engl J Med.* (2003) 349:2527–39. doi: 10.1056/NEJMra023226
57. Golde DW, Territo M, Finley TN, Cline MJ. Defective lung macrophages in pulmonary alveolar proteinosis. *Ann Intern Med.* (1976) 85:304–9. doi: 10.7326/0003-4819-85-3-304
58. Gonzalez-Rothi RJ, Harris JO. Pulmonary alveolar proteinosis. Further evaluation of abnormal alveolar macrophages. *Chest.* (1986) 90:656–61. doi: 10.1378/chest.90.5.656
59. Punatar AD, Kusne S, Blair JE, Seville MT, Vikram HR. Opportunistic infections in patients with pulmonary alveolar proteinosis. *J Infect.* (2012) 65:173–9. doi: 10.1016/j.jinf.2012.03.020
60. Crum-Cianflone NF, Lam PV, Ross-Walker S, Rosen LB, Holland SM. Autoantibodies to granulocyte-macrophage colony-stimulating factor associated with severe and unusual manifestations of *Cryptococcus gattii* infections. *Open Forum Infect Dis.* (2017) 4:ofx211. doi: 10.1093/ofid/ofx211
61. Schroder K, Hertzog PJ, Ravasi T, Hume DA. Interferon-gamma: an overview of signals, mechanisms and functions. *J Leukoc Biol.* (2004) 75:163–89. doi: 10.1189/jlb.0603252
62. Hercus TR, Thomas D, Guthridge MA, Ekert PG, King-Scott J, Parker MW, et al. The granulocyte-macrophage colony-stimulating factor receptor: linking its structure to cell signaling and its role in disease. *Blood.* (2009) 114:1289–98. doi: 10.1182/blood-2008-12-164004
63. Czaja CA, Merkel PA, Chan ED, Lenz LL, Wolf ML, Alam R, et al. Rituximab as successful adjunct treatment in a patient with disseminated nontuberculous mycobacterial infection due to acquired anti-interferon-gamma autoantibody. *Clin Infect Dis.* (2014) 58:e115–8. doi: 10.1093/cid/cit809
64. Browne SK, Zaman R, Sampaio EP, Jutivorakool K, Rosen LB, Ding L, et al. Anti-CD20 (rituximab) therapy for anti-IFN-gamma autoantibody-associated nontuberculous mycobacterial infection. *Blood.* (2012) 119:3933–9. doi: 10.1182/blood-2011-12-395707
65. Lutt JR, Pisculli ML, Weinblatt ME, Deodhar A, Winthrop KL. Severe nontuberculous mycobacterial infection in 2 patients receiving rituximab for refractory myositis. *J Rheumatol.* (2008) 35:1683–5.
66. Soyez B, Borie R, Menard C, Cadranel J, Chavez L, Cottin V, et al. Rituximab for auto-immune alveolar proteinosis, a real life cohort study. *Respir Res.* (2018) 19:74. doi: 10.1186/s12931-018-0780-5
67. Kumar A, Abdelmalak B, Inoue Y, Culver DA. Pulmonary alveolar proteinosis in adults: pathophysiology and clinical approach. *Lancet Respir Med.* (2018) 6:554–65. doi: 10.1016/S2213-2600(18)30043-2
68. Tazawa R, Trapnell BC, Inoue Y, Arai T, Takada T, Nasuhara Y, et al. Inhaled granulocyte/macrophage-colony stimulating factor as therapy for pulmonary alveolar proteinosis. *Am J Respir Crit Care Med.* (2010) 181:1345–54. doi: 10.1164/rccm.200906-0978OC

3

Application of Flow Cytometry in Primary Immunodeficiencies: Experience From India

Manisha Rajan Madkaikar, Snehal Shabrish, Manasi Kulkarni, Jahnavi Aluri, Aparna Dalvi, Madhura Kelkar and Maya Gupta*

Department of Paediatric Immunology and Leukocyte Biology, National Institute of Iummunohematology (ICMR), Mumbai, India

***Correspondence:**
Manisha Rajan Madkaikar
madkaikarmanisha@gmail.com

Primary immunodeficiency diseases (PID) are a clinically and immunologically heterogeneous group of disorders of immune system. Diagnosis of these disorders is often challenging and requires identification of underlying genetic defects, complemented by a comprehensive evaluation of immune system. Flow cytometry, with its advances in the last few decades, has emerged as an indispensable tool for enumeration as well as characterization of immune cells. Flow cytometric evaluation of the immune system not only provides clues to underlying genetic defects in certain PIDs and helps in functional validation of novel genetic defects, but is also useful in monitoring immune responses following specific therapies. India has witnessed significant progress in the field of flow cytometry as well as PID over last one decade. Currently, there are seven Federation of Primary Immunodeficiency Diseases (FPID) recognized centers across India, including two Indian Council of Medical research (ICMR) funded centers of excellence for diagnosis, and management of PIDs. These centers offer comprehensive care for PIDs including flow cytometry based evaluation. The key question which always remains is how one selects from the wide array of flow cytometry based tests available, and whether all these tests should be performed before or after the identification of genetic defects. This becomes crucial, especially when resources are limited and patients have to pay for the investigations. In this review, we will share some of our experiences based on evaluation of a large cohort of hemophagocytic lymphohistiocytosis, severe combined immunodeficiency, and chronic granulomatous disease, and the lessons learned for optimum use of this powerful technology for diagnosis of these disorders.

Keywords: flow cytometry, primary immunodeficiency disorders, familial HLH, severe combined immunodeficiency (SCID), chronic granulomatous disease (CGD)

INTRODUCTION

Primary immunodeficiency diseases (PID) are an heterogeneous inherited group of disorders of different components within the immune system, resulting from genetic defects (1). PIDs are clinically and immunologically diverse and require a wide array of diagnostic tools for their accurate diagnosis. Flow cytometry, with the advances that have occurred in the last few decades, has emerged as an indispensable tool for evaluation of the immune system (2). It helps in enumeration as well as characterization of immune cells, and thus helps in the diagnosis of large number of PIDs.

It has now become widely available and is increasingly used for diagnostic purposes. In India, we have nearly 2000 installations of different flow cytometers across the country. The majority of them are being utilized for the measurement of CD4 counts in HIV infected patients and leukemia immunophenotyping. However, in the last decade there has been significant progress in the field of PID in India; currently there are two "Indian Council of Medical research-Centre of Excellence (COE) for PID" and seven Federation of Primary Immunodeficiency (FPID) centers across India. Both the COEs not only focus their work on setting up diagnostic facilities for PIDs in India, but also on understanding the immunopathogenesis of certain rare PIDs.

Due to the complexity of the immune system, multiple assays, which are expensive, are often required for comprehensive evaluation of the immune system. Moreover, they may not always give a definite diagnosis in spite of extensive evaluation. Furthermore, for final confirmation of diagnosis one always requires identification of the underlying genetic defect. With recent progress in the genetics field and increasing accessibility to Next Generation sequencing (NGS) based analysis, NGS is often used as a preferred modality for the diagnosis of PIDs. However, one needs to remember the utility and limitations of both genetic testing as well as phenotypic analysis. It is important that for all the genetic defects identified, corresponding immunological consequences are demonstrated, which are most often based on flow cytometry.

UTILITY OF FLOW CYTOMETRY FOR DIAGNOSIS OF PIDS- EXPERIENCE AT ICMR-NIIH

ICMR-NIIH is one of the few centers in India providing comprehensive workup for patients suspected with PID. To determine the utility of flow cytometry in the diagnosis of PIDs, we retrospectively correlated findings of flow cytometry based assays and molecular confirmation of the disorder. In the last 10 years, we have diagnosed 753 PID patients by using flow cytometry based assays including immunophenotyping, specific protein detection, and functional analysis. Of these patients, we could molecularly characterize 319 PID patients; 232 (73%) by using direct Sanger sequencing and 87 (27%) by using NGS.

In our experience, perforin deficiency (FHL-2) LAD-I and CGD were among the PIDs in which flow cytometry based assays provided a direct clue for the underlying genetic defect. Sanger sequencing of the respective genes correlated in >90% of the patients (LAD-I: 100%; FHL2 (Perforin deficiency): 97%; CGD: 90%). Thus, for molecular confirmation of these disorders, one should first perform Sanger sequencing of the respective genes rather than directly proceeding for NGS. This approach will be less time consuming and cost-effective.

However, for some PIDs, especially HLH with defective degranulation mechanism and SCID, multiple genes are involved. Flow cytometry based degranulation assay helps in identifying HLH patients with defective degranulation assay, and lymphocyte subset assay, T cell proliferation, and naïve T cell markers help in identifying SCID patients. Though flow cytometry based assays help in the diagnosis of these disorders, they are not sufficient for identifying specific genes involved in causing the disorder. Thus, these assays may be utilized as screening tests for diagnosing the disorders and molecular confirmation targeted at NGS is essential (**Supplementary Table 1**).

At ICMR-NIIH, we have maximum experience of using flow cytometry based assays in three disorders included under PIDs: familial hemophagocytic lymphohistiocytosis (FHL); severe combined immunodeficiency diseases (SCID); and chronic granulomatous diseases (CGD). We have reviewed the use of flow cytometry in these diseases systematically and shared some of our important practical experiences for the further, improved utility of flow cytometry in diagnosis of these disorders.

FAMILIAL HEMOPHAGOCYTIC LYMPHOHISTIOCYTOSIS (FHL)

Hemophagocytic lymphohistiocytosis (HLH) is a life-threatening hyperinflammatory syndrome, characterized by excessive activation of macrophages and T cells, resulting from defective cytotoxicity. It presents as a severe systemic illness with persistent high-grade fever, progressive cytopenias, and hepatosplenomegaly.

HLH can either be genetic (due to inherited defects in NK cell function) or acquired HLH (HLH resulting from secondary causes like infections, malignancy, etc.). Genetic HLH can be classified as familial HLH (FHL) and lymphoproliferative syndromes and FHL is then further sub-classified as with and without hypopigmentation. Till now, based on the mutated gene, FHL is classified as FHL2 (*PRF1*), FHL3 (*UNC13D*), FHL4 (*STX11*), and FHL5 (*STXBP2*) encoding for Perforin, Munc13-4, Syntaxin11, and Syntaxin binding protein 2, respectively (3).

FHL1 (9q21.3-22) was identified by homozygosity mapping of four inbred families of Pakistani origin (4), however, the disease-causing gene has so far not been identified in this locus. The incidence of the four types varies significantly in different ethnic groups. FHL with hypopigmentation includes Griscelli syndrome type 2 (GS2) (*Rab27a*), Chediak-Higashi syndrome (CHS) (*LYST*), and Hermansky-Pudlak syndrome type 2 (*AP3B1*). Exposure to EBV or other viruses can trigger HLH associated with lymphoproliferative syndromes, which can either be X-linked (XLP and XMEN) or autosomal recessive (*ITK* deficiency and CD27 deficiency).

Clinical and laboratory features of HLH overlap with those of severe infection and other inflammatory diseases, leading to either misdiagnosis or delay in the diagnosis of HLH. Unless specific genetic defect is identified, no single laboratory test is specific for HLH. Thus, in 1991, the Histiocyte society established guidelines for HLH diagnosis which collectively included clinical manifestations and laboratory findings. These criteria were revised in 2007 (5). Five of the eight criteria are required for diagnosis of HLH. Though these criteria help in the diagnosis of HLH, it does not help in differentiating genetic HLH from acquired HLH.

Both genetic and acquired HLH patients have impaired NK cells and CTL cells function. However, genetic HLH patients have inherited defect in the granule mediated cytotoxicity, while acquired HLH patients have transient defect. Thus, evaluating NK cell and CTL cell function in HLH patients helps in identifying genetic HLH patients.

Reduced NK cell cytotoxicity is one of the eight HLH diagnostic criteria (5) used for identifying HLH patients. New flow cytometry based assays have been developed in recent years, for evaluating NK cell and CTL cell functions by detection of intracellular perforin levels and degranulation assays (determined by upregulation of CD107a expression). Granule release assay (GRA) is a screening test for diagnosing FHL3, FHL4, and FHL5 patients, and helps in discriminate primary HLH with degranulation defects from secondary HLH. Whereas, detection of intracellular perforin levels helps in identifying FHL2 patients. Flow cytometry based assays, for determination of intracellular SAP and XIAP expression, helps in the diagnosis of XLP-1 and XLP-2, respectively.

In 2017, Rubin et al. retrospectively studied the diagnostic accuracy of NK cell cytotoxicity, intracellular perforin expression, and CD107a upregulation in a large cohort of HLH patients. In this, the sensitivity and specificity of these assays were evaluated in HLH patients. The authors concluded, firstly, the protocols used for NK cell cytotoxicity assay are labor intensive, usually involving radioactivity, and are not widely available. Secondly, the assay does not discriminate between primary and secondary HLH and, therefore, is not useful for differential diagnosis of HLH subtypes. It also proposes that perforin and CD107a tests are more sensitive and no less specific, compared with NK-cell cytotoxicity testing when screening for genetic HLH, and should be considered as an addition to current HLH criteria (6).

PERFORIN AND GRANZYME EXPRESSION

Apoptosis of target cells recognized by NK cells and CTLs is induced by the synergistic action of perforin and granzymes. Perforin deficiency caused by mutation in the *PRF1* gene causes FHL2 and accounts for 20 to 50% of all FHL cases (5, 7). Whereas, elevated granzyme B in NK cells and CTLs is reported as a signature of immune activation in HLH patients, regardless of underlying genetic defect (8).

Flow cytometric detection of perforin in NK cells and CTLs has been reported in literature and is found to be a rapid and sensitive approach for the detection of perforin deficiency (9). Two antibody clones, δG9 and B-D48, are available for the

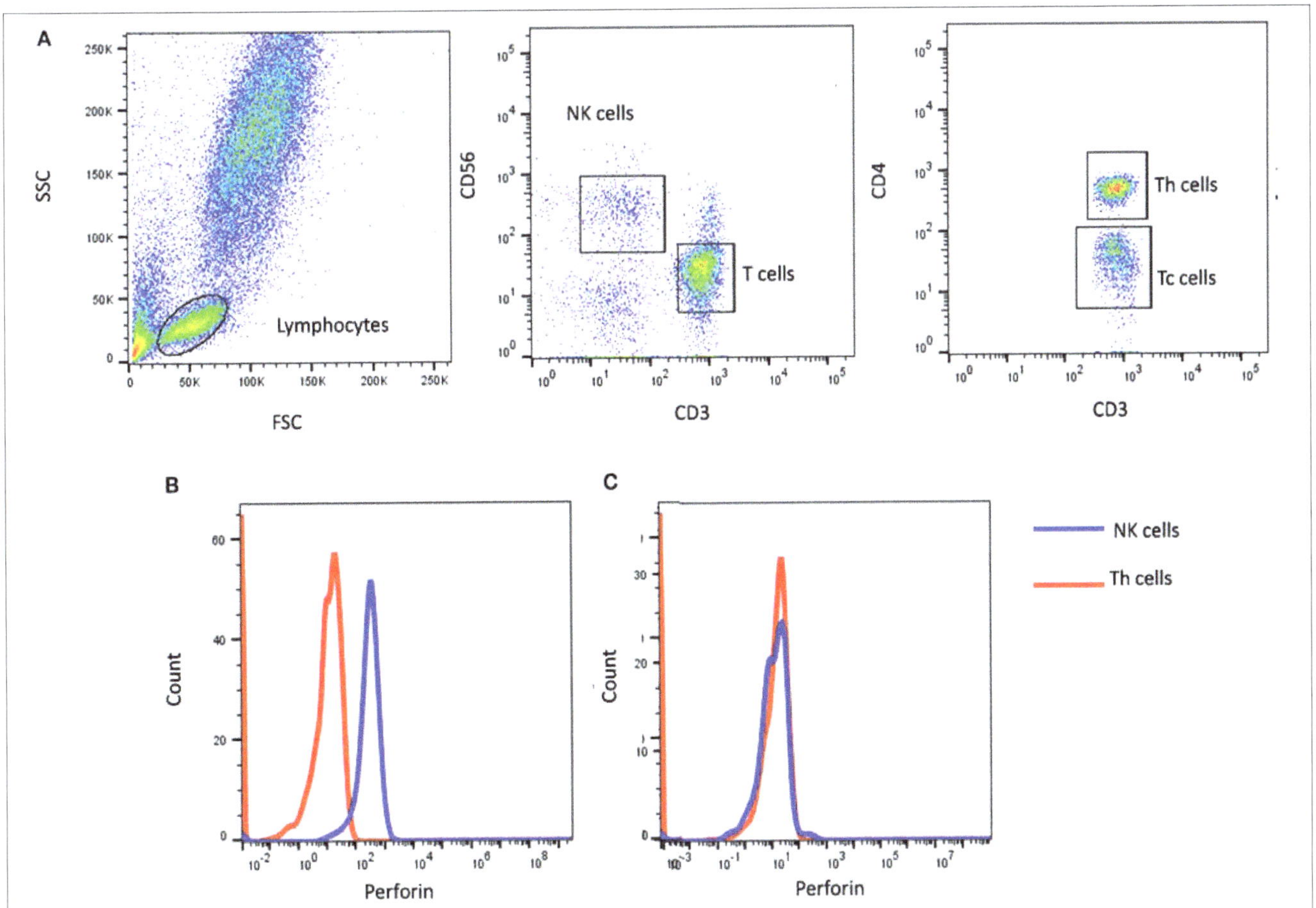

FIGURE 1 | Perforin expression on NK cells. **(A)** Samples were analyzed by flow cytometry, gating on lymphocytes by forward/side scatter. Perforin expression was analyzed on natural killer (NK) cells (CD56+CD3-) (blue histogram) using T helper cells as internal negative control (red histogram). Perforin expression results are shown from **(B)** a healthy control and **(C)** FHL2 (Perforin deficient) patient.

detection of perforin. Clone δG9 detects the form of perforin found in the acidic milieu of the granules and clone B-D48 recognizes both the late form of perforin as well as its newly synthesized form. For clinical flow cytometric screening of perforin in HLH patients, clone δG9 is used unanimously (6, 9–11), whereas, clone B-D48 is used in *in-vitro* assays, especially in cytokine-staining (ICS) assays (12).

In healthy individuals, perforin expression in NK cells is reported to be more than 80%, irrespective of age; however, that increases with age in CTLs (9, 13). Our data is also in agreement of these findings. In perforin deficient patients, both NK cells and CTLs have either absent or partial perforin expression and need further confirmation by molecular testing of *PRF1* gene. The most detrimental *PRF1* gene mutations are usually associated with minimal or no protein expression, while compound heterozygous *PRF1* gene missense mutations may encode partially active perforin and are predominantly detected in older patients with milder clinical manifestations probably due to the residual perforin protein (7, 14, 15). In a study by Kogawa et al. (9), perforin expression in parents (heterozygous carriers) of perforin deficient patients was evaluated. It was observed that they had normal perforin expression in NK cells but with reduced mean fluorescent intensity. CTLs, though, had reduced perforin expression (9). However, the reason for this reduced perforin expression in heterozygous carriers of *PRF1* mutations remains unclear.

In our institute, we have evaluated more than 600 HLH patients of which we have identified 39 perforin deficient patients. We could perform molecular characterization on *PRF1* gene in 36 patients and identified mutation in 34 patients (95%) (10) (**Figure 1**). Also, one HLH patient with normal perforin expression (78% on NK cells) harbored a mutation in the *PRF1* gene; thus highlighting that normal perforin expression does not rule out defect in functionally or structurally abnormal protein. In a recent report by Abdalgani et al. (11), where accuracy of perforin expression by flow cytometry was evaluated, it was concluded that, compared to patients with biallelic*PRF1* mutations, patients with monoallelic mutations, variants of uncertain clinical significance, and a minority of HLH patients without *PRF1* mutations, had normal perforin expression but lower mean fluorescence intensity (MFI) (11). Thus, while analyzing perforin expression, both frequency and MFI should also be considered. Overall literature and our experience support the fact that clinical flow cytometric screening for perforin deficiency is sensitive and is associated with a low false-negative rate.

Elevated granzyme B expression in NK cells and CTLs is a signature of immune activation in HLH patients, irrespective of genetic background. While assessing perforin expression, intracellular granzyme B staining is routinely utilized as an internal control in some laboratories. In 2013, Sabine reported granzyme B as a useful biomarker of disease activity (8). However, further studies including patients with MAS, autoinflammatory disorder, autoimmune diseases, sepsis, etc., are essential for understanding the utility of granzyme B in the diagnosis of HLH.

NK CELL AND CTL DEGRANULATION ASSAY

Flow cytometry based granule release assay (GRA) is a rapid assay for the evaluation of granule exocytosis pathway. CD107a, a lysosomal protein, is present on the surface of cytolytic granules in NK cells and CTLs and is not expressed on the cell surface. After stimulation of these cells the lytic granules fuse with the plasma membrane of cytotoxic lymphocytes and CD107a is expressed on the cell surface. Abnormal degranulation after stimulation suggests defect in the degranulation mechanism, which includes cytolytic granule migration, docking, priming, or fusion.

This assay is a screening test for diagnosing FHL3, FHL4, and FHL5 patients, and helps in discriminating primary HLH with degranulation defects from secondary HLH.

In literature, various protocols for evaluating degranulation mechanism in NK cells and CTLs have been reported. These protocols mainly differ in the stimuli used, the initial sample used purified cells or whole blood cells and the use of a cytolytic content secretion inhibitor, monensin. Here we have reviewed the different protocols reported in literature and also shared our experience.

Different stimuli having specific mechanisms for activating CTLs and NK cells have been reported, including K562 (NK cell specific MHC I devoid target cells), PMA/ionomycin (protein kinase C activator), PHA (mitogen receptor), and anti-CD3 plus anti-CD-28 (TCR/CD3 complex). Although PMA/Ionomycin, PHA, and anti-CD3 plus anti-CD28 can all activate lymphocytes, PMA/ionomycin is reported to be the best one for short-term stimulation (16, 17). PMA is a substitute for diacylglycerol (DAG), one of the adaptor proteins required for the activation of protein kinase C, and Ionomycin increases intracellular calcium levels. Therefore, the combination of PMA/Ionomycin facilitates the activation of protein kinase C and an influx of intracellular calcium which are the necessary signaling events for degranulation.

Conventionally these assays use either PBMC or pure cell populations, however, this requires additional steps of cell purification and more volume of blood. In 2009, Claus M reported comprehensive analysis of NK cell function in whole blood samples (18). In this report, the CD107a surface expression was evaluated by stimulating NK cells with K562 cells using whole blood sample and no significant difference in the results were observed.

In our previous publication (19), we have also reported NK cell degranulation assay using whole blood and stimulation with PMA/Ionomycin (**Figure 2**). We had compared PBMC and whole blood and also K562 and PMA/Ionomycin stimuli. The results of whole blood with PMA/Ionomycin stimuli showed comparable results to the conventional methods. In this modified assay, whole blood is used and no cell line is needed thus it requires reduced blood volume, is cost-effective, less time consuming, and avoids necessity for specialized laboratory for cell culture, which makes it applicable in routine clinical set-up.

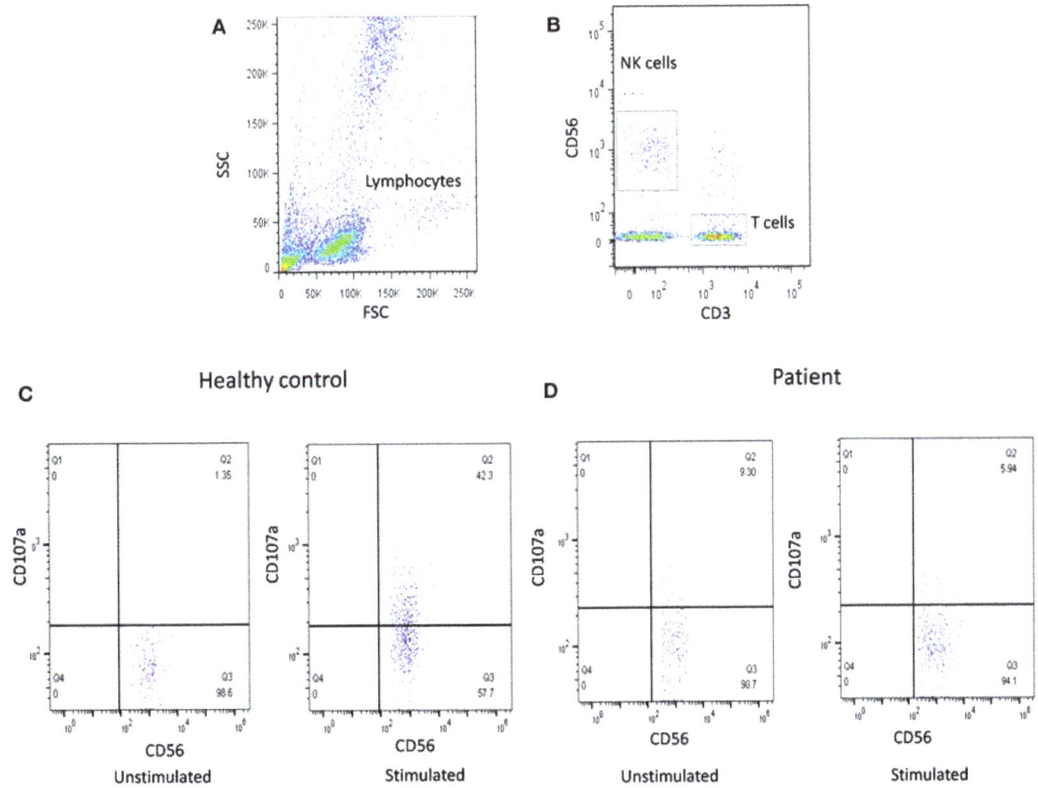

FIGURE 2 | NK cell degranulation assay results. **(A)** Samples were analyzed by flow cytometry, gating on lymphocytes by forward/side scatter. **(B)** NK cells were gated based on (CD56+CD3-). CD107a expression was analyzed on unstimulated and Ca-I + PMA stimulated natural killer (NK) cells (CD56+CD3-). Degranulation assay results are shown from **(C)** healthy control (representative plot) and **(D)** FHL patients with degranulation defect.

After degranulation, once CD107a is expressed on the cell surface it becomes internalized by endocytosis. To prevent the degradation of internalized CD107a monensin is usually added. Monensin is a polyether ionophore that blocks the acidification of endocytic vesicles. However, such ionophores may disturb cellular signaling and function and should be avoided in experiments studying NK cell function. Moreover, in assays lasting 2 h or less, the internalization of surface expressed CD107a on resting NK cells is negligible (20, 21). Assays using monensin require 4–6 h of incubation, as reported by Bryceson YT (21); this was supported by our experience of CD107a expression as using a 2 h assay without monensin was observed to have comparable results to that reported in literature using monensin (19, 21).

Different reported studies have revealed that the results of degranulation on NK-cell and CTLs are in accordance with each other for the correct diagnosis of patients (22–24). However, in a recent report by Hori et al (25), it is suggested that, rather than NK-cell based assays, CD57+ CTL degranulation assay more effectively identified FHL-3 patients. Earlier studies have shown that CTL expressing CD57 has a high cytotoxic potential, and CD57 expression on CTL can be used as a measure of their degranulation capacity (25). This study concludes that NK cell degranulation assay detects FHL-3 patients with high sensitivity (100%) but low specificity (71%), whereas CD57+ CTL degranulation assay has high sensitivity and specificity (both 100%).

A low number of NK cells during active HLH episode often results in the interpretation of the assay result challenging. In such conditions, the CD107a degranulation on CTL for the diagnosis of HLH can be tested, as CTL numbers are usually much higher than NK cell numbers, even in patients with lymphopenia. Although limited studies are available in the literature on degranulation on CTLs as compared to NK cell mediated degranulation, a selective few reports suggest utilization of CTL degranulation for the characterization of FHL-3, FHL-4, and FHL-5 *in vitro* and *in vivo* (22, 25).

At our own institute, we have compared CD107a degranulation of NK-cells and CTL for the diagnosis of HLH in a small patient cohort (unpublished data). In our cohort, CD107a degranulation both on NK-cells and CTLs correlated in all patients. In nine patients we observed severe lymphopenia (absolute lymphocyte count <500/μl), all of whom had very low NK cell numbers (<25 cell/mm^3); hence, performing NK cell degranulation was not feasible. These patients had normal CTL degranulation assays. Observations from our small cohort suggest that, in addition to decreased NK-cell degranulation being a diagnostic criterion for HLH, CTL degranulation assays can be used in those patients with a low NK cell number, although validation in large study cohort is needed for confirmation.

SAP AND XIAP EXPRESSION

For diagnosis of XLP-1 and XLP-2, all male patients should be additionally investigated for the expression of SAP (*SH2D1A*) and XIAP, respectively, (*BIRC4*).

XLP-1 and XLP-2 patients demonstrate low or absent SAP and XIAP expression, respectively (26–28). Since these are X-linked disorders, the bimodal pattern of SAP or XIAP expression in flow cytometric analysis can be used for the detection of carrier status, especially in mothers of affected patients (26). In carrier mothers, interestingly bimodal distribution of XIAP is seen to be skewed toward XIAP-expressing cells in all subsets, indicating a likely survival advantage for XIAP-expressing cells (28). *De novo* mutations in *SH2D1A* as well as *BIRC4* are also observed and in such cases bimodal pattern of respective protein might not be observed in carrier mothers.

However, molecular characterization of *SH2D1A* and *BIRC4* gene is essential for confirmation of diagnosis.

ALGORITHM FOR DIAGNOSIS OF HLH

Based on our experience, and also as reported in literature (29–33), perforin deficiency and granule release assay defect is observed to be more or less equally present and, hence, in our algorithm we suggest to perform perforin estimation and GRA simultaneously, which saves much time in diagnosis (**Figure 3**). It is also important to screen all suspected HLH patients using the flow cytometry based assays and all male patients for SAP and XIAP expression irrespective of age and clinical presentations.

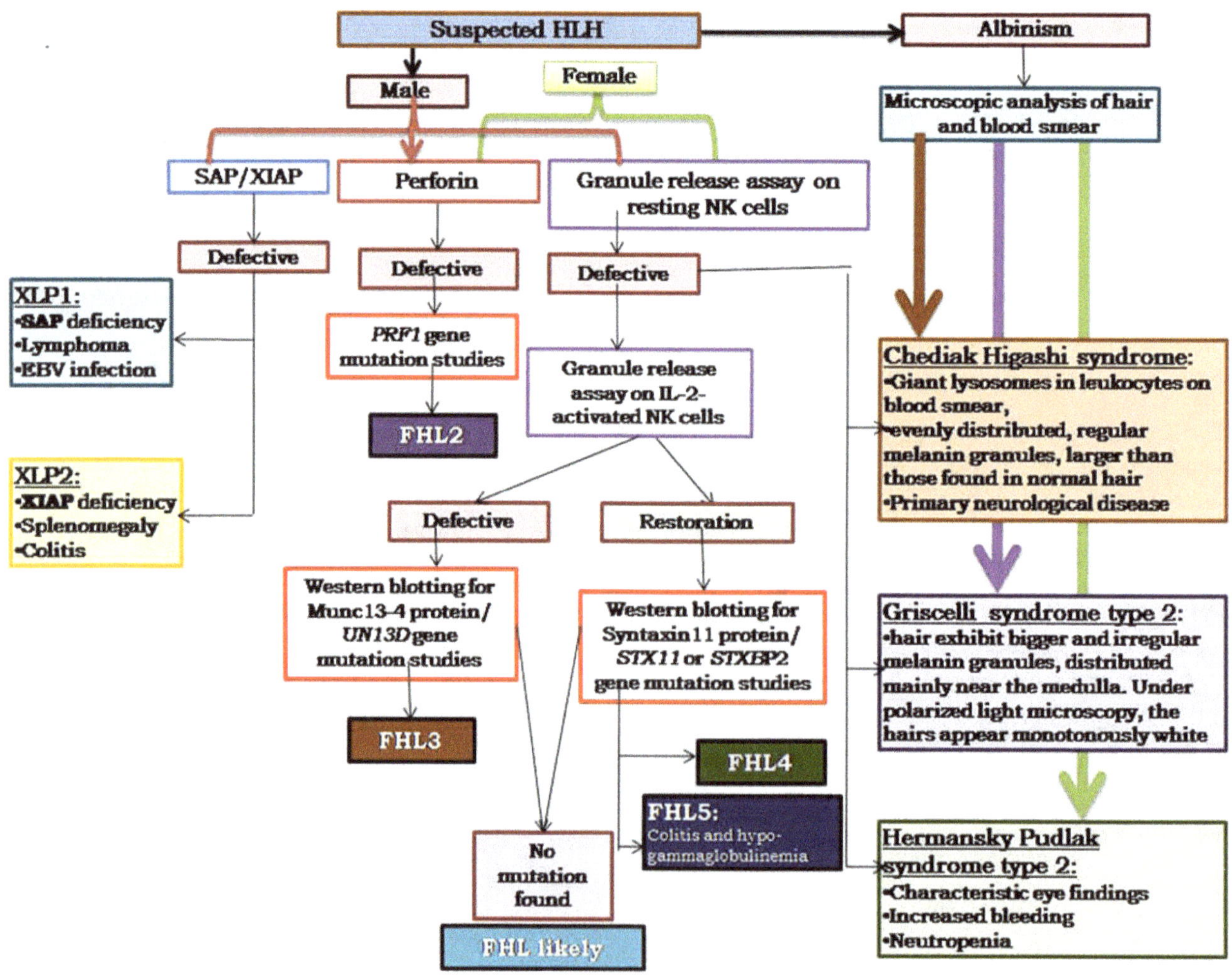

FIGURE 3 | Illustrates the HLH algorithm based on the flow cytometric assays. All the patients fitting into HLH criteria, irrespective of age, and clinical presentations, should be screened for perforin expression and Granule release assay. All the male patients should be screened for SAP and XIAP expression. For patients clinically presenting with albinism, microscopic analysis of hair, and blood smear is essential for differential diagnosis of Chediak Higashi, Griscelli syndrome, and Hermansky-Pudlak syndrome. Based on the defect in expression of a particular protein identified, molecular characterization for the respective gene should be performed for confirmation of diagnosis (33).

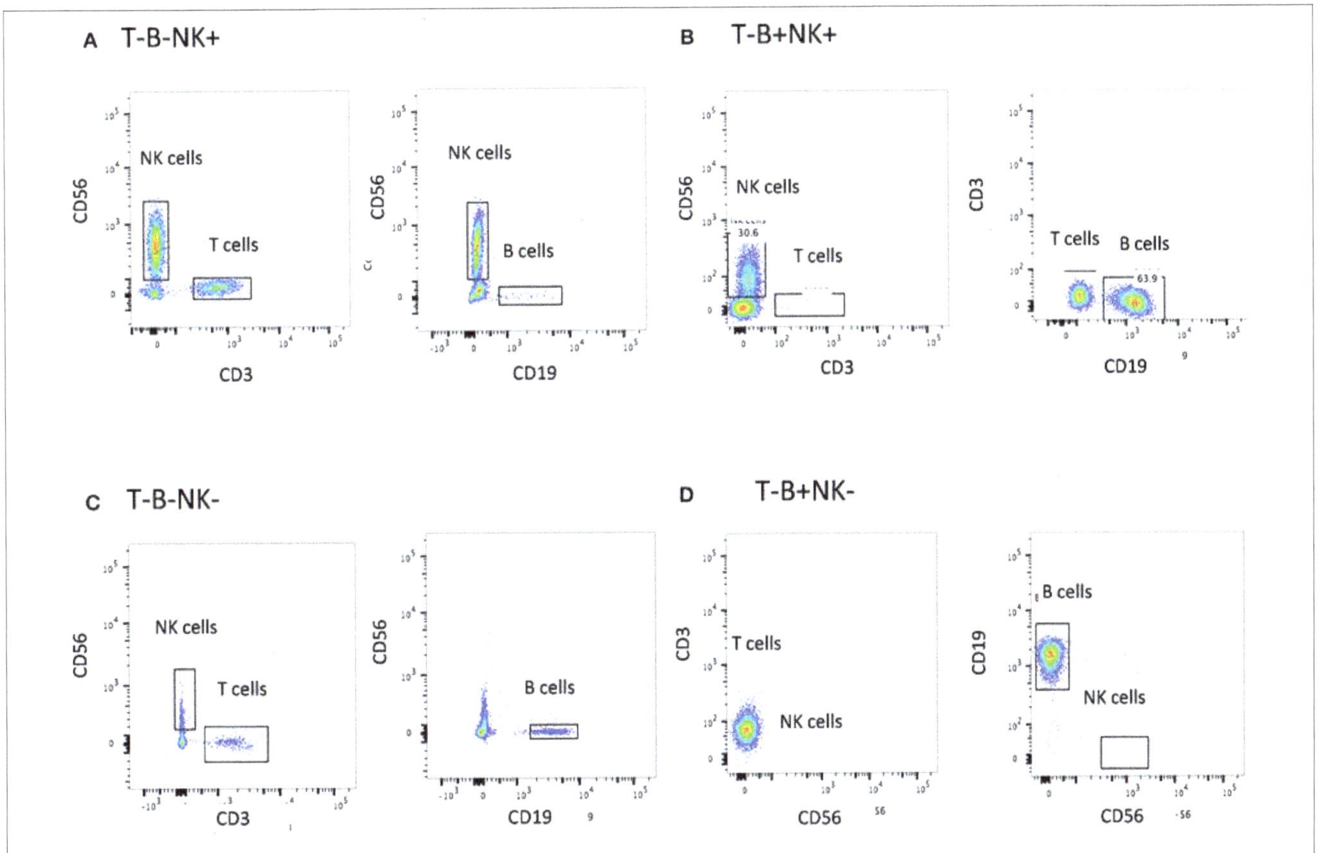

FIGURE 4 | Lymphocyte subset analysis for SCID. Samples were analyzed by flow cytometry, gating on lymphocytes by forward/side scatter and gating T cells (CD3+), B cells (CD19+), and NK cells (CD56+CD3-) **(A)** T-B-NK+ **(B)** T-B-NK+ **(C)** T-B-NK- **(D)** T-B+NK- SCID, respectively.

SEVERE COMBINED IMMUNODEFICIENCY DISEASES (SCID)

Severe combined immunodeficiency (SCID) is a highly complex and heterogeneous group of primary immunodeficiency disorders (PID). More than 30 different genetic defects can lead to SCID (34). A unifying feature of all the different forms of SCID is a defect in the T cell compartment. Depending on the genetic defect, the B cell, NK cell numbers, and/or function may also be affected.

The first step in diagnosis of SCID is the study of lymphocyte subsets (T, Th, Tc, B, NK) by flow cytometry for preliminary classification of SCID into T-B+NK+ SCID, T-B-NK+ SCID, T-B+NK- SCID, and T-B-NK- SCID (**Figure 4**). Typical SCIDs have absent/reduced (<300 cells/μl) T cell counts (35). In cases with residual CD3+T cells (>300 cells/μL), the study of subsets that reflect their naïve/memory and activation state using CD45RA, CD45RO, and HLA-DR aids in the diagnosis of Leaky SCID and Omenn Syndrome. The different T cell transition states can be studied using a combination of CD45RA with CD62L or CD31 to study the naïve ($C45RA^{+}CD62L^{+}$), central memory ($C45RA^{-}CD62L^{+}$), and effector memory ($C45RA^{-}CD62L^{-}$) cells (**Figure 5**). The typical SCIDs lack the naïve T cell markers and both Leaky SCID and Omenn Syndrome patients have a predominance of CD45RO+ T cells. Varying display of the naive cell markers on CD4 and CD8 T cells may also give a clue to conditions with isolated T cell defects, such as selective deficiency of naïve Th cells in MHC class II deficiency. A highly activated state of the T cell hints at Omenn syndrome or maternal engraftment. Studying the lack of HLA-DR expression on T cells, B cells, and monocytes serve as a useful panel for the rapid identification of patients with MHC class II deficiency.

Genetic diagnosis of SCID is not straightforward because of an immunophenotypic overlap between different categories of SCID. A child with T-B+ SCID can have a defect in either *IL2RG*, *IL7RA*, or *JAK3* gene. Hence, in such cases, flow cytometric analysis of specific protein expressions may serve as a rapid tool to narrow down the list of possible genetic defect.

A flow cytometry panel that defines subsets like CD132 (IL2RG), CD127 (IL7RA), CD3, and CD19 helps in classification of T-B+ SCID patients into X-Linked SCID or IL7RA deficient SCID (**Figure 6**). However, in cases with zero T cells, studying the T cell specific markers like CD127 holds a limited utility. Also, a reduced CD127 expression needs to be further evaluated for IL7 receptor internalization as high circulating levels of IL7 in lymphopenic patients can cause the down regulation of CD127. Flow cytometry also enables the study of intracellular proteins

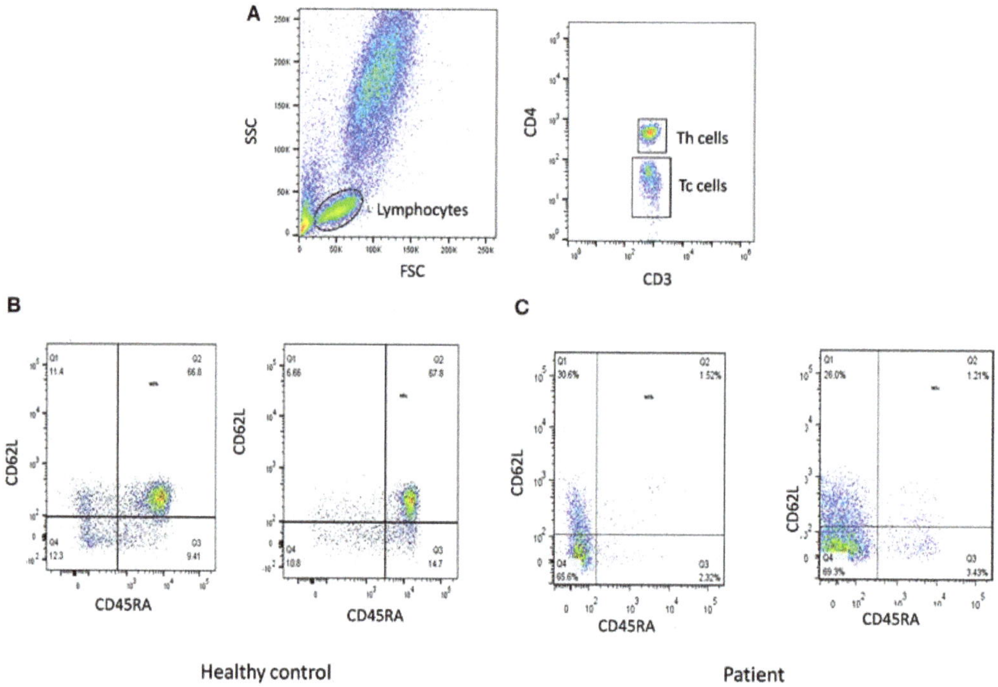

FIGURE 5 | Naïve T cells analysis. **(A)** Samples were analyzed by flow cytometry, gating on lymphocytes by forward/side scatter. Tc and Th cells were gated as CD3+CD8+ and CD3+CD4+, respectively. Naïve T cells were gated as CD45RA+CD62L+ on Th cells and Tc cells. Figure represents Naïve T cell population in **(B)** healthy control **(C)** SCID patient. SCID patients had low percentages of naïve T cells.

like phosphor-STATs. IL-2 stimulated JAK3-pSTAT5 expression on T cells helps identify JAK3 deficient SCID forms.

In our experience with the immunological characterization of SCID patients, almost 65% of our B^+ SCID cohort had absent T cells. Hence, both CD127 and phospho-STAT5 assays had a limited utility in our study and we had to rely on genetic analysis to identify the defect (36). Exploiting the fact that CD132 is expressed on all the lymphocyte sub-populations, studying its expression on B cells helps rule out X-SCID. For patients that lack T cells, the use of IL-21 stimulant and analyzing the JAK3-pSTAT3 expression on B cells serves as an alternative method for the identification of JAK3 deficiency.

Generally, a T-B-NK- immunophenotypic pattern leads to a suspicion of Adenosine deaminase (ADA) deficiency. A flow cytometry based approach to assess the intracellular ADA levels can be performed to identify ADA deficient patients (37). The other possible defect is reticular dysgenesis (RD), which is suspected in the case of a defect in both the lymphoid and myeloid development. In our experience, we also identified a Purine nucleoside phosphorylase deficient (PNP) SCID child with an immunophenotypic pattern of T-B-NK-.

Within the T-B-NK+ SCID, it is extremely important to determine if the patient is sensitive to ionizing radiations. Recently, a flow cytometry based approach has been described which involves analysis of γH2AX as a useful marker for classifying patients with radiosensitive SCID (38).

Hypomorphic mutation in SCID genes leads to the generation of a residual number of T cells. In such cases, the basic flow studies have to be supported by T cell functional studies. These involve flow based assays, which use dyes like CFSE to monitor the T cell response to various stimulants like Phytohemagglutinin (PHA), anti-CD3, and anti-CD28 (39). Such assays are also useful in a setting of isolated T cells defects like ZAP70 deficiency, where patients lack CD8+ T cells but have normal CD4 cells which do not respond to CD3 stimulation.

The results of a T cell proliferation assay or tests that look for phosphor proteins is highly affected by the quality of the sample, especially when samples are shipped to a reference laboratory from different parts of the country. To demonstrate that the test results are not affected by the quality of the sample, it is mandatory to process the patient's sample along with a shipped healthy control sample. In cases where the result on healthy control sample seems inconclusive, a repeat testing needs to be performed on a fresh blood sample. In our experience, with samples that took 24–48 h to reach our laboratory it was difficult to establish a diagnosis in almost 20% of cases.

Another assay that holds importance in SCID patients with circulating T cells is the evaluation of T cell receptor diversity. This can be done by a PCR based approach called T-cell spectratyping, or a flow cytometry–based method that tests the Vβ repertoire. A restricted TCR repertoire is highly suggestive of SCID. In a few cases, testing for the TCRαβ+ T cells and TCRγδ+ T cells also helps identify specific defects in the development of T cells; for example, defects in the TCRa constant gene (TRAC), which show an impaired surface expression of TCRαβ complex (40). Similarly, flow based studies to look for specific CD3 subunits like CD3 zeta, help identify CD3 complex subunit deficiencies.

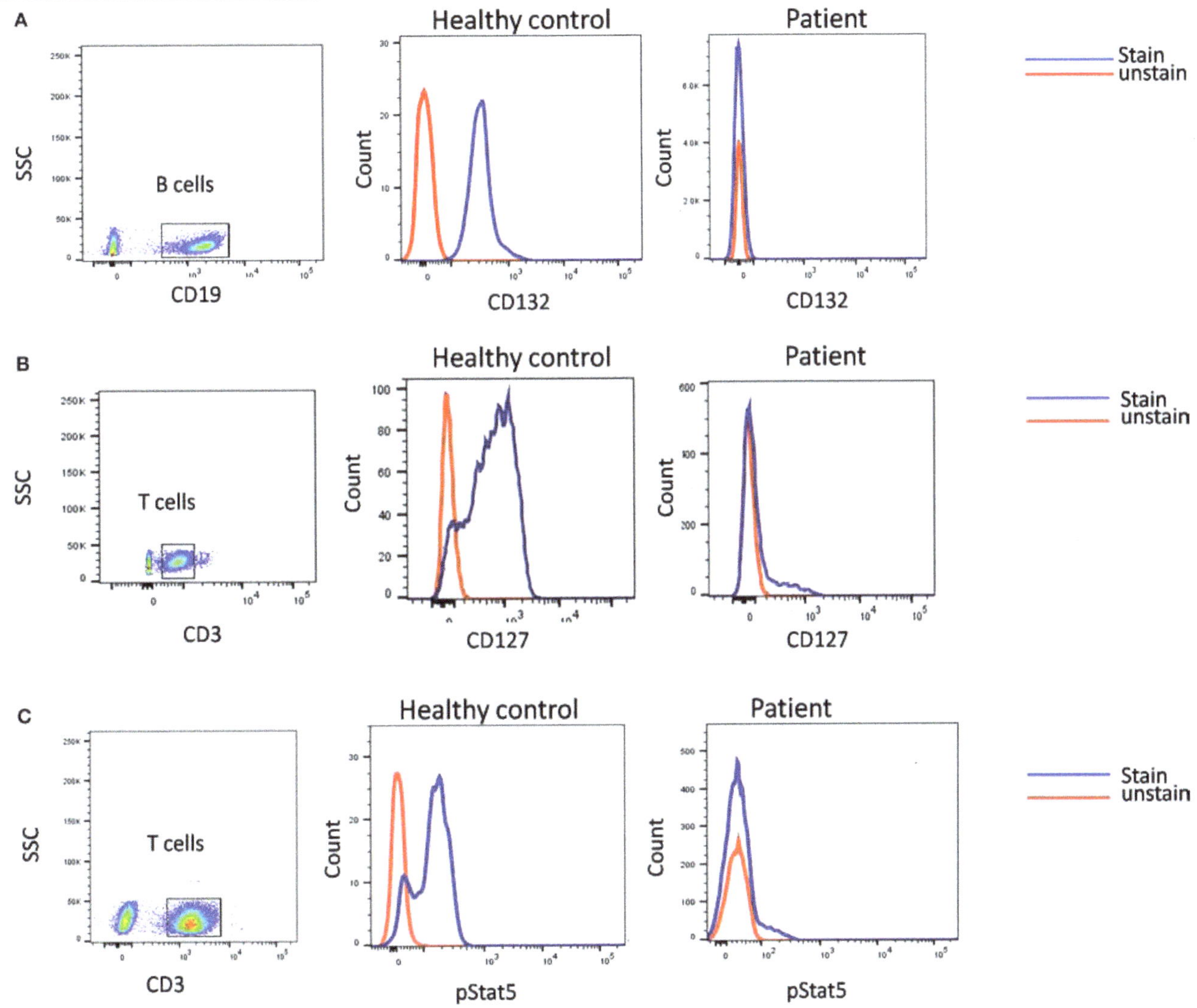

FIGURE 6 | Samples were analyzed by flow cytometry, for **(A)** the common gamma chain (γc) (Or CD132), also known as interleukin-2 receptor subunit gamma or IL-2RG on CD19 cells. **(B)** IL7Ra (CD 127) expression on CD3 cells. CD132 and CD127 expression was absent in patient indicative of X –SCID and AR- IL7Rα. **(C)** Flow cytometric evaluation of STAT5 phosphorylation following IL-2 stimulation. Patient cells fail to respond. Healthy control (Blue histogram) and SCID patient (Red histogram).

Overall, flow cytometry holds a great role in the immunological characterization of SCID by allowing enumeration of lymphocyte sub-populations, assessing thymic capabilities and the TCR diversity, measuring specific receptor expression, studying downstream molecules, and testing T cell function. It also serves as useful guide to determining the probable genetic defect involved in SCID pathogenesis (**Figure 7**).

CHRONIC GRANULOMATOUS DISEASES (CGD)

Chronic Granulomatous Disease (CGD), a rare (1: 200,000), inherited primary immunodeficiency disorder (PID), is caused due to a defect in components of NADPH oxidase complex (41, 42). Variability is observed in the pattern of underlying genetic defect with regards to the ethnicity and consanguinity. Overall, X-linked (XL)-CGD (due to mutations in *CYBB* gene) is the most prevalent (65%) type of CGD (42, 43). However, a higher rate of autosomal recessive (AR)-CGD (due to mutations in *CYBA, NCF1, NCF2, NCF4 genes*) is reported in the regions where consanguineous marriage is more common (44, 45). It is characterized by the inability of phagocytes to form reactive oxygen species (ROS) upon interaction with bacterial or fungal pathogens (46). The patients are susceptible to recurrent bacterial and fungal infections because of reduced or absent superoxide (47). The overlapping clinical manifestations and generic patterns in diagnostic tests sometimes mask the underlying genotype of CGD during an initial diagnosis.

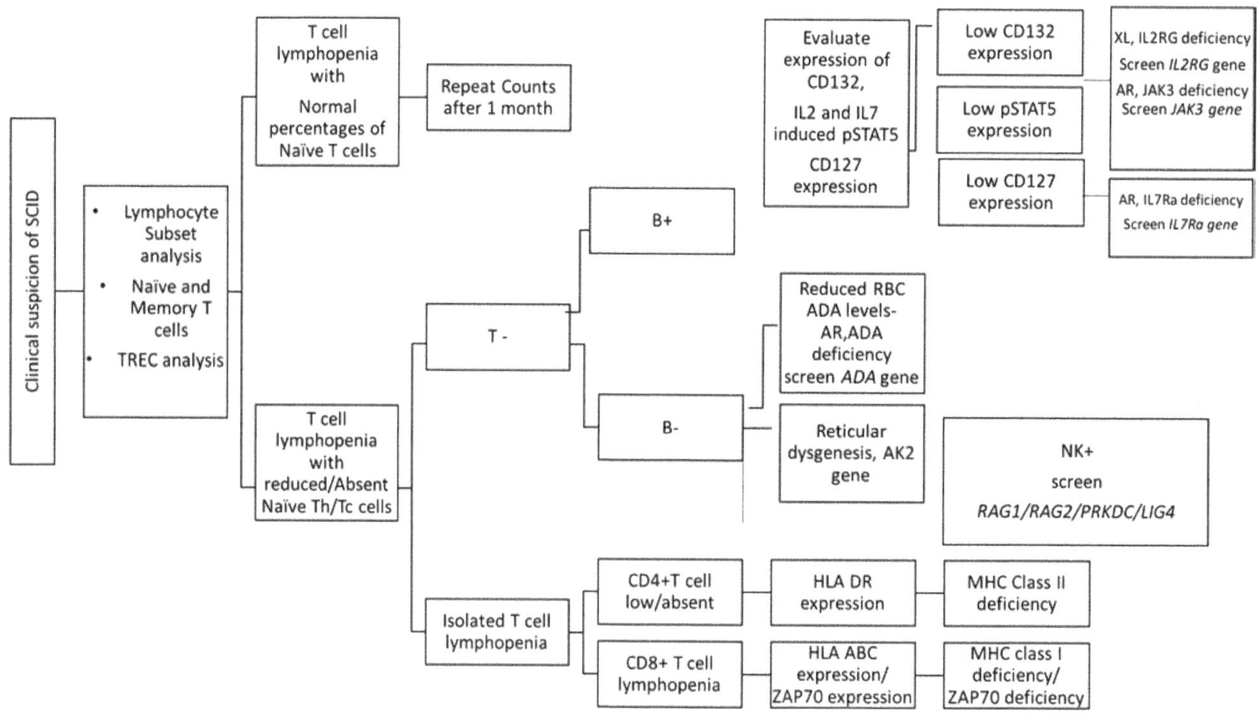

FIGURE 7 | Diagnostic algorithm for diagnosis of SCID patients using flow cytometry based assays.

Significant differences are observed in age at diagnosis, residual superoxide activity, clinical course, and mean survival age among the CGD subtypes (41, 44, 48, 49).

Primary diagnosis of CGD involves laboratory screening tests that demonstrate an insufficiency of phagocytes to generate reactive oxygen species during respiratory burst activity. Nitroblue tetrazolium test (NBT) is a basic and most commonly used diagnostic test for CGD. However, it is now largely substituted with dihydrorhodamine assay (DHR) because of its sensitivity and specificity in providing rapid results (50). Both these tests are based on the principle of superoxide generation upon stimulation with agonists such as phorbolmyristate acetate (PMA) and N-Formyl-Met-Leu-Phe (FMLP), among others. DHR assay is performed by flow cytometry where formation of the reactive oxygen species (ROS) is monitored by fluorescence generated due to the oxidation of DHR 123 dye. It involves an indirect measurement of an ROS such as hydrogen peroxide (51, 52). The fluorescence generated after stimulation is quantitated by the mean peak channel fluorescence. The results are expressed as a stimulation index (SI) of neutrophils, which is a ratio of the mean fluorescence of stimulated neutrophils to the mean fluorescence of unstimulated neutrophils. Although, neutrophils are the cells of interest, when studying oxidative burst, monocytes serve as a low-level control and lymphocytes serve as a negative control. The SI value and coefficient of variation (CV) of the peak after the stimulation is extremely important to distinguish between the two genotypes, $p47^{phox}$ deficiency and $gp91^{phox}$ deficiency. The DHR assay is sensitive enough to detect trace amounts of residual superoxide activity which is retained in $p47^{phox}$ deficiency. Hence, increased fluorescence (SI value or broad CV) is observed in $p47^{phox}$ deficiency patients as compared to $gp91^{phox}$ deficiency (50, 53). Thus, flow cytometry helps to identify the genotype-dependent variability in the evaluation of NADPH oxidase activity. It has been observed that autosomal recessive (AR-CGD) subtypes (*CYBA, NCF1, NCF2,* and *NCF4*gene defects) have slightly higher amounts of residual superoxide activity compared with the X-linked recessive (XL-CGD) subtype (*CYBB* gene defect) patients (48, 54). This mainly affects the severity of the clinical progression. However, previous studies have also shown that the amount of residual superoxide activity is dependent on the type of mutation in the affected gene (44, 48, 55). These diagnostic tests do not help to identify the exact genotype (except for the XL-CGD where mother is the carrier of the disease). In cases of AR-CGD and others where mothers do not show carrier pattern (~10%), additional tests are required to identify the genotype of CGD.

Additionally, the functional analysis of NADPH oxidase complex involves component expression analysis by western blotting or flow cytometric evaluation, which involves the use of specific monoclonal antibodies (mAbs) against each of its components. Of the five components, $gp91^{phox}$ and $p22^{phox}$ form a heterodimer, which is expressed on the transmembrane. Other cytoplasmic components ($p47^{phox}$, $p67^{phox}$, and $p40^{phox}$) form a heterotrimer and are translocated to the membrane upon activation (56). The study of specific protein expression by flow

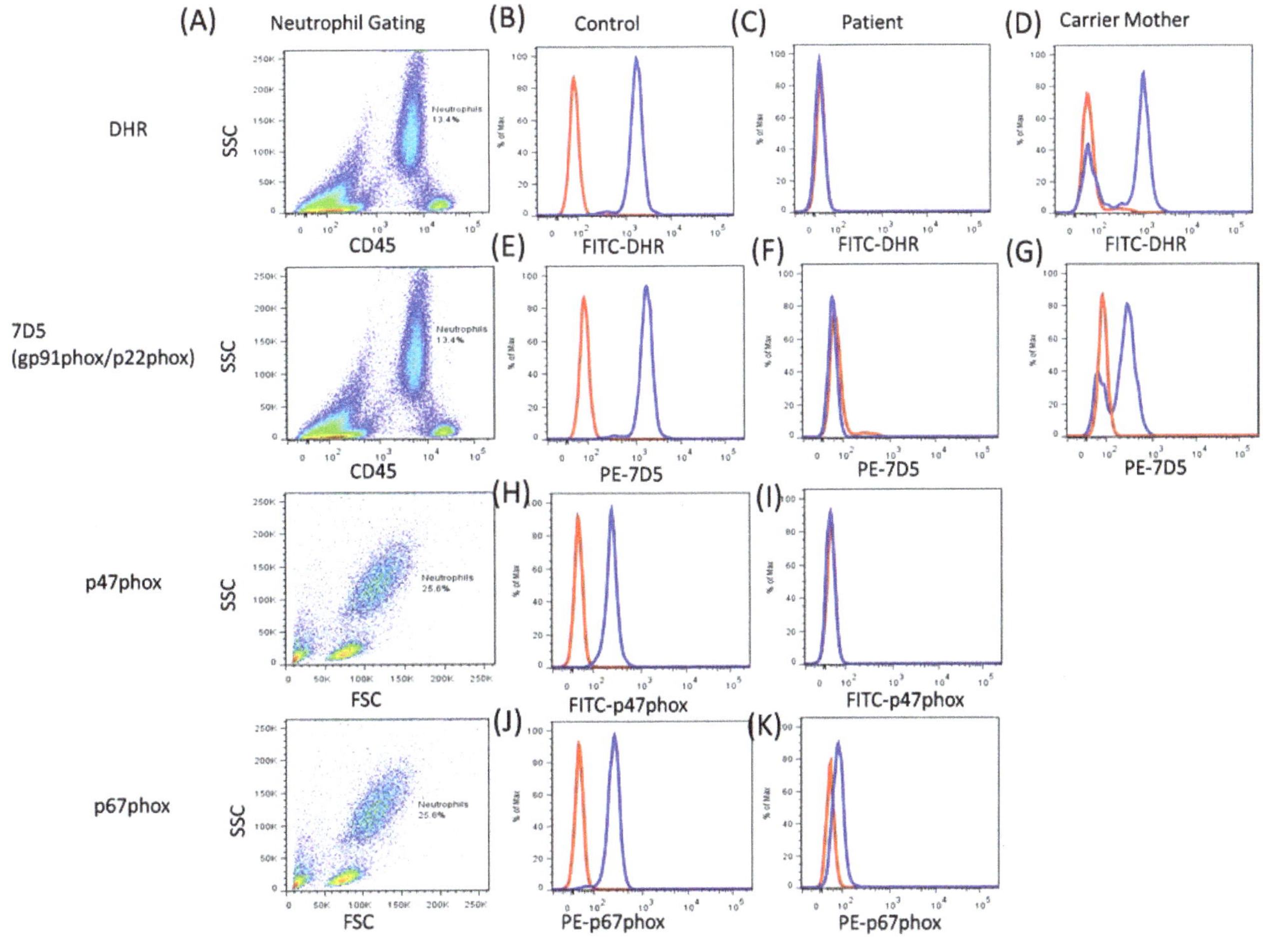

FIGURE 8 | CGD analysis. **(A)** Samples were analyzed by flow cytometry, gating on neutrophils by forward/side scatter and/or CD45/side scatter. **(B)** a healthy control, **(C)** Abnormal DHR expression in CGD patient, **(D)** X-linked carrier mother-mosaic pattern. NADPH oxidase component expression (7D5 for anti-gp91phox/p22phox, anti-p47phox, and anti-p67phox) was analyzed on neutrophils cells. **(E)** a healthy control, **(F)** Abnormal expression of gp91phox (*CYBB* gene) or p22phox (*CYBA* gene) in CGD patient, **(G)** X-linked carrier mother-mosaic pattern. **(H)** a healthy control, **(I)** Abnormal expression of p47phox (*NCF1* gene) in CGD patient, **(J)** a healthy control, **(K)** Abnormal expression of p67phox (*NCF2* gene) in CGD patient.

cytometry helps to identify defective protein components and also the underlying defective genotype (**Figure 8**).

The expression pattern of each of the component on neutrophils is studied, however, monocytes and B cells show low levels of expression, while T cells do not show any expression (57). The 7D5 mAb binds to an extracellular domain of $gp91^{phox}$, as expressions of $gp91^{phox}$ and $p22^{phox}$ are dependent on each other for mature and stable expression. Hence, if any one of these proteins is defective then loss of expression of the other protein is also observed (58). Abnormal 7D5 expression can thus be inferred as a defect in the *CYBB* or *CYBA* gene, and requires further investigation or molecular confirmation. Similarly, an abnormal expression of other antibodies also suggests a defect in respective genes which further requires validation by sequencing the respective gene. One needs to keep in mind that the presence of protein expression does not necessarily implicate the presence/generation of a functional protein (45, 53). In this way, flow cytometry offers an opportunity to evaluate protein expression at a single cell level and is a secondary, helpful tool for further characterization of CGD patients.

Carrier detection is a very important aspect for genetic counseling and in prenatal diagnosis. Carriers of the XL-CGD could be detected by NBT and DHR analysis of mother's sample, which is not applicable in the case of AR-CGD (59). Additionally, the samples traveled from long distances or an old sample (more than 24 h old) make the analysis more difficult, due to non-viable neutrophils (60, 61). Studies by Kulkarni et al. (62) and Kuhns et al. (63) have described the use of flow cytometric NADPH oxidase component analysis for identification of the carriers of *NCF1* gene defect. Although molecular confirmation is the most preferred method to confirm the carrier status in both XL-CGD and AR-CGD, a quick identification of CGD patients and carriers is possible with NADPH oxidase component expression. The information on this is not conclusive due to limited data and there is a need for large patient cohort analyses.

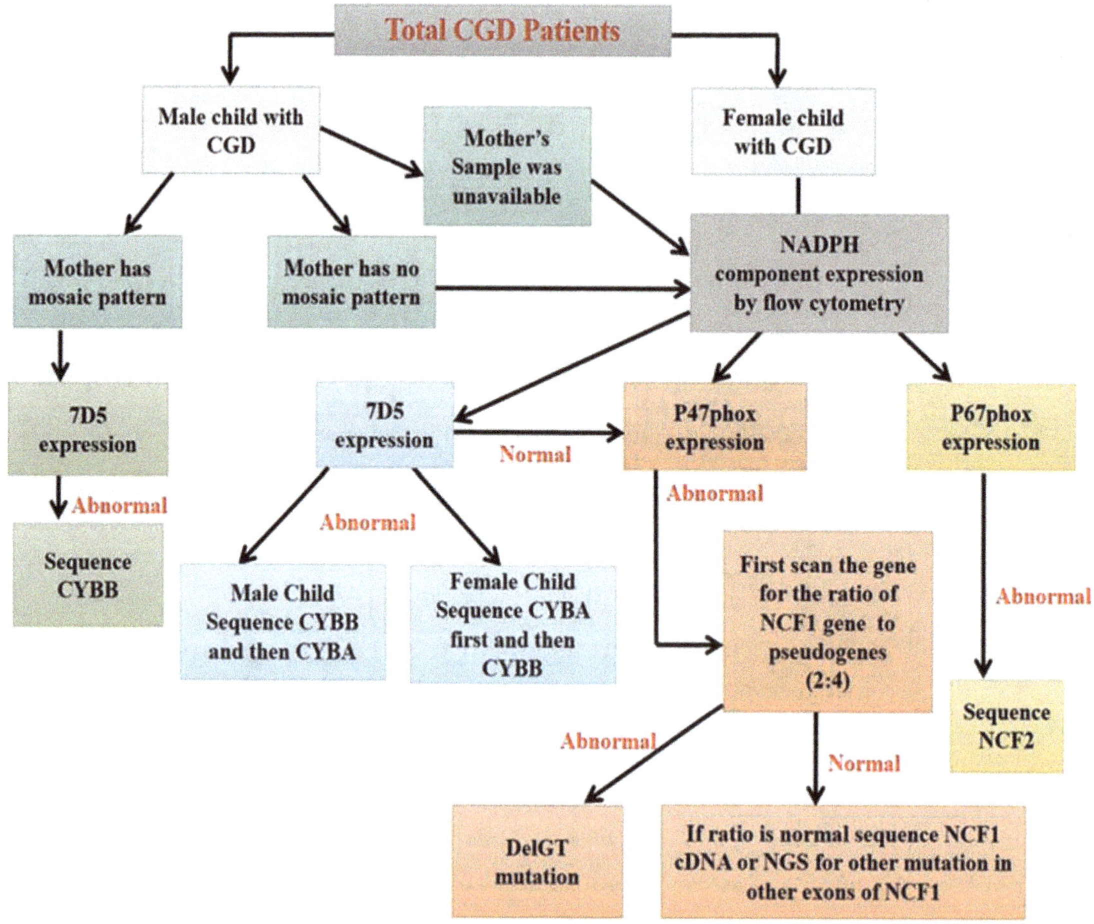

FIGURE 9 | Algorithm for diagnosis of CGD patients using flow cytometry based assays (44).

Molecular confirmation is definitive diagnosis of CGD, however, it could be time-consuming and laborious to analyze each and every exon with the help of Sanger sequencing. The current technological advances, such as Next Generation Sequencing (NGS), could overcome these difficulties using targeted panel sequencing or Whole Exome Sequencing (WES) methods. Still, the factors such as long turn-around time and complication in data analysis due to presence of pseudogenes, big gene deletion, and/or GC rich regions are some of the challenges that makes it unsuitable as a routine diagnostic method (64, 65). Particularly, *NCF1* gene has two pseudogenes (>99% homology), which are difficult to analyze by either the Sanger or NGS method, and require a simple Gene Scan analysis to identify the most common Del GT mutation (at the beginning of exon 2) (66). In such cases, flow cytometric evaluation could play an important role in making the choice of appropriate method for further molecular characterization of CGD patients (44, 67).

This strategy was used in molecular characterization of 90 Indian patients, where only 12% (11 out of 90) of the patients required NGS analysis. Among them, a genotype could not be identified using flow cytometric evaluation in two patients. In a country like India with limited resources, the predominance of AR-CGD type, and a high frequency of consanguineous marriages, the flow cytometric classification of CGD patients remains a vital tool in the early diagnosis and guide for molecular characterization (by suggesting appropriate method) (44, 68) (**Figure 9**).

PRENATAL DIAGNOSIS USING FLOW CYTOMETRY

Though, over the years, understanding of the pathogenesis of PIDs has improved, the management of these disorders still remains challenging. As these are inherited disorders, hematopoietic stem cell transplantation (HSCT) is essential for long term survival of majority of these patients. However, in country like India transplantation is often not feasible either due to lack of HLA-matched donor or the prohibitive cost of therapy. Thus, in such a scenario, genetic counseling with the possibility of carrier detection and prenatal diagnosis in affected families remains an important part of management.

Molecular diagnosis may not be possible or available in all affected cases; thus, phenotypic prenatal diagnosis by cordocentesis for families with an index case having an immunophenotypically well-characterized PID is an apt alternative. Thus, phenotypic prenatal diagnosis by flow cytometry offers a simple and rapid tool compared to molecular characterization (68, 69).

At ICMR-NIIH, we have established the normal ranges for the diagnostic parameters for a selected few PIDs, which include SCID, CGD, LAD-I, and XLA. In the last 10 years, using flow cytometry based assays, we offered prenatal diagnosis to 26 affected families (8 CGD, 9 SCID, 7 LAD-I, 1 XLA, and 1 MHC-II deficient) using a flow cytometry based assay of which five fetuses were affected with disease (unpublished data).

However, for utilizing flow cytometry as tool for prenatal diagnosis, there are few points one has to consider. Firstly, at the appropriate gestational age, the marker used for prenatal diagnosis should be expressed by a larger cell population. Secondly, gestational age-defined cut-off or range for the cell subset or marker of interest should be well-defined. Thirdly, the presence of a particular protein does not rule out functional defects and, hence, it can be used as a diagnostic marker in only those cases where the index case shows absent protein expression. And finally, one has to keep in mind that the use of flow cytometry based prenatal diagnosis has to be restricted to those PIDs in which diagnosis based on the markers and cells has been analyzed.

CONCLUSION

Primary immunodeficiency disorders (PIDs) are an heterogeneous group of inherited disorders of the immune system. As the spectrum of PIDs is expanding, it is often difficult to diagnose PIDs based on clinical and conventional laboratory findings alone. Genetic analysis helps in the confirmation of diagnosis of a PID, however, they are expensive and time consuming. Flow cytometry, with its advances in the last few decades has emerged as an indispensable tool for enumeration and characterization of immune cells. Thus, this review has comprehensively evaluated our experience of the utility of flow cytometry in the diagnosis of PIDs, and concludes that flow cytometry serves as a bridge between clinical diagnosis and molecular testing, aiding rapid, and highly sensitive tools for the evaluation of PIDs. It not only provides clues to underlying genetic defects in certain PIDs, but also helps in the functional validation of novel genetic defects.

AUTHOR CONTRIBUTIONS

MM, SS, MKu, JA, AD, MKe, MG were involved in performing laboratory investigations and writing the manuscript. MM and SS compiled the data and reviewed the manuscript.

REFERENCES

1. Bousfiha A, Jeddane L, Picard C, Ailal F, Bobby Gaspar H, Al-Herz W, et al. The 2017 IUIS phenotypic classification for primary immunodeficiencies. *J Clin Immunol.* (2018) 38:129–43. doi: 10.1007/s10875-017-0465-8
2. Kanegane H, Hoshino A, Okano T, Yasumi T, Wada T, Takada H, et al. Flow cytometry-based diagnosis of primary immunodeficiency diseases. *Allergol Int.* (2018) 67:43–54. doi: 10.1016/j.alit.2017.06.003
3. Janka GE. Familial and acquired hemophagocytic lymphohistiocytosis. *Annu Rev Med.* (2012) 63:233–46. doi: 10.1146/annurev-med-041610-134208
4. Ohadi M, Lalloz MR, Sham P, Zhao J, Dearlove AM, Shiach C, et al. Localization of a gene for familial hemophagocytic lymphohistiocytosis at chromosome 9q21.3-22 by homozygosity mapping. *Am J Hum Genet.* (1999) 64:165–71. doi: 10.1086/302187
5. Filipovich AH. Hemophagocytic lymphohistiocytosis (HLH) and related disorders. *Hematology.* (2009) 2009:127–31. doi: 10.1182/asheducation-2009.1.127
6. Rubin TS, Zhang K, Gifford C, Lane A, Choo S, Bleesing JJ, et al. Perforin and CD107a testing is superior to NK cell function testing for screening patients for genetic HLH. *Blood.* (2017) 129:2993–9. doi: 10.1182/blood-2016-12-753830
7. Stepp SE, Dufourcq-Lagelouse R, Le Deist F, Bhawan S, Certain S, Mathew PA, et al. Perforin gene defects in familial hemophagocytic lymphohistiocytosis. *Science.* (1999) 286:1957–9. doi: 10.1126/science.286.5446.1957
8. Mellor-Heineke S, Villanueva J, Jordan MB, Marsh R, Zhang K, Bleesing JJ, et al. Elevated granzyme B in cytotoxic lymphocytes is a signature of immune activation in hemophagocytic lymphohistiocytosis. *Front Immunol.* (2013) 4:72. doi: 10.3389/fimmu.2013.00072
9. Kogawa K, Lee SM, Villanueva J, Marmer D, Sumegi J, Filipovich AH. Perforin expression in cytotoxic lymphocytes from patients with hemophagocytic lymphohistiocytosis and their family members. *Blood.* (2002) 99:61–6. doi: 10.1182/blood.V99.1.61
10. Mhatre S, Madkaikar M, Desai M, Ghosh K. Spectrum of perforin gene mutations in familial hemophagocytic lymphohistiocytosis (FHL) patients in India. *Blood Cells Mol Dis.* (2015) 54:250–7. doi: 10.1016/j.bcmd.2014.11.023
11. Abdalgani M, Filipovich AH, Choo S, Zhang K, Gifford C, Villanueva J, et al. Accuracy of flow cytometric perforin screening for detecting patients with FHL due to PRF1 mutations. *Blood.* (2015) 8 126:1858–60. doi: 10.1182/blood-2015-06-648659
12. Hersperger AR, Makedonas G, Betts MR. Flow cytometric detection of perforin upregulation in human CD8 T cells. *Cytometry.* (2008) 73:1050–7. doi: 10.1002/cyto.a.20596
13. Rutella S, Rumi C, Lucia MB, Etuk B, Cauda R, Leone G. Flow cytometric detection of perforin in normal human lymphocyte subpopulations defined by expression of activation/differentiation antigens. *Immunol Lett.* (1998) 60:51–5. doi: 10.1016/S0165-2478(97)00132-6
14. Trizzino A, zur Stadt U, Ueda I, Risma K, Janka G, Ishii E, et al. Genotype-phenotype study of familial haemophagocytic lymphohistiocytosis due to perforin mutations. *J Med. Gen.* (2008) 45:15–21. doi: 10.1136/jmg.2007.052670
15. Chia J, Yeo KP, Whisstock JC, Dunstone MA, Trapani JA, Voskoboinik I. Temperature sensitivity of human perforin mutants unmasks subtotal loss of cytotoxicity, delayed FHL, and a predisposition to cancer. *Proc Natl Acad Sci USA.* (2009) 106:9809–14. doi: 10.1073/pnas.0903815106
16. Hou H, Zhou Y, Yu J, Mao L, Bosco MJ, Wang J, et al. Establishment of the reference intervals of lymphocyte function in healthy adults based

on IFN-γ secretion assay upon phorbol-12-myristate-13-acetate/ionomycin stimulation. *Front Immunol.* (2018) 9:172. doi: 10.3389/fimmu.2018.00172
17. Alter G, Malenfant JM, Altfeld M. CD107a as a functional marker for the identification of natural killer cell activity. *J Immunol Methods.* (2004) 294:15–22. doi: 10.1016/j.jim.2004.08.008
18. Claus M, Greil J, Watzl C. Comprehensive analysis of NK cell function in whole blood samples. *J Immunol. Methods.* (2009) 341:154–64. doi: 10.1016/j.jim.2008.11.006
19. Shabrish S, Gupta M, Madkaikar M. A modified NK cell degranulation assay applicable for routine evaluation of NK cell function. *J Immunol Res.* (2016) 2016:3769590. doi: 10.1155/2016/3769590
20. Bryceson YT, March ME, Barber DF, Ljunggren H-G, Long EO. Cytolytic granule polarization and degranulation controlled by different receptors in resting NK cells. *J Exp Med.* (2005) 202:1001–12. doi: 10.1084/jem.20051143
21. Bryceson YT, Fauriat C, Nunes JM, Wood SM, Björkström NK, Long EO, et al. Functional analysis of human NK cells by flow cytometry. In: Campbell K, editor. *Natural Killer Cell Protocols. Methods in Molecular Biology.* Clifton, NJ: Humana Press (2010) p. 335–52. doi: 10.1007/978-1-60761-362-6_23
22. Bryceson YT, Pende D, Maul-Pavicic A, Gilmour KC, Ufheil H, Vraetz T, et al. A prospective evaluation of degranulation assays in the rapid diagnosis of familial hemophagocytic syndromes. *Blood.* (2012) 119:2754–63. doi: 10.1182/blood-2011-08-374199
23. D'Orlando O, Zhao F, Kasper B, Orinska Z, Müller J, Hermans-Borgmeyer I, et al. Syntaxin 11 is required for NK and $CD8^+$ T-cell cytotoxicity and neutrophil degranulation. *Eur J Immunol.* (2013) 43:194–208. doi: 10.1002/eji.201142343
24. Cruikshank M, Anoop P, Nikolajeva O, Rao A, Rao K, Gilmour K, et al. Screening assays for primary haemophagocytic lymphohistiocytosis in children presenting with suspected macrophage activation syndrome. *Pediatr Rheumatol.* (2015) 13:48. doi: 10.1186/s12969-015-0043-7
25. Hori M, Yasumi T, Shimodera S, Shibata H, Hiejima E, Oda H, et al. A CD57+ CTL degranulation assay effectively identifies familial hemophagocytic lymphohistiocytosis type 3 patients. *J Clin Immunol.* (2017) 37:92–9. doi: 10.1007/s10875-016-0357-3
26. Tabata Y, Villanueva J, Lee SM, Zhang K, Kanegane H, Miyawaki T, et al. Rapid detection of intracellular SH2D1A protein in cytotoxic lymphocytes from patients with X-linked lymphoproliferative disease and their family members. *Blood.* (2005) 105:3066–71. doi: 10.1182/blood-2004-09-3651
27. Rigaud S, Fondanèche M-C, Lambert N, Pasquier B, Mateo V, Soulas P, et al. XIAP deficiency in humans causes an X-linked lymphoproliferative syndrome. *Nature.* (2006) 444:110–4. doi: 10.1038/nature05257
28. Marsh RA, Bleesing JJ, Filipovich AH. Flow cytometric measurement of SLAM-associated protein and X-linked inhibitor of apoptosis. *Methods Mol Biol.* (2013) 979:189–97. doi: 10.1007/978-1-62703-290-2_15
29. Göransdotter Ericson K, Fadeel B, Nilsson-Ardnor S, Söderhäll C, Samuelsson A, Janka G, et al. Spectrum of perforin gene mutations in familial hemophagocytic lymphohistiocytosis. *Am J Hum Genet.* (2001) 68:590–7. doi: 10.1086/318796
30. Molleran Lee S, Villanueva J, Sumegi J, Zhang K, Kogawa K, Davis J, et al. Characterisation of diverse PRF1 mutations leading to decreased natural killer cell activity in North American families with haemophagocytic lymphohistiocytosis. *J Med Genet.* (2004) 41:137–44. doi: 10.1136/jmg.2003.011528
31. Ishii E, Ohga S, Imashuku S, Yasukawa M, Tsuda H, Miura I, et al. Nationwide survey of hemophagocytic lymphohistiocytosis in Japan. *Int J Hematol.* (2007) 86:58–65. doi: 10.1532/IJH97.07012
32. Jordan MB, Allen CE, Weitzman S, Filipovich AH, McClain KL. How I treat hemophagocytic lymphohistiocytosis. *Blood.* (2011) 118:4041–52. doi: 10.1182/blood-2011-03-278127
33. Madkaikar M, Shabrish S, Desai M. Current updates on classification, diagnosis and treatment of hemophagocytic lymphohistiocytosis (HLH). *Indian J Pediatr.* (2016) 83:434–43. doi: 10.1007/s12098-016-2037-y
34. Cossu F. Genetics of SCID. *Italian J Pediatr.* (2010) 36:76. doi: 10.1186/1824-7288-36-76
35. Shearer WT, Dunn E, Notarangelo LD, Dvorak CC, Puck JM, Logan BR, et al. Establishing diagnostic criteria for severe combined immunodeficiency disease (SCID), leaky SCID, and omenn syndrome: the primary immune deficiency treatment consortium experience. *J Allergy Clin Immunol.* (2014) 133:1092–8. doi: 10.1016/j.jaci.2013.09.044
36. Aluri J, Desai M, Gupta M, Dalvi A, Terance A, Rosenzweig SD, et al. Clinical, immunological, and molecular findings in 57 patients with severe combined immunodeficiency (SCID) from India. *Front Immunol.* (2019) 10:23. doi: 10.3389/fimmu.2019.00023
37. Otsu M, Yamada M, Nakajima S, Kida M, Maeyama Y, Hatano N, et al. Outcomes in two Japanese adenosine deaminase-deficiency patients treated by stem cell gene therapy with no cytoreductive conditioning. *J Clin Immunol.* (2015) 35:384–98. doi: 10.1007/s10875-015-0157-1
38. Buchbinder D, Smith MJ, Kawahara M, Cowan MJ, Buzby JS, Abraham RS. Application of a radiosensitivity flow assay in a patient with DNA ligase 4 deficiency. *Blood Adv.* (2018) 2:1828–32. doi: 10.1182/bloodadvances.2018016113
39. Rosenzweig SD, Fleisher TA. Laboratory evaluation for T-cell dysfunction. *J Allergy Clin Immunol.* (2013) 131:622–3.e1-4. doi: 10.1016/j.jaci.2012.11.018
40. Morgan NV, Goddard S, Cardno TS, McDonald D, Rahman F, Barge D, et al. Mutation in the TCRα subunit constant gene (TRAC) leads to a human immunodeficiency disorder characterized by a lack of TCRαβ+ T cells. *J Clin Invest.* (2011) 121:695–702. doi: 10.1172/JCI41931
41. Wolach B, Gavrieli R, de Boer M, van Leeuwen K, Berger-Achituv S, Stauber T, et al. Chronic granulomatous disease: clinical, functional, molecular, and genetic studies. The Israeli experience with 84 patients: research article. *Am J Hematol.* (2017) 92:28–36. doi: 10.1002/ajh.24573
42. Winkelstein JA, Marino MC, Johnston RB, Boyle J, Curnutte J, Gallin JI, et al. Chronic granulomatous disease. Report on a national registry of 368 patients. *Medicine.* (2000) 79:155–69. doi: 10.1097/00005792-200005000-00003
43. Zhou Q, Hui X, Ying W, Hou J, Wang W, Liu D, et al. A cohort of 169 chronic granulomatous disease patients exposed to BCG vaccination: a retrospective study from a single center in Shanghai, China (2004–2017). *J Clin Immunol.* (2018) 38:260–72. doi: 10.1007/s10875-018-0486-y
44. Kulkarni M, Hule G, de Boer M, van Leeuwen K, Kambli P, Aluri J, et al. Approach to molecular diagnosis of chronic granulomatous disease (CGD): an experience from a large cohort of 90 indian patients. *J Clin Immunol.* (2018) 38:898–916. doi: 10.1007/s10875-018-0567-y
45. Köker MY, Camcioglu Y, van Leeuwen K, Kiliç SS, Barlan I, Yilmaz M, et al. Clinical, functional, and genetic characterization of chronic granulomatous disease in 89 Turkish patients. *J Allergy Clin Immunol.* (2013) 132:1156–1163.e5. doi: 10.1016/j.jaci.2013.05.039
46. Baehner RL, Nathan DG. Leukocyte oxidase: defective activity in chronic granulomatous disease. *Science.* (1967) 155:835–6. doi: 10.1126/science.155.3764.835
47. Holland SM. Chronic granulomatous disease. *Clin Rev Allergy Immunol.* (2010) 38:3–10. doi: 10.1007/s12016-009-8136-z
48. Kuhns DB, Alvord WG, Heller T, Feld JJ, Pike KM, Marciano BE, et al. Residual NADPH oxidase and survival in chronic granulomatous disease. *N Engl J Med.* (2010) 363:2600–10. doi: 10.1056/NEJMoa1007097
49. Marciano BE, Spalding C, Fitzgerald A, Mann D, Brown T, Osgood S, et al. Common severe infections in chronic granulomatous disease. *Clin Infect Dis.* (2015) 60:1176–83. doi: 10.1093/cid/ciu1154
50. Vowells SJ, Fleisher TA, Sekhsaria S, Alling DW, Maguire TE, Malech HL. Genotype-dependent variability in flow cytometric evaluation of reduced nicotinamide adenine dinucleotide phosphate oxidase function in patients with chronic granulomatous disease. *J Pediatr.* (1996) 128:104–7. doi: 10.1016/S0022-3476(96)70437-7
51. O'Gorman MR, Corrochano V. Rapid whole-blood flow cytometry assay for diagnosis of chronic granulomatous disease. *Clin Diagnos Lab Immunol.* (1995) 2:227–32.

52. O'Gorman MRG, Zollett J, Bensen N. Flow cytometry assays in primary immunodeficiency diseases. *Methods Mol Biol.* (2011) 699:317–35. doi: 10.1007/978-1-61737-950-5_15
53. Jirapongsananuruk O, Malech HL, Kuhns DB, Niemela JE, Brown MR, Anderson-Cohen M, et al. Diagnostic paradigm for evaluation of male patients with chronic granulomatous disease, based on the dihydrorhodamine 123 assay. *J Allergy Clin Immunol.* (2003) 111:374–9. doi: 10.1067/mai.2003.58
54. Al-Riyami AZ, Al-Zadjali S, Al-Mamari S, Al-Said B, Al-Qassabi J, Al-Tamemi S. Correlation between flow cytometry and molecular findings in autosomal recessive chronic granulomatous disease: a cohort study from Oman. *Int J Lab Hematol.* (2018) 40:592-96. doi: 10.1111/ijlh.12873
55. Rawat A, Singh S, Suri D, Gupta A, Saikia B, Minz RW, et al. Chronic granulomatous disease: two decades of experience from a tertiary care centre in North West India. *J Clin Immunol.* (2014) 34:58–67. doi: 10.1007/s10875-013-9963-5
56. Diebold BA, Bokoch GM. Molecular basis for Rac2 regulation of phagocyte NADPH oxidase. *Nat Immunol.* (2001) 2:211–5. doi: 10.1038/85259
57. Wada T, Muraoka M, Toma T, Imai T, Shigemura T, Agematsu K, et al. Rapid detection of intracellular p47phox and p67phox by flow cytometry; useful screening tests for chronic granulomatous disease. *J Clin Immunol.* (2013) 33:857–64. doi: 10.1007/s10875-012-9859-9
58. Kawai C, Yamauchi A, Kuribayashi F. Monoclonal antibody 7D5 recognizes the R147 epitope on the gp91 ^{phox}, phagocyte flavocytochrome b_{558} large subunit: macrophages, dendritic cells, and leukocytes. *Microbiol Immunol.* (2018) 62:269–80. doi: 10.1111/1348-0421.12584
59. He J-X, Yin Q-Q, Tong Y-J, Liu X-Y, Xu B-P, Zhao S-Y, et al. Diagnosis and carrier screening of X-linked chronic granulomatous disease by DHR 123 flow cytometry. *Chin J Contemp Pediatri.* (2014) 16:81–4.
60. Roesler J. Remarks on the article genetics and immunopathology of chronic granulomatous disease by Marie José Stasia and Xing Jun Li. *Semin Immunopathol.* (2008) 30:365. doi: 10.1007/s00281-008-0129-0
61. Mauch L, Lun A, O'Gorman MRG, Harris JS, Schulze I, Zychlinsky A, et al. Chronic granulomatous disease (CGD) and complete myeloperoxidase deficiency both yield strongly reduced dihydrorhodamine 123 test signals but can be easily discerned in routine testing for CGD. *Clin Chem.* (2007) 53:890–6. doi: 10.1373/clinchem.2006.083444
62. Kulkarni M, Desai M, Gupta M, Dalvi A, Taur P, Terrance A, et al. Clinical, immunological, and molecular findings ofpatients with p47phox defect chronic granulomatous disease (CGD) in Indian families. *J Clin Immunol.* (2016) 36:774–84. doi: 10.1007/s10875-016-0333-y
63. Kuhns DB, Hsu AP, Sun D, Lau K, Fink D, Griffith P, et al. NCF1 (p47phox)-deficient chronic granulomatous disease: comprehensive genetic and flow cytometric analysis. *Blood Adv.* (2019) 3:136–47. doi: 10.1182/bloodadvances.2018023184
64. Mousallem T, Urban TJ, McSweeney KM, Kleinstein SE, Zhu M, Adeli M, et al. Clinical application of whole-genome sequencing in patients with primary immunodeficiency. *J Allergy Clin Immunol.* (2015) 136:476–479.e6. doi: 10.1016/j.jaci.2015.02.040
65. Roos D. Chronic granulomatous disease. *Br Med Bull.* (2016) 118:50–63. doi: 10.1093/bmb/ldw009
66. Richardson AM, Moyer AM, Hasadsri L, Abraham RS. Diagnostic tools for inborn errors of human immunity (Primary Immunodeficiencies and Immune Dysregulatory Diseases). *Curr Allergy Asthma Rep.* (2018) 18:19. doi: 10.1007/s11882-018-0770-1
67. Meshaal S, El Hawary R, Abd Elaziz D, Alkady R, Galal N, Boutros J, et al. Chronic granulomatous disease: review of a cohort of Egyptian patients. *Allergol Immunopathol.* (2015) 43:279–85. doi: 10.1016/j.aller.2014.11.003
68. Kulkarni M, Gupta M, Madkaikar M. Phenotypic prenatal diagnosis of chronic granulomatous disease: a useful tool in the absence of molecular diagnosis. *Scand J Immunol.* (2017) 86:486–90. doi: 10.1111/sji.12621
69. Mishra A, Gupta M, Dalvi A, Ghosh K, Madkaikar M. Rapid flow cytometric prenatal diagnosis of primary immunodeficiency (PID) disorders. *J Clin Immunol.* (2014) 34:316–22. doi: 10.1007/s10875-014-9993-7

4

Current Flow Cytometric Assays for the Screening and Diagnosis of Primary HLH

Samuel Cern Cher Chiang[1*], Jack J. Bleesing[1,2] and Rebecca A. Marsh[1,2*]

[1] Division of Bone Marrow Transplantation and Immune Deficiency, Cincinnati Children's Hospital Medical Center, Cincinnati, OH, United States, [2] Department of Pediatrics, University of Cincinnati, Cincinnati, OH, United States

***Correspondence:**
Samuel Cern Cher Chiang
sam.chiang@cchmc.org
Rebecca A. Marsh
rebecca.marsh@cchmc.org

Advances in flow cytometry have led to greatly improved primary immunodeficiency (PID) diagnostics. This is due to the fact that patient blood cells in suspension do not require further processing for analysis by flow cytometry, and many PIDs lead to alterations in leukocyte numbers, phenotype, and function. A large portion of current PID assays can be classified as "phenotyping" assays, where absolute numbers, frequencies, and markers are investigated using specific antibodies. Inherent drawbacks of antibody technology are the main limitation to this type of testing. On the other hand, "functional" assays measure cellular responses to certain stimuli. While these latter assays are powerful tools that can be used to detect defects in entire pathways and distinguish variants of significance, it requires samples with robust viability and also skilled processing. In this review, we concentrate on hemophagocytic lymphohistiocytosis (HLH), describing the principles and accuracies of flow cytometric assays that have been proven to assist in the screening diagnosis of primary HLH.

Keywords: flow cytometry, HLH, hemophagocytic lymphohistiocytosis, primary immunodeficiencies, clinical diagnostics, diagnostic accuracy, clinical laboratory tests, XLP

INTRODUCTION

Hemophagocytic lymphohistiocytosis (HLH) can be described as a systemic hyperinflammatory syndrome. It is most often thought to be caused by an inability to clear an inciting infectious or other immunologic trigger. This leads to pathologic immune activation and a positive feedback loop of ever increasing cytokine secretion and cellular cytotoxicity that ultimately results in self harm (1, 2). HLH can be classified as "primary" or "secondary" depending on whether it occurs as a result of an inborn error leading to a dysfunctional immune system like perforin deficiency, or occurs in settings such as infection, malignancy, rheumatologic, or other disease without a known underlying inherited defect in the immune system (3–5). Primary HLH can be caused by mutations in a number of genes which affect cytotoxic lymphocyte granule-mediated cytotoxicity including *PRF1, UNC13D, STX11, STXBP2, RAB27A* (Griscelli Syndrome), *AP3B1* (Hermansky-Pudlak syndrome type 2), and *LYST* (Chediak-Higashi Syndrome). Primary HLH can also include other genetic diseases such as XIAP deficiency, which is characterized by inflammasome dysregulation, and SAP deficiency which has a complicated mechanism of disease, though these diseases are usually classified as X-linked lymphoproliferative diseases (XLP) type 1 and type 2, respectively. Regardless, the classification of HLH into primary or secondary groups is sometimes difficult due to the varied phenotype presented and delays or limitations in obtaining genetic results. This has necessitated the development of faster diagnostic screening assays. Many excellent reviews exist on the subject of primary HLH and cytotoxic lymphocyte function, and the reader would be wise to refer to them for a deeper understanding on the subject (1, 6–10). In this review, we will focus on summarizing the laboratory assays currently used to screen for genetic abnormalities in primary HLH linked genes and explore their accuracy. We will also briefly discuss possible pitfalls and future directions in diagnosing diseases typically associated with HLH.

PERFORIN DEFICIENCY

NK cells and cytotoxic T lymphocytes are often grouped together as cytotoxic lymphocytes. Their primary role is to kill virus infected or malignant cells (11, 12). Perforin, the pore forming protein, is encoded by the gene *PRF1* and is a key player in this process as well as the archetypical example of primary HLH (13). *PRF1* is also historically the first primary HLH gene to be identified and is often referred to as familial hemophagocytic lymphohistiocytosis type 2 (FHL2) (14). Perforin is stored within cytotoxic granules. Once secreted from cytotoxic lymphocyte granules, perforin oligomerizes on the surface of target cells to create pores which allow the penetration of contents such as granzymes into the target. Perforin is easily stained for intracellularly in NK cells using a conjugated monoclonal antibody. Perforin has been shown to be absent or highly reduced in persons with biallelic mutations for *PRF1* gene. Staining can be performed using fresh whole blood or peripheral blood mononuclear cell (PBMC). First, the various lymphocyte lineages are extracellularly stained followed by cell fixation and permeabilization. Intracellular perforin is then stained for and the cells finally analyzed on a flow cytometer (15). To note, while freshly isolated NK cells contain perforin and are routinely used for perforin analysis, only a minority of cytotoxic T cells in "healthy" individuals express perforin. Perforin expression in resting bulk $CD8^+$ cells thus varies greatly between individuals. To overcome this, *bona fide* effector T cells can be gated using CD57 if evaluation of perforin in resting T cells is desired (16, 17). This can greatly help in individuals with poor NK cell counts.

The diagnostic accuracy of perforin expression in NK cells for detecting biallelic *PRF1* mutations has recently been published and is highly accurate with sensitivity of 96.6% and specificity of 89.5% for an overall area under the curve (AUC) of 0.971 (**Table 1**) (18, 20). These and other reports have also shown that *PRF1* mutation carriers (a mutation in only one allele) often have clearly reduced perforin expression arguing for an allele dependent perforin expression (19, 26, 27).

The A91V alteration in *PRF1* is unique. Having a high prevalence of 0.22 to 3.9% depending on the population studied, it has been assumed to be less pathologic (**Figure 1**) (28–31). However, *in vitro* studies have shown that A91V leads to reduced perforin function (32, 33). Individuals with A91V in both compound heterozygous and homozygous state can be identified by laboratory assays and show low to no residual protein expression, and such results may be indiscriminable from other pathologic *PRF1* mutations (30, 34, 35).

The lack of perforin leads to an inability to kill target cells. This functional defect can be detected by lowered chromium release using the radioactive chromium cytotoxicity assay (36). Because the chromium release assay shows suboptimal accuracy, many have turned to screening for primary HLH diseases with perforin staining coupled with the degranulation/exocytosis/CD107a assay in place of or in addition to chromium release NK cell function testing. The CD107a assay examines if cytotoxic lymphocytes (NK cells and CTL) can release secretory lysosomes as described below, but this assay does not report if target cells are killed. Samples from patients with perforin deficiency will not show any degranulation abnormalities but is nonetheless often run to confirm normal degranulation. Typical perforin deficiency can thus be confidently diagnosed based on the lack of perforin staining, deficient NK cell cytotoxicity, but normal degranulation.

SECRETORY GRANULE EXOCYTOSIS DEFICIENCY

Autosomal recessive mutations in *UNC13D*, *STX11*, or *STXBP2* have been linked to primary HLH disease. These encode the proteins Munc13-4, syntaxin-11, or Munc18-2, and as diseases are known as FHL3, FHL4, or FHL5, respectively. The proteins encoded are crucial for perforin-containing secretory lysosome exocytosis, a process more commonly referred to as degranulation. Defects in *RAB27A*, *LYST*, and *AP3B1*, leading to Griscelli syndrome type 2 (GS2), Chediak-Higashi syndrome (CHS), and Hermansky-Pudlak syndrome type *2* (HPS2), respectively, also cause defective degranulation. These latter patients often manifest with HLH and usually, but not always, occulocutaneous albinism (22, 37–42). Together, these 6 genes can be grouped for diagnostic screening as they show a similar cellular phenotype of failed secretory lysosome content release and failure to kill target cells.

At this juncture, it is important to differentiate between the terms "NK cell degranulation" and "NK cell function," as they are often thought to be one and the same. The NK degranulation assay, also known as CD107a or NK exocytosis assay, evaluates if CD107a containing secretory lysosomes are able to release their content and thus deposit CD107a on the external cell membrane where it is measured as a surrogate for degranulation (**Figure 2**). Under the microscope, CD107a and perforin often co-localize and so it is assumed that when granules bearing CD107a are externalized, perforin would also most likely be released at the immune synapse (43, 44). In the case of perforin deficiency, the CD107a assay is not useful as a screening tool because secretory lysosomes without perforin are still released and CD107a still expressed on the cell membrane. The CD107a assay is also unable to detect whether granules are headed toward the immune synapse where the target cell is being engaged. When stimulating NK cells *in vitro* with anti-CD16 antibody, the release of secretory lysosomes are non-polarized which would not be efficient for target cell elimination (43). The CD107a assay has been found useful for the diagnosis of FHL3-5, GS2, CHS, and HPS2, and possibly ORAI1, STIM1, and HPS10 (45–48),

TABLE 1 | Sensitivity and specificity results for the diagnosis of primary HLH and related diseases extrapolated from various studies using a range of immunological assays.

References	Gene(s) studied	Assay description	Sensitivity, specificity (%)	Number of primary cases
Abdalgani et al. (18)	*PRF1*	Direct Intracellular staining of NK or CTL	97, 90	48
Tesi et al. (19)	*PRF1*	Direct Intracellular staining of NK or CTL	100, 100	14
	PRF1	NK cytotoxicity (chromium release) upon K562 stimulation	100, 95	14
Rubin et al. (20)	*PRF1*	Direct Intracellular staining of NK or CTL	97, 83	29
	PRF1, UNC13D, STX11, STXBP2, RAB27A, LYST, AP3B1	NK cytotoxicity (chromium release) upon K562 stimulation	60, 72	84
	UNC13D, STX11, STXBP2, RAB27A, LYST, AP3B1	NK degranulation (CD107a) upon K562 stimulation	94, 73	32
Bryceson et al. (21)	*UNC13D, STX11, STXBP2, RAB27A, LYST*	NK degranulation (CD107a) upon K562 stimulation	96, 88	90
Chiang et al. (16)	*UNC13D, STX11, STXBP2*	NK degranulation (CD107a) upon K562 stimulation	94, 84	16
	UNC13D, STX11, STXBP2	NK degranulation (CD107a) upon anti-CD16 antibody stimulation	88, 98	16
	UNC13D, STX11, STXBP2	CTL degranulation (CD107a) upon anti-CD3 antibody stimulation	88, 98	16
Chiang et al. (22)	*LYST*	NK degranulation (CD107a) upon K562 stimulation	85, 75	20
	LYST	NK degranulation (CD107a) upon anti-CD16 antibody stimulation	86, 96	21
	LYST	CTL degranulation (CD107a) upon anti-CD3 antibody stimulation	90, 90	20
	LYST	NK cytotoxicity (chromium release) upon K562 stimulation	89, 94	18
Hori et al. (23)	*UNC13D*	NK degranulation (CD107a) upon K562 stimulation	100, 71	6
	UNC13D	CTL degranulation (CD107a) upon anti-CD3 antibody stimulation	100, 100	6
Gifford et al. (24)	*SH2D1A*	Direct Intracellular staining of NK or CTL	87, 89	15
	XIAP/BIRC4	Direct Intracellular staining of NK or CTL	95, 61	19
Ammann et al. (25)	*XIAP/BIRC4*	Monocyte activation (TNF) upon L-18MDP stimulation	100, 100	12

because in all these cases, secretory lysosomes are unable reach the cell membrane or fail to fuse with the cell membrane leading to the absence of surface CD107a after relevant stimulation. But, in cases of preserved detection of CD107a upregulation, additional testing to evaluate NK cell killing may be needed, as lysosome degranulation does not necessarily equate to the death of target cells.

As such, the often crowned "gold standard" chromium release assay still holds relevance since described in the 1960s (49, 50). In this assay, K562 cells (ATCC, CCL-243) first preloaded with radioactive chromium-51 will be killed by NK cells and the extent to which the stored chromium is freed is taken to represent the percentage of K562 killed (51–53). No published data exists exploring the accuracies of NK cytotoxicity assay in diagnosing each subtype of primary HLH, possibly due to sample number limitations. Only one recent study attempted to systematically quantify the accuracy of the chromium release NK cell function assay when used in the clinical lab setting for diagnosing *PRF1*, *UNC13D*, *STX11*, *STXBP2*, *RAB27A*, *LYST*, and *AP3B1* mutations, and found it lacking with a sensitivity of 60% and specificity of 72% (**Table 1**) (20).

The low accuracy of this assay, often used during acute phase HLH, may be partly blamed on the assay's dependency on the NK cell percentage in the sample. HLH patients normally experience large expansions of CD8 T cells, and stressed blood samples from these patients often leave large numbers of RBC and cell debris in the peripheral blood mononuclear cell (PBMC) suspension after ficoll. This leads to an artificially low NK cell percentage which is often unaccounted for, giving an impression of reduced NK function when in fact it is due to the overwhelming number of other cells in the mix. Because the assay is sensitive as such, care must be taken when interpreting poor NK cytotoxicity results especially during acute HLH as it could indicate poor sample quality rather than dysfunctional NK cells. While this assay has many limitations, the result distinctly demonstrates whether or not target cells are finally killed (**Figure 2**) (54). Numerous flow-, colorimetric-, and imaging-based cytotoxicity assays have been touted as possible chromium release assay replacements but no large cohort of primary HLH cases has been validated on any of these platforms (55–59). Pending such reports, the chromium release assay is still the only published clinical standard for NK functional studies.

Therefore, we currently rely on the CD107a NK cell degranulation assay for the screening diagnosis of primary HLH related to mutations in *UNC13D*, *STX11*, *STXBP2*, *RAB27A*, *LYST*, and *AP3B1*. The most commonly used NK degranulation

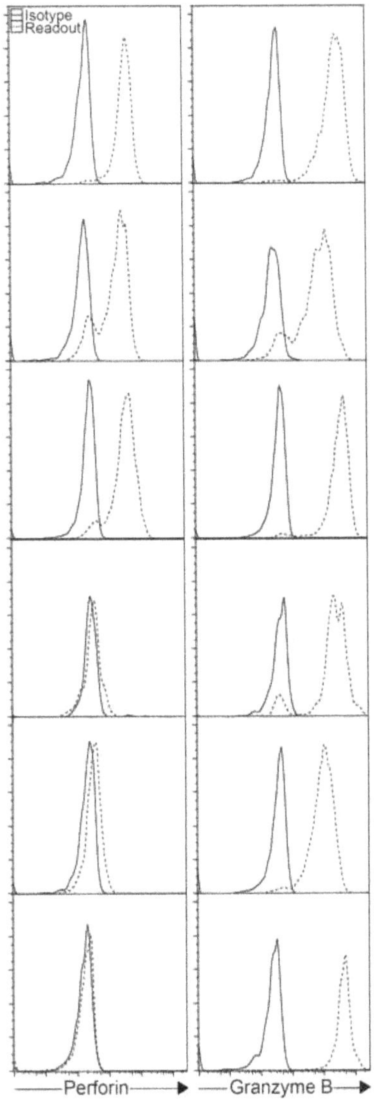

FIGURE 1 | Intracellular staining of perforin and granzyme B in different individuals. Histograms represent gated NK cells showing varying levels of perforin expression as a consequence of the different *PRF1* variants as shown.

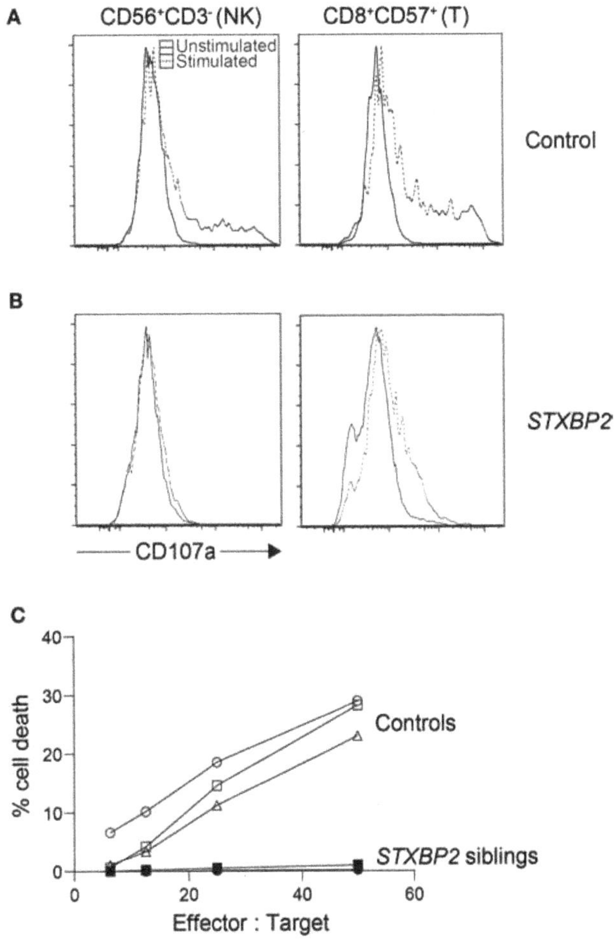

FIGURE 2 | Cytotoxic lymphocyte evaluation of an *STXBP2* patient. We performed NK cytotoxicity as well as NK and T cell degranulation using fresh PBMC from a case with homozygous c.1430C>T (p.Pro477Leu) mutations. While **(A)** control NK cells and CD8$^+$CD57$^+$ T cells degranulated as expected when stimulated, respectively with K562 or anti-CD3 antibody, **(B)** the patient's cytotoxic lymphocytes did not. **(C)** NK cytotoxicity was also evaluated via ^{51}Cr release and found deficient. In addition, we included cytotoxicity data from a sibling carrying the same homozygous mutation.

assay tests rested PBMC stimulated with the myelogenous leukemia cell line K562 (21). After co-incubation for several hours, the percentage of NK cells bearing surface CD107a or the fluorescence intensity of CD107a positive NK cells is then evaluated. Persons with a defect in secretory lysosome transport or membrane fusion will show greatly reduced surface CD107a levels (**Figure 2**). A pan European study found 97% of FHL3-5 and 85% of GS2 and CHS cases had abnormal percentage of NK cell degranulation (<5% CD107a$^+$ NK cells) to give an overall sensitivity of 96% and specificity of 88% in diagnosing a genetic degranulation disorder (**Table 1**) (21). A follow-up study on a North American cohort evaluated CD107a mean channel fluorescence (MCF) of NK cells instead of percentage of degranulating cells (20). It found 93.8% of patients with biallelic mutations in an HLH-associated degranulation gene with lowered CD107a MCF but only 60.4% of individuals without biallelic mutations in relevant genes with normal CD107a levels, giving an overall area under the curve of 0.86. More recently, a cohort of 21 CHS cases has likewise confirmed the CD107a assay is able to accurately identify primary defects in NK degranulation (22). In the first two studies, a sizable portion of controls were found to have lowered NK degranulation. This could be due to technical issues, stress during blood sample transport, medications leading to reduced lymphocyte reaction, or epigenetic changes resulting in NK cells with a particularly skewed functional response (60–63). So while better than the chromium release assay, the NK-K562 degranulation assay, like all diagnostic assays, is not perfect.

To overcome the shortcomings stemming from an overreliance on any single test, NK degranulation can also be evaluated through other means, for example, via stimulation using PMA, activating antibodies such as anti-CD16 targeting the Fc receptor, or activation of synergistic NK receptors (16, 64, 65). Preliminary data has found Fc stimulation induced degranulation returns 88% sensitivity and 98% specificity in a cohort of 16 FHL3-5 (**Table 1**) (16). We can thus infer that both NK cell natural cytotoxicity and antibody-dependent cellular cytotoxicity are defective in classical primary HLH. This is an important point to note as immunodeficiencies could affect only one specific pathway. For instance, a certain CD16 (FcγRIIIA) mutation was found to impair natural NK cytotoxicity but Fc specific function was intact (66). Current standard clinical tests limited to only K562 stimulation would be insufficient for detecting abnormalities in such cases.

Cytotoxic T lymphocytes have also been found defective in degranulation in the context of primary HLH due to mutations in the genes required for normal degranulation. Previously, T cell blasts had to be grown up over weeks in order to sufficiently stimulate perforin production in T cells and generate enough cell numbers for experimentation (21). More recently, it was noticed that specific populations of T cells, namely $CD3^{+}CD8^{+}CD57^{+}$ contain perforin and granzymes *ex vivo* without prior need for stimulation (17). This population of *bone fide* effector cells, by virtue of perforin expression, was found to efficiently degranulate upon anti-CD3 antibody stimulation. Crucial to our context, when tested on primary HLH samples, $CD3^{+}CD8^{+}CD57^{+}$ T cell degranulation was defective to a similar level as in NK cells (16). A small confirmatory study found high sensitivity with a cohort of biallelic pathogenic *UNC13D* variants (23). With multiple ways to induce degranulation on multiple cell types, we could speculate on possible undiscovered immunodeficiencies that affect only NK cells or T cells and detectable only with a combination of various degranulation assays.

Like perforin, it is possible to directly detect Munc13-4, syntaxin11, Munc18-2, and Rab27a with antibodies (67–69). However, this is usually performed with western blot. One exception is Munc13-4 detection in platelets with flow cytometry (70, 71). Although this assay has been found to be highly accurate for predicting *UNC13D* mutations, the antibody used is polyclonal and not commercially available.

Taken together, when primary HLH is suspected, performing the triad of perforin staining, NK and/or T cell degranulation, and NK cytotoxicity will give a more complete evaluation of cytotoxic cell activity and improve HLH diagnosis. While all the assays are individually accurate, we suggest moving toward a "multiplexing" of degranulation assays in the future to increase confidence in diagnosis, provide security should any one cell population be poorly represented, and pave the way for detecting degranulation deficiencies in specific pathways or cell types. Additionally, validating a radioactivity-free killing assay that accounts for effector cell counts would be highly useful for true assessment of cytotoxic lymphocyte function.

X-LINKED DISEASES

The genes *SH2D1A* and *XIAP/BIRC4* encode the proteins SAP and XIAP, respectively. Deficiencies in these proteins lead to X-linked lymphoproliferative disease type (XLP) 1 and 2 (72, 73). As their names imply, both genes are X-linked and often manifest HLH with Epstein-Barr virus (EBV) infection (74–76) but beyond that, XLP1 and XLP2 have quite different phenotypes and share little functional or structural similarities (77).

Similar to perforin, SAP and XIAP monoclonal antibodies exist and have been validated clinically for direct intracellular protein detection (**Figures 3, 4**) (78–80). However, care must be taken when reading such reports as certain pathologic variants have been found to preserve antibody binding leading to false negative (false normal) results (81–83). Also, while the absence of binding can be equated with the absence of that protein and thus strongly suggests a defect, the binding of an antibody to its antigen says nothing about the function of the protein bound. As such, patients expressing normal SAP and XIAP levels, or for that matter all direct antibody phenotyping tests, should still be sequenced if clinically suspicious. Bimodal staining patterns are also useful in identifying female carriers as well as estimating the level of chimerism for transplant monitoring (24, 79). For XIAP, there has been reports of non-random X inactivation in some female carriers. Lymphocytes bearing the wild-type allele have been seen selected in some while others show the opposite, skewing toward the defective X chromosome at risk for disease manifestations (73, 84, 85). Direct screening of SAP returns 87% sensitivity and 89% specificity for the prediction of pathologic mutations in *SH2D1A* while direct screening of XIAP gives 95% sensitivity and 61% specificity (**Table 1**) (24, 86).

It has been demonstrated that both SAP and XIAP are required for the development of normal invariant NKT (iNKT) cells and for normal T cell restimulation-induced cell death (RICD) (73, 76, 87, 88). As such, iNKT quantification and RICD assays can be performed for cases where direct staining is inconclusive, or if further supporting data is desired (**Figure 3**). A more sophisticated cytotoxic assay looking at inhibitory 2B4 signaling in NK cells has also been reported to discriminate functional SAP deficiency (89). Likewise, a functional test exists where XIAP function is investigated downstream of NOD2 stimulation on monocytes. Following stimulation with L18-MDP, TNF is normally produced by CD14 positive cells. However, patients with pathologic mutations in XIAP, even where XIAP protein staining was found normal or in patients with milder clinical phenotype, all had equally defective TNF production and could easily be discriminated (**Figure 4**) (25). A cutoff of 10% TNF-producing monocytes perfectly distinguished 12 XIAP patients from 29 healthy controls and 6 female carriers (**Table 1**). Subsequent reports demonstrated the assay's usefulness in diagnosing inflammatory bowel disease (IBD) cases with novel XIAP mutations (90, 91). By performing phenotyping as well as functional assays side by side, it is hoped that future cases might be more accurately identified.

OTHER PRIMARY IMMUNODEFICIENICES

A host of patients with other diseases such as ALPS, CGD, CVID, and SCID, as well as variants in genes including *BTK*,

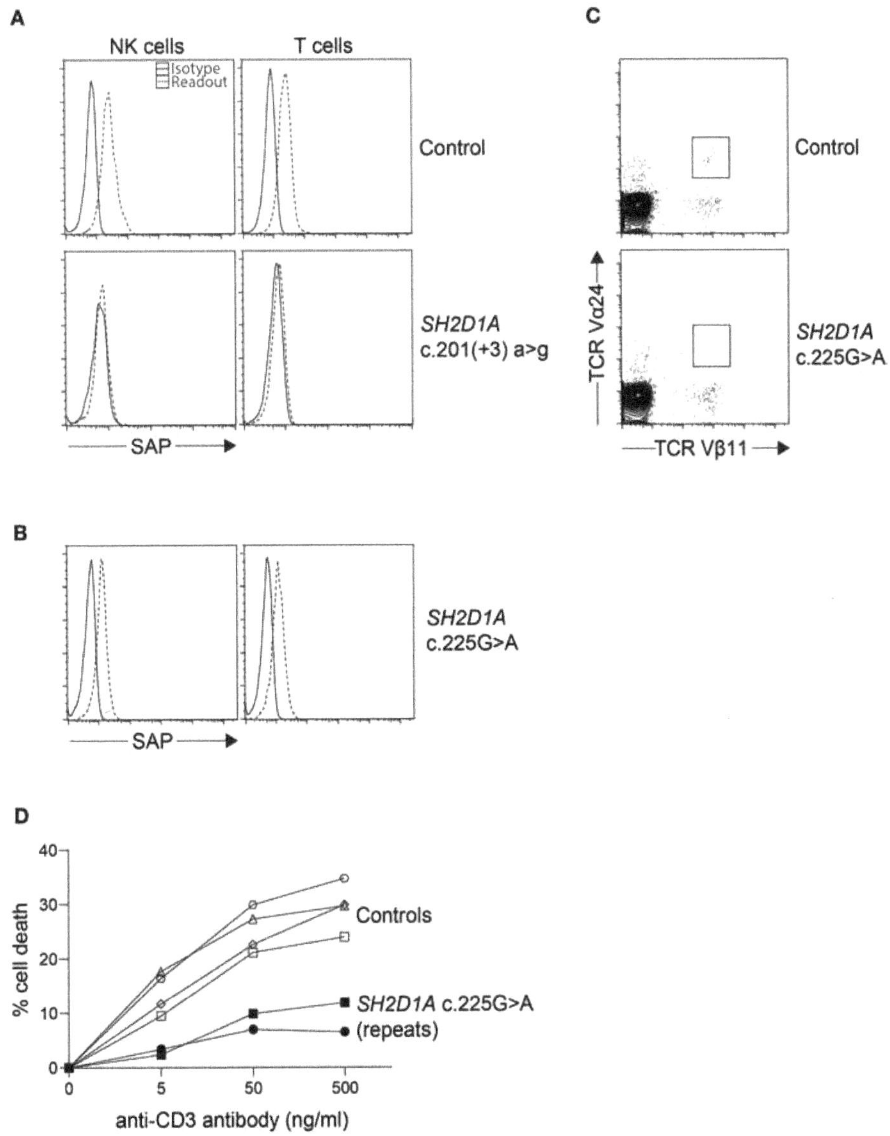

FIGURE 3 | Indirect diagnosis of XLP1. **(A)** While most *SH2D1A* mutations result in absent or lowly expressing SAP protein levels, we found **(B)** a clinically suspicious patient with c.125 G > A (p.Cys42Tyr) missense mutation with only a slight reduction in SAP protein expression by flow cytometry. The patient was thus further evaluated for **(C)** iNKT numbers on bulk $CD3^+$ cells and **(D)** restimulation-induced cell death (RICD) via anti-CD3 antibody repeated on two occasions. The low iNKT counts and reduced cell death upon TCR restimulation provided evidence that the missense *SH2D1A* variant found was indeed pathological.

CARMIL2, CD27, ITK, LRBA, MAGT1, NEMO, PIK3CD, RAG2, WAS, NLR genes, and STAT genes, have been implicated with possible HLH (92–94). The assays described so far including NK cell degranulation and cytotoxicity will be of little diagnostic use here except to rule out defective secretory lysosome transport. For some genes, there exist flow cytometric assays that can assist with diagnosis. For example T, B, and NK specific subset phenotyping panels can pick up ALPS (increased double negative T cells), X-linked agammaglobulinemia due to mutations in *BTK* (low B cell counts or BTK expression), mutations in *CD27* (absent surface expression of CD27), mutations in *MAGT1* (lowered NKG2D expression), and a variety of SCID disorders (very low B, T, and/or NK counts, reduced recent thymic emigrants and CD45RA expression) (95). The neutrophil oxidative burst assay is an excellent assay for the diagnosis of CGD (96). WAS can be accurately diagnosed through direct staining of intracellular WAS protein (97). Multiple excellent reviews exist for PID diagnostics (98, 99).

A second group of primary immunodeficiency genes demonstrate defective NK cell activity without pronounced HLH. However, before suggesting that NK degranulation and cytotoxicity assays could be used in helping with the diagnosis of these PIDs, larger cohorts of patients must be collected for

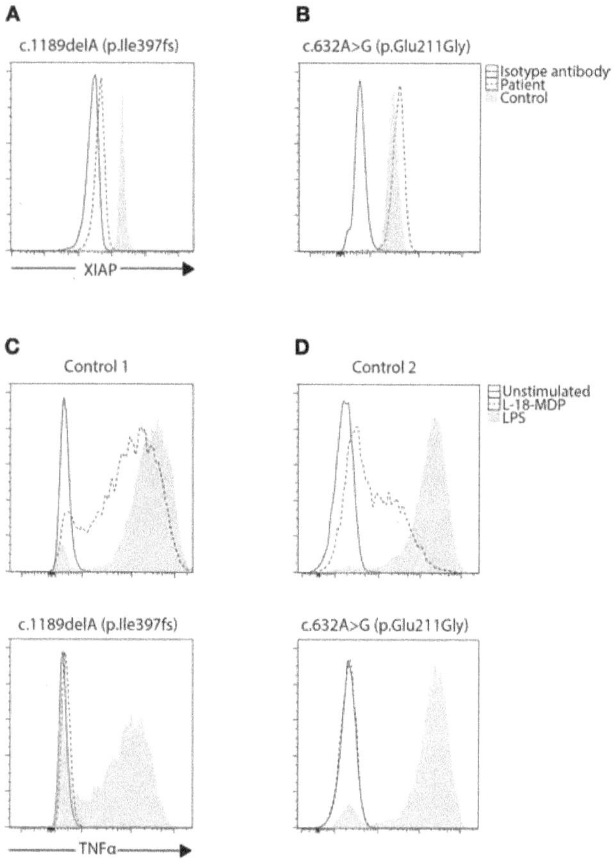

FIGURE 4 | Phenotyping and functional evaluation for XLP2. **(A)** While a majority of *BIRC4* mutations present with absent or lowly expressing XIAP protein levels, we found **(B)** a patient with c.632A>G (p.Glu211Gly) variant of uncertain significance (VUCS) with only a slight reduction in XIAP protein expression by flow cytometry. Functional evaluation of XIAP can be done through stimulation of NOD2 with L18-MDP. This signaling pathway requires XIAP for TNF transcription through NF-κB. **(C,D)** When examined, both these cases show equally defective TNF production regardless of XIAP expression revealing the VUCS is in fact a damaging mutation. LPS acts as a positive control that signals through TLR4 demonstrating preserved cellular function in patient cells.

evaluation to confirm and explore cytotoxic lymphocytes further including: whether or not both NK and CTL are affected, if both degranulation and cytotoxicity are defective, and if the majority of mutations in that gene share the same phenotype. Genes in this group include *AP3D1*, *CTSC*, *FERMT3*, *GATA2*, *IRF8*, *MYH9*, *ORAI1*, and *STIM1* (45, 47, 48, 100–107). From this list, we know that not all persons for whom NK cell function is defective should be labeled primary HLH. Moreover, a thorough evaluation is hampered as many of publications lack NK degranulation or cytotoxicity data, something we hope future endeavors will address. These genes are thus currently not grouped together with the "classical" primary HLH family because clinical HLH is not usually the outstanding feature. Most are also very rare leading to difficulty in performing large cohort evaluations of cytotoxic lymphocyte activity.

THE FUTURE OF HLH DIAGNOSTICS

The HLH field has come some ways since the HLH-2004 criteria were established (108). A European cohort of cases with clinical HLH and PID other than defects in cytotoxicity found 63 cases, 80% of which were CGD and CID (109). Across the Atlantic, another HLH cohort was comprised of only 19% primary HLH disorders, with 58% of patients having other PIDs including genes associated with inflammasome function (92). We reason the high percentage of "non-classical-HLH" cases is a reflection of improved HLH awareness within the community and should be looked upon positively. These and other studies looking into specific sensitivities of various HLH-2004 criteria have found them wanting (110–112). The concern often cited is the inability to distinguish between primary HLH, secondary HLH, and other PIDs. A simple solution that can easily be adopted today is increased screening. As can be concluded from **Table 1**, many subtypes of primary HLH can be diagnosed with good accuracy. As such, the fulfillment of HLH criteria should act as an actionable gateway to seriously consider PID by performing various laboratory tests as discussed. This in tandem with advanced sequencing should more often than not provide conclusive diagnosis for all the common primary HLH cases. As previously mentioned, we believe the field of HLH diagnostics will move toward a "multiplexing" of screening assays to more quickly screen for multiple defects simultaneously.

The evaluation of gene expression signatures is an exciting development that could help untangle some of the primary vs. secondary HLH questions going forward. Unique interferon-stimulated gene signatures have been found in systemic lupus erythematosus differentiating it from rheumatoid arthritis and control samples (113, 114). Other studies successfully used the interferon score to identify various Mendelian Type-I IFN-mediated autoinflammatory diseases (115, 116). Preliminary work to define a HLH signature has also been performed with favorable results (117, 118). While research on this area is in its infancy today, we postulate a future where specific gene expression fingerprints from tens or hundreds of genes would be elucidated for the various shades of HLH. We could then quickly and accurately segregate HLH into several subcategories as well as deduce their disease status. The signatures could not only act as a "precision" diagnostic tool but also afford us a deeper cellular mechanistic understanding on the pathobiology of various closely related diseases, and thus opportunities for "precision" therapeutics. We are excited to see what the future holds in terms of HLH diagnostics.

AUTHOR CONTRIBUTIONS

RM initiated the manuscript which SC wrote and JB edited.

ACKNOWLEDGMENTS

The authors wish to thank Kathryn Quinn, Carrie Gifford, Joyce Collett, and the entire staff of the Diagnostic Immunology Laboratory.

REFERENCES

1. Janka GE, Lehmberg K. Hemophagocytic syndromes–an update. *Blood Rev.* (2014) 28:135–42. doi: 10.1016/j.blre.2014.03.002
2. Jenkins MR, Rudd-Schmidt JA, Lopez JA, Ramsbottom KM, Mannering SI, Andrews DM, et al. Failed CTL/NK cell killing and cytokine hypersecretion are directly linked through prolonged synapse time. *J Exp Med.* (2015) 212:307–17. doi: 10.1084/jem.20140964
3. Bracaglia C, Prencipe G, De Benedetti F. Macrophage activation syndrome: different mechanisms leading to a one clinical syndrome. *Pediatr Rheumatol Online J.* (2017) 15:5. doi: 10.1186/s12969-016-0130-4
4. Machowicz R, Janka G, Wiktor-Jedrzejczak W. Similar but not the same: differential diagnosis of HLH and sepsis. *Crit Rev Oncol Hematol.* (2017) 114:1–12. doi: 10.1016/j.critrevonc.2017.03.023
5. Wang H, Xiong L, Tang W, Zhou Y, Li F. A systematic review of malignancy-associated hemophagocytic lymphohistiocytosis that needs more attentions. *Oncotarget.* (2017) 8:59977–85. doi: 10.18632/oncotarget.19230
6. Ham H, Billadeau DD. Human immunodeficiency syndromes affecting human natural killer cell cytolytic activity. *Front Immunol.* (2014) 5:2. doi: 10.3389/fimmu.2014.00002
7. Marsh RA, Haddad E. How i treat primary haemophagocytic lymphohistiocytosis. *Br J Haematol.* (2018) 182:185–99. doi: 10.1111/bjh.15274
8. Marsh RA, Jordan MB, Talano JA, Nichols KE, Kumar A, Naqvi A, et al. Salvage therapy for refractory hemophagocytic lymphohistiocytosis: a review of the published experience. *Pediatr Blood Cancer.* (2017) 2017:64. doi: 10.1002/pbc.26308
9. Risma KA, Marsh RA. Hemophagocytic lymphohistiocytosis: clinical presentations and diagnosis. *J Allergy Clin Immunol Pract.* (2019) 7:824–32. doi: 10.1016/j.jaip.2018.11.050
10. Sepulveda FE, de Saint Basile G. Hemophagocytic syndrome: primary forms and predisposing conditions. *Curr Opin Immunol.* (2017) 49:20–6. doi: 10.1016/j.coi.2017.08.004
11. Ljunggren HG, Karre K. In search of the 'missing self': MHC molecules and NK cell recognition. *Immunol Today.* (1990) 11:237–44. doi: 10.1016/0167-5699(90)90097-S
12. Prager I, Watzl C. Mechanisms of natural killer cell-mediated cellular cytotoxicity. *J Leukoc Biol.* (2019) 105:1319–29. doi: 10.1002/JLB.MR0718-269R
13. Voskoboinik I, Trapani JA. Perforinopathy: a spectrum of human immune disease caused by defective perforin delivery or function. *Front Immunol.* (2013) 4:441. doi: 10.3389/fimmu.2013.00441
14. Stepp SE, Dufourcq-Lagelouse R, Le Deist F, Bhawan S, Certain S, Mathew PA, et al. Perforin gene defects in familial hemophagocytic lymphohistiocytosis. *Science.* (1999) 286:1957–9. doi: 10.1126/science.286.5446.1957
15. Chiang S, Bryceson Y. Measurement of NK cell phenotype and activity in humans. In: Detrick B, Schmitz J, Hamilton R, editors. *Manual of Molecular and Clinical Laboratory Immunology*, Eighth Edition. Washington, DC: ASM Press (2016). p. 300–9.
16. Chiang SC, Theorell J, Entesarian M, Meeths M, Mastafa M, Al-Herz W, et al. Comparison of primary human cytotoxic T-cell and natural killer cell responses reveal similar molecular requirements for lytic granule exocytosis but differences in cytokine production. *Blood.* (2013) 121:1345–56. doi: 10.1182/blood-2012-07-442558
17. Chattopadhyay PK, Betts MR, Price DA, Gostick E, Horton H, Roederer M, et al. The cytolytic enzymes granyzme A, granzyme B, and perforin: expression patterns, cell distribution, and their relationship to cell maturity and bright CD57 expression. *J Leukoc Biol.* (2009) 85:88–97. doi: 10.1189/jlb.0208107
18. Abdalgani M, Filipovich AH, Choo S, Zhang K, Gifford C, Villanueva J, et al. Accuracy of flow cytometric perforin screening for detecting patients with FHL due to PRF1 mutations. *Blood.* (2015) 126:1858–60. doi: 10.1182/blood-2015-06-648659
19. Tesi B, Chiang SC, El-Ghoneimy D, Hussein AA, Langenskiold C, Wali R, et al. Spectrum of atypical clinical presentations in patients with biallelic PRF1 missense mutations. *Pediatr Blood Cancer.* (2015) 62:2094–100. doi: 10.1002/pbc.25646
20. Rubin TS, Zhang K, Gifford C, Lane A, Choo S, Bleesing JJ, et al. Perforin and CD107a testing is superior to NK cell function testing for screening patients for genetic HLH. *Blood.* (2017) 129:2993–9. doi: 10.1182/blood-2016-12-753830
21. Bryceson YT, Pende D, Maul-Pavicic A, Gilmour KC, Ufheil H, Vraetz T, et al. A prospective evaluation of degranulation assays in the rapid diagnosis of familial hemophagocytic syndromes. *Blood.* (2012) 119:2754–63. doi: 10.1182/blood-2011-08-374199
22. Chiang SCC, Wood SM, Tesi B, Akar HH, Al-Herz W, Ammann S, et al. Differences in granule morphology yet equally impaired exocytosis among cytotoxic T Cells and NK cells from chediak-higashi syndrome patients. *Front Immunol.* (2017) 8:426. doi: 10.3389/fimmu.2017.00426
23. Hori M, Yasumi T, Shimodera S, Shibata H, Hiejima E, Oda H, et al. A CD57(+) CTL Degranulation Assay Effectively Identifies Familial Hemophagocytic Lymphohistiocytosis Type 3 Patients. *J Clin Immunol.* (2017) 37:92–9. doi: 10.1007/s10875-016-0357-3
24. Gifford CE, Weingartner E, Villanueva J, Johnson J, Zhang K, Filipovich AH, et al. Clinical flow cytometric screening of SAP and XIAP expression accurately identifies patients with SH2D1A and XIAP/BIRC4 mutations. *Cytometry B Clin Cytom.* (2014) 86:263–71. doi: 10.1002/cyto.b.21166
25. Ammann S, Elling R, Gyrd-Hansen M, Duckers G, Bredius R, Burns SO, et al. A new functional assay for the diagnosis of X-linked inhibitor of apoptosis (XIAP) deficiency. *Clin Exp Immunol.* (2014) 176:394–400. doi: 10.1111/cei.12306
26. Hussein AA, Hamadah T, Qandeel M, Sughayer M, Amarin R, Mansour A, et al. Hematopoietic stem cell transplantation of an adolescent with neurological manifestations of homozygous missense PRF1 mutation. *Pediatr Blood Cancer.* (2014) 61:2313–5. doi: 10.1002/pbc.25166
27. Kim JY, Shin JH, Sung SI, Kim JK, Jung JM, Ahn SY, et al. A novel PRF1 gene mutation in a fatal neonate case with type 2 familial hemophagocytic lymphohistiocytosis. *Korean J Pediatr.* (2014) 57:50–3. doi: 10.3345/kjp.2014.57.1.50
28. Martinez-Pomar N, Lanio N, Romo N, Lopez-Botet M, Matamoros N. Functional impact of A91V mutation of the PRF1 perforin gene. *Hum Immunol.* (2013) 74:14–7. doi: 10.1016/j.humimm.2012.10.011
29. Santoro A, Cannella S, Trizzino A, Lo Nigro L, Corsello G, Arico M. A single amino acid change A91V in perforin: a novel, frequent predisposing factor to childhood acute lymphoblastic leukemia? *Haematologica.* (2005) 90:697–8.
30. Tesi B, Lagerstedt-Robinson K, Chiang SC, Ben Bdira E, Abboud M, Belen B, et al. Targeted high-throughput sequencing for genetic diagnostics of hemophagocytic lymphohistiocytosis. *Genome Med.* (2015) 7:130. doi: 10.1186/s13073-015-0244-1
31. Zur Stadt U, Beutel K, Weber B, Kabisch H, Schneppenheim R, Janka G. A91V is a polymorphism in the perforin gene not causative of an FHLH phenotype. *Blood.* (2004) 104:1909; author reply 10. doi: 10.1182/blood-2004-02-0733
32. Voskoboinik I, Sutton VR, Ciccone A, House CM, Chia J, Darcy PK, et al. Perforin activity and immune homeostasis: the common A91V polymorphism in perforin results in both presynaptic and postsynaptic defects in function. *Blood.* (2007) 110:1184–90. doi: 10.1182/blood-2007-02-072850
33. Voskoboinik I, Thia MC, Trapani JA. A functional analysis of the putative polymorphisms A91V and N252S and 22 missense perforin mutations associated with familial hemophagocytic lymphohistiocytosis. *Blood.* (2005) 105:4700–6. doi: 10.1182/blood-2004-12-4935
34. Mancebo E, Allende LM, Guzman M, Paz-Artal E, Gil J, Urrea-Moreno R, et al. Familial hemophagocytic lymphohistiocytosis in an adult patient homozygous for A91V in the perforin gene, with tuberculosis infection. *Haematologica.* (2006) 91:1257-60.
35. Sanchez IP, Leal-Esteban LC, Alvarez-Alvarez JA, Perez-Romero CA, Orrego JC, Serna ML, et al. Analyses of the PRF1 gene in individuals with hemophagocytic lymphohystiocytosis reveal the common haplotype R54C/A91V in Colombian unrelated families associated with late onset disease. *J Clin Immunol.* (2012) 32:670–80. doi: 10.1007/s10875-012-9680-5
36. Trizzino A, zur Stadt U, Ueda I, Risma K, Janka G, Ishii E, et al. Genotype-phenotype study of familial haemophagocytic

lymphohistiocytosis due to perforin mutations. *J Med Genet.* (2008) 45:15–21. doi: 10.1136/jmg.2007.052670
37. Enders A, Zieger B, Schwarz K, Yoshimi A, Speckmann C, Knoepfle EM, et al. Lethal hemophagocytic lymphohistiocytosis in Hermansky-Pudlak syndrome type II. *Blood.* (2006) 108:81–7. doi: 10.1182/blood-2005-11-4413
38. Fontana S, Parolini S, Vermi W, Booth S, Gallo F, Donini M, et al. Innate immunity defects in Hermansky-Pudlak type 2 syndrome. *Blood.* (2006) 107:4857–64. doi: 10.1182/blood-2005-11-4398
39. Wood SM, Meeths M, Chiang SC, Bechensteen AG, Boelens JJ, Heilmann C, et al. Different NK cell-activating receptors preferentially recruit Rab27a or Munc13-4 to perforin-containing granules for cytotoxicity. *Blood.* (2009) 114:4117–27. doi: 10.1182/blood-2009-06-225359
40. Netter P, Chan SK, Banerjee PP, Monaco-Shawver L, Noroski LM, Hanson IC, et al. A novel Rab27a mutation binds melanophilin, but not Munc13-4, causing immunodeficiency without albinism. *J Allergy Clin Immunol.* (2016) 138:599–601 e3. doi: 10.1016/j.jaci.2015.12.1337
41. Tesi B, Rascon J, Chiang SCC, Burnyte B, Lofstedt A, Fasth A, et al. A RAB27A 5' untranslated region structural variant associated with late-onset hemophagocytic lymphohistiocytosis and normal pigmentation. *J Allergy Clin Immunol.* (2018) 142:317–21 e8. doi: 10.1016/j.jaci.2018.02.031
42. Dell'Acqua F, Saettini F, Castelli I, Badolato R, Notarangelo LD, Rizzari C. Hermansky-Pudlak syndrome type II and lethal hemophagocytic lymphohistiocytosis: Case description and review of the literature. *J Allergy Clin Immunol Pract.* (2019). doi: 10.1016/j.jaip.2019.04.001. [Epub ahead of print].
43. Bryceson YT, March ME, Barber DF, Ljunggren HG, Long EO. Cytolytic granule polarization and degranulation controlled by different receptors in resting NK cells. *J Exp Med.* (2005) 202:1001–12. doi: 10.1084/jem.200 51143
44. Krzewski K, Gil-Krzewska A, Nguyen V, Peruzzi G, Coligan JE. LAMP1/CD107a is required for efficient perforin delivery to lytic granules and NK-cell cytotoxicity. *Blood.* (2013) 121:4672-83. doi: 10.1182/blood-2012-08-453738
45. Ammann S, Schulz A, Krageloh-Mann I, Dieckmann NM, Niethammer K, Fuchs S, et al. Mutations in AP3D1 associated with immunodeficiency and seizures define a new type of Hermansky-Pudlak syndrome. *Blood.* (2016) 127:997–1006. doi: 10.1182/blood-2015-09-671636
46. Fuchs S, Rensing-Ehl A, Speckmann C, Bengsch B, Schmitt-Graeff A, Bondzio I, et al. Antiviral and regulatory T cell immunity in a patient with stromal interaction molecule 1 deficiency. *J Immunol.* (2012) 188:1523-33. doi: 10.4049/jimmunol.1102507
47. Klemann C, Ammann S, Heizmann M, Fuchs S, Bode SF, Heeg M, et al. Hemophagocytic lymphohistiocytosis as presenting manifestation of profound combined immunodeficiency due to an ORAI1 mutation. *J Allergy Clin Immunol.* (2017) 140:1721-4. doi: 10.1016/j.jaci.2017. 05.039
48. Maul-Pavicic A, Chiang SC, Rensing-Ehl A, Jessen B, Fauriat C, Wood SM, et al. ORAI1-mediated calcium influx is required for human cytotoxic lymphocyte degranulation and target cell lysis. *Proc Natl Acad Sci U.S.A.* (2011) 108:3324-9. doi: 10.1073/pnas.1013285108
49. Brunner KT, Mauel J, Cerottini JC, Chapuis B. Quantitative assay of the lytic action of immune lymphoid cells on 51-Cr-labelled allogeneic target cells *in vitro*; inhibition by isoantibody and by drugs. *Immunology.* (1968) 14:181–96.
50. Wigzell H. Quantitative titrations of mouse H-2 antibodies using Cr-51-labelled target cells. *Transplantation.* (1965) 3:423–31. doi: 10.1097/00007890-196505000-00011
51. Bryant J, Day R, Whiteside TL, Herberman RB. Calculation of lytic units for the expression of cell-mediated cytotoxicity. *J Immunol Methods.* (1992) 146:91–103. doi: 10.1016/0022-1759(92)90052-U
52. Pross HF, Maroun JA. The standardization of NK cell assays for use in studies of biological response modifiers. *J Immunol Methods.* (1984) 68:235–49. doi: 10.1016/0022-1759(84)90154-6
53. Whiteside TL, Bryant J, Day R, Herberman RB. Natural killer cytotoxicity in the diagnosis of immune dysfunction: criteria for a reproducible assay. *J Clin Lab Anal.* (1990) 4:102–14. doi: 10.1002/jcla.1860040207
54. Pollock RE, Zimmerman SO, Fuchshuber P, Lotzova E. Lytic units reconsidered: pitfalls in calculation and usage. *J Clin Lab Anal.* (1990) 4:274–82. doi: 10.1002/jcla.1860040408
55. Fassy J, Tsalkitzi K, Goncalves-Maia M, Braud VM. A Real-time cytotoxicity assay as an alternative to the standard chromium-51 release assay for measurement of human NK and T Cell cytotoxic activity. *Curr Protoc Immunol.* (2017) 118:7 42 1–7:12. doi: 10.1002/cpim.28
56. He L, Hakimi J, Salha D, Miron I, Dunn P, Radvanyi L. A sensitive flow cytometry-based cytotoxic T-lymphocyte assay through detection of cleaved caspase 3 in target cells. *J Immunol Methods.* (2005) 304:43–59. doi: 10.1016/j.jim.2005.06.005
57. Piriou L, Chilmonczyk S, Genetet N, Albina E. Design of a flow cytometric assay for the determination of natural killer and cytotoxic T-lymphocyte activity in human and in different animal species. *Cytometry.* (2000) 41:289–97. doi: 10.1002/1097-0320(20001201)41:4<289::AID-CYTO7>3.0.CO;2-5
58. Zaritskaya L, Shurin MR, Sayers TJ, Malyguine AM. New flow cytometric assays for monitoring cell-mediated cytotoxicity. *Expert Rev Vaccines.* (2010) 9:601-16. doi: 10.1586/erv.10.49
59. van der Haar Avila I, Marmol P, Cany J, Kiessling R, Pico de Coana Y. Evaluating antibody-dependent cell-mediated cytotoxicity by flow cytometry. *Methods Mol Biol.* (2019) 1913:181–94. doi: 10.1007/978-1-4939-8979-9_13
60. Meehan AC, Mifsud NA, Nguyen TH, Levvey BJ, Snell GI, Kotsimbos TC, et al. Impact of commonly used transplant immunosuppressive drugs on human NK cell function is dependent upon stimulation condition. *PLoS ONE.* (2013) 8:e60144. doi: 10.1371/journal.pone.0060144
61. Schlums H, Cichocki F, Tesi B, Theorell J, Beziat V, Holmes TD, et al. Cytomegalovirus infection drives adaptive epigenetic diversification of NK cells with altered signaling and effector function. *Immunity.* (2015) 42:443–56. doi: 10.1016/j.immuni.2015.02.008
62. Theorell J, Gustavsson AL, Tesi B, Sigmundsson K, Ljunggren HG, Lundback T, et al. Immunomodulatory activity of commonly used drugs on Fc-receptor-mediated human natural killer cell activation. *Cancer Immunol Immunother.* (2014) 63:627–41. doi: 10.1007/s00262-014-1539-6
63. Wai LE, Fujiki M, Takeda S, Martinez OM, Krams SM. Rapamycin, but not cyclosporine or FK506, alters natural killer cell function. *Transplantation.* (2008) 85:145-9. doi: 10.1097/01.tp.0000296817.28053.7b
64. Bryceson YT, March ME, Ljunggren HG, Long EO. Synergy among receptors on resting NK cells for the activation of natural cytotoxicity and cytokine secretion. *Blood.* (2006) 107:159–66. doi: 10.1182/blood-2005-04-1351
65. Cruikshank M, Anoop P, Nikolajeva O, Rao A, Rao K, Gilmour K, et al. Screening assays for primary haemophagocytic lymphohistiocytosis in children presenting with suspected macrophage activation syndrome. *Pediatr Rheumatol Online J.* (2015) 12 Suppl 1:48. doi: 10.1186/s12969-015-0043-7
66. Grier JT, Forbes LR, Monaco-Shawver L, Oshinsky J, Atkinson TP, Moody C, et al. Human immunodeficiency-causing mutation defines CD16 in spontaneous NK cell cytotoxicity. *J Clin Invest.* (2012) 122:3769-80. doi: 10.1172/JCI64837
67. Menasche G, Pastural E, Feldmann J, Certain S, Ersoy F, Dupuis S, et al. Mutations in RAB27A cause Griscelli syndrome associated with haemophagocytic syndrome. *Nat Genet.* (2000) 25:173–6. doi: 10.1038/76024
68. zur Stadt U, Schmidt S, Kasper B, Beutel K, Diler AS, Henter JI, et al. Linkage of familial hemophagocytic lymphohistiocytosis (FHL) type-4 to chromosome 6q24 and identification of mutations in syntaxin 11. *Hum Mol Genet.* (2005) 14:827–34. doi: 10.1093/hmg/ddi076
69. Cote M, Menager MM, Burgess A, Mahlaoui N, Picard C, Schaffner C, et al. Munc18-2 deficiency causes familial hemophagocytic lymphohistiocytosis type 5 and impairs cytotoxic granule exocytosis in patient NK cells. *J Clin Invest.* (2009) 119:3765–73. doi: 10.1172/JCI40732
70. Murata Y, Yasumi T, Shirakawa R, Izawa K, Sakai H, Abe J, et al. Rapid diagnosis of FHL3 by flow cytometric detection of intraplatelet Munc13-4 protein. *Blood.* (2011) 118:1225–30. doi: 10.1182/blood-2011-01-329540
71. Shibata H, Yasumi T, Shimodera S, Hiejima E, Izawa K, Kawai T, et al. Human CTL-based functional analysis shows the reliability of a munc13-4 protein expression assay for FHL3 diagnosis. *Blood.* (2018) 131:2016–25. doi: 10.1182/blood-2017-10-812503
72. Purtilo DT, Cassel CK, Yang JP, Harper R. X-linked recessive progressive combined variable immunodeficiency (Duncan's disease). *Lancet.* (1975) 1:935–40. doi: 10.1016/s0140-6736(75)92004-8

73. Rigaud S, Fondaneche MC, Lambert N, Pasquier B, Mateo V, Soulas P, et al. XIAP deficiency in humans causes an X-linked lymphoproliferative syndrome. *Nature.* (2006) 444:110–4. doi: 10.1038/nature05257
74. Marsh RA. Epstein-Barr Virus and Hemophagocytic Lymphohistiocytosis. *Front Immunol.* (2017) 8:1902. doi: 10.3389/fimmu.2017.01902
75. Seemayer TA, Gross TG, Egeler RM, Pirruccello SJ, Davis JR, Kelly CM, et al. X-linked lymphoproliferative disease: twenty-five years after the discovery. *Pediatr Res.* (1995) 38:471–8. doi: 10.1203/00006450-199510000-00001
76. Snow AL, Pandiyan P, Zheng L, Krummey SM, Lenardo MJ. The power and the promise of restimulation-induced cell death in human immune diseases. *Immunol Rev.* (2010) 236:68–82. doi: 10.1111/j.1600-065X.2010.00917.x
77. Filipovich AH, Zhang K, Snow AL, Marsh RA. X-linked lymphoproliferative syndromes: brothers or distant cousins? *Blood.* (2010) 116:3398–408. doi: 10.1182/blood-2010-03-275909
78. Kanegane H, Yang X, Zhao M, Yamato K, Inoue M, Hamamoto K, et al. Clinical features and outcome of X-linked lymphoproliferative syndrome type 1 (SAP deficiency) in Japan identified by the combination of flow cytometric assay and genetic analysis. *Pediatr Allergy Immunol.* (2012) 23:488–93. doi: 10.1111/j.1399-3038.2012.01282.x
79. Marsh RA, Bleesing JJ, Filipovich AH. Using flow cytometry to screen patients for X-linked lymphoproliferative disease due to SAP deficiency and XIAP deficiency. *J Immunol Methods.* (2010) 362:1–9. doi: 10.1016/j.jim.2010.08.010
80. Zhao M, Kanegane H, Kobayashi C, Nakazawa Y, Ishii E, Kasai M, et al. Early and rapid detection of X-linked lymphoproliferative syndrome with SH2D1A mutations by flow cytometry. *Cytometry B Clin Cytom.* (2011) 80:8–13. doi: 10.1002/cyto.b.20552
81. Erdos M, Uzvolgyi E, Nemes Z, Torok O, Rakoczi E, Went-Sumegi N, et al. Characterization of a new disease-causing mutation of SH2D1A in a family with X-linked lymphoproliferative disease. *Hum Mutat.* (2005) 25:506. doi: 10.1002/humu.9339
82. Morra M, Simarro-Grande M, Martin M, Chen AS, Lanyi A, Silander O, et al. Characterization of SH2D1A missense mutations identified in X-linked lymphoproliferative disease patients. *J Biol Chem.* (2001) 276:36809–16. doi: 10.1074/jbc.M101305200
83. Speckmann C, Lehmberg K, Albert MH, Damgaard RB, Fritsch M, Gyrd-Hansen M, et al. X-linked inhibitor of apoptosis (XIAP) deficiency: the spectrum of presenting manifestations beyond hemophagocytic lymphohistiocytosis. *Clin Immunol.* (2013) 149:133–41. doi: 10.1016/j.clim.2013.07.004
84. Yang X, Hoshino A, Taga T, Kunitsu T, Ikeda Y, Yasumi T, et al. A female patient with incomplete hemophagocytic lymphohistiocytosis caused by a heterozygous XIAP mutation associated with non-random X-chromosome inactivation skewed towards the wild-type XIAP allele. *J Clin Immunol.* (2015) 35:244–8. doi: 10.1007/s10875-015-0144-6
85. Holle JR, Marsh RA, Holdcroft AM, Davies SM, Wang L, Zhang K, et al. Hemophagocytic lymphohistiocytosis in a female patient due to a heterozygous XIAP mutation and skewed X chromosome inactivation. *Pediatr Blood Cancer.* (2015) 62:1288–90. doi: 10.1002/pbc.25483
86. Marsh RA, Villanueva J, Zhang K, Snow AL, Su HC, Madden L, et al. A rapid flow cytometric screening test for X-linked lymphoproliferative disease due to XIAP deficiency. *Cytometry B Clin Cytom.* (2009) 765):334–44. doi: 10.1002/cyto.b.20473
87. Nichols KE, Hom J, Gong SY, Ganguly A, Ma CS, Cannons JL, et al. Regulation of NKT cell development by SAP, the protein defective in XLP. *Nat Med.* (2005) 11:340–5. doi: 10.1038/nm1189
88. Pasquier B, Yin L, Fondaneche MC, Relouzat F, Bloch-Queyrat C, Lambert N, et al. Defective NKT cell development in mice and humans lacking the adapter SAP, the X-linked lymphoproliferative syndrome gene product. *J Exp Med.* (2005) 201:695–701. doi: 10.1084/jem.20042432
89. Meazza R, Tuberosa C, Cetica V, Falco M, Parolini S, Grieve S, et al. Diagnosing XLP1 in patients with hemophagocytic lymphohistiocytosis. *J Allergy Clin Immunol.* (2014) 134:1381–7 e7. doi: 10.1016/j.jaci.2014.04.043
90. Cifaldi C, Chiriaco M, Di Matteo G, Di Cesare S, Alessia S, De Angelis P, et al. Novel X-linked inhibitor of apoptosis mutation in very early-onset inflammatory bowel disease child successfully treated with HLA-haploidentical hemapoietic stem cells transplant after removal of alphabeta(+) T and B cells. *Front Immunol.* (2017) 8:1893. doi: 10.3389/fimmu.2017.01893
91. Girardelli M, Arrigo S, Barabino A, Loganes C, Morreale G, Crovella S, et al. The diagnostic challenge of very early-onset enterocolitis in an infant with XIAP deficiency. *BMC Pediatr.* (2015) 15:208. doi: 10.1186/s12887-015-0522-5
92. Chinn IK, Eckstein OS, Peckham-Gregory EC, Goldberg BR, Forbes LR, Nicholas SK, et al. Genetic and mechanistic diversity in pediatric hemophagocytic lymphohistiocytosis. *Blood.* (2018) 132:89–100. doi: 10.1182/blood-2017-11-814244
93. Mukda E, Trachoo O, Pasomsub E, Tiyasirichokchai R, Iemwimangsa N, Sosothikul D, et al. Exome sequencing for simultaneous mutation screening in children with hemophagocytic lymphohistiocytosis. *Int J Hematol.* (2017) 106:282–90. doi: 10.1007/s12185-017-2223-3
94. Pasic S, Micic D, Kuzmanovic M. Epstein-Barr virus-associated haemophagocytic lymphohistiocytosis in Wiskott-Aldrich syndrome. *Acta Paediatr.* (2003) 92:859–61. doi: 10.1111/j.1651-2227.2003.tb02548.x
95. Abraham RS, Aubert G. Flow cytometry, a versatile tool for diagnosis and monitoring of primary immunodeficiencies. *Clin Vaccine Immunol.* (2016) 23:254–71. doi: 10.1128/CVI.00001-16
96. Epling CL, Stites DP, McHugh TM, Chong HO, Blackwood LL, Wara DW. Neutrophil function screening in patients with chronic granulomatous disease by a flow cytometric method. *Cytometry.* (1992) 13:615–20. doi: 10.1002/cyto.990130609
97. Chiang SCC, Vergamini SM, Husami A, Neumeier L, Quinn K, Ellerhorst T, et al. Screening for Wiskott-Aldrich syndrome by flow cytometry. *J Allergy Clin Immunol.* (2018) 142:333-5 e8. doi: 10.1016/j.jaci.2018.04.017
98. Boldt A, Bitar M, Sack U. Flow Cytometric Evaluation of Primary Immunodeficiencies. *Clin Lab Med.* (2017) 37:895-913. doi: 10.1016/j.cll.2017.07.013
99. Kanegane H, Hoshino A, Okano T, Yasumi T, Wada T, Takada H, et al. Flow cytometry-based diagnosis of primary immunodeficiency diseases. *Allergol Int.* (2018) 67:43–54. doi: 10.1016/j.alit.2017.06.003
100. Gruda R, Brown AC, Grabovsky V, Mizrahi S, Gur C, Feigelson SW, et al. Loss of kindlin-3 alters the threshold for NK cell activation in human leukocyte adhesion deficiency-III. *Blood.* (2012) 120:3915-24. doi: 10.1182/blood-2012-02-410795
101. Mace EM, Bigley V, Gunesch JT, Chinn IK, Angelo LS, Care MA, et al. Biallelic mutations in IRF8 impair human NK cell maturation and function. *J Clin Invest.* (2017) 127:306–20. doi: 10.1172/JCI86276
102. Pham CT, Ivanovich JL, Raptis SZ, Zehnbauer B, Ley TJ. Papillon-Lefevre syndrome: correlating the molecular, cellular, and clinical consequences of cathepsin C/dipeptidyl peptidase I deficiency in humans. *J Immunol.* (2004) 173:7277-81. doi: 10.4049/jimmunol.173.12.7277
103. Schaballie H, Rodriguez R, Martin E, Moens L, Frans G, Lenoir C, et al. A novel hypomorphic mutation in STIM1 results in a late-onset immunodeficiency. *J Allergy Clin Immunol.* (2015) 136:816–9 e4. doi: 10.1016/j.jaci.2015.03.009
104. Andzelm MM, Chen X, Krzewski K, Orange JS, Strominger JL. Myosin IIA is required for cytolytic granule exocytosis in human NK cells. *J Exp Med.* (2007) 204:2285–91. doi: 10.1084/jem.20071143
105. Sanborn KB, Mace EM, Rak GD, Difeo A, Martignetti JA, Pecci A, et al. Phosphorylation of the myosin IIA tailpiece regulates single myosin IIA molecule association with lytic granules to promote NK-cell cytotoxicity. *Blood.* (2011) 118:5862–71. doi: 10.1182/blood-2011-03-344846
106. Mace EM, Hsu AP, Monaco-Shawver L, Makedonas G, Rosen JB, Dropulic L, et al. Mutations in GATA2 cause human NK cell deficiency with specific loss of the CD56(bright) subset. *Blood.* (2013) 121:2669-77. doi: 10.1182/blood-2012-09-453969
107. Meade JL, de Wynter EA, Brett P, Sharif SM, Woods CG, Markham AF, et al. A family with Papillon-Lefevre syndrome reveals a requirement for cathepsin C in granzyme B activation and NK cell cytolytic activity. *Blood.* (2006) 107:3665–8. doi: 10.1182/blood-2005-03-1140
108. Henter JI, Horne A, Arico M, Egeler RM, Filipovich AH, Imashuku S, et al. HLH-2004: Diagnostic and therapeutic guidelines for

hemophagocytic lymphohistiocytosis. *Pediatr Blood Cancer.* (2007) 48:124-31. doi: 10.1002/pbc.21039

109. Bode SF, Ammann S, Al-Herz W, Bataneant M, Dvorak CC, Gehring S, et al. The syndrome of hemophagocytic lymphohistiocytosis in primary immunodeficiencies: implications for differential diagnosis and pathogenesis. *Haematologica.* (2015) 100:978–88. doi: 10.3324/haematol.2014.121608
110. Gupta A, Tyrrell P, Valani R, Benseler S, Weitzman S, Abdelhaleem M. The role of the initial bone marrow aspirate in the diagnosis of hemophagocytic lymphohistiocytosis. *Pediatr Blood Cancer.* (2008) 51:402–4. doi: 10.1002/pbc.21564
111. Otrock ZK, Hock KG, Riley SB, de Witte T, Eby CS, Scott MG. Elevated serum ferritin is not specific for hemophagocytic lymphohistiocytosis. *Ann Hematol.* (2017) 96:1667–72. doi: 10.1007/s00277-017-3072-0
112. Schram AM, Campigotto F, Mullally A, Fogerty A, Massarotti E, Neuberg D, et al. Marked hyperferritinemia does not predict for HLH in the adult population. *Blood.* (2015) 125:1548–52. doi: 10.1182/blood-2014-10-602607
113. El-Sherbiny YM, Psarras A, Md Yusof MY, Hensor EMA, Tooze R, Doody G, et al. A novel two-score system for interferon status segregates autoimmune diseases and correlates with clinical features. *Sci Rep.* (2018) 8:5793. doi: 10.1038/s41598-018-24198-1
114. Zhang R, Yang X, Wang J, Han L, Yang A, Zhang J, et al. Identification of potential biomarkers for differential diagnosis between rheumatoid arthritis and osteoarthritis via integrative genomewide gene expression profiling analysis. *Mol Med Rep.* (2019) 19:30-40. doi: 10.3892/mmr.2018.9677
115. Kim H, de Jesus AA, Brooks SR, Liu Y, Huang Y, VanTries R, et al. Development of a validated interferon score using nanostring technology. *J Interferon Cytokine Res.* (2018) 38:171-85. doi: 10.1089/jir.2017.0127
116. Rice GI, Melki I, Fremond ML, Briggs TA, Rodero MP, Kitabayashi N, et al. Assessment of type I interferon signaling in pediatric inflammatory disease. *J Clin Immunol.* (2017) 37:123–32. doi: 10.1007/s10875-016-0359-1
117. Sumegi J, Nestheide S, Aronow B, Fletcher D, Keddache M, Villanueva J, et al. MicroRNA activation signature in patients with hemophagocytic lymphohistiocytosis and reversibility with disease-specific therapy. *J Allergy Clin Immunol.* (2016) 137:309-12. doi: 10.1016/j.jaci.2015.06.006
118. Sumegi J, Nestheide SV, Barnes MG, Villanueva J, Zhang K, Grom AA, et al. Gene-expression signatures differ between different clinical forms of familial hemophagocytic lymphohistiocytosis. *Blood.* (2013) 121:e14-24. doi: 10.1182/blood-2012-05-425769

5

EuroFlow-Based Flowcytometric Diagnostic Screening and Classification of Primary Immunodeficiencies of the Lymphoid System

Jacques J. M. van Dongen[1†], Mirjam van der Burg[2,3†], Tomas Kalina[4†], Martin Perez-Andres[5,6†], Ester Mejstrikova[4], Marcela Vlkova[7], Eduardo Lopez-Granados[8], Marjolein Wentink[2], Anne-Kathrin Kienzler[9], Jan Philippé[10], Ana E. Sousa[11], Menno C. van Zelm[2,12], Elena Blanco[5,6] and Alberto Orfao[5,6†] on behalf of the EuroFlow Consortium*

[1] Department of Immunohematology and Blood Transfusion, Leiden University Medical Center, Leiden, Netherlands, [2] Department of Immunology, Erasmus MC, Rotterdam, Netherlands, [3] Department of Pediatrics, Leiden University Medical Center, Leiden, Netherlands, [4] Department of Pediatric Hematology and Oncology, University Hospital Motol, Charles University, Prague, Czechia, [5] Department of Medicine, Cancer Research Centre (IBMCC, USAL-CSIC), Cytometry Service (NUCLEUS), University of Salamanca (USAL), Institute of Biomedical Research of Salamanca (IBSAL), Salamanca, Spain, [6] Biomedical Research Networking Centre Consortium of Oncology (CIBERONC), CB/16/12/00233, Instituto Carlos III, Madrid, Spain, [7] Institute of Clinical Immunology and Allergology, St. Anne's University Hospital Brno, Masaryk University, Brno, Czechia, [8] Department of Immunology, Hospital Universitario La Paz, Madrid, Spain, [9] Experimental Medicine Division, Nuffield Department of Medicine, University of Oxford, Oxford, United Kingdom, [10] Department of Laboratory Medicine, University Hospital Ghent, Ghent, Belgium, [11] Faculdade de Medicina, Instituto de Medicina Molecular, Universidade de Lisboa, Lisbon, Portugal, [12] Department of Immunology and Pathology, Central Clinical School, Alfred Hospital, Monash University, Melbourne, VIC, Australia

***Correspondence:**
Jacques J. M. van Dongen
j.j.m.van_dongen@lumc.nl

† These authors have contributed equally to this work

Guidelines for screening for primary immunodeficiencies (PID) are well-defined and several consensus diagnostic strategies have been proposed. These consensus proposals have only partially been implemented due to lack of standardization in laboratory procedures, particularly in flow cytometry. The main objectives of the EuroFlow Consortium were to innovate and thoroughly standardize the flowcytometric techniques and strategies for reliable and reproducible diagnosis and classification of PID of the lymphoid system. The proposed EuroFlow antibody panels comprise one orientation tube and seven classification tubes and corresponding databases of normal and PID samples. The 8-color 12-antibody PID Orientation tube (PIDOT) aims at identification and enumeration of the main lymphocyte and leukocyte subsets; this includes naïve pre-germinal center (GC) and antigen-experienced post-GC memory B-cells and plasmablasts. The seven additional 8(-12)-color tubes can be used according to the EuroFlow PID algorithm in parallel or subsequently to the PIDOT for more detailed analysis of B-cell and T-cell subsets to further classify PID of the lymphoid system. The Pre-GC, Post-GC, and immunoglobulin heavy chain (IgH)-isotype B-cell tubes aim at identification and enumeration of B-cell subsets for evaluation of B-cell maturation blocks and specific defects in IgH-subclass production. The severe combined immunodeficiency (SCID) tube and T-cell memory/effector subset tube aim at identification and enumeration of T-cell subsets for assessment of T-cell defects, such as SCID. In case of suspicion of antibody deficiency, PIDOT is preferably directly combined with the IgH isotype tube(s) and in case of SCID suspicion (e.g., in newborn screening programs) the PIDOT is preferably directly combined with the SCID T-cell tube. The proposed ≥8-color antibody panels and corresponding reference databases combined with the EuroFlow PID algorithm are designed to provide fast, sensitive and cost-effective flowcytometric diagnosis of PID of the lymphoid system, easily applicable in multicenter diagnostic settings world-wide.

Keywords: immunodeficiency, immunophenotyping, flow cytometry, diagnosis, classification, EuroFlow, standardization

INTRODUCTION

Primary immunodeficiencies (PID) are inherited disorders of the immune system, generally presenting with recurrent, sometimes life-threatening infections. To date, more than 350 genes have been identified that can be mutated in PID patients (1–3). Depending on the genetic defect, one part of the immune system or one cell type can be absent, decreased or dysfunctional. The majority of PID patients (60–65%) have a defect in the lymphoid system, involving B- and/or T-cells alone or in combination with other cells (1–5). Flowcytometric immunophenotyping plays a central role in the diagnostic workup of patients suspected of PID, particularly those involving lymphoid cells (1, 6). An accurate immunophenotypic diagnosis is essential for guiding further functional testing as well as for genetic testing, whether Sanger sequencing or next generation sequencing (NGS) targeted to specific genes, whole exome sequencing (WES), whole genome sequencing (WGS) or combinations thereof (2, 5, 7–10). Considering the clinical heterogeneity in genetically homogeneous disease entities, immunophenotyping has an additional role in understanding the clinical heterogeneity in disease presentation and outcome (11–13). Immunophenotyping can also support treatment decisions and monitoring, such as in case of immunoglobulin (Ig) replacement therapy, hematopoietic stem cell transplantation, and gene therapy (7, 8, 14–18).

In complex diseases with high numbers of affected genes and still many genes to be discovered, some investigators recommend the "Genetics First" approach via targeted NGS, WES, and/or WGS, already at an early phase in the diagnostic process (19, 20). Indeed, in absence of other in-depth diagnostic methods, the "Genetics First" approach has clearly contributed to better classification and more insight in some well-defined disease categories with high genetic diagnosis yields, such as in intellectual disability syndrome, hereditary spastic paraplegias, and neuromuscular disorders (21–24). However, in the complex field of PID most targeted NGS and/or WES studies have genetic diagnosis yields varying from 15 to 30% (25–29), sometimes increasing to 40% or higher, depending on the number of targeted genes (varies from 170 to 571), young age (higher yield in children), high frequency of X-linked diseases, high frequency of families with PID history, and highly consanguineous populations with high frequencies of autosomal recessive diseases, such as in the Middle East and North Africa region (9, 30–34). Importantly, virtually all above-mentioned NGS and/or WES studies did not apply the "Genetics First" approach, because the included PID patients were defined according to the guidelines of the European Society for Immunodeficiencies (ESID) and the International Union of Immunological Societies (IUIS), which include flowcytometric immunophenotyping (2, 5, 6). In fact, the genetic diagnosis yield in immunophenotypically defined PID (sub)categories ranges from >95% in severe combined immunodeficiency (SCID), 85–90% in well-defined agammaglobulinemia patients, ~75% in Hyper IgM syndrome, down to 10–20% among the most frequently occurring PID, such as common variable immunodeficiency (CVID) and immunoglobulin (Ig) isotype deficiencies (5, 35–38).

Clearly, adequate clinical and immunophenotypic characterization of PID patients should guide the diagnostic process; this is supported by the diagnosis and classification guidelines of ESID, IUIS, and Clinical Immunology Society (CIS) (2, 6, 39). Compared to other organ systems, many different genes are involved in the immune system, particularly in mature B-cells during and after germinal center (GC) responses. Use of WES and WGS will detect many allelic immune gene variants, which might not be causally related to disease, implying that significant efforts in immunobiological validation studies will be needed. Furthermore, in-depth immunological and functional studies are essential to define the consequences of genetic defects for the immune system. At least part of these studies will be based on flow cytometry. Especially in case of hypomorphic defects, flow cytometry can help to better understand the effects of the genetic defect on the composition of the lymphoid compartment (11–13, 40, 41). Finally, flow cytometry is an important tool for monitoring of targeted therapies, including cellular therapies (15, 16, 18, 42).

Many PID centers have developed their own local multi-color flowcytometric protocols and antibody panels for diagnosis and classification of PID (8, 14, 43–45). These single-center initiatives have led to a great variability in sample processing, antibody panels, immunostaining procedures, instrument setup, sample measurement and data analysis. In addition, the low incidence and the clinical-immunological heterogeneity of PID hamper prospective multicenter diagnostic validation in large patient series and age-matched healthy controls (43–45). As a consequence, the typical but rare immunophenotypic PID patterns are difficult to compare between centers at the national and international level.

Whilst several recent international efforts have tried to harmonize flowcytometric diagnostics of PID (43–48), they have only been partially successful, mainly because these efforts have been restricted to parts of the full pathway of pre-analytical, analytical and post-analytical procedures, frequently focusing on the antibody panels only. Most proposed antibody panels aim at identification of severe defects in B and T lymphocytes, NK-cells, and/or diagnostic screening for a specific inherited disorder or a specific subgroup of disorders. Examples of such disease-oriented antibody panels are meant for: (i) diagnostic screening and classification of SCID based on quantification of B-, T- and NK-cells with CD3, CD19, and CD56 or CD16; (ii) diagnostic screening of congenital agammaglobulinemia, merely based on enumeration of blood B lymphocytes; (iii) classification of common variable immunodeficiency (CVID) according to the proportion of transitional, non-switched/marginal zone-like (smIgMD^{+}) and class-switched (smIgMD^{-}), and CD21^{dim} B lymphocytes; (iv) diagnostic screening of DiGeorge patients based on relative blood counts of recent thymic emigrant (RTE) CD4^{+} T-cells, and; (v) quantification of CD4/CD8-double negative TCR$\alpha\beta^{+}$ T-cells (DNT) for screening of autoimmune lymphoproliferative syndrome (ALPS) (49, 50). Consequently, such antibody panels do not provide a complete overview of the many distinct subsets of circulating leukocytes, as required for fast, efficient, and cost-effective PID diagnostics.

Several initiatives in other fields of clinical immunology have also lead to consensus antibody panels for harmonized flowcytometric immune monitoring, such as the CLIP study (51), the NIH study (52), the ONE study (53), the Pasteur initiative (54), and the NATURIMMUN consortium (55). These antibody panels allow identification of several subpopulations of B-, T-, and NK-cells (e.g., naïve vs. memory, activated cells, TCR$\gamma\delta$ vs. TCR$\alpha\beta$) together with the identification of monocytes, dendritic cells, and granulocytes. However, the proposed antibody combinations do not provide the fully integrated information as needed for diagnosis and classification of PID.

Here we describe newly designed, fully validated EuroFlow procedures and tools for comprehensive immunophenotypic diagnostic screening and classification of PID of the lymphoid system. The proposed EuroFlow PID approach relies on: 1. Optimized and validated ≥8-color antibody panels; 2. Standardized procedures for sample preparation, immunostaining, acquisition, and analysis of up to millions of cells per sample; 3. Automated gating procedures for reproducible identification of the many different immune cell subsets in blood and bone marrow (BM). A diagnostic algorithm and age-related reference values are provided for guiding the flowcytometric PID diagnosis and classification process; the entries in the EuroFlow diagnostic algorithm are based on available clinical information and basic laboratory data (**Figure 1A**), followed by stepwise application of the newly designed antibody combinations with age-related reference values of lymphocyte subsets in absolute counts (**Figures 1A,B**).

This report describes the overall EuroFlow PID approach, while detailed validation and reference value studies, including healthy subjects and PID patient series, are provided per PID tube (set) in separate EuroFlow PID reports (56–60).

METHODS

Design of the EuroFlow-PID Study

The design of the EuroFlow PID study took advantage of the experience built in the field of leukemia and lymphoma diagnosis, classification, and monitoring (61–65) and the previously developed EuroFlow pre-analytical and analytical standard operating procedures (SOPs) for sample collection, transportation and staining of $\geq 10^6$ nucleated cells (63, 64), together with EuroFlow 8-color instrument set-up and calibration procedures (62), extended to ≥12-color flow cytometry (56). Multicenter evaluation of the performance of antibody panels was done in consecutive cycles of design-testing-evaluation-redesign in large series of healthy controls and patient samples in 10 EuroFlow centers, experienced in PID diagnostics (56–59). For this purpose we used EuroFlow multivariate analytical tools (66), incorporated in the Infinicyt software and developed by Cytognos SL (Salamanca, Spain).

Stepwise application of newly-designed and validated antibody combinations and available clinical and laboratory information resulted in an algorithm for guiding immunophenotypic diagnosis and classification of PID. The final versions of the EuroFlow PID tubes were used to build EuroFlow databases of normal and patient samples, for automated classification of cell populations (i.e., automated gating) and disease profiles (i.e., orientation of PID diagnosis and classification), as described in detail elsewhere (64, 65, 67).

The multiple cycles of design-testing-evaluation-redesign started in 2012 and took a total of 6 years and 20 in-person EuroFlow PID meetings to reach the final results. No single EuroFlow laboratory could have afforded the above described efforts on its own. Solely thanks to intensive collaboration and frequent exchange of results and information during the EuroFlow meetings, the here described results could be achieved, supported by local funds and by royalty income from pre-existing EuroFlow patents in the leukemia-lymphoma field.

Flow Cytometers and Instrument Settings and Calibration

Most laboratories (9 out of 10) used FACSCanto-II flowcytometers (BD Biosciences, San Jose, CA), one laboratory used a Navios flowcytometer (Beckman-Coulter, Hialeah, FL). Standardized EuroFlow SOPs for instrument set-up and calibration were used for both instruments, as provided in detail via the EuroFlow website (www.EuroFlow.org) and by Kalina et al. (62). With such protocols, fully comparable results are obtained as previously demonstrated for both FACSCanto II, Navios, and other ≥8-color instruments, even when run by different operators (68).

For condensing sets of two 8-color tubes into single 12-color tubes, BD LSR Fortessa X-20 or FACSLyric instruments (BD Biosciences) were used in four centers where the EuroFlow

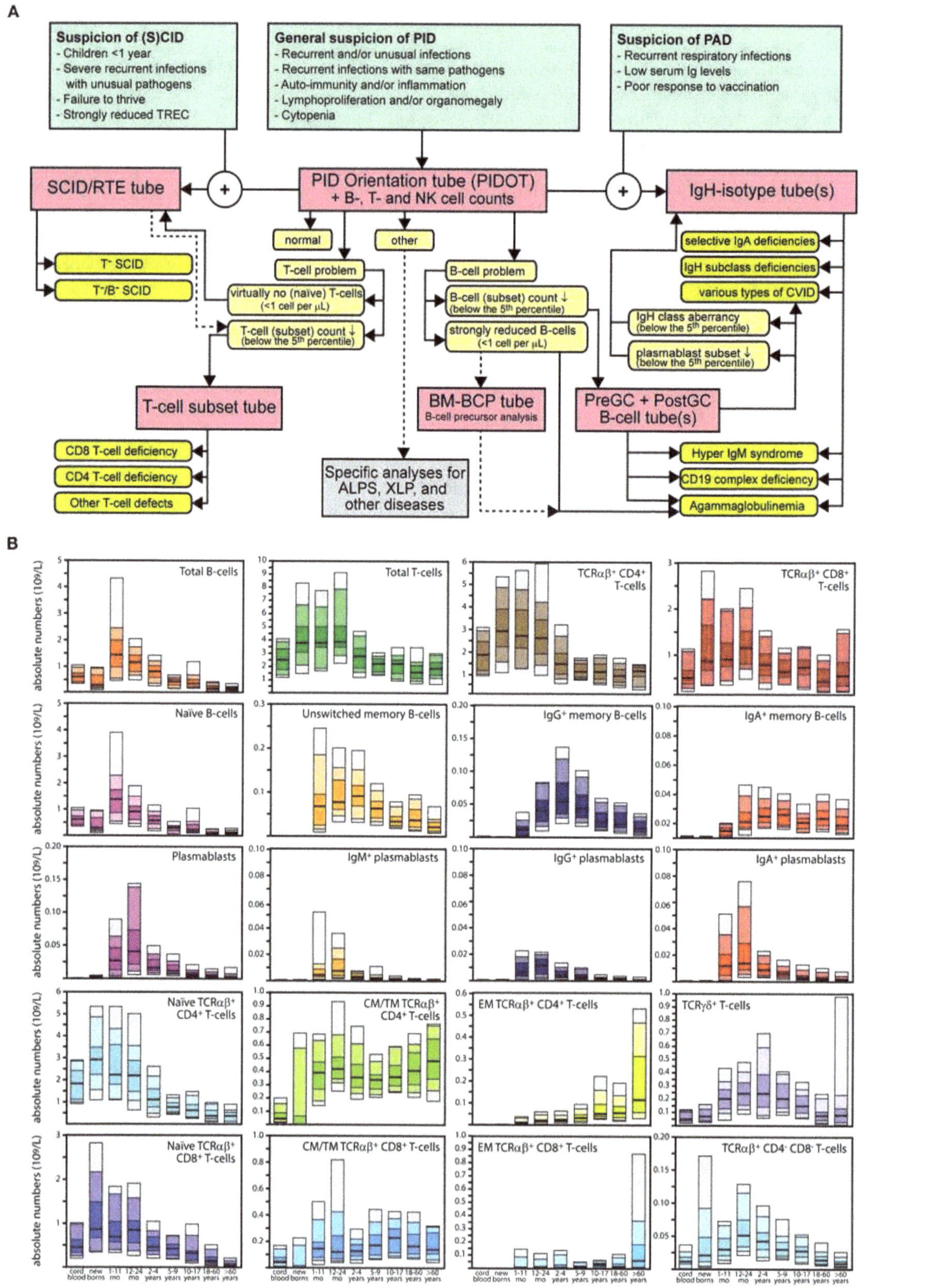

FIGURE 1 | Continued

FIGURE 1 | Strategy for flowcytometric immunophenotyping for screening and classification of lymphoid PID. **(A)** EuroFlow algorithm. On the basis of several entries of clinical and laboratory parameters, blood samples of patients suspected to have PID are screened with the 8-color (or 10-color) PID Orientation tube (PIDOT). Based on the obtained results, additional 8-color or 10-color T- and/or B-cell classification tubes are applied in a stepwise fashion, including the BM B-cell precursor (BM-BCP) tube. In case of suspicion of PAD, both the PIDOT and the IgH-isotype tube(s) should be applied together. In case of suspicion of (S)CID and cases with strongly reduced TRECs, both the PIDOT and the SCID/RTE tube can be applied together. See text for detailed description of the stepwise application of the EuroFlow PID tubes. GC, germinal center; PAD, predominantly antibody deficiency; RTE, recent thymic emigrant; SCID, severe combined immunodeficiency. **(B)** Age-related reference values. Absolute counts of all lymphocyte subsets are provided in the format of age-related percentile bars (median; 25–75 percentiles; 10–90 percentiles; 5–95 percentiles). The age groups are: cord blood ($n = 15$), newborns ($n = 16$), 1–11 months ($n = 19$), 12–23 months ($n = 30$), 2–4 years ($n = 35$), 5–9 years ($n = 28$), 10–17 years ($n = 33$), 18–60 years ($n = 79$), and >60 years ($n = 66$). In case of naïve TCRαβ$^+$CD4$^+$ T-cells, CM/TM TCRαβ$^+$CD4$^+$ T-cells, EM TCRαβ$^+$ CD4$^+$ T-cells, TCRγδ$^+$ T-cells, naïve TCRαβ$^+$CD8$^+$, CM/TM TCRαβ$^+$CD8$^+$ T-cells, EM TCRαβ$^+$CD8$^+$ T-cells, TCRαβ$^+$CD4$^-$CD8$^-$ T-cells, IgM$^+$ plasmablasts, IgG$^+$ plasmablasts, and IgA$^+$ plasmablasts, the age groups of 10–17 years and >60 years contained only $n = 18$ and $n = 21$ individuals, respectively. The original data set with the age-related reference values will be available via the EuroFlow website (www.EuroFlow.org) and will continuously be updated when more data become available, also for other leukocyte subsets.

instrument set-up and calibration SOPs were extended for the required extra colors, as described elsewhere (56, 58) and on the EuroFlow website (www.EuroFlow.org).

EuroFlow Standard Operating Procedures for Sample Preparation and Acquisition of High Cell Numbers

To gain detailed insight into the composition of the lymphocyte compartment, including robust identification of small cell populations such as plasmablasts subsets, EuroFlow developed SOPs for acquisition of high cell numbers ($\geq$1–5 × 10^6 total nucleated cells) and/or large sample volumes (up to 2 mL per tube) (56, 63, 64). These procedures can be used for fresh (<36 h, preferably <24 h) blood and BM samples (69).

For acquisition of high cell numbers, the EuroFlow bulk-lysis-and-stain technique is recommended (56, 64), as described also on the EuroFlow website (www.EuroFlow.org). Briefly, the sample (up to 2 mL) is diluted in a total volume of 50 mL of an ammonium chloride hypotonic solution (1:25 mL vol:vol per 50 mL tube), gently mixed and incubated for 15 min in a roller. Then, nucleated cells were centrifuged and washed twice in phosphate buffered saline (PBS) containing 0.5% bovine serum albumin (BSA). Subsequently, the surface membrane markers on nucleated cells are stained with the corresponding antibody mixtures. Overall, $\geq$1–5 × 10^6 nucleated cells were measured for each antibody combination.

Construction of Antibody Panels

Antibody panels were designed for unequivocal identification and full dissection of lymphocyte subsets and their maturation-associated pathways, in parallel to other leukocyte subpopulations, which might show uniquely altered patterns in different PID categories. Specific combinations of fluorochrome-conjugated reagents were selected based on the need for brightness, stability, limited fluorescence spill-over and compensation requirements, as described elsewhere (58, 62, 70). These antibody combinations were evaluated in parallel in multiple centers (at least 4 centers per testing round) and they were optimized via multiple consecutive cycles of design-testing-evaluation-redesign. In each testing cycle, the Infinicyt software was used to identify antibodies for optimal recognition and clear-cut separation of the target cell subsets, while other antibodies were discarded because of insufficient separation of target cell subsets, poor contribution and/or redundancy, as exemplified for the PIDOT in Van der Burg et al. (59). Once optimal recognition and separation of the different target cell subsets was achieved with high reproducibility among the different laboratories, the antibody combination was frozen for final validation in large series of normal and PID patient samples (56, 59, 60). This included an intra-laboratory and inter-laboratory coefficient of variation (CV) for the identification of different minor and major lymphoid subsets of <10 and <30%, respectively, as described for example for the PIDOT (60) and the IgH-isotype tube (57).

Optimal recognition and clear-cut separation of target cell populations avoids arbitrary marker settings between cell populations with vague cutoff values, which easily vary between different laboratories, particularly when different antibody clones and fluorochrome conjugates are used. Therefore, the above described procedures are essential for obtaining reproducible results, which allow comparison of flowcytometric patterns of PID patients between centers at the international level.

Patients and Age-Matched Healthy Controls

The proposed antibody panels were extensively evaluated in multicenter studies by analyzing blood ($n = 541$) and BM ($n = 43$) samples. Blood samples from healthy controls ($n = 300$) included different age groups: cord blood ($n = 15$), newborns ($n = 16$), 1–11 months ($n = 19$), 12–23 months ($n = 30$), 2–4 years ($n = 35$), 5–9 years ($n = 28$), 10–17 years ($n = 33$), 18–60 years ($n = 79$), and >60 years ($n = 66$).

The PID patients included in the study were all genetically-defined cases, except for the most frequent subgroups of predominantly antibody deficiencies (CVID, Ig-subclass deficiencies), for which the ESID and IUIS diagnostic and classification criteria (1, 5) were applied. The PID patients ($n = 241$) concerned: SCID ($n = 24$), CVID ($n = 66$), DiGeorge syndrome ($n = 6$), ALPS ($n = 5$), Wiskott-Aldrich Syndrome ($n = 3$), selective IgA-deficiency ($n = 68$), BTK-deficiency ($n = 10$), CD40L-deficiency ($n = 6$), other less profound CID ($n = 6$), other CID with syndromic features ($n = 11$), and several other PID subgroups ($n = 36$), such as IgG subclass deficiency with IgA deficiency ($n = 10$), PI3K delta syndrome ($n = 5$), GATA2 deficiency ($n = 5$), other diseases of immune dysregulation ($n = 4$), together with other PID patients not classified as primary defects of the lymphoid system, e.g., chronic granulomatous disease ($n = 5$), defects of innate immunity ($n = 3$) and complement deficiencies ($n = 4$) (59).

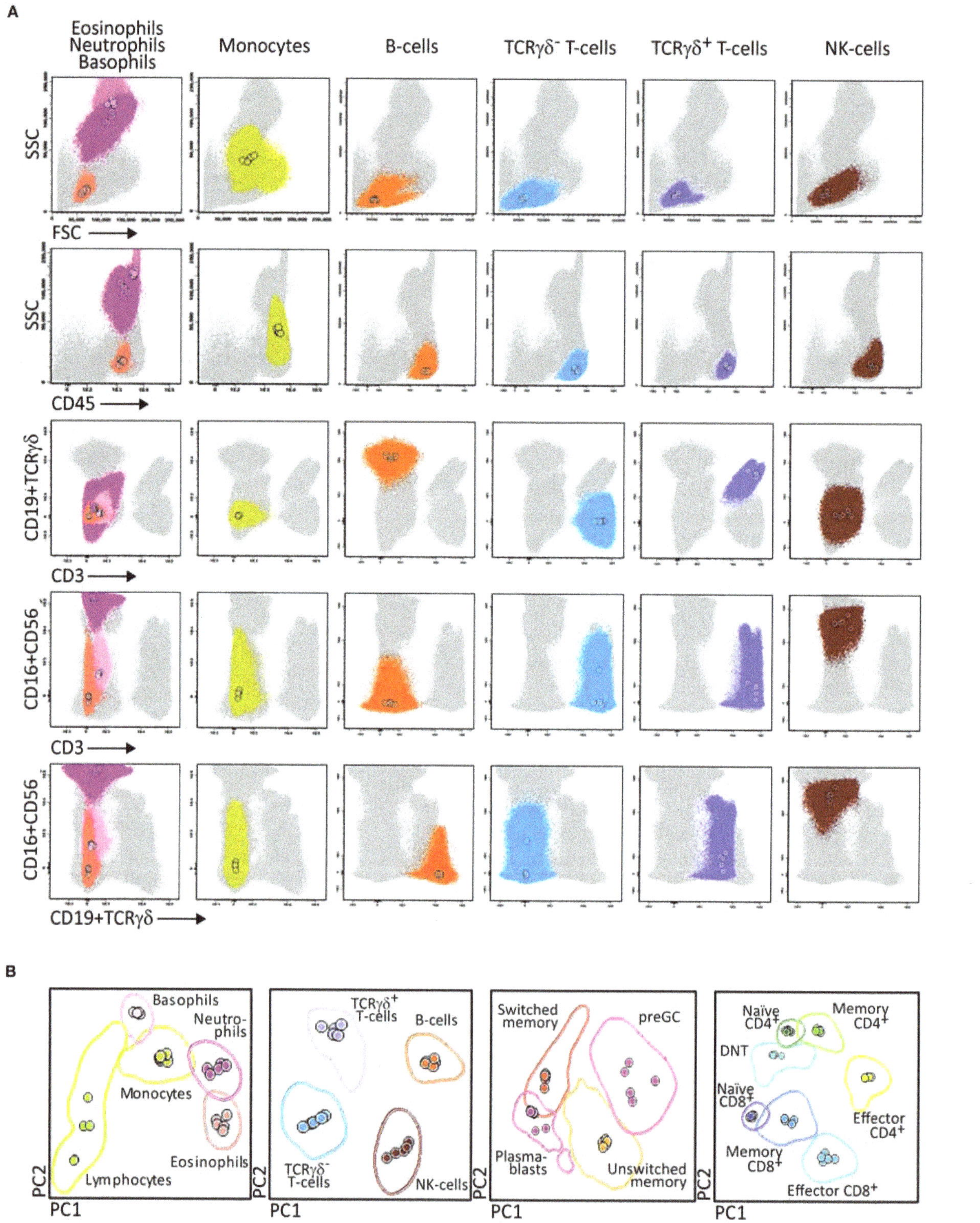

FIGURE 2 | Generation of a reference principal component analysis 1 (PCA1) vs. PCA2 representation in an n-dimensional space for discrimination of the lymphocytes subsets identified with PIDOT. **(A)** Data files from 5 healthy donors were merged and lymphocyte subsets of interest identified using bivariate plots. **(B)** The merged data were used to define an n-dimensional space with the best principal component analysis 1 (PC1) vs. PC2 representation to discriminate these subsets. The PCA representation of the data is resumed in 2 × Standard Deviation (SD) curves to be used as a reference for supervised automatic analysis of the samples.

Normal blood samples were obtained from healthy adult volunteers or from children upon informed consent of the parents. The BM samples concerned remaining cell material of sibling BM stem cell transplantation donors who consented to participate in the study. All normal and patient samples were collected in tubes containing EDTA as anti-coagulant and processed within 24 h after sampling (69).

Ethical approval and informed consent procedures were according to the local ethical guidelines of the participating EuroFlow institutions and the Declaration of Helsinki (University of Salamanca, Salamanca, Spain; Charles University, Prague, Czech Republic; La Paz Hospital, Madrid, Spain; Erasmus MC, Rotterdam, The Netherlands; University Hospital Ghent, Belgium; and St. Anne's University, Brno, Czech Republic). The study was approved by the local ethics committees of the participating centers: University of Salamanca, Salamanca, Spain (USAL CSIC 20-02-2013); Charles University, Prague, Czech Republic (15-28541A); Erasmus MC, Rotterdam, The Netherlands (MEC-2013-026); University Hospital Ghent, Belgium (B670201523515); and St. Anne's University, Brno, Czech Republic (METC 1G2015).

Data Acquisition and Data Analysis With EuroFlow Software Tools

Data acquisition was performed at low-medium speed (5,000–10,000 cells/s) using either FACSDiva (version 8) or the Navios software. For data analysis, the Infinicyt software (version 2.0) was used. Briefly, standardized Boolean gating strategies were defined and used for manual gating of the distinct cell populations identified in each tube. The merge function of the Infinicyt software was used to merge data files into reference databases. For each cell population its relative distribution among all nucleated cells, lymphocytes, and the corresponding B-, T-, and NK-cell subsets, were calculated and the MFI values per marker reported for each cell subset identified. In addition, absolute lymphocyte counts were calculated using a CD45PerCP, CD3FITC, CD19APC, and CD16$^+$CD56PE TruCOUNT tube (BD Biosciences) following the instructions of the manufacturer.

For automated identification of the cell populations present in the PID tubes, PID databases were built, containing normal blood samples stained with the same antibody combination(s). Reference ranges with abnormality alarms were set per age-group, based on the analysis of a large cohort of 250 healthy control samples: cord blood ($n = 15$), childhood <18 years ($n = 146$), and adults ≥18 years ($n = 89$).

Multicenter Validation of PID Tubes

In order to ensure full comparability between the MFI per marker per cell subset in different samples stained at distinct centers, all EuroFlow centers were trained in the EuroFlow instrument set-up and calibration as well as sample preparation SOPs. Afterward, each center was enrolled in the EuroFlow Quality Assurance program (71, 72). EuroFlow QA program showed that overall QA results of EuroFlow laboratories showed CVs below 30% in more than 90 and 70% of cell populations in 59/72 (82%) and in 71/72 (99%) QA sets, irrespectively of the flowcytometer used and the participant.

In addition, normal blood samples stained with the PID Orientation tube upon strictly following the EuroFlow SOPs,

TABLE 1 | Composition of the 8-color PID Orientation tube and technical information on reagents.

BV421	BV510	FITC	PE	PerCPCy5.5	PECy7	APC	APCH7
CD27	CD45RA	CD8 and SmIgD	CD16 and CD56	CD4 and SmIgM	CD19 and TCRγδ	CD3	CD45

Marker	Fluorochrome	Clone	Source	Catalog number	Application in EuroFlow panel	μl/test
CD3	APC	SK7	BD Biosciences	345767	Orientation, SCID/RTE, T cell subset tubes	2.5
CD4	PerCPCy5.5	SK3	BD Biosciences	332772	Orientation tube	7
CD8	FITC	SK1	BD Biosciences	345772	Orientation tube	5
CD16	PE	3G8	BD Biosciences	555407	Orientation tube	5
CD19	PECy7	J3-119	Beckman Coulter	IM3628	Orientation, BM-BCP, Pre-GC, Post-GC, IgH-isotype tubes	5
CD27	BV421	M-T271	BD Biosciences	562513	Orientation, Pre-GC, Post-GC, T cell subset tubes	1
*CD27**	*BV421*	*O323*	*BioLegend*	*302824*	Orientation, Pre-GC, Post-GC, T cell subset tubes	1
CD45	APCH7	2D1	BD Biosciences	641417	Orientation tube	2
CD45RA	BV510	HI100	BD Biosciences	563031	Orientation tube	2.5
*CD45RA**	*BV510*	*HI100*	*BioLegend*	*304142*	Orientation tube	2.5
CD56	PE	C5.9	Cytognos	CYT-56PE	Orientation tube	5
*CD56**	*PE*	*Leu11c*	*BD Biosciences*	*332779*	Orientation tube	5
SmIgD	FITC	IA6-2	BioLegend	348205	Orientation tube	1.25
SmIgM	PerCPCy5.5	MHM-88	BioLegend	314511	Orientation tube	2
TCRγδ	PECy7	11F2	BD Biosciences	655410	Orientation, SCID/RTE, T cell subset tubes	1

**Alternative reagents tested to provide same results.*

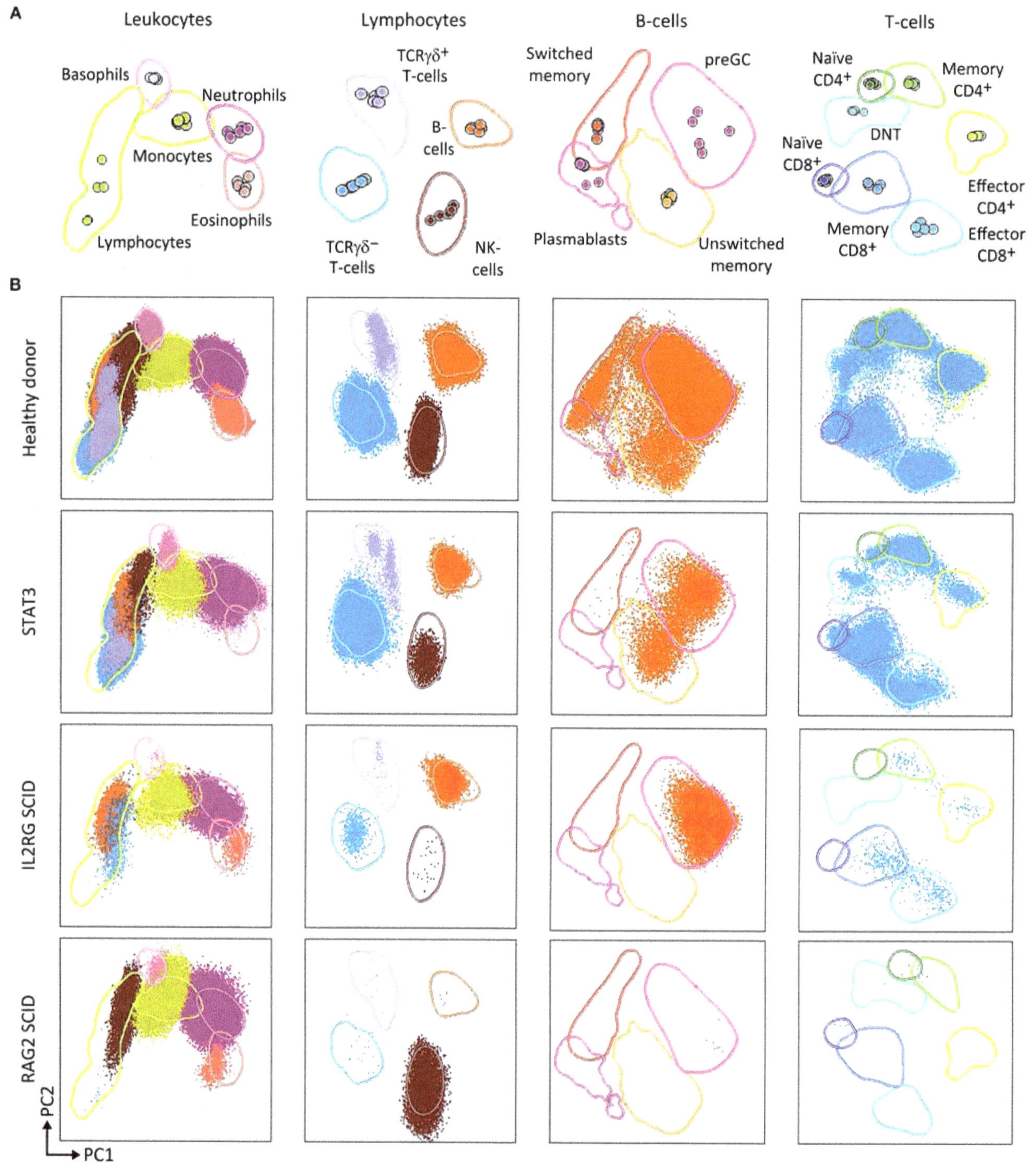

FIGURE 3 | PCA representation of PIDOT results, showing the distinct blood leukocyte subsets in the reference data file and supervised analysis of blood samples from a healthy donor and three different PID patients. **(A)** Reference principal component analysis. PCA1 vs. PCA2 representation was generated from five healthy donors data files, analyzed with the EuroFlow PIDOT. **(B)** Different patient samples were analyzed against the healthy donor PCA reference. Blood samples from a healthy donor, a patient with mutated STAT3, a SCID patient with IL2 receptor gamma chain (IL2RG) deficiency, and a SCID patient with recombination activating gene 2 (RAG2) deficiency were stained and acquired under identical/comparable conditions. The STAT3 deficient patient shows the typical pattern of reduced naïve T-cells, virtually no IgH-class switched B-cells, and no eosinophils. The IL2RG deficient SCID patient has virtually no T-cells, particularly no naïve T-cells (<1 cell/μL; see **Figure 1B**), B-cells are present, but no memory B-cells or plasmablasts, and NK-cells are virtually absent. The RAG2 deficient SCID patient has no B-cells and no T-cells, while NK-cells are present in normal numbers. DNT, double negative T-cells, negative for CD4 and CD8, but positive for CD3.

showed ≤1% abnormality alarms for the normal lymphocyte and myeloid cell populations.

RESULTS

EuroFlow Algorithm for PID Diagnosis and Classification

Suspicious patient features, such as recurrent and unusual infections, particularly with the same pathogen, auto-immunity, inflammation, lymphoproliferation, and/or organomegaly are triggers for application of the "PID Orientation tube" (PIDOT). In line with the EuroFlow PID algorithm (**Figure 1A**), the results of the PIDOT will guide the next steps:

- When the PIDOT identifies *strongly reduced B-cell counts* (<1 cell/μL; see **Figure 1B**) in the absence of a T-cell problem, the diagnosis of agammaglobulinemia is likely. In such case analysis of the B-cell precursor (BCP) compartment in BM with the PID-BCP tube might be informative to define the position and degree of blockade in early B-cell development, which differs between different genetic defects (37, 38).

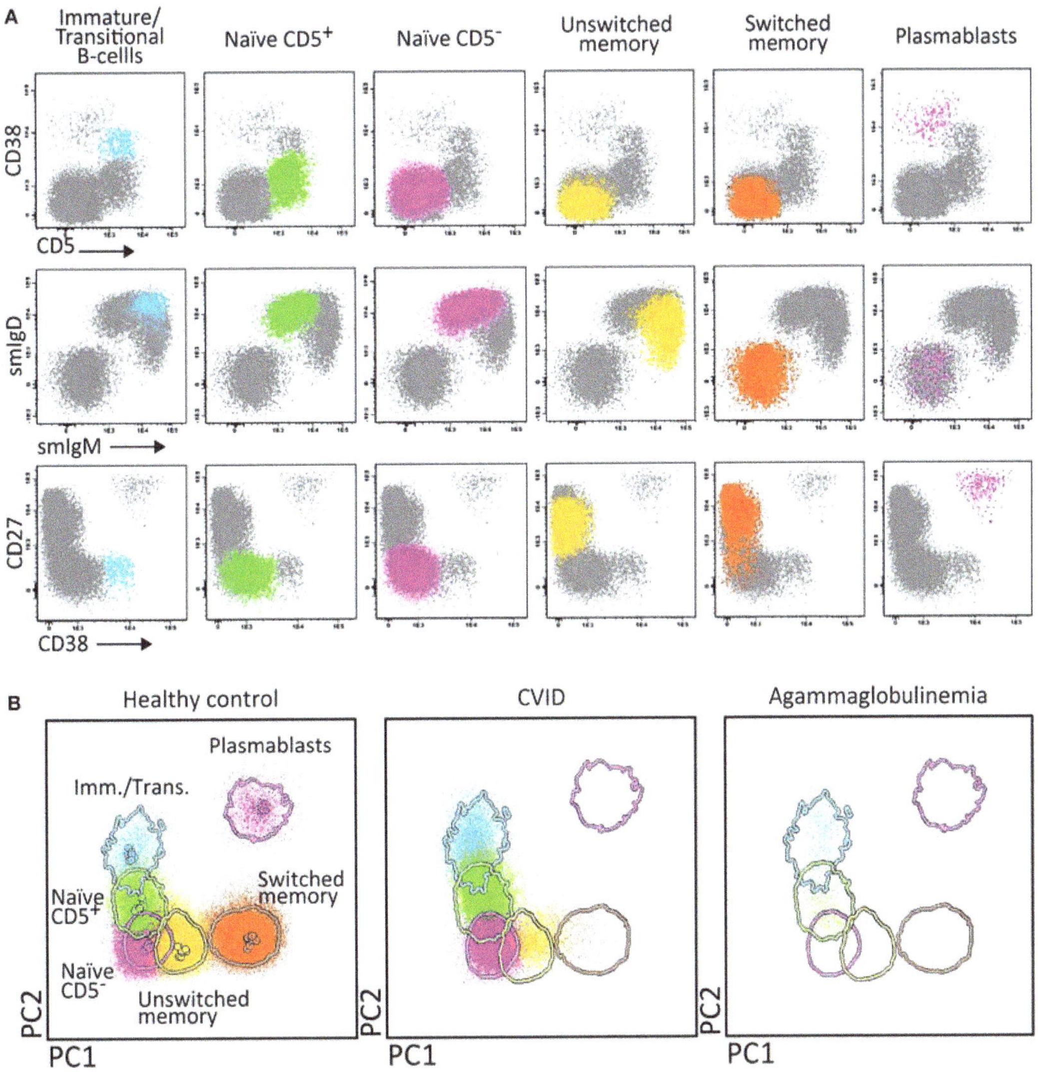

FIGURE 4 | Application of the Pre-GC tube, showing the major B-cell subsets in blood of healthy controls, and PID patients using classical 2-dimensional plots vs. n-dimensional PCA. Analysis of circulating B-cell subsets (FS/SS^{lo}CD19^{+}) identified within 2 × 10^6 blood leukocytes using the markers from the Pre-GC tube: Immature (CD5^{+} CD27^{-} CD38^{++} smIgM^{++} smIgD^{+}), CD5^{+} and CD5^{-} naïve B-cells (CD27^{-} CD38^{+d} smIgM^{+} smIgD^{++}), Ig non-switched and Ig-switched memory B-cells (CD5^{-} CD27^{+} CD38^{-} smIgM^{+} smIgD^{++} and CD5^{-} CD27$^{+/-}$ CD38^{-} smIgM^{-} smIgD^{-}, respectively), and plasmablasts (CD5^{-} CD27^{++} CD38^{+++}). **(A)** The identification of biologically relevant subsets of B-cells using the minimum number of bivariate plots required for a 5 marker-combination (three bivariate plots/cell population). **(B)** The same data via PC1 vs. PC2 representation of a 5-dimensional space in blood of six healthy controls (left panel), in blood of a patient with common variable immunodeficiency (CVID; middle) and in blood of a patient with agammaglobulinemia (right), all stained with the Pre-GC tube under comparable conditions. The CVID patient lacks plasmablasts in blood (<0.01 cell/μL blood) and has reduced IgH-class switched MBC. The agammaglobulinemia patient has no plasmablasts, no MBC, and also the naïve B-cell compartment is strongly reduced.

- In case the PIDOT reveals *reduced B-cell (subset) counts* (<5th percentile ≈ <2 SD values; see **Figure 1B**), application of the "Pre- and Post-GC B-cell tubes" is advised.
- The results of the "Pre- and Post-GC B-cell tubes" might directly support the diagnosis of Hyper IgM syndrome or CD19 complex deficiency (**Figure 1A**).
- If the "Pre- and Post-GC B-cell tubes" do not detect plasmablasts in blood (<0.01 cell/μL; see **Figure 1B**), in the presence of reduced memory B-cell subsets, the CVID diagnosis should be considered (57). The IgH isotype tube can further support such diagnosis (57).
- If the "Pre- and Post-GC B-cell tubes" reveal IgH class aberrancies in memory B-cell subsets or plasmablast subsets (<5th percentile ≈ <2 SD values; see **Figure 1B**), application of the IgH isotype tubes is advised.
- When the PIDOT tube identifies *virtually no (naïve) T-cells* (<1 cell/μL; see **Figure 1B**), application of the "SCID/recent thymic emigrant (RTE)" tube is advised to confirm the lack of T-cell production. It should be noted that SCID patients might have normal or reduced T-cell counts in the virtual absence of naïve T-cells (<1 cell/μL; see **Figure 1B**) with T-cell "right shifts" to more mature T-cell subsets; this is typically seen in subgroups of SCID patients such as "leaky SCID" and Omen syndrome (59) and generally appear to concern oligoclonal expansions of mature T-cells (73, 74).
- In case of *reduced T-cell (subset) counts* (<5th percentile ≈ <2 SD values; see **Figure 1B**), application of the T-cell subset tube is proposed.

The combined results of all ($n = 241$) evaluated PID patients demonstrated that in *patients with suspicion of predominantly antibody deficiency, e.g., recurrent respiratory infections, low serum Ig levels, and poor antibody response to vaccination*, the PID Orientation tube should (at diagnostic screening) directly be combined with the "*IgH-isotype B-cell tubes*".

Similarly, in case of *infants with failure to thrive and severe recurrent infections with unusual pathogens*, the "SCID/RTE tube" should directly be combined with the PID Orientation tube at diagnostic screening. Such combined SCID/RTE + PIDOT tube approach will also be useful for positive cases from newborn screening (NBS) programs, i.e., cases with strongly reduced T-cell receptor excision circles (TRECs) in blood (14, 75–77).Whenever *specific diseases such as ALPS or XLP are suspected* (e.g., increased $CD4^-/CD8^-$ counts or increased total T-cells counts; **Figure 1B**) additional studies need to be performed (not addressed in this manuscript).

PID Orientation Tube

The PID Orientation tube has been designed for full dissection of all major blood leukocyte (sub)populations ($n = 27$) in a single tube (**Figure 2**). The choice of markers, corresponding antibodies and fluorochromes aim at reliable detection and quantitation of these blood leukocyte subsets and their potential alterations.

After four cycles of design-testing-evaluation-redesign, the final version of the 8-color PID Orientation tube consisted of 12 markers: CD27, CD45RA, CD8, IgD, CD16, CD56, CD4, IgM, CD19, CD3, CD45, and either TCRαβ or preferably TCRγδ, wherein the following antibody pairs CD8/IgD, CD16/CD56, CD4/IgM, and CD19/TCRγδ or CD19/TCRαβ are conjugated to the same fluorochrome (**Table 1**). These reagents aim at detailed dissection of eight major blood leukocyte subsets (**Figure 2**): B-cells, T-cells, NK-cells, monocytes (including non-classical $CD16^+$ monocytes), dendritic cells, basophils, neutrophils and eosinophils. Additionally, B-cells and T-cells can be classified into a total of four and twelve different maturation pathway-associated subsets, respectively. Accordingly, B-cells are divided into pre-GC B-cells (including both immature/transitional and naïve B-cells), unswitched (including IgM^+IgD^+, IgM-only and IgD-only) and Ig-switched memory B-cells (MBC) and generally also plasmablasts (**Figure 2**). The T-cell compartment can be divided into different functional subsets according to the TCRγδ or TCRαβ lineage and according to CD4 and CD8 expression. These T-cell subsets can be further subdivided according to their maturation stage into naïve, central/transitional memory, and effector memory/terminally differentiated T-cells (**Figure 2**).

Therefore, the PID Orientation tube detects defects in the production of B-cells, T-cells and NK-cells, together with alterations (defective but also increase) in the production of monocytes, dendritic cells, neutrophils, eosinophils, and basophils. Three typical PID patient examples (STAT3, IL2RG, and RAG2 deficiency) are shown in **Figure 3** to illustrate the disease-associated immunophenotypic profiles. However, in most cases the PID Orientation tube does not allow precise (sub)classification of the T-cell and B-cell defects, implying that further characterization is required with additional B-cell and T-cell tubes, according to the EuroFlow PID algorithm (**Figure 1A**), as described below [see also (59)].

Some diagnostic laboratories in the PID field use a simple B-T-NK tube as first screening step, while most laboratories use several 4- to 6-color tubes in parallel to perform initial screening (generally using 12–18 antibodies with multiple repeats). The here proposed 8-color tube with 12 antibodies provides information on up to 20 different leukocyte (sub)populations, clearly separated in multidimensional principal component analysis (**Figures 2, 3**), thereby providing the basis for further classification of PID of the lymphoid system.

B-Cell Tubes

For antibody deficiencies and combined T/B-cell defects, detailed analysis of the B-cell compartment in blood and BM is required. B-cells originate from the BCP differentiation pathway in BM into immature and naïve B-cells that enter the periphery, including blood. In the periphery, the B-cells encounter antigen which induces a GC reaction. Consequently, blood contains naïve B-cells that did not yet undergo a GC reaction (pre-GC B-cells) or that have already been exposed to antigen, such as antigen-experienced memory B-cells (MBC), plasmablasts and plasma cells. The antigen-experienced subsets can be further subdivided according to class switching of their IgH-isotypes (and subclasses): IgM, IgD, IgE, IgG (including IgG1, IgG2, IgG3, IgG4), and IgA (including IgA1, IgA2).

TABLE 2 | Composition of the 8-color B-cell tubes and technical information on reagents.

	BV421	BV510	FITC	PE	PerCPCy5.5	PECy7	APC	APCAF750
Pre-GC	CD27	SmIgM	CD38	CD5	SmIgD	CD19	CD21	CD24
Post-GC	CD27	SmIgM	SmIgE and SmIgA	SmIgG and SmIgA	SmIgD	CD19	CD21	CD38
IgH-isotype-I	CD27	SmIgM	SmIgG4 and SmIgG2	SmIgG1 and SmIgG2	SmIgD	CD19	CD21	CD38
IgH-isotype-II	CD27	SmIgM	SmIgG3 and SmIgA1	SmIgA2 and SmIgA1	SmIgD	CD19	CD21	CD38

Marker	Fluorochrome	Clone	Source	Catalog number	Application in EuroFlow-PID panel	μl/test
CD5	PE	UCHT-2	BioLegend	300608	Pre-GC tube	5
CD19	PECy7	J3-119	Beckman Coulter	IM3628	Orientation, BM-BCP, Pre-GC, Post-GC, IgH-isotype tubes	5
CD21	APC	B-ly4	BD Biosciences	559867	Pre-GC, Post-GC, IgH-isotype tubes	10
CD24	APCAF750	ALB9	Beckman Coulter	B10738	Pre-GC,	5
CD27	BV421	M-T271	BD Biosciences	562513	Orientation, Pre-GC, Post-GC, IgH-isotype, T-cell subset tubes	1 (Pre/Post-GC)/2 (IgH-isotype)
CD38	FITC	HB7	BD Biosciences	340909	Pre-GC tube	5
CD38	APCH7	HB7	BD Biosciences	656646	Post-GC tube, IgH-isotype	3
SmIgA	FITC	IS11-8E10	Miltenyi	130-093-071	Post-GC tube	1
SmIgA	PE	IS11-8E10	Miltenyi	130-093-128	Post-GC tube	1
SmIgA1	FITC	SAA1	Cytognos	CYT-IGA1F	IgH-isotype tube	3
SmIgA1	PE	SAA1	Cytognos	CYT-IGA1PE	IgH-isotype tube	3
SmIgA2	PE	SAA2	Cytognos	CYT-IGA2PE	IgH-isotype tube	3
SmIgD	PerCPCy5.5	IA6-2	BioLegend	348208	Pre-GC, Post-GC, IgH-isotype tubes	1.5
SmIgE	FITC	polyclonal	Life Technologies	H15701	Post-GC tube	2
SmIgG	PE	G18-145	BD Biosciences	555787	Post-GC tube	20
SmIgG1	PE	SAG1	Cytognos	CYT-IGG1PE	IgH-isotype tube	3
SmIgG2	FITC	SAG2	Cytognos	CYT-IGG2F	IgH-isotype tube	3
SmIgG2	PE	SAG2	Cytognos	CYT-IGG2F	IgH-isotype tube	3
SmIgG3	FITC	SAG3	Cytognos	CYT-IGG3F	IgH-Isotype tube	3
SmIgG4	FITC	SAG4	Cytognos	CYT-IGG4F	IgH-isotype tube	3
SmIgM	BV510	MHM-88	BioLegend	314521	Pre-G, Post-GC, IgH-isotype tubes	1.3 (Pre/Post-GC)/2 (IgH-isotype)

Therefore two 8-color panels were designed for the identification of (i) different pre-GC B-cell subsets, including immature/transitional, naïve CD5$^+$ and naïve CD5$^-$ B-cells, and (ii) antigen-experienced subsets, including MBC and plasmablasts (**Figure 4**). The latter panel includes sub-classification of both MBC and PC according to IgH-isotype (IgM, IgD, IgG, IgA, IgE). Further IgH subsetting according to the specific subclasses (IgM, IgD, IgG1, IgG2, IgG3, IgG4, IgA1, and IgA2) was designed in a combination of two separate 8-color tubes or a single 10 or 12-color tube (56).

Accordingly, the EuroFlow 8-color PID B-cell tube set consists of five tubes for detailed subsetting of blood pre-GC B-cells (Pre-GC B-cell tube), antigen-experienced B-cells (Post-GC B-cell tube), including detailed IgH-isotype and subclass analysis of MBC and plasmablasts (IgH-isotype B-cell tubes 1 and 2), and BM BCP analysis (BCP tube) (**Figure 1A**).

Briefly, the **"Pre-GC B-cell tube"** contains CD27, IgM, CD38, CD5, IgD, CD19, CD21, and CD24 markers (**Table 2**), which allows detection of immature/transitional B-cells, CD5$^+$ and CD5$^-$ naïve B-cells (including their CD21 and CD24 subsets), unswitched (including IgM$^+$IgD$^+$, IgM-only, and IgD-only) and switched MBC and PC. The **"Post-GC B-cell tube"** contains CD27, IgM, IgA, IgG, IgD, CD19, CD21, CD38, and optionally IgE, wherein two distinctly labeled antibodies against IgA allow to have the IgE/IgA pair and IgG/IgA pair conjugated to the same fluorochrome (**Table 2**) (78). The **"IgH-Isotype B-cell tube-1 and tube-2"** (**Figure 5A**) both contain CD27, IgM, IgD, CD19, CD21, and CD38 together with IgG4, IgG2, IgG1, or with IgA2, IgA1, IgG3, respectively. In this composition two distinctly labeled antibodies against IgG2 and IgA1 are used, wherein the antibodies within the pairs IgG1/IgG2 and IgG2/IgG4 or IgA1/IgG3 and IgA1/IgA2 are conjugated to the same fluorochrome (**Table 2**).

Finally, the **BCP-BM tube** consists of the seven cell surface membrane markers CD20, IgM, CD38, IgD, CD19, CD34, and CD10 and the three intracellular markers cyIgμ, nuTdT, and cyCD79a (**Table 3**). This combination of markers allows detailed analysis of the BM-BCP compartment from the CD19-negative stage until the naïve B-cells and can visualize complete and partial

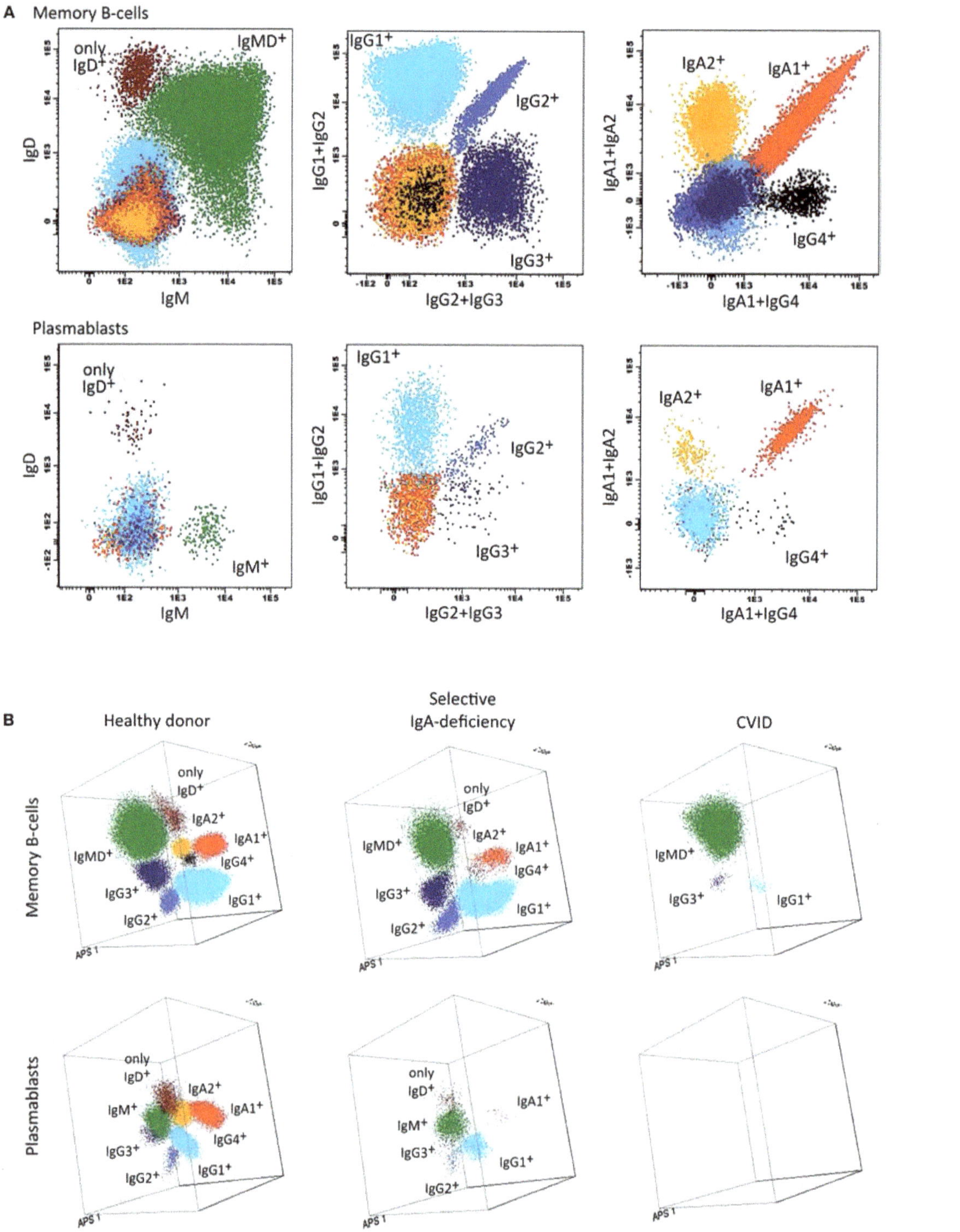

FIGURE 5 | Application of the IgH-isotype tube for the dissection of switched memory B-cells and plasmablasts in blood from healthy donors and PID patients. **(A)** Bivariate plots showing the distribution of switched memory B-cells (smIgMD^{-}CD19^{+}CD38^{-}) and plasmablasts (CD19^{+}CD27^{++}CD38^{+++}) according to the surface membrane expression of the different IgH-isotypes (IgG1, IgG2, IgG3, IgG4, IgA1, and IgA2) in 5×10^6 peripheral blood leukocytes analyzed with the IgH-isotype tubes in samples from a healthy adult. **(B)** Three dimensional PCA representation of IgH-isotype subsets in memory B-cells (top) and plasmablasts (lower) in a healthy adult donor (left), a selective IgA-deficient patient (middle), and a CVID patient (right). No plasmablasts were detected in blood from the CVID patient (count of <0.01 cells/μL blood), while variable defects were detected in the memory B-cell compartment, particularly involving switched memory B-cells. The defects in the IgA-deficient patient mainly concerned the IgA-class-switched plasmablasts.

TABLE 3 | Composition of the 10-color BM-BCP tube and technical information on reagents.

PacB	BV510	BV605	FITC	PE	PECF594	PerCPCy5.5	PECY7	APC	APCC750
CD20	SmIgM	CD38	nuTdT	CyCD79a	SmIgD	CyIgM	CD19	CD34	CD10

Marker	Fluorochrome	Clone	Source	Catalog number	Application in EuroFlow-PID panel	µl/test
CD10	APCC750	HI10a	Cytognos	CYT-10AC750	BM-BCP	3
CD19	PECy7	J3-119	Beckman Coulter	IM3628	Orientation, BM-BCP, Pre-GC, Post-GC, IgH-isotype tubes	5
CD20	PacB	2H7	Biolegend	302320	BM-BCP tube	1
CD34	APC	8G12	BD Biosciences	345804	BM-BCP tube	5
CD38	BV605	HIT2	Biolegend	303532	BM-BCP tube	
CyCD79a	PE	HM57	Dako	R7159	BM-BCP tube	3
SmIgD	PECF594	IA6-2	BD Biosciences	562540	BM-BCP tube	5
SmIgM	BV510	MHM-88	BioLegend	314521	BM-BCP, Pre-GC, Post-GC, IgH-isotype tubes	2
CyIgM	PerCPCy5.5	MHM-88	BioLegend	314512	BM-BCP tube	2
nuTdT	FITC	HT-6	Dako	F7139	BM-BCP tube	10

blocks in BCP differentiation as well as aberrant expression profiles (Wentink et al., unpublished results).

For reasons of efficiency, the two IgH-isotype tubes can be combined into a single 10-color IgH-isotype tube with CD27, IgM, IgG3, IgG2, IgG1, IgD, CD19, CD21, CD38, IgA1, IgA2, and IgG4, with two distinctly labeled antibodies against IgG2 and two distinctly labeled antibodies against IgA1 ("10-color IgH-isotype tube"). Preferably, the four blood B-cell tubes (Pre-GC, Post-GC, and the two IgH-isotype tubes) can be combined into a single 12-color tube by the further addition of CD5 and CD24 ("12-color IgH-isotype B-cell tube") (56, 57).

In summary, the Pre-GC and Post-GC tubes can visualize blockades in differentiation of transitional to mature naïve B-cells in e.g., a subset of XLA patients, and variable defects in IgH-switched MBC and plasmablasts, such as in patients with Hyper IgM syndrome, CD19 complex deficiencies, IgH class aberrancies, and CVID with almost systematic absence of plasmablasts (<0.01 cell/uL) (**Figures 1B, 4B**) (57). In addition, the IgH-isotype tubes can uncover more subtle defects in IgH-class switching e.g., in selective IgA- and IgG-subclass deficiencies (**Figure 5B**) (57). Finally, the BCP tube detects early blockades in BCP maturation in BM.

T-Cell Tubes

In many cases with suspicion of PID of the lymphoid system, analysis of T-cell subsets is an essential part of making a correct diagnosis. If the PID Orientation tube indicates reduced T-cell (subset) counts or abnormal T-cell maturation, further investigation of the blood T-cell compartment is recommended. The SCID/RTE tube is meant for cases with strongly reduced (naïve) T-cell production (<1 cell/µL; see **Figure 1B**), whereas the T-cell subset tube should be applied when the PID orientation tubes reveals an imbalanced composition of the memory and effector T-cell compartments.

In case of high suspicion of SCID in children of <1 year with severe recurrent infections by unusual pathogens and failure to thrive, the SCID/RTE tube should be directly applied in combination with the PID Orientation tube (**Figures 1A, 6**). In such patients the detected blood T-cells might be (non-autologous) transplacentally-derived maternal T-cells. The predominant presence of (activated) memory T-cells (either autologous or maternal) in the absence of T-cells recently emigrated from the thymus (RTE), further supports the SCID diagnosis (**Figure 6**).

Upfront identification of the major TCRγδ, TCRαβ, CD4, and CD8 T-cell lineages is required for further detailed dissection of their maturation pathways into ($CD31^+$) RTE, naïve, memory and effector subsets, including activated ($HLA\text{-}DR^+$) T-cells (**Figure 6**). The T-cell subset tube further dissects the blood T-cell lineages into central memory (CM), transitional memory (TM), effector memory (EM), terminal differentiated (TD), and terminal effector (TE) subsets (**Figure 7**).

Briefly, two 8-color T-cell tubes have been designed: (i) the **SCID/RTE tube** with the five backbone markers CD3, CD4, CD8, CD45RO, and TCRαβ or TCRγδ, supplemented with the subsetting markers CD31, CD62L, HLA-DR for identification of RTEs and activated T-cells (**Table 4**); and (ii) the **T-cell subset tube** with the same five backbone markers, combined with CD27, CD28, and CCR7 (**Table 4**) for detailed dissection of the above mentioned memory and effector compartments (**Figures 6, 7**).

In summary, while the first tube identifies major defects in T-cell production, the second tube focusses on milder defects in T-cell production and/or altered T-cell responses (**Figures 6, 7**).

EuroFlow Reference Databases as Essential Tool for Easy, Fast, and Reproducible Analysis of Patient Samples

Similarly to the EuroFlow leukemia-lymphoma diagnosis and monitoring databases (64–66), reference databases have been generated for the EuroFlow PID tubes to facilitate: 1. Automated gating of all leukocyte subsets; 2. Identification of PID-associated immune cell profiles vs. normal age-matched reference values

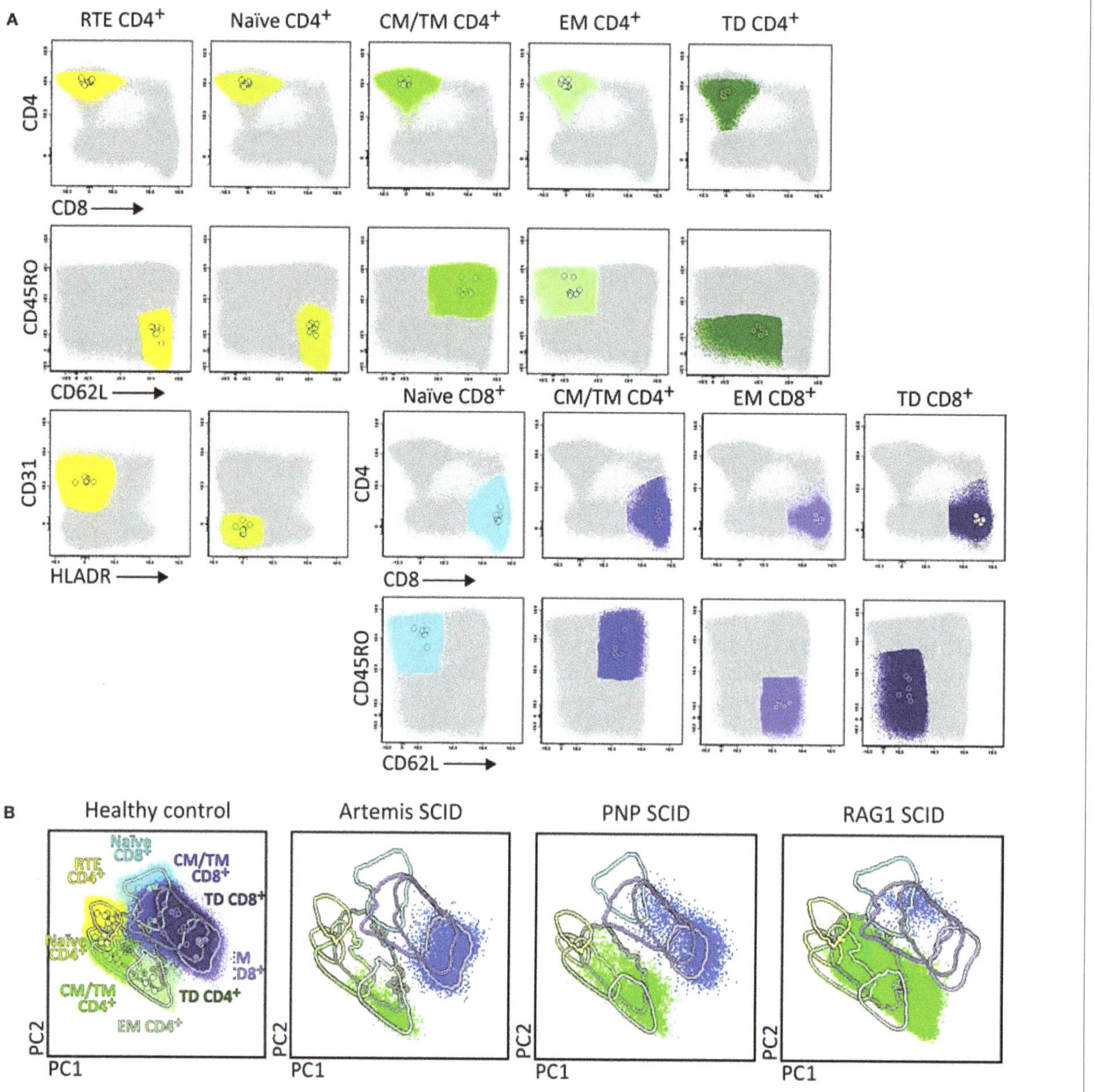

FIGURE 6 | Application of the RTE-SCID tube in healthy controls and T-cell defects. Analysis of circulating T-cell subsets (FS/SS^{lo}CD3$^+$) identified within 1x10^6 blood leukocytes using the markers from the RTE-SCID tube: Recent Thymic Emigrants (RTE) CD4$^+$ T-cells (CD4$^+$ CD8$^-$ CD45RO$^-$ CD62L$^+$ CD31$^+$ HLA-DR$^-$), and naïve (CD45RO$^-$ CD62L$^+$ CD31$^+$ HLA-DR$^-$), Central/Transitional Memory (CM/TM) (CD45RO$^+$ CD62L$^+$), Effector Memory (EM) (CD45RO$^+$ CD62L$^-$), and Terminally Differentiated (TD) (CD45RO$^-$ CD62L$^-$) CD4$^+$ and CD8$^+$ T-cells. **(A)** The identification of biologically relevant T-cell subsets in six healthy controls using the minimum number of bivariate plots required for a 6 marker-combination (three bivariate plots/cell population). **(B)** Comparable T-cell data via PCA1 vs. PCA2 representation of a 6-dimensional space in six healthy controls (left) as well as in three severe combined immunodeficiency (SCID) patients, diagnosed with Artemis, PNP and RAG-1 defects, all stained with the RTE/SCID tube under comparable conditions. All three SCID patients show "leakiness" with virtually complete absence of naïve T-cells (<1 cell/μL blood) and clear "right shift" to mature CM/TM, EM, and TD T-cells in both the CD4 and CD8 lineages.

and phenotypes; and 3. Further sub-classification of PID cases into distinct diagnostic categories (**Figures 2–7**).

Stepwise application of the EuroFlow PID tubes according to the proposed algorithm (**Figure 1A**) supports the diagnosis of many PID evaluated so far ($n = 233$), and provides further classification of most lymphoid PID cases into distinct diagnostic categories according to altered flowcytometric immune cell profiles (**Table 5**). For example, the PIDOT together with the IgH-isotype tubes (**Figure 8**) support the diagnosis of virtually all IgA- and IgG-subclass deficiencies and CVID patients, including their detailed characterization (57). **Figure 9** shows an example of combined application of the PIDOT, the Pre-GC tube and

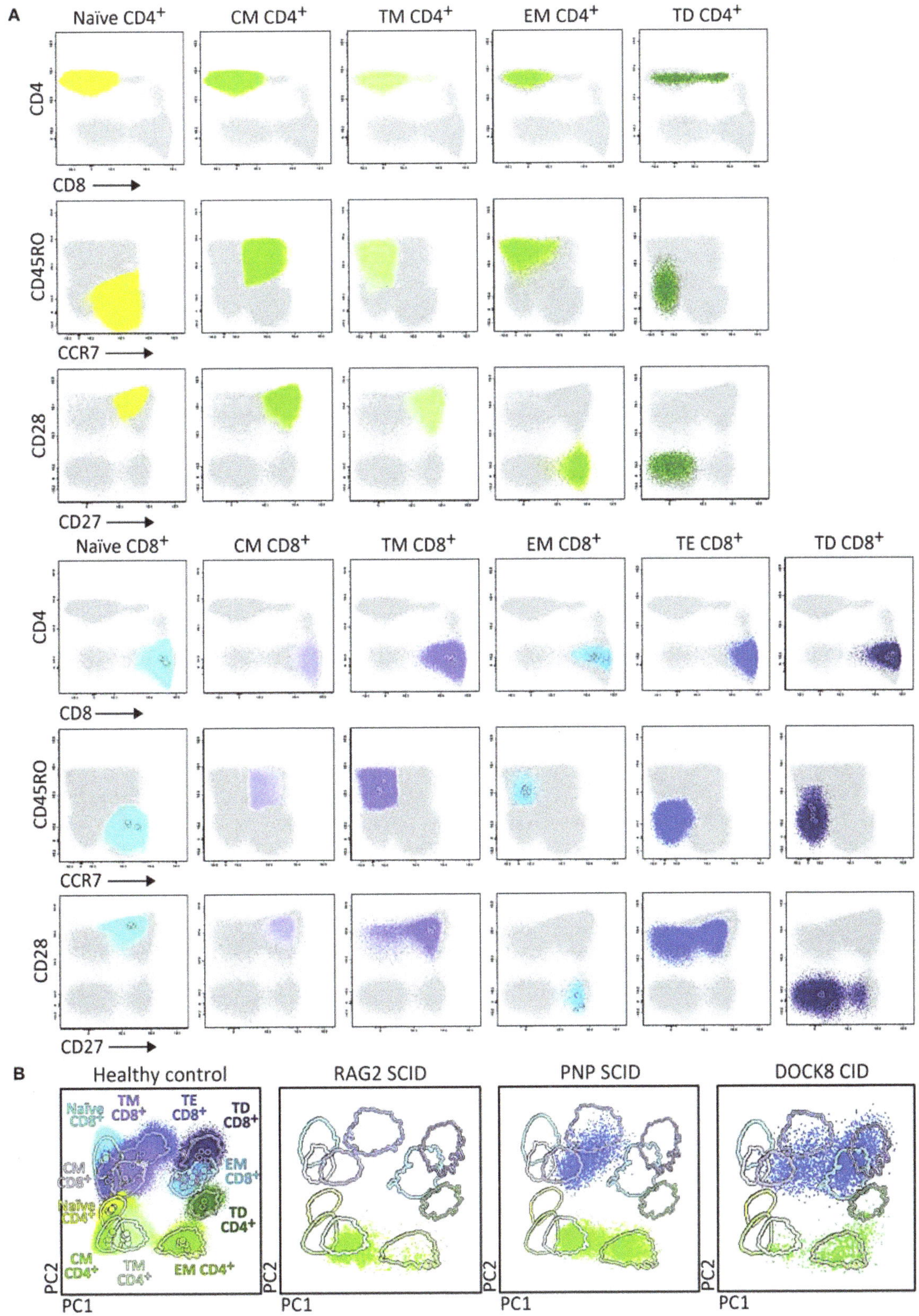

FIGURE 7 | Application of the T-cell panel tube in healthy controls and PID patients with T-cell defects. Analysis of circulating T-cell subsets (FS/SS^{lo}CD3^{+}) identified within 1 × 10^{6} blood leukocytes using the markers from the T-cell panel tube: naïve (CD45RO^{-} CCR7^{+} CD27^{+} CD28^{+}), Central Memory (CM) (CD45RO^{+} CCR7^{+}

(Continued)

FIGURE 7 | CD27$^+$ CD28$^+$), Transitional Memory (TM) (CD45RO$^+$ CCR7$^-$ CD27$^+$ CD28$^{+/-}$), Effector Memory (EM) (CD45RO$^+$ CCR7$^-$ CD27$^-$ CD28$^+$), Terminal Effector (TE) (CD45RO$^-$ CCR7$^-$ CD27$^+$ CD28$^{+/-}$), and Terminally Differentiated (TD) (CD45RO$^-$ CCR7$^-$ CD27$^-$ CD28$^{+/-}$) CD4$^+$ and CD8$^+$ T-cells. **(A)** The identification of biologically relevant subsets of T-cells in six healthy controls using the minimum number of bivariate plots required for a 6 marker-combination (three bivariate plots/cell population). **(B)** Comparable data via PCA1 vs. PCA2 representation of a 6-dimensional space in blood of six healthy controls (left) as compared to blood samples of three severe combined immunodeficiency (SCID) patients, diagnosed with RAG2, PNP, and DOCK8 defects, all stained with the RTE/SICD tube under comparable conditions. The SCID patients show "leakiness" with absence of naïve T-cells (<1 cell/μL blood) and variable "right shift" to mature CM/TM, EM, and TD T-cells in the CD4 lineage (all 3 SCID patients) and CD8 lineage (PNP and DOCK8 defects).

TABLE 4 | Composition of the 8-color BM-BCP tube and technical information on reagents.

	BV421	BV510	FITC	PE	PerCPCy5.5	PECy7	APC	APCAF750
SCID/RTE panel	CD62L	CD4	CD45RO	CD31	HLA-DR	TCRγδ	CD3	CD8
T-cell panel	CD27	CD4	CD45RO	CD197	CD28	TCRγδ	CD3	CD8

Marker	Fluorochrome	Clone	Source	Catalog number	Application in EuroFlow panel	μl/test
CD3	APC	SK7	BD Biosciences	345767	Orientation, SCID/RTE, T cell subset tubes	2.5
CD4	BV510	OKT4	BioLegend	317443	Orientation, SCID/RTE, T cell subset tubes	1.5
CD8	APCAF750	B9.11	Beckman Coulter	A94683	Orientation, SCID/RTE, T cell subset tubes	1.5
CD27	BV421	M-T271	BD Biosciences	562513	Orientation, Pre-GC, Post-GC, T cell subset tubes	1
*CD27**	*BV421*	*O323*	*BioLegend*	*302824*	Orientation, Pre-GC, Post-GC, T cell subset tubes	1
CD28	PerCPCy5.5	CD28.2	BioLegend	302921	T-cell subset tube	4
CD31	PE	MEM-05	Exbio	1P-273-T100	SCID/RTE tube	5
CD45RO	FITC	UCHL1	Exbio	1F-498-T100	SCID/RTE, T cell subset tube	10
CD62L	BV421	DREG-56	Biolegend	304827	SCID/RTE tube	2
CD197	PE	FR 11-11E8	Miltenyi	130-093-621	T cell subset tube	5
HLADR	PerCPCy5.5	L243	Biolegend	307629	SCID/RTE tube	1.5
TCRγδ	PECy7	11F2	BD Biosciences	649806	Orientation, SCID/RTE, T cell subset tubes	1

**Alternative reagent tested to provide same results.*

the T-cell subset tube in a patient with a WASp defect, showing several aberrancies in T-cell subsets.

More detailed results on the application of the individual EuroFlow PID tubes and their corresponding reference databases and age-matched reference values are provided in separate publications (57, 59) and are implemented in the EuroFlow-based Infinicyt software, respectively.

DISCUSSION

Diagnosis and classification of rare diseases deserves well-defined strategies that are efficient and easily accessible, providing a diagnosis at an early stage, in order to prevent diagnostic delays with higher chances of irreversible organ damage. In case of PID, this requires awareness of general practitioners and pediatricians about the most efficient and cost-effective diagnostic pathways as proposed by ESID and IUIS (2, 5, 6). These diagnostic pathways include flowcytometric immunophenotyping at an early stage, which can guide other diagnostic tests such as functional assays and genetic studies.

Specialized reference centers are required for full diagnostics and clinical management of rare diseases such as PID. Broad and easy access to fast diagnostic screening strategies and linkage to these highly specialized PID reference centers of excellence shall reduce morbidity and mortality of PID patients. The medical indications for testing of PID are well-defined ("***the 10 warning signs of PID***") and several consensus reports on stepwise diagnostic strategies have been proposed (2, 5, 7, 79, 80). However practical implementation of these consensus proposals has only partially been achieved. This is mainly due to lack of standardization in the pre-analytical and analytical laboratory procedures, particularly in flow cytometry and NGS/WES (9, 10, 43–45). At least in part, this lack of standardization is caused by the fast technological developments in both fields, which has led to great variability in technical procedures and assays between individual laboratories, thereby hampering comparability of diagnostic results, even among reference PID centers.

The main objectives of the EuroFlow Consortium were to innovate and standardize the flowcytometric techniques and strategies, applied in the diagnosis and classification of PID of the lymphoid system and to generate reliable and reproducible results across laboratories and countries, for guiding both functional testing and genetic testing in flowcytometrically-defined PID subgroups. To achieve these objectives, the EuroFlow Consortium took advantage of its concepts, technologies, tools and experience from the field of leukemia and lymphoma diagnosis, classification and monitoring (61–65). Consequently, we sequentially (i) developed 8-color tubes (and one 12-color BM tube) for efficient diagnostic testing and classification of PID in multiple multicenter cycles of design-testing-evaluation-redesign, following strict rules for selection of optimal combinations of antibody clones and their fluorochrome conjugates; (ii) validated the approved antibody tubes in healthy controls and PID patient series (56–59);

TABLE 5 | Application of EuroFlow PID tubes for the primary immunodeficiency disease categories.

Disease category (IUIS 2017) (1)	**EuroFlow PID tubes**						
	Orientation	**Pre-GC**	**Post-GC**	**IgH-isotypes**	**SCID/RTE**	**T-cell subset tube**	**Frequency correct diagnosis**
Immunodeficiency affecting cellular and humoral immunity ($n = 36$)	Diagnostic screening	Exploratory	Exploratory	Exploratory	Clinical classification	Clinical classification	100%
5CID with associated or syndromic features ($n = 20$)	Diagnostic screening	Exploratory	Exploratory	Exploratory	Clinical classification	Clinical classification	75%*
Predominantly antibody deficiencies ($n = 150$)	Diagnostic screening	Clinical classification	Clinical classification	Diagnostic screening and classification	Exploratory	Exploratory	100%
Diseases of immune dysregulation ($n = 10$)	Diagnostic screening	Exploratory	Exploratory	Exploratory	Exploratory	Exploratory	90%
Congenital defects of phagocyte numbers or functions ($n = 10$)	Immuno-evaluation	Exploratory	Exploratory	Exploratory	Exploratory	Exploratory	70%
Defects in intrinsic and innate immunity ($n = 3$)	Immuno-evaluation	Exploratory	Exploratory	Exploratory	Exploratory	Exploratory	67%
Autoinflammatory disorders ($n = 0$)	Immuno-evaluation	Exploratory	Exploratory	Exploratory	Exploratory	Exploratory	–
Complement deficiencies ($n = 4$)	Immuno-evaluation	Exploratory	Exploratory	Exploratory	Exploratory	Exploratory	0%

**60% of cases showing normal blood lymphocyte subset counts were DiGeorge Syndrome patients. Diagnostic screening: mandatory for the diagnosis and management of the patient according to international classifications (1, 2, 5, 40). Clinical classification: required for identification of subgroups of patients with different disease presentation and outcome, including guiding genetic testing (1, 2, 5, 41, 43). Immuno-evaluation: provides information indicated for treatment decision and patients monitoring (11–13). Exploratory: not required for clinical management, might provide relevant immune information; CID, Combined Immunodeficiency.*

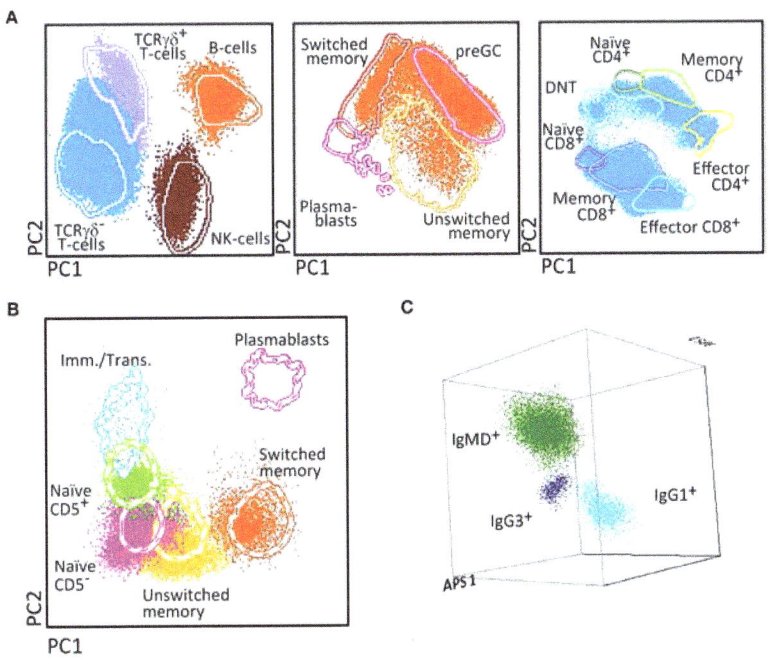

FIGURE 8 | PCA representation of the biologically relevant subsets in a patient diagnosed with IgG2 subclass deficiency with IgA deficiency (40 years). The distribution of the biologically relevant PB lymphocyte subsets has been represented using multidimensional reference plots. The supervised analysis of the PID orientation tube using PC1 vs. PC2 reference plots **(A)** shows that plasmablasts were undetectable in the patient sample after acquiring 1×10^6 cells. Lack of plasma cells was confirmed in the analysis of the Pre-GC and Post-GC B-cell tubes **(B)**. In addition, three dimensional PCA representation of IgH-isotype subsets in memory B-cells **(C)** showed that although the counts of total switched memory B-cells was normal in the previous tubes, the subsets of IgG2$^+$, IgA1$^+$, and IgA2$^+$ were undetectable with a sensitivity of 10 cells in a mL of peripheral blood (0.01 cells/μL).

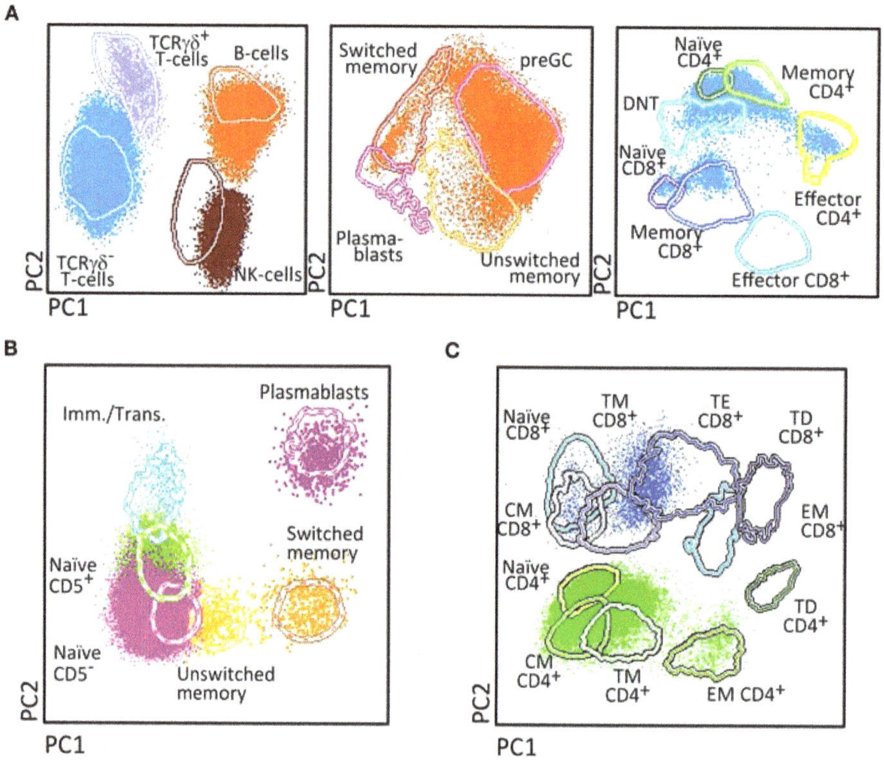

FIGURE 9 | PCA representation of the biologically relevant subsets in a patient diagnosed with a WASp defect (5 years-old). The distribution of the biologically relevant PB lymphocyte subsets has been represented using multidimensional reference plots. The supervised analysis of the PID orientation tube using PC1 vs. PC2 reference plots **(A)** shows that low numbers of total and naïve CD8$^+$ T-cells, and unswitched and switched memory B-cells, were detected in the patient sample after acquiring 1×10^6 cells. Decreased counts of unswitched memory B-cells was confirmed in the analysis of the B-cell tubes **(B)**. In addition, PCA1 vs. PCA2 representation of the T-cell tube **(C)** confirmed that naïve CD8$^+$ T-cells were decreased.

(iii) constructed reference databases of normal samples and well-annotated patient samples, which can serve as templates for prospective data analysis; and (iv) provided the basis for standardized interpretation of the results obtained in individual laboratories, which apply the same EuroFlow methods and tools.

As evaluated in more than 240 PID patients, the stepwise application of the proposed tubes according to the EuroFlow PID algorithm (**Figure 1A**) provides efficient and cost-effective flowcytometric diagnostic screening and classification of virtually all PID of the lymphoid system, based on fast, sensitive, easy, and reproducible identification and enumeration of all relevant subsets (**Figure 1**). The B-cell tubes have proven to more accurately dissect the blood memory B-cell and plasmablast compartments than achieved previously, thereby providing new possibilities to better diagnose and classify antibody deficiencies, including IgH-subclass deficiencies and CVID (57). In patients suspected of SCID (e.g., in the TREC-based NBS programs), the combined application of the PIDOT and SCID tubes will be highly informative (14, 75–77). Furthermore, the diagnostic procedures for secondary immunodeficiencies might profit as well from the proposed PID tubes and tools (81). Still several subsets of PID patients might present with no or minimally altered lymphoid subset numbers, such as in some DiGeorge patients and part of ALPS, Nijmegen breakage syndrome and ataxia telangiectasia patients at young age. In such cases functional and genetic testing are more informative. Finally, in this study not all types of lymphoid PID could be studied in large series, implying that more cases of the rare diagnostic PID categories should be evaluated. This will be a continuous process to further support the clinical use of the proposed PID tubes; the EuroFlow Consortium will continue to contribute to this process.

Based on our experience in the leukemia and lymphoma field, we believe that the provided standardized strategies, tools, and reference databases are cost-effective and can easily be implemented, not only in specialized PID reference centers, but in any medical immunology laboratory equipped with an 8-color flow cytometer in any PID center in the world. However, it should be noted that standardized flow cytometry, although critical for PID evaluation, does not replace and has to be coupled to immunological functional and genetic testing in order to reach a final diagnosis in most cases.

AUTHOR'S NOTE

All authors wish to stress that they are scientifically independent and have full freedom to act without any obligation to industry other than scientific advice to companies in the context of licensed patents. The selection of antibodies by the EuroFlow consortium is always explicitly based on quality, relevance, and continuous availability. Consequently all proposed antibody panels consist of mixtures of antibodies from many different companies (see **Tables 1–4**).

AUTHOR CONTRIBUTIONS

JvD, MvdB, TK, MP-A, MvZ, and AO contributed conception and design of the study. TK, MP-A, EM, MV, EL-G, MW, A-KK, JP, AS, and EB performed the data acquisition and data analysis. MP-A and EB organized the database. JvD, MP-A, and AO wrote the manuscript. All authors contributed to manuscript revision, read, and approved the submitted version.

FUNDING

The coordination and innovation processes of this study were financially supported and coordinated by the EuroFlow Consortium (Chairmen: JvD and AO). MvZ is supported by Senior Research Fellowship GNT1117687 from the Australian National Health and Medical Research Council. TK and EM were supported by projects 15-28541A from Ministry of Health, LO1604 from Ministry of Education, Youth and Sports and GBP302/12/G101 from Grant Agency of the Czech Republic. MP-A, EB, and AO were supported by a grant from the Junta de Castilla y León (Fondo Social Europeo, ORDEN EDU/346/2013, Valladolid, Spain) and the CB16/12/00400 grant (CIBER/ONC, Instituto de Salud Carlos III, Ministerio de Economía y Competitividad, -Madrid, Spain- and FONDOS FEDER), the FIS PI12/00905-FEDER grant (Fondo de Investigación Sanitaria of Instituto de Salud Carlos III, Madrid, Spain), and a grant from Fundación Mutua Madrileña (Madrid, Spain).

ACKNOWLEDGMENTS

We thank our EuroFlow colleagues Christina Grosserichter, Quentin Lecrevisse, and Sandra Posthumus, Ingrid Pico for their technical support in performing the PID studies and our clinical colleagues Sonia de Arriba-Mendez, Ana Remesal, Noemi Puig, Cristina Serrano, Susana Silva, and Carolien Bonroy for recruiting PID patients and control sample donations, and W. Marieke Bitter for her continuous support in the management of the EuroFlow Consortium.

REFERENCES

1. Picard C, Bobby Gaspar H, Al-Herz W, Bousfiha A, Casanova JL, Chatila T, et al. International Union of Immunological Societies: 2017 Primary Immunodeficiency Diseases Committee Report on Inborn Errors of Immunity. *J Clin Immunol.* (2018) 38:96–128. doi: 10.1007/s10875-017-0464-9
2. Bousfiha A, Jeddane L, Picard C, Ailal F, Bobby Gaspar H, Al-Herz W, et al. The 2017 IUIS phenotypic classification for primary immunodeficiencies. *J Clin Immunol.* (2018) 38:129–43. doi: 10.1007/s10875-017-0465-8
3. ESID. *European Society for Immunodeficiencies: ESID Database Statistics 2004-2014*. Available online at: https://esid.org/Working-Parties/Registry/ESID-Database-Statistics (accessed May 25, 2019)
4. Kindle G, Gathmann B, Grimbacher B. The use of databases in primary immunodeficiencies. *Curr Opin Aller Clin Immunol.* (2014) 14:501–8. doi: 10.1097/ACI.0000000000000113
5. ESID. *European Society for Immunodeficiencies: ESID Registry - Clinical diagnosis criteria of PID*. Available online at: https://esid.org/Working-Parties/Registry/Diagnosis-criteria (accessed May 25, 2019)
6. de Vries E. Patient-centred screening for primary immunodeficiency, a multi-stage diagnostic protocol designed for non-immunologists: 2011 update. *Clin Exp Immunol.* (2012) 167:108–19. doi: 10.1111/j.1365-2249.2011.04461.x
7. Bonilla FA, Khan DA, Ballas ZK, Chinen J, Frank MM, Hsu JT, et al. Practice parameter for the diagnosis and management of primary immunodeficiency. *J Allergy Clin Immunol.* (2015) 136:1186–205.e1-78. doi: 10.1016/j.jaci.2015.04.049
8. Dorsey MJ, Dvorak CC, Cowan MJ, Puck JM. Treatment of infants identified as having severe combined immunodeficiency by means of newborn screening. *J Allergy Clin Immunol.* (2017) 139:733-42. doi: 10.1016/j.jaci.2017.01.005
9. Stray-Pedersen A, Sorte HS, Samarakoon P, Gambin T, Chinn IK, Coban Akdemir ZH, et al. Primary immunodeficiency diseases: Genomic approaches delineate heterogeneous Mendelian disorders. *J Allergy and clinical immunology.* (2017) 139:232-45. doi: 10.1016/j.jaci.2016.05.042
10. Abolhassani H, Chou J, Bainter W, Platt CD, Tavassoli M, Momen T, et al. Clinical, immunologic, and genetic spectrum of 696 patients with combined immunodeficiency. *J Allergy Clin Immunol.* (2018) 141:1450-8. doi: 10.1016/j.jaci.2017.06.049
11. Schuetz C, Pannicke U, Jacobsen EM, Burggraf S, Albert MH, Honig M, et al. Lesson from hypomorphic recombination-activating gene (RAG) mutations: Why asymptomatic siblings should also be tested. *J Allergy Clin Immunol.* (2014) 133:1211-5. doi: 10.1016/j.jaci.2013.10.021
12. Volk T, Pannicke U, Reisli I, Bulashevska A, Ritter J, Bjorkman A, et al. DCLRE1C (ARTEMIS) mutations causing phenotypes ranging from atypical severe combined immunodeficiency to mere antibody deficiency. *Hum Mol Genet.* (2015) 24:7361–72. doi: 10.1093/hmg/ddv437
13. IJspeert H, Driessen GJ, Moorhouse MJ, Hartwig NG, Wolska-Kusnierz B, Kalwak K, et al. Similar recombination-activating gene (RAG) mutations result in similar immunobiological effects but in different clinical phenotypes. *J Allergy Clin Immunol.* (2014) 133:1124–33. doi: 10.1016/j.jaci.2013.11.028
14. Kwan A, Abraham RS, Currier R, Brower A, Andruszewski K, Abbott JK, et al. Newborn screening for severe combined immunodeficiency in 11 screening programs in the United States. *JAMA.* (2014) 312:729–38. doi: 10.1001/jama.2014.9132
15. Ogonek J, Kralj Juric M, Ghimire S, Varanasi PR, Holler E, Greinix H, et al. Immune Reconstitution after Allogeneic Hematopoietic Stem Cell Transplantation. *Front Immunol.* (2016) 7:507. doi: 10.3389/fimmu.2016.00507
16. Heimall J, Logan BR, Cowan MJ, Notarangelo LD, Griffith LM, Puck JM, et al. Immune reconstitution and survival of 100 SCID patients post-hematopoietic cell transplant: a PIDTC natural history study. *Blood.* (2017) 130:2718–27. doi: 10.1182/blood-2017-05-781849
17. Ameratunga R, Woon ST, Gillis D, Koopmans W, Steele R. New diagnostic criteria for common variable immune deficiency (CVID), which may assist with decisions to treat with intravenous or subcutaneous immunoglobulin. *Clin Exp Immunol.* (2013) 174:203-11. doi: 10.1111/cei.12178

18. Barmettler S, Price C. Continuing IgG replacement therapy for hypogammaglobulinemia after rituximab-for how long? *J Allergy Clin Immunol.* (2015) 136:1407–9. doi: 10.1016/j.jaci.2015.06.035
19. Rabbani B, Mahdieh N, Hosomichi K, Nakaoka H, Inoue I. Next-generation sequencing: impact of exome sequencing in characterizing Mendelian disorders. *J Hum Genet.* (2012) 57:621–32. doi: 10.1038/jhg.2012.91
20. Stessman HA, Bernier R, Eichler EE. A genotype-first approach to defining the subtypes of a complex disease. *Cell.* (2014) 156:872–7. doi: 10.1016/j.cell.2014.02.002
21. Jansen S, Hoischen A, Coe BP, Carvill GL, Van Esch H, Bosch DGM, et al. A genotype-first approach identifies an intellectual disability-overweight syndrome caused by PHIP haploinsufficiency. *Eur J Hum Genet.* (2018) 26:54-63. doi: 10.1038/s41431-017-0039-5
22. D'Amore A, Tessa A, Casali C, Dotti MT, Filla A, Silvestri G, et al. Next generation molecular diagnosis of hereditary spastic paraplegias: an Italian cross-sectional study. *Front Neurol.* (2018) 9:981. doi: 10.3389/fneur.2018.00981
23. Chae JH, Vasta V, Cho A, Lim BC, Zhang Q, Eun SH, et al. Utility of next generation sequencing in genetic diagnosis of early onset neuromuscular disorders. *J Med Genet.* (2015) 52:208–16. doi: 10.1136/jmedgenet-2014-102819
24. Waldrop MA, Pastore M, Schrader R, Sites E, Bartholomew D, Tsao CY, et al. Diagnostic utility of whole exome sequencing in the neuromuscular clinic. *Neuropediatrics.* (2019) 50):96–102. doi: 10.1055/s-0039-1677734
25. Al-Mousa H, Abouelhoda M, Monies DM, Al-Tassan N, Al-Ghonaium A, Al-Saud B, et al. Unbiased targeted next-generation sequencing molecular approach for primary immunodeficiency diseases. *J Allergy Clin Immunol.* (2016) 137:1780–7. doi: 10.1016/j.jaci.2015.12.1310
26. Gallo V, Dotta L, Giardino G, Cirillo E, Lougaris V, D'Assante R, et al. Diagnostics of primary immunodeficiencies through next-generation sequencing. *Front Immunol.* (2016) 7:466. doi: 10.3389/fimmu.2016.00466
27. Stoddard JL, Niemela JE, Fleisher TA, Rosenzweig SD. Targeted NGS: A cost-effective approach to molecular diagnosis of PIDs. *Front Immunol.* (2014) 5:531. doi: 10.3389/fimmu.2014.00531
28. Chi ZH, Wei W, Bu DF, Li HH, Ding F, Zhu P. Targeted high-throughput sequencing technique for the molecular diagnosis of primary immunodeficiency disorders. *Medicine.* (2018) 97:e12695. doi: 10.1097/MD.0000000000012695
29. Cifaldi C, Brigida I, Barzaghi F, Zoccolillo M, Ferradini V, Petricone D, et al. Targeted NGS platforms for genetic screening and gene discovery in primary immunodeficiencies. *Front Immunol.* (2019) 10:36. doi: 10.3389/fimmu.2019.00316
30. Rae W, Ward D, Mattocks C, Pengelly RJ, Eren E, Patel SV, et al. Clinical efficacy of a next-generation sequencing gene panel for primary immunodeficiency diagnostics. *Clin Genet.* (2018) 93:647–55. doi: 10.1111/cge.13163
31. Abolhassani H, Kiaee F, Tavakol M, Chavoshzadeh Z, Mahdaviani SA, Momen T, et al. Fourth update on the iranian national registry of primary immunodeficiencies: integration of molecular diagnosis. J Clin Immunol. (2018) 38:816–32. doi: 10.1007/s10875-018-0556-1
32. Al-Herz W, Chou J, Delmonte OM, Massaad MJ, Bainter W, Castagnoli R, et al. Comprehensive genetic results for primary immunodeficiency disorders in a highly consanguineous population. *Front Immunol.* (2018) 9:3146. doi: 10.3389/fimmu.2018.03146
33. Xia Y, He T, Luo Y, Li C, Lim CK, Abolhassani H, et al. Targeted next-generation sequencing for genetic diagnosis of 160 patients with primary immunodeficiency in south China. *Pediatr Allergy Immunol.* (2018) 29:863–72. doi: 10.1111/pai.12976
34. Al-Mousa H, Al-Saud B. Primary immunodeficiency diseases in highly consanguineous populations from middle east and north Africa: epidemiology, diagnosis, and care. *Front Immunol.* (2017) 8:678. doi: 10.3389/fimmu.2017.00678
35. Bogaert DJ, Dullaers M, Lambrecht BN, Vermaelen KY, De Baere E, Haerynck F. Genes associated with common variable immunodeficiency: one diagnosis to rule them all? *J Med Genet.* (2016) 53:575–90. doi: 10.1136/jmedgenet-2015-103690
36. Mahlaoui N, Picard C, Bach P, Costes L, Courteille V, Ranohavimparany A, et al. Genetic diagnosis of primary immunodeficiencies: a survey of the French national registry. *J Allergy Clin Immunol.* (2019) 143:1646–9. doi: 10.1016/j.jaci.2018.12.994
37. van der Burg M, van Zelm MC, Driessen GJ, van Dongen JJ. New frontiers of primary antibody deficiencies. *Cell Mol Life Sci.* (2012) 69:59–73. doi: 10.1007/s00018-011-0836-x
38. van der Burg M, van Zelm MC, Driessen GJ, van Dongen JJ. Dissection of B-cell development to unravel defects in patients with a primary antibody deficiency. *Adv Exp Med Biol.* (2011) 697:183–96. doi: 10.1007/978-1-4419-7185-2_13
39. Heimall JR, Hagin D, Hajjar J, Henrickson SE, Hernandez-Trujillo HS, Tan Y, et al. Use of Genetic testing for primary immunodeficiency patients. *J Clin Immunol.* (2018) 38:320–9. doi: 10.1007/s10875-018-0489-8
40. Abolhassani H, Wang N, Aghamohammadi A, Rezaei N, Lee YN, Frugoni F, et al. A hypomorphic recombination-activating gene 1 (RAG1) mutation resulting in a phenotype resembling common variable immunodeficiency. *J Allergy Clin Immunol.* (2014) 134:1375–80. doi: 10.1016/j.jaci.2014.04.042
41. Notarangelo LD, Kim MS, Walter JE, Lee YN. Human RAG mutations: biochemistry and clinical implications. *Nat Rev Immunol.* (2016) 16:234–46. doi: 10.1038/nri.2016.28
42. Rao VK, Webster S, Dalm V, Sediva A, van Hagen PM, Holland S, et al. Effective "activated PI3Kdelta syndrome"-targeted therapy with the PI3Kdelta inhibitor leniolisib. *Blood.* (2017) 130:2307–16. doi: 10.1182/blood-2017-08-801191
43. O'Gorman MR, Zollett J, Bensen N. Flow cytometry assays in primary immunodeficiency diseases. *Methods Mol Biol.* (2011) 699:317–35. doi: 10.1007/978-1-61737-950-5_15
44. Boldt A, Borte S, Fricke S, Kentouche K, Emmrich F, Borte M, et al. Eight-color immunophenotyping of T-, B-, and NK-cell subpopulations for characterization of chronic immunodeficiencies. *Cytom B Clincytom.* (2014) 86:191–206. doi: 10.1002/cytob.21162
45. Takashima T, Okamura M, Yeh TW, Okano T, Yamashita M, Tanaka K, et al. Multicolor flow cytometry for the diagnosis of primary immunodeficiency diseases. *J Clin Immunol.* (2017) 37:486–95. doi: 10.1007/s10875-017-0405-7
46. Abraham RS, Aubert G. Flow cytometry, a versatile tool for diagnosis and monitoring of primary immunodeficiencies. *Clinical Vacc Immunol.* (2016) 23:254–71. doi: 10.1128/CVI.00001-16
47. Oliveira JB, Notarangelo LD, Fleisher TA. Applications of flow cytometry for the study of primary immune deficiencies. *Curr Opinion Allergy Clin Immunol.* (2008) 8:499–509. doi: 10.1097/ACI.0b013e328312c790
48. Kanegane H, Hoshino A, Okano T, Yasumi T, Wada T, Takada H, et al. Flow cytometry-based diagnosis of primary immunodeficiency diseases. *Allergol Int.* (2018) 67:43–54. doi: 10.1016/j.alit.2017.06.003
49. Warnatz K, Wehr C, Drager R, Schmidt S, Eibel H, Schlesier M, et al. Expansion of CD19(hi)CD21(lo/neg) B cells in common variable immunodeficiency (CVID) patients with autoimmune cytopenia. *Immunobiology.* (2002) 206:502–13. doi: 10.1078/0171-2985-00198
50. Wehr C, Kivioja T, Schmitt C, Ferry B, Witte T, Eren E, et al. The EUROclass trial: defining subgroups in common variable immunodeficiency. *Blood.* (2008) 111:77–85. doi: 10.1182/blood-2007-06-091744
51. Biancotto A, Fuchs JC, Williams A, Dagur PK, McCoy JP, Jr. High dimensional flow cytometry for comprehensive leukocyte immunophenotyping (CLIP) in translational research. *J Immunol Method.* (2011) 363:245–61. doi: 10.1016/j.jim.2010.06.010
52. Maecker HT, McCoy JP, Nussenblatt R. Standardizing immunophenotyping for the human immunology project. *Nat Rev Immunol.* (2012) 12:191–200. doi: 10.1038/nri3158
53. Streitz M, Miloud T, Kapinsky M, Reed MR, Magari R, Geissler EK, et al. Standardization of whole blood immune phenotype monitoring for clinical trials: panels and methods from the ONE study. *Transplant Res.* (2013) 2:17. doi: 10.1186/2047-1440-2-17
54. Duffy D, Rouilly V, Libri V, Hasan M, Beitz B, David M, et al. Functional analysis via standardized whole-blood stimulation systems defines the boundaries of a healthy immune response to complex stimuli. *Immunity.* (2014) 40:436–50. doi: 10.1016/j.immuni.2014.03.002
55. Veluchamy JP, Delso-Vallejo M, Kok N, Bohme F, Seggewiss-Bernhardt R, van der Vliet HJ, et al. Standardized and flexible eight colour flow cytometry panels

harmonized between different laboratories to study human NK cell phenotype and function. *Sci Rep.* (2017) 7:43873. doi: 10.1038/srep43873

56. Blanco E, Perez-Andres M, Arriba-Mendez S, Contreras-Sanfeliciano T, Criado I, Pelak O, et al. Age-associated distribution of normal B-cell and plasma cell subsets in peripheral blood. *J Allergy Clin Immunol.* (2018) 141:2208–19.e16. doi: 10.1016/j.jaci.2018.02.017
57. Blanco E, Perez-Andres M, Arriba-Mendez S, Serrano C, Criado I, Pino-Molina LD, et al. Defects in memory B-cell and plasma cell subsets expressing different immunoglobulin-subclasses in CVID and Ig-subclass deficiencies. *J Allergy Clin Immunol.* (2019). doi: 10.1016/j.jaci.2019.02.017. [Epub ahead of print].
58. Blanco E, Perez-Andres M, Sanoja-Flores L, Wentink M, Pelak O, Martin-Ayuso M, et al. Selection and validation of antibody clones against IgG and IgA subclasses in switched memory B-cells and plasma cells. *J. Immunol Method.* (2017). doi: 10.1016/j.jim.2017.09.008. [Epub ahead of print].
59. van der Burg M, Kalina T, Perez-Andres M, Vlkova M, Lopez-Granados E, Blanco E, et al. The EuroFlow PID orientation tube for flow cytometric diagnostic screening of primary immunodeficiencies of the lymphoid system. *Front Immunol.* (2019) 10:246. doi: 10.3389/fimmu.2019.00246
60. van der Velden VH, Flores-Montero J, Perez-Andres M, Martin-Ayuso M, Crespo O, Blanco E, et al. Optimization and testing of dried antibody tube: The EuroFlow LST and PIDOT tubes as examples. *J Immunol Method.* (2017). doi: 10.1016/j.jim.2017.03.011. [Epub ahead of print].
61. van Dongen JJ, Lhermitte L, Bottcher S, Almeida J, van der Velden VH, Flores-Montero J, et al. EuroFlow antibody panels for standardized n-dimensional flow cytometric immunophenotyping of normal, reactive and malignant leukocytes. *Leukemia.* (2012) 26:1908–75. doi: 10.1038/leu.2012.120
62. Kalina T, Flores-Montero J, van der Velden VH, Martin-Ayuso M, Bottcher S, Ritgen M, et al. EuroFlow standardization of flow cytometer instrument settings and immunophenotyping protocols. *Leukemia.* (2012) 26:1986–2010. doi: 10.1038/leu.2012.122
63. Theunissen P, Mejstrikova E, Sedek L, van der Sluijs-Gelling AJ, Gaipa G, Bartels M, et al. Standardized flow cytometry for highly sensitive MRD measurements in B-cell acute lymphoblastic leukemia. *Blood.* (2017) 129:347–57. doi: 10.1182/blood-2016-07-726307
64. Flores-Montero J, Sanoja-Flores L, Paiva B, Puig N, Garcia-Sanchez O, Bottcher S, et al. Next generation flow for highly sensitive and standardized detection of minimal residual disease in multiple myeloma. *Leukemia.* (2017) 31:2094–103. doi: 10.1038/leu.2017.29
65. Lhermitte L, Mejstrikova E, van der Sluijs-Gelling AJ, Grigore GE, Sedek L, Bras AE, et al. Automated database-guided expert-supervised orientation for immunophenotypic diagnosis and classification of acute leukemia. *Leukemia.* (2018) 32:874-81. doi: 10.1038/leu.2017.313
66. Pedreira CE, Costa ES, Lecrevisse Q, van Dongen JJ, Orfao A. Overview of clinical flow cytometry data analysis: recent advances and future challenges. *Trends Biotechnol.* (2013) 31:415–25. doi: 10.1016/j.tibtech.2013.04.008
67. van Dongen JJ, van der Velden VH, Bruggemann M, Orfao A. Minimal residual disease diagnostics in acute lymphoblastic leukemia: need for sensitive, fast, and standardized technologies. *Blood.* (2015) 125:3996–4009. doi: 10.1182/blood-2015-03-580027
68. Novakova M, Glier H, Brdickova N, Vlkova M, Santos AH, Lima M, et al. How to make usage of the standardized EuroFlow 8-color protocols possible for instruments of different manufacturers. *J Immunol Method.* (2017). doi: 10.1016/j.jim.2017.11.007. [Epub ahead of print].
69. Diks, A. M., Bonroy, C., Teodosio, C., Groenland, R. J., De Mooij, B., De Maertelaere, E., et al. (in press). Impact of blood storage and sample handling on quality of high dimensional flow cytometric data in multicenter clinical research. *J. Immunol. Method.* doi: 10.1016/j.jim.2019.06.007
70. Bottcher S, van der Velden VHJ, Villamor N, Ritgen M, Flores-Montero J, Murua Escobar H, et al. Lot-to-lot stability of antibody reagents for flow cytometry. *J Immunol Method.* (2017). doi: 10.1016/j.jim.2017.03.018. [Epub ahead of print].
71. Kalina T, Flores-Montero J, Lecrevisse Q, Pedreira CE, van der Velden VH, Novakova M, et al. Quality assessment program for EuroFlow protocols: summary results of four-year (2010–2013) quality assurance rounds. *Cytom A.* (2015) 87:145–56. doi: 10.1002/cyto.a.22581
72. Kalina T, Brdickova N, Glier H, Fernandez P, Bitter M, Flores-Montero J, et al. Frequent issues and lessons learned from EuroFlow QA. Journal of immunological methods. (2018). doi: 10.1016/j.jim.2018.09.008. [Epub ahead of print].
73. Frenkel J, Neijens HJ, den Hollander JC, Wolvers-Tettero IL, van Dongen JJ. Oligoclonal T cell proliferative disorder in combined immunodeficiency. *Pediatric Res.* (1988) 24:622–7. doi: 10.1203/00006450-198811000-00017
74. Harville TO, Adams DM, Howard TA, Ware RE. Oligoclonal expansion of CD45RO+ T lymphocytes in Omenn syndrome. *J Clin Immunol.* (1997) 17:322–32. doi: 10.1023/A:1027330800085
75. Chan K, Puck JM. Development of population-based newborn screening for severe combined immunodeficiency. *J Allergy Clin Immunol.* (2005) 115:391–8. doi: 10.1016/j.jaci.2004.10.012
76. Brown L, Xu-Bayford J, Allwood Z, Slatter M, Cant A, Davies EG, et al. Neonatal diagnosis of severe combined immunodeficiency leads to significantly improved survival outcome: the case for newborn screening. *Blood.* (2011) 117:3243–6. doi: 10.1182/blood-2010-08-300384
77. Thakar MS, Hintermeyer MK, Gries MG, Routes JM, Verbsky JW. A practical approach to newborn screening for severe combined immunodeficiency using the t cell receptor excision circle assay. *Front Immunol.* (2017) 8:1470. doi: 10.3389/fimmu.2017.01470
78. Berkowska MA, Heeringa JJ, Hajdarbegovic E, van der Burg M, Thio HB, van Hagen PM, et al. Human IgE(+) B cells are derived from T cell-dependent and T cell-independent pathways. *J Allergy Clin Immunol.* (2014) 134:688–97.e6. doi: 10.1016/j.jaci.2014.03.036
79. JMF. *Jeffrey Modell Foundation: 4 Stages of Testing for Primary Immunodeficiency.* Available online at: http://downloads.info4pi.org/pdfs/Physician-Algorithm-2-.pdf (accessed May 25, 2019)
80. ESID. *European Society for Immunodeficiencies: The 6 ESID Warning Signs for ADULT Primary Immunodeficiency Diseases.* Available online at: https://esid.org/Education/6-Warning-Signs-for-PID-in-Adults (accessed May 25, 2019)
81. Criado I, Blanco E, Rodriguez-Caballero A, Alcoceba M, Contreras T, Gutierrez ML, et al. Residual normal B-cell profiles in monoclonal B-cell lymphocytosis versus chronic lymphocytic leukemia. *Leukemia.* (2018) 32:2701–5. doi: 10.1038/s41375-018-0164-3

6

The EuroFlow PID Orientation Tube for Flow Cytometric Diagnostic Screening of Primary Immunodeficiencies of the Lymphoid System

Mirjam van der Burg[1,2†], Tomas Kalina[3†], Martin Perez-Andres[4,5†], Marcela Vlkova[6], Eduardo Lopez-Granados[7], Elena Blanco[4,5], Carolien Bonroy[8], Ana E. Sousa[9], Anne-Kathrin Kienzler[10], Marjolein Wentink[1], Ester Mejstríková[3], Vendula Šinkorova[3], Jan Stuchly[3], Menno C. van Zelm[11], Alberto Orfao[4,5] and Jacques J. M. van Dongen[1,12] on behalf of the EuroFlow PID consortium*

[1] *Department of Immunology, Erasmus MC, Rotterdam, Netherlands,* [2] *Department of Pediatrics, Laboratory for Immunology, Leiden University Medical Center, Leiden, Netherlands,* [3] *Department of Paediatric Haematology and Oncology, Second Faculty of Medicine, Charles University and University Hospital Motol, Prague, Czechia,* [4] *Department of Medicine, Cancer Research Centre (IBMCC, USAL-CSIC), Cytometry Service (NUCLEUS), University of Salamanca (USAL), Institute of Biomedical Research of Salamanca (IBSAL), Salamanca, Spain,* [5] *Biomedical Research Networking Centre Consortium of Oncology (CIBERONC), Instituto de Salud Carlos III, Madrid, Spain,* [6] *Institute of Clinical Immunology and Allergology, St Anne's University Hospital, Brno, Czechia,* [7] *Immunology, Universitario La Paz, Madrid, Spain,* [8] *Laboratory for Clinical Biology and Hematology, University Hospital Ghent, Ghent, Belgium,* [9] *Faculdade de Medicina, Instituto de Medicina Molecular, Universidade de Lisboa, Lisbon, Portugal,* [10] *BRC-Translational Immunology Lab, University of Oxford, Oxford, United Kingdom,* [11] *Department of Immunology and Pathology, Central Clinical School, Monash University, Melbourne, VIC, Australia,* [12] *Department of Immunohematology and Blood Transfusion, Leiden University Medical Center, Leiden, Netherlands*

***Correspondence:**
Jacques J. M. van Dongen
j.j.m.van_dongen@lumc.nl

† *These authors have contributed equally to this work*

In the rapidly evolving field of primary immunodeficiencies (PID), the EuroFlow consortium decided to develop a PID orientation and screening tube that facilitates fast, standardized, and validated immunophenotypic diagnosis of lymphoid PID, and allows full exchange of data between centers. Our aim was to develop a tool that would be universal for all lymphoid PIDs and offer high sensitivity to identify a lymphoid PID (without a need for specificity to diagnose particular PID) and to guide and prioritize further diagnostic modalities and clinical management. The tube composition has been defined in a stepwise manner through several cycles of design-testing-evaluation-redesign in a multicenter setting. Equally important appeared to be the standardized pre-analytical procedures (sample preparation and instrument setup), analytical procedures (immunostaining and data acquisition), the software analysis (a multidimensional view based on a reference database in Infinicyt software), and data interpretation. This standardized EuroFlow concept has been tested on 250 healthy controls and 99 PID patients with defined genetic defects. In addition, an application of new EuroFlow software tools with multidimensional pattern recognition was designed with inclusion of maturation pathways in multidimensional patterns (APS plots). The major advantage of the EuroFlow approach is that data can be fully exchanged between different laboratories in any country of the world, which is especially of interest for the PID field, with generally low numbers of cases per center.

Keywords: flow cytometric immunophenotyping, primary immunodeficiencies, automated gating strategy, standardization, EuroFlow

INTRODUCTION

Primary immunodeficiencies (PID) of the lymphoid system are rare inherited disorders with heterogeneous clinical presentations (1, 2). Most patients have clinical manifestations of immune dysfunction such as recurrent infections (early in life), and autoimmunity frequently causing irreversible organ damage in case of delayed diagnosis. As a consequence fast and efficient diagnostic screening is required. Advanced multicolor flow cytometry serves on this need. Flow cytometric immunophenotyping of T, B, and NK cells is the classically recommended method in the diagnostic work-up in case of a suspicion of PID of the lymphoid system. The complete diagnosis and classification consists of stepwise screening and subsequent characterization for numerical alterations in lymphocyte (sub) populations, detection of functional defects, and functional assays. However, lack of standardization and the rarity of PID has so far complicated a common strategy in PID diagnostics.

The introduction and the availability of next generation sequencing (NGS) based on targeted panel sequencing or whole exome sequencing (WES) with a filter for PID genes has an important impact on PID diagnostics in identification of the variants in known PID genes (3, 4). Moreover, it contributes to the broadening of the clinical spectrum of known PIDs. Finally, WES and whole genome sequencing (WGS) allows the identification of genetic defects in new PID candidate genes. However, the turnaround time is relatively long (i.e., a couple of months in a routine diagnostic setting) in contrast to flow cytometry, which already provides complete insight into the composition of the lymphoid compartment within a day. For correct interpretation of NGS data, it is crucial that the immunophenotype is known. Furthermore, flow cytometry can play an important role in the functional validation of genetic variants to evaluate the impact on the immune system. Altogether, this illustrates that both NGS and flow cytometry are valuable tools in PID diagnostics.

In this study, we developed a PID screening and orientation tube which allows fast and robust detection and enumeration of the lymphocyte subsets. It is important to notice that more than 70% of all PID concern inborn defects in the lymphoid system. Orientation in an early phase of the diagnostic process forms the basis for consecutive diagnostics, treatment, and clinical management. Therefore, we need a PID screening and orientation tube (PIDOT) which allows dissection of especially the lymphoid compartment in peripheral blood with full standardization to allow international comparability of results.

METHODS

Patient and Control Samples

Peripheral blood samples were collected from 250 healthy controls divided into 14 age groups: cord blood ($n = 15$), neonatal blood ($n = 16$), 1-5 month ($n = 12$), 5-11 m ($n = 7$), 12-24 m ($n = 30$), 2-4 years ($n = 35$), 5-9y ($n = 28$), 10-17y ($n = 18$), 18-29y ($n = 31$), 30-39y ($n = 15$), 40-49y ($n = 12$), 50-59y ($n = 10$), 60-69y ($n = 10$), >70y ($n = 11$). Healthy controls were selected as having no signs or suspicion of immunological or hematological diseases (including an abnormal infection rate or a known history of allergies). All individuals were vaccinated following similar national vaccination schedules (European Center for Disease Prevention and Control; *http://vaccine-schedule.ecdc.europa.eu/Pages/Scheduler.aspx*). They were enrolled at the different EuroFlow laboratories after informed consent was provided by each subject, their legal representatives, or both, according to the Declaration of Helsinki. In addition 99 patients with a genetically defined PID were collected according to the local medical ethics regulations of the participating centers. All samples were collected after informed consent was provided by the subjects, their legal representatives, or both, according to the Declaration of Helsinki. The study was approved by the local ethics committees of the participating centers [University of Salamanca, Salamanca, Spain (USAL-CSIC 20-02-2013); Charles University, Prague, Czech Republic (15-28541A); Erasmus MC, Rotterdam, The Netherlands (MEC-2013-026); University Hospital Ghent, Belgium (B670201523515) and St Anne's University, Brno, Czech Republic(METC 1G2015)].

Assessment of Absolute Numbers of B, T, and NK Cells

The absolute number of lymphocytes (B, T, and NK cells) was determined either in a separate TrueCount (BD) tube with anti-CD45 PerCP alone or BD Multitest™ CD3/CD16+CD56/CD45/CD19 or it was determined by hematological analyser as a part of a diagnostic workup.

Design of the PID Screening Tube

The PID screening tube was designed to assess the composition of the lymphoid compartment in a single 8-color labeling for guiding diagnosis of PID patients via detecting all relevant subpopulations. To this end, at certain fluorochrome positions two markers, i.e., a B-cell and a T-cell marker were combined of which is absolutely secured that they are exclusively expressed on only one of the subsets. So, two similarly labeled antibodies defining two distinct populations are mixed. CD19 was combined with TCRγδ, CD4 with IgM, and CD8 with IgD. CD16 and CD56 were already combined on the same channel for detection of NK cells. In addition to the above mentioned markers, we included CD3, CD45, CD27, and CD45RA. The optimal combination of clones and fluorochromes was reached after four rounds of testing in the participating centers (**Supplementary Table 1**). In order to achieve higher sensitivity to low abundant cell types, we used a lyse-stain-wash-fix protocol and the antibody staining time was increased to 30 min (6). This optimized staining procedure yielded more acquired cells (lymphocyte event counts were in average 2.89×10^{e5} in healthy controls and 1.32×10^{e5} in PID patients) per sample with less non-leukocyte particles (less debris), and yielded higher median fluorescence intensity (MFI) patterns for several antibodies (**Figure S1**). The data were acquired on BD LSRII or BD FACSCanto II instruments with the standard EuroFlow instrument settings (7). For data analysis, the Infinicyt software (Cytognos SL, Salamanca, Spain) was used in parallel to local data analysis software programs FACS Diva (BD) and FlowJo (FlowJo, LLC, Ashland, OR, USA). Infinicyt software is a commercially available product from Cytognos SL

(Salamanca Spain) and a free-dowload demo version is available at www.infinicyt.com.

Analysis of Lymphocyte Subsets in Healthy Controls

The lymphoid PID screening tube was used for analysis of 250 healthy controls of different ages to define the patterns and to set the reference for the database. All samples were analyzed in conventional analysis software programs (FlowJo and FACSDiva) and using Infinicyt Software. In both software packages the same analysis strategy was followed for definition of the lymphocyte subsets. Percentile ranges were calculated for each age group, for unified overview in **Figure S2** values in patients compared to two or five standard deviations of controls were used.

Analysis of Genetically Defined PID Patients

Next we tested the lymphoid PID screening tube on 99 genetically defined PID patients. The patients were classified according to the IUIS classification, which divides PID into 8 categories. First, the absolute number and relative frequencies of the lymphocyte subset populations were determined in all patients. This data set formed the basis for development of our new approach for flow cytometry in PID.

Statistical Analyses

Mean and range values were calculated for all continuous variables using the SPSS statistical software (SPSS software v23, IBM, Armonk, NY). Data files from 50 healthy donors were merged and lymphocytes subsets of interest identified using bivariate plots (Figure). This analysis was used to define in an n-dimensional space the best principal component analysis 1 (PC1) vs. PC2 representation to discriminate these subsets using the Infinicyt software. The PCA representation of the data is graphically summarized in 2 × Standard Deviation (SD) curves to be used as a reference for supervised automatic analysis of the samples (APS view; **Figures 3–5**). In order to graphically display an overview of abnormalities found in a PID group adjusted to age, we calculated a relative distance from age matched healthy controls for each value in each PID case as a number of standard deviations (SD) from healthy controls. Values below−2 SD or above 2 SD are considered abnormal. Repeatedly abnormal values (in a given PID disease group) are plotted in supplementary figures. Calculations and graphic displays of the discriminating parameters (**Supplementary Figure 2**) were created using R-project/ Bioconductor *http://www.r-project.org* and Microsoft Excel for Mac 2011 (Redmont, WA, USA).

RESULTS

Multidimensional Analysis of the EuroFlow PID Orientation Tube

In this study, we aimed to advance flow cytometric immunophenotyping of PID patients by linking the flow cytometric data to potential immunological defects and by incorporating this approach into the diagnostic process. To this end, we designed a PID orientation tube (PIDOT) (8 colors; 14 parameters) that allowed the analysis of all main lymphocyte subpopulations in a single standardized and validated tube (**Table 1**, **Figure 1**). After gating leukocytes as CD45+ and lymphocytes on FSc and SSc, the markers CD3,

TABLE 1 | Composition of the EuroFlow PID Screening tube and information of monoclonal antibodies used in the PID screening tube including volumes, clones, and suppliers.

BV421	BV510	FITC	PE	PerCP-Cy5,5	PC7/PE-Cy7	APC	APC-H7
CD27	CD45RA	CD8	CD16	CD4	CD19	CD3	CD45
		IgD	CD56	IgM	TCRgd		

Marker	Fluorochrome	Clone	Source	Catalog number	µl/test
CD3	APC	SK7	BD Biosciences	345767	2.5
CD4	PerCPC5.5	SK3	BD Biosciences	332772	7
CD8	FITC	SKI	BD Biosciences	345772	5
CD16	PE	3G8	BD Biosciences	555407	5
CD19	PECy7	J3-119	Beckman Coulter	IM3628	5
CD27	BV421	M-T271	BD Biosciences	562513	1
CD27 alternative	BV421	O323	BioLegend	302823	1
CD45	APCH7	2D1	BD Biosciences	641417	2
CD45RA	BV510	HI100	BD Biosciences	563031	2.5
CD45RA alternative	BV510	HI100	Biolegend	304141	2.5
CD56	PE	C5.9	Cytognos	CYT-56PE	5
SmIgD	FITC	IA6-2	BioLegend	348205	1.25
SmIgM	PerCPCy5.5	MHM-88	BioLegend	314511	2
TCRγδ	PECy7	11F2	BD Biosciences	649806	1

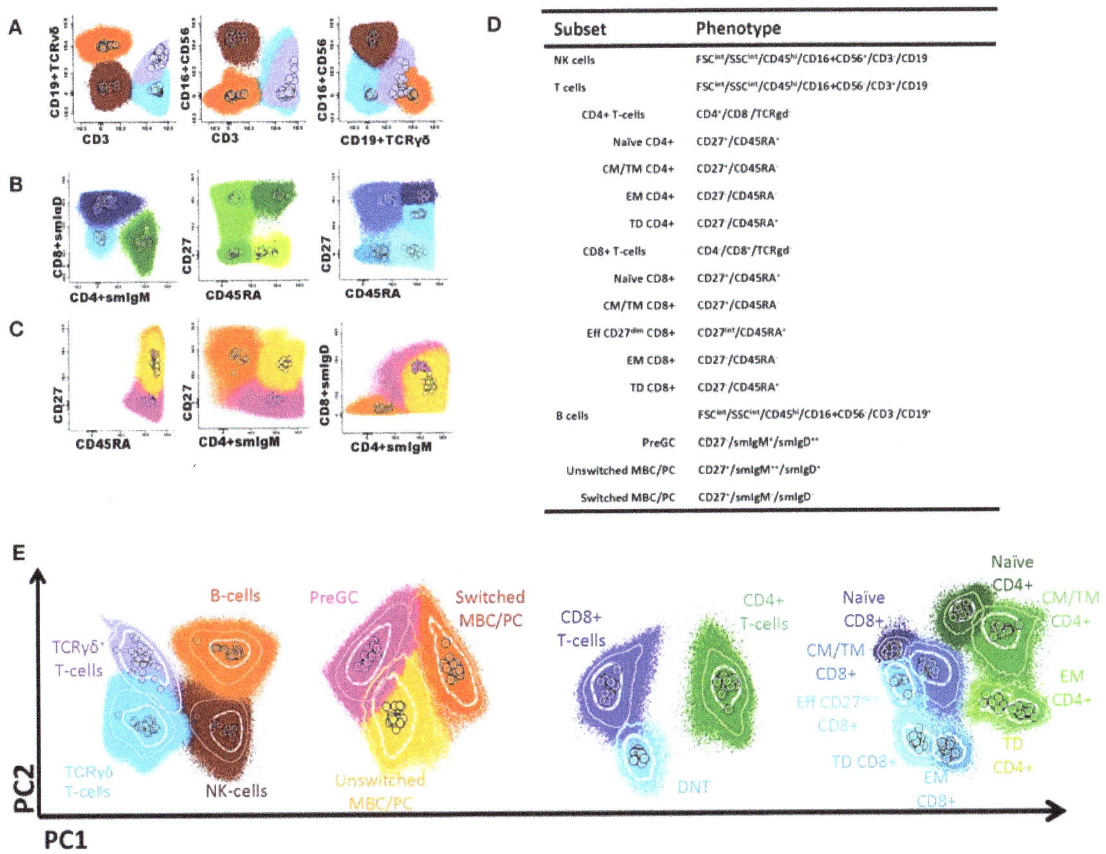

Subset	Phenotype
NK cells	$FSC^{int}/SSC^{int}/CD45^{hi}/CD16{+}CD56^{+}/CD3^{-}/CD19^{-}$
T cells	$FSC^{int}/SSC^{int}/CD45^{hi}/CD16{+}CD56^{-}/CD3^{+}/CD19^{-}$
CD4+ T-cells	$CD4^{+}/CD8^{-}/TCRgd^{-}$
Naïve CD4+	$CD27^{+}/CD45RA^{+}$
CM/TM CD4+	$CD27^{+}/CD45RA^{-}$
EM CD4+	$CD27^{-}/CD45RA^{-}$
TD CD4+	$CD27^{-}/CD45RA^{+}$
CD8+ T-cells	$CD4^{-}/CD8^{+}/TCRgd^{-}$
Naïve CD8+	$CD27^{+}/CD45RA^{+}$
CM/TM CD8+	$CD27^{+}/CD45RA^{-}$
Eff $CD27^{dim}$ CD8+	$CD27^{int}/CD45RA^{+}$
EM CD8+	$CD27^{-}/CD45RA^{-}$
TD CD8+	$CD27^{-}/CD45RA^{+}$
B cells	$FSC^{int}/SSC^{int}/CD45^{hi}/CD16{+}CD56^{-}/CD3^{-}/CD19^{+}$
PreGC	$CD27^{-}/smIgM^{+}/smIgD^{++}$
Unswitched MBC/PC	$CD27^{+}/smIgM^{++}/smIgD^{+}$
Switched MBC/PC	$CD27^{+}/smIgM^{-}/smIgD^{-}$

FIGURE 1 | Flow cytometric analysis of B- and T-cell populations using the EuroFlow PID screening tube, 50 healthy controls are shown in the same plot, median of each gated subset is shown as a circle. **(A)** After gating leukocytes as CD45+ and lymphocytes on FSc and SSc, the markers CD3, CD19 in combination with TCRγδ and CD16+56 were used to define B-cells (orange); TCRγδ+ T-cells (lilac); TCRγδ- T-cells (blue); and NK cells (brown). **(B)** The T-cell subsets were further subdivided into naïve (CD27+CD45RA+; dark green), central memory/transitional memory (CM/TM; CD27+CD45RA-; bright green), effector memory (EM; CD27-CD45RA-; green) and terminally differentiated (TD; CD27-CD45RA+; light green) CD4+ T cells and into naïve (CD27+CD45RA+; purple), CM/TM (CD27+CD45RA-; dark blue), EM (CD27-CD45-; pale blue), and TD (CD27-CD45RA+; turqoise) CD8+ T cells. Also, as previously reported (5), some effector CD8+ T-cells showed dim CD27 positivity (EffCD27dim; CD27int-CD45RA+; blue). CD4/CD8 double negative T-cells are indicated in light blue. **(C)** B-cell subsets could be further subdivided into pre germinal center (PreGC; $IgM^{+}IgD^{+}CD27^{-}$; orange) unswitched memory B-cells/plasma cells (Unswitched MBC/PC; $IgM^{+}IgD^{+/-}CD27^{+}$; yellow), switched memory MBC/PC ($IgM^{-}IgD^{-}CD27^{+}$; pink). **(D)** Definition and hierarchy of the defined subsets. **(E)** Multidimensional view (APS view) based on the most discriminating parameters for lymphocytes, B-cell, T-cells, and T-cell subsets.

CD19 in combination with TCRγδ and CD16+56 were used to define B-cells, TCRγδ+ or TCRγδ- T-cells and NK cells (**Figure 1A**). The T-cell subsets were further subdivided into naïve, central memory (CM)/transitional memory (TM), effector memory and terminally differentiated (TD) CD4+/CD8+ T cells (**Figures 1B,D**); for CD8+ T-cells one extra population, effector $CD27^{dim}$ was defined. Also CD4-CD8- (double negative) T-cells were defined (5). B-cell subsets were further subdivided into pre germinal center B-cells (PreGC), unswitched memory B-cells (MBC) or plasma cells (PC), and switched MBC **Figures 1C,D**) (8, 9). The total set and hierarchy of lymphocyte subsets that was identified is listed in **Figure 1D**.

To offer intuitive and fast interpretation of the complete lymphoid compartment we developed a new analysis and visualization strategy for the PIDOT using a principle component analysis based multidimensional view (APS graph). First, reference plots were generated using a set of 30 samples of healthy donors in Infinicyt software. The lymphocyte populations were manually analyzed and subsequently, the most discriminating projection into a single APS graph was determined (**Figure 1E**).

Reference Values and Database

Subsequently, this analysis strategy and visualization was tested on 250 healthy controls in 14 different age ranges, which resulted in a unique reference data set of all lymphocyte subsets. All values of this reference data set are displayed as bar graphs representing the median, minimum, maximum, and p10, p25, p75, and p90 percentiles in **Figure 2**. Finally, 99 genetically defined PID patients were analyzed to study the performance of the EuroFlow PIDOT (**Table 2**).

PID With Absence or Strong Reduction in One or More Lymphocyte Subsets

The two main categories of PID with absence or strong reduction in one or more lymphocyte subsets are SCID and agammaglobulinemia with absent T (NK) and/or B-cells.

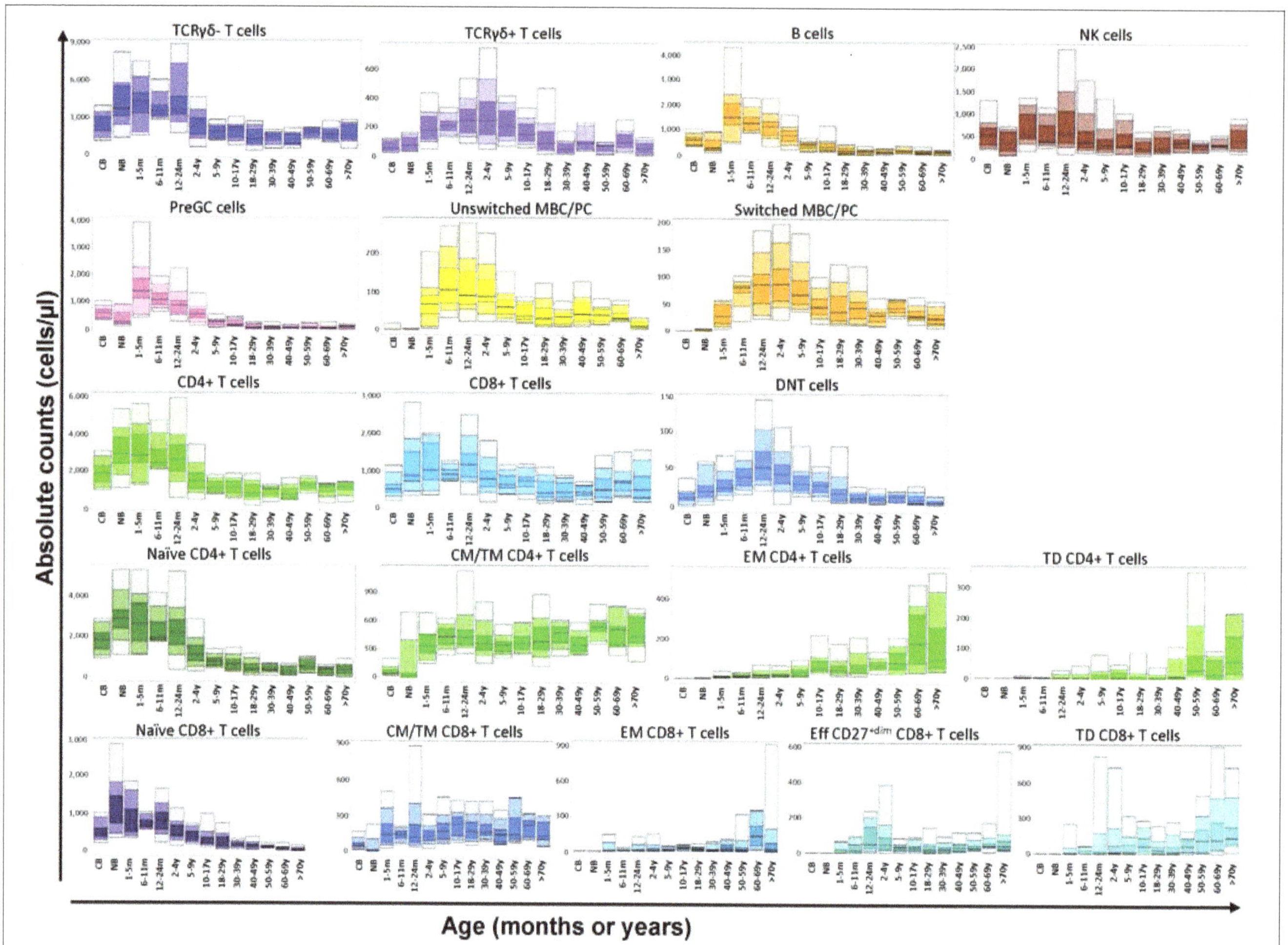

FIGURE 2 | Flow cytometric analysis of B- and T-cell populations using the EuroFlow PIDOT in 250 healthy controls in 14 different age ranges. All values of this reference data set are displayed as bar graphs representing the median, minimum, maximum, and p10, p25, p75, and p90 percentiles. For data visualization package gplot2 for the statistical language R was used (10).

SCID

Absence or strong reduction of lymphocyte subsets (B, NK, CD4, and CD8 T-cells) can be easily established by comparison of absolute numbers of lymphocyte subsets of patient vs. age-matched reference values. We analyzed patients with RAG1 ($n = 8$), RAG2 ($n = 5$), Artemis ($n = 3$), IL2RG ($n = 6$), IL7RA ($n = 1$), and ZAP70 ($n = 3$) deficiencies. In all patients the CD3-positive T-cells were strongly reduced, except for one patient with a RAG2 deficiency who presented with a high number of T-cells. In ZAP70 deficient patients, CD8-positive T-cells were reduced and in one of them also the CD4-positive T-cells, although to a lesser extent. NK cells, however, show a more heterogenous/variable pattern. This illustrates that NK cell numbers cannot straightforwardly be used for classification and it supports the idea to leave out NK cells for classification (11, 12). In addition to evaluation of the absolute counts, the APS views provide insight into the distribution of the lymphocyte subsets. RAG deficiencies can give a broad spectrum of clinical and immunological phenotypes. This partly depends on the type of mutation and the residual V(D)J recombinase activity (13–15). On top of that, the same mutation can also be associated with clinical heterogeneity (14). This phenomenon is also reflected in the APS profiles of RAG deficiencies (**Figure 3A**). RAG1, RAG2 as well as Artemis deficiencies with a null mutation will result in complete absence of B and T cells (RAG-1 patient A in **Figure 3A**). However, in case of a leaky or hypomorphic mutation T-cells are present (RAG-1 patient B in **Figure 3A**), which are in this case all TCRγδ- and had a memory or effector T-cell phenotype. In such situation the origin of T-cells need to be determined to investigate whether these T-cells are autologous or from maternal origin. A third pattern that can be seen is the presence of both T and B cells (RAG patient C and D). In both cases both TCRγδ- and TCRγδ+ T-cells are present (with a memory or effector phenotype) and the B-cells were mainly naïve or natural effector. No switched memory B cells or plasma cells were detected. So, the hallmark for RAG deficiencies with residual T-cells, which is characteristic for Omenn Syndrome, is absence or strong reduction of naïve CD4 and CD8 T-cells.

TABLE 2 | Frequency of patients with inborn errors of immunity showing defects of the major subsets identified in the EF PIDOT, as compared to age-reference values (Summary of **Supplementary Tables 2, 3**).

	Any T cell subset	Any B cells subset	NK cells	Any of them
SCID (*n* = 24)	100%	100%	25%	100%
IL2Rg	6/6	6/6	5/6	6/6
IL7R	1/1	1/1	0/1	1/1
RAG1	8/8	8/8	1/8	8/8
RAG2	5/5	5/5	0/5	5/5
DCLRE1C	3/3	3/3	0/3	3/3
NHEJI	1/1	1/1	0/1	1/1
CID (*n* = 12)	58%	83%	25%	100%
CD40L	1/6	6/6	0/6	6/6
ZAP70	3/3	1/3	0/3	3/3
DOCK8	2/2	2/2	2/2	2/2
BCL10	1/1	1/1	1/1	1/1
CID with syndromic features (*n* = 20)	70%	60%	10%	75%
WASp	3/3	3/3	0/3	3/3
ATM	5/6	4/6	0/6	5/6
Di George	3/6	1/6	0/6	3/6
STAT3	1/2	2/2	1/2	2/2
NEMO	1/2	1/2	0/2	1/2
PNP	1/1	1/1	1/1	1/1
PAD (*n* = 16)	31%	100%	25%	100%
BTK	1/10	10/10	1/10	10/10
PIK3CD	4/5	5/5	3/5	5/5
AID	0/1	1/1	0/1	1/1
Disease of immune dysregulation (*n* = 10)	70%	60%	10%	90%
Syntaxin	1/1	1/1	0/1	1/1
FAS	5/5	2/5	1/5	5/5
XLP	0/1	1/1	0/1	1/1
CD27	1/1	1/1	0/1	1/1
CTPS1	0/2	1/2	0/2	1/2
Defects of phagocytes or function (*n* = 10)	30%	60%	40%	70%
CGD	1/5	3/5	1/5	3/5
GATA2	2/5	3/5	3/5	4/5
Defects innate immunity (*n* = 3)	67%	67%	33%	67%
STAT1	1/1	1/1	1/1	1/1
WHIM	1/1	1/1	0/1	1/1
IRAK4	0/1	0/1	0/1	0/1
Complement deficiencies (*n* = 4)	0%	0%	0%	0%

Results expressed as percentage of patients showing absolute counts below the lower limit of normality, compared to age-reference values obtained from 250 healthy donors analyzed with the same protocol. SCID, Severe Combined Immunodeficiency; CID, Combined Immunodeficiency; PAD, Predominantly Antibody Deficiency.

In IL2RG, IL7RA and ZAP70 deficiencies B-cell numbers were normal. IL2RG and IL7RA deficiency have in common that all B-cells have a naïve phenotype, which is in line with the fact that T-cell help is lacking for further differentiation (**Figure 3B**). In the ZAP70 deficiency some natural effector and switched memory B-cells are present. In case T-cells were present in patients with IL2RG deficiency, they had a memory phenotype (IL2RG B and C, **Figure 3B**).

Agammaglobulinemia

A second clear cut example in which lymphocyte subset analysis is highly informative in PID diagnostics is absence of B-cells in the 10 patients with X-linked agammaglobulinemia. The absolute number of B-cells is strongly reduced or the B-cells are even absent. As shown by the APS plots, if B-cells are present, they only have a naive phenotype (**Figure 4A**). The advantage of this approach is that on top of the maturation pathway that can be visualized with the APS plots, novel information can be obtained. The expression level within the naïve B-cells is shifted, indicating that the phenotype of this population also differs from normal.

Disturbed Distribution Patterns of Lymphocyte Subsets in PID

In certain PID a specific distribution of lymphocyte subsets can be observed, which serves as a hallmark of the disease. A genetic defect in CD40L results in disturbed B-T interaction and consequently in reduced generation of (switched) memory B-cells that are T-cell dependent (16). As shown in a representative case, patients with CD40L deficiency have normal numbers of total B-cells, but they mainly consist of naïve or unswitched memory B-cells (**Figure 4A**). A second example is autoimmune lymphoproliferative disease (ALPS) mainly caused by mutations in FAS and FASL, which is characterized by the presence of a high frequency of TCRαβ+CD4-CD8- T-cells (i.e., double negative T-cells) (**Figure 4A, Figure S2**). Disturbed distributions of lymphocyte subsets or combinations of lymphocyte subsets can also be observed in other PID cases such as patients with WAS, ATM, DOCK8 deficiency, or DiGeorge syndrome (**Figure 4B**). However, these altered distribution profiles must be interpreted in the context of age-matched healthy controls. Therefore, correct interpretation relies on both patterns and absolute numbers.

We integrated the data of the total cohort of genetically-defined PID patients and the total set of healthy controls to define which lymphocyte subsets were abnormal (i.e., the absolute counts below the lower limit of normal, compared to age-reference values) and calculated the percentage of patients showing abnormal values (**Table 2** and **Supplementary Tables 2, 3**). Per disease category the frequency of patients with defects in any of the lymphoid subsets detected with the EuroFlow PIDOT was determined. Naïve CD4, naïve CD8, and swiched memory B-cells were the most frequently aberrant populations (**Figure S2**). For example, in the category SCID all patients had aberrancies in any of the T-cell subpopulations or in any of the B-cell populations. More specifically, in all patients naïve T cells as well as unswitched and switched memory B-cells were reduced. **Supplementary Tables 2, 3** give a further break down per T and B-cell subset. In other PID categories similar characteristic abnormalities were observed. For CID and PAD it was expected that aberrancies in lymphoid subsets are expected, but this dataset shows that also in patients with immune dysregulation

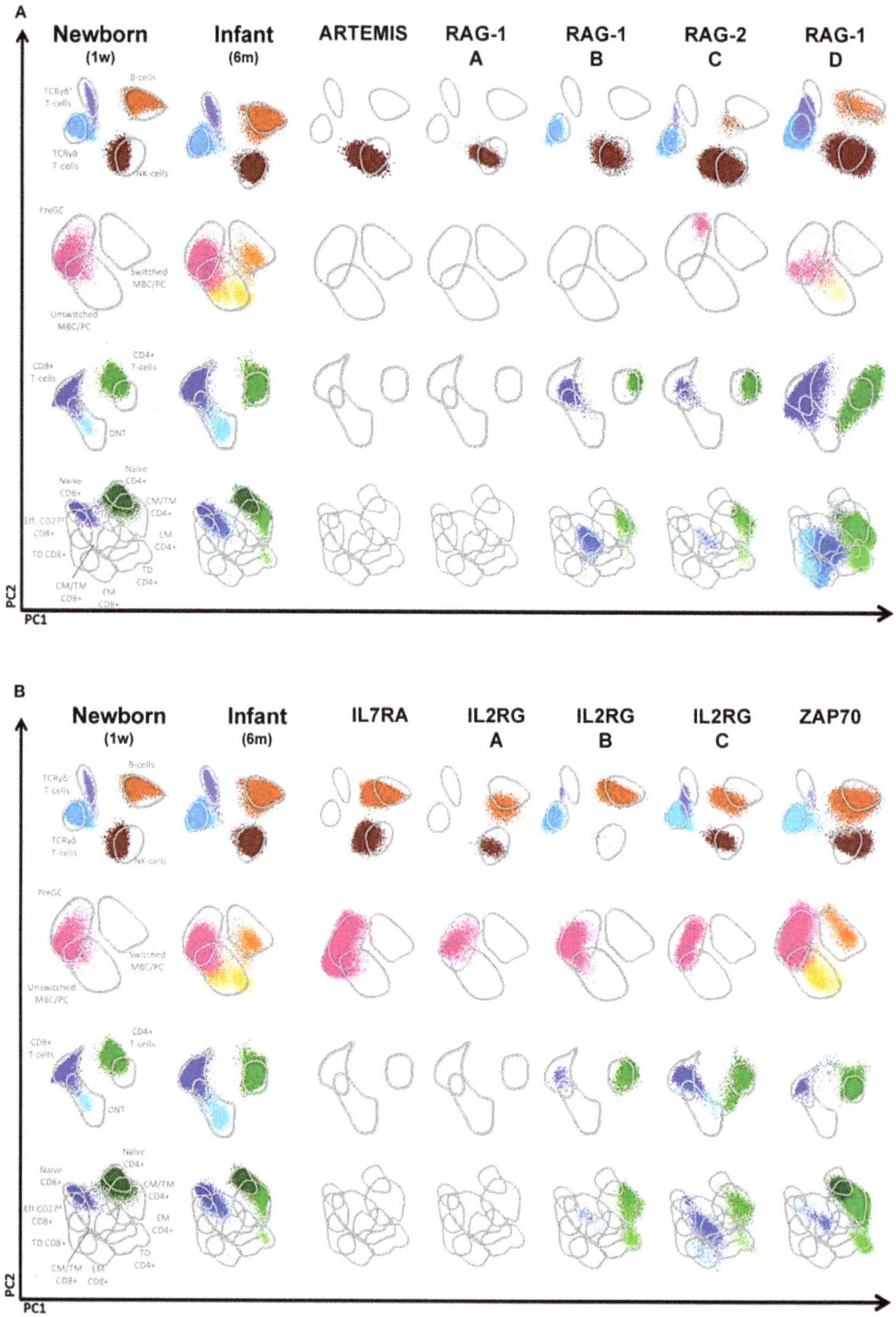

FIGURE 3 | Flowcytometric analysis of B- and T-cell populations using the EuroFlow PID screening tube on controls and patients with SCID. From the top down, APS plots of gated lymphocytes, B-cells, CD3+ T cells and TCRgd- T cells are shown. Lines depict a 2 standard deviation boundary of all controls combined. **(A)** Multidimensional views of all lymphocyte subsets of a newborn, an infant, one Artemis-deficient and four RAG-deficient SCID patients. **(B)** Multidimensional views of all lymphocyte subsets of a newborn, one IL7RA-deficient, three IL2RG-deficient and a ZAP70-deficient patient.

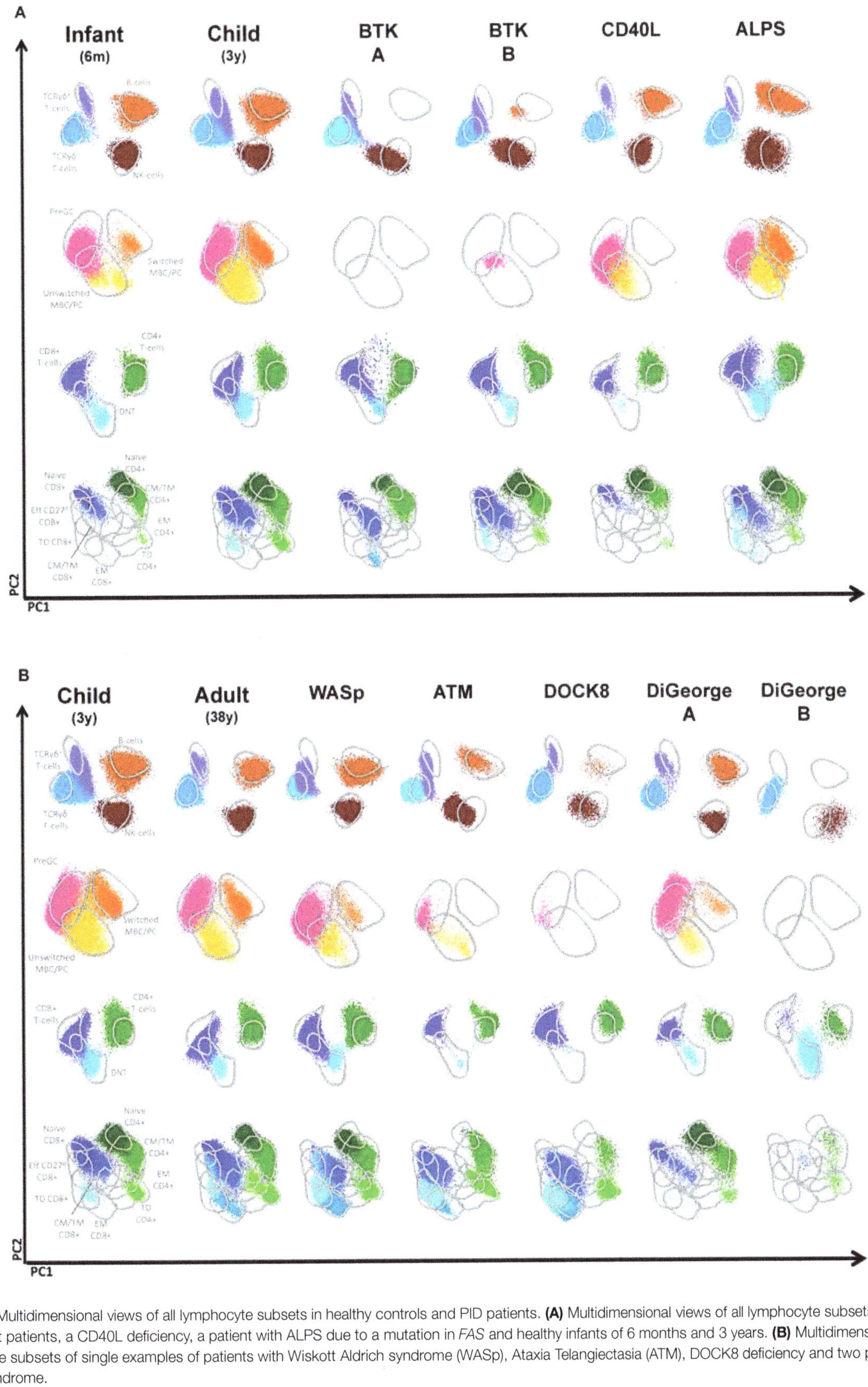

FIGURE 4 | Multidimensional views of all lymphocyte subsets in healthy controls and PID patients. **(A)** Multidimensional views of all lymphocyte subsets of two BTK-deficient patients, a CD40L deficiency, a patient with ALPS due to a mutation in *FAS* and healthy infants of 6 months and 3 years. **(B)** Multidimensional views of all lymphocyte subsets of single examples of patients with Wiskott Aldrich syndrome (WASp), Ataxia Telangiectasia (ATM), DOCK8 deficiency and two patients with DiGeorge syndrome.

and defects in phagocyte and innate immunity aberrancies were found with high frequencies. This illustrates that the PIDOT is a powerful tool to detect aberrancies in a broad range of PID with lymphocyte defects. As expected the PIDOT did not give any abnormalities in complement deficiencies, since these PIDs do not display any lymphocytes' derangement.

Automated Analysis

The advantage of the large reference data set of normal samples and well-annotated PID patient samples is that it can serve as templates for prospective data analysis. In the Infinicyt software program, an automatic analysis option has been included, which can be applied on all samples provided that the samples were processed, stained and measured according to the standardized EuroFlow protocols. Also in case the lyophilized version of the PIDOT is used, the data can be analyzed via this strategy (17). This new feature provides per patient the multidimensional APS plot, the absolute values of the lymphocyte subsets plotted in the age-matched bar graph and the numerical table with values for direct uploading in the electronic laboratory management and patient systems. For a patient with APDS and GATA2 the output is visualized in **Figure 5**. For the APDS patient this representation clearly shows the combination of low level of B-cells–preGC and especially (switched) memory B-cells, low naïve CD4 and CD8 cells and an expansion of the memory CD8 cell fractions, which is characteristic for APDS (18). Also for the GATA2-deficient patient displayed, the combined data show some characteristic features: reduced B and NK cells in combination with numbers of T-cell subsets which were below median but still within the normal range. **Table 2** and **Supplementary Tables 2, 3** can be consulted to verify how representative an immunophenotype is for a given genetically defined PID. This new application of EuroFlow software tools support diagnosis of PID.

DISCUSSION

In this study, we designed a single flow cytometry staining tube, PIDOT, for analysis of defined B and T cell subsets and validated its sensitivity performance on 250 healthy controls and 99 genetically-defined and IUIS-classified PID patients. This tube is fully standardized with the aim to have fully comparable data for international exchange of data and to support diagnosis of PID. With the multicenter EuroFlow approach, the PIDOT was designed over multiple rounds of design, testing in multiple labs, evaluation, and redesign. In addition, an application of new EuroFlow software tools with multidimensional pattern recognition was designed with inclusion of maturation pathways in multidimensional patterns (APS plots). Finally, we created a reference data base for automated data analysis, which can be implemented in diagnostic laboratories for routine

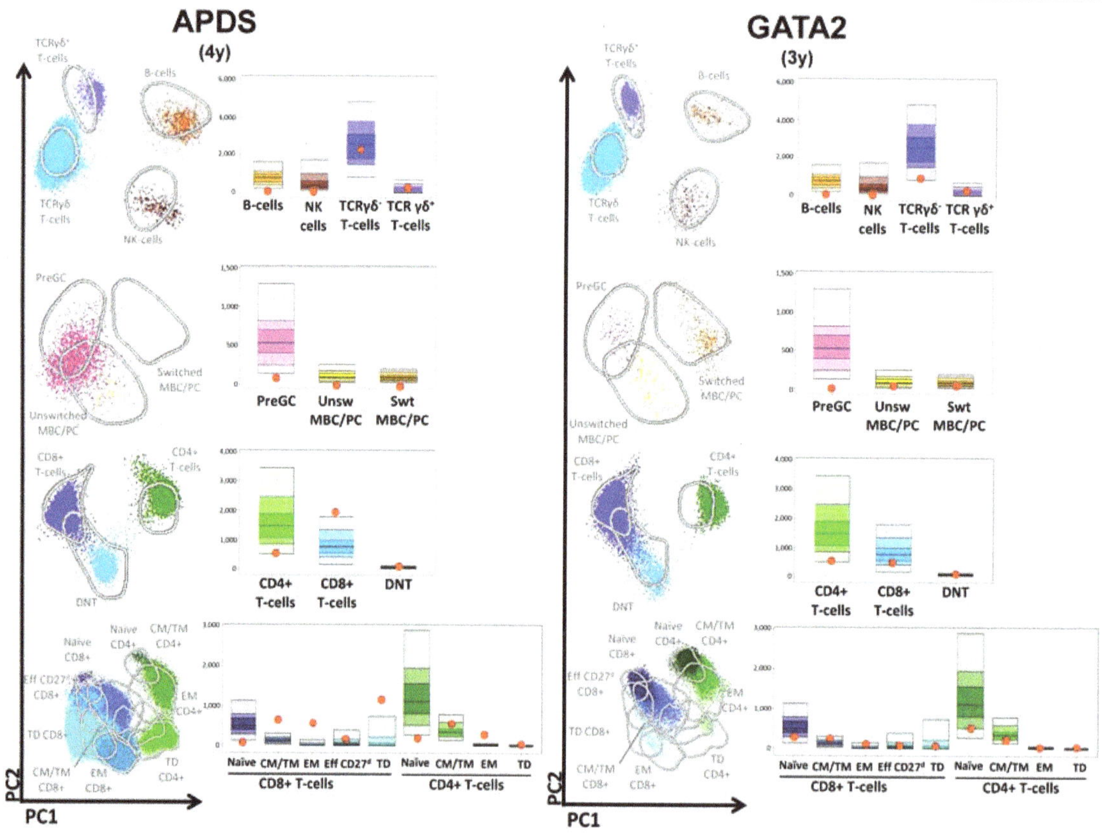

FIGURE 5 | Multidimensional views of all lymphocyte subsets in combination with the absolute values of all subpopulations plotted as red dots in the age-matched reference bar graphs after automated analysis. **(APDS)** Patients with activated PI3K delta syndrome (APDS). **(GATA2)** Patient with GATA2 deficiency.

diagnostics of patients suspected for PID. With this PIDOT, we could analyze all major lymphocyte subsets and the important lymphocyte subpopulations allowing the generation of data on the absolute counts and frequency of the lymphocyte subsets and a lymphocyte profile as APS view with a single tube. This tube can readily be implemented in the diagnostics of PID.

The PIDOT serves as the central tube in the EuroFlow algorithm for PID. Based on the results of the PIDOT other tubes shall be used for more detailed analysis of B- and/or T-cell subsets. For example, for patients with SCID the PIDOT is a strong screening tool, that in combination with the immunophenotyping of recent thymic emigrants in cases with present yet abnormal T-cells can provide diagnostic information with direct clinical consequences (Kalina et al. manuscript in preparation, in this issue). In the PIDOT tube we choose CD27 and CD45RA as a marker for naïve T cells (CD27+CD45RA+), while CD62L is used in the so called SCID-RTE tube together with CD45RO and CD31 to confirm the absence of recent thymic emigrants [Kalina et al. Manuscript in preparation, (19)]. Based on the flow cytometric results the treatment strategy can be initiated even prior to the result of genetic testing. The presence of T-cells in case of a clinical suspicion of SCID should be interpreted with care. It is known that especially RAG1 and RAG2 deficiencies can present with T-cells. The presence of T-cells in a patient clinically presenting as SCID can be due to hypomorphic mutation (with residual activity) (20) Alternatively, T-cells can be of maternal origin (21). In rare cases the presence of T-cells can be the result of reversion mutations (22). In these cases, we recommend additional labeling for SCID including CD31, CD62L, HLA-DR, and CD45RO for further typing of T-cells (Kalina et al. manuscript in preparation). For some PID disease categories, e.g., Common Variable Immunodeficiency (CVID) it might be necessary to have a more detailed phenotyping of the T- and B-cell subsets, e.g., with respect to certain subsets expressing specific Ig subclasses (8, 23).

If the PIDOT is used as screening tube to test whether the patient suffer from a PID, relative frequencies of naive CD4+ cells, as well as CD4 and CD8 effector memory cells were most frequently aberrant. We propose that this approach is used in any patient with a clinical suspicion of PID, because multiple and clear abnormal values are indicative of severe PID that requires adequate clinical management. In other, less pronounced phenotypes, PID screening tube can direct further evaluation including prioritization for NGS or gene panel evaluation). In PIDs that do not affect the lymphoid compartment (CGD, IRAK4 and complement deficiencies) no aberrant populations were identified, indicating that this tube is not useful for these categories. It will be of great value to prospectively collect the data of PID analyzed with the PIDOT to better define the characteristic pattern of aberrant subsets in a large cohort of genetically defined PID. Moreover, in combination with the clinical presentation and the exact mutation, the spectrum of PID can be better defined.

Recently, a lyophilized version of the PID screening tube has been developed and has proven to give the same results as when antibodies are used the liquid form and are added separately to the mixture. The advantage of using dried tubes is that it is not only time-saving and less prone to operational mistakes, but that it also significantly reduces the time spent in antibody inventory management (ordering of reagents and acceptance testing of antibodies (one single tube vs. 12 individual antibodies), including all the corresponding registrations (17), thus making the process suitable for any clinical laboratory. The major advantage of the EuroFlow approach using standardized protocols and flowcytometer instruments setting is that the generated data can be fully exchanged between laboratories and diagnostic centers, and will allow the generation of databases of patient that are extremely rare. Standardized EuroFlow multicolor flow cytometry is relatively easy to adopt, as EuroFlow has created standard operating protocols, published them on a eurofow.org website and commented on their use in the literature. In order to support the widespread adoption in reasonable quality EuroFlow educational meetings are organized as well as Quality Assessment (24).

Availability of the fully standardized PIDOT and accessibility to EuroFlow reference data base allows any lab in the world to perform standardized PID diagnostic, also in non-Western countries, because all over the world 8-color flow cytometers are now available, thanks to the HIV diagnostics and leukemia and lymphoma diagnostics. In addition, the multidimensional data analysis strategy and visualization will disclose new information, which is otherwise lost if only frequencies and absolute numbers of separate lymphocyte subsets are taken in consideration. With these developments, a new dimension is added to flow cytometry in the PID field in which the number of newly identified PIDs is still increasing.

AUTHOR CONTRIBUTIONS

MvdB, TK, MP-A, MvZ, AO, and JvD contributed to the conception and design of the study. TK, MP-A, MV, EL-G, EB, CB, AS, A-KK, MW, EM, VS, and JS performed the data acquisition and data analysis. MP-A and EB organized the database; MvdB, TK, AO, and JvD wrote the manuscript. All authors contributed to manuscript revision, read and approved the submitted version.

FUNDING

The coordination and innovation processes of this study were supported by the EuroFlow Consortium (Chairmen: MvdB and AO). MvZ is supported by Senior Research Fellowship GNT1117687 from the Australian National Health and Medical Research Council. TK and EM were supported by projects 15-28541A from Ministry of Health, LO1604 from Ministry of Education, Youth and Sports and GBP302/12/G101 from Grant Agency of the Czech Republic. MP-A, EB, and AO were supported by a grant from the Junta de Castilla y León (Fondo Social Europeo, ORDEN EDU/346/2013, Valladolid, Spain) and the CB16/12/00400 grant (CIBER/ONC, Instituto de Salud Carlos III, Ministerio de Economía y Competitividad, - Madrid, Spain- and FONDOS FEDER), the FIS PI12/00905-FEDER grant

(Fondo de Investigación Sanitaria of Instituto de Salud Carlos III, Madrid, Spain) and AP119882013 grant (Fundación Mutua Madrileña, Madrid, Spain). Publishing costs for this article were covered by the International Union of Immunological Societies (IUIS).

REFERENCES

1. Picard C, Bobby Gaspar H, Al-Herz W, Bousfiha A, Casanova JL, Chatila T, et al. International union of immunological societies: 2017 primary immunodeficiency diseases committee report on inborn errors of immunity. *J Clin Immunol.* (2018) 38:96–128. doi: 10.1007/s10875-017-0464-9
2. Bousfiha A, Jeddane L, Picard C, Ailal F, Bobby Gaspar H, Al-Herz W, et al. The 2017 IUIS phenotypic classification for primary immunodeficiencies. *J Clin Immunol.* (2018) 38:129–43. doi: 10.1007/s10875-017-0465-8
3. Gallo V, Dotta L, Giardino G, Cirillo E, Lougaris V, D'Assante R, et al. Diagnostics of primary immunodeficiencies through next-generation sequencing. *Front Immunol.* (2016) 7:466. doi: 10.3389/fimmu.2016.00466
4. Seleman M, Hoyos-Bachiloglu R, Geha RS, Chou J. Uses of next-generation sequencing technologies for the diagnosis of primary immunodeficiencies. *Front Immunol.* (2017) 8:847. doi: 10.3389/fimmu.2017.00847
5. Mahnke YD, Brodie TM, Sallusto F, Roederer M, Lugli E. The who's who of T-cell differentiation: human memory T-cell subsets. *Eur J Immunol.* (2013) 43:2797–809. doi: 10.1002/eji.201343751
6. Kalina T, Flores-Montero J, Lecrevisse Q, Pedreira CE, van der Velden VH, Novakova M, et al. Quality assessment program for EuroFlow protocols: summary results of four-year (2010-2013) quality assurance rounds. *Cytometry A.* (2015) 87:145–56. doi: 10.1002/cyto.a.22581
7. Kalina T, Flores-Montero J, van der Velden VH, Martin-Ayuso M, Bottcher S, Ritgen M, et al. EuroFlow standardization of flow cytometer instrument settings and immunophenotyping protocols. *Leukemia.* (2012) 26:1986–2010. doi: 10.1038/leu.2012.122
8. Blanco E, Perez-Andres M, Arriba-Mendez S, Contreras-Sanfeliciano T, Criado I, Pelak O, et al. Age-associated distribution of normal B-cell and plasma cell subsets in peripheral blood. *J Allergy Clin Immunol.* (2018) 141:2208–19. doi: 10.1016/j.jaci.2018.02.017
9. Perez-Andres M, Paiva B, Nieto WG, Caraux A, Schmitz A, Almeida J, et al. Human peripheral blood B-cell compartments: a crossroad in B-cell traffic. *Cytometry B Clin Cytom.* (2010) 78 (Suppl. 1):S47–60. doi: 10.1002/cyto.b.20547
10. Wickham H. *Elegant Graphics for Data Analysis.* New York, NY; Springer-Verlag (2016).
11. Fuchs S, Rensing-Ehl A, Erlacher M, Vraetz T, Hartjes L, Janda A, et al. Patients with T(+)/low NK(+) IL-2 receptor gamma chain deficiency have differentially-impaired cytokine signaling resulting in severe combined immunodeficiency. *Eur J Immunol.* (2014) 44:3129–40. doi: 10.1002/eji.201444689
12. Yao CM, Han XH, Zhang YD, Zhang H, Jin YY, Cao RM, et al. Clinical characteristics and genetic profiles of 44 patients with severe combined immunodeficiency (SCID): report from Shanghai, China (2004-2011). *J Clin Immunol.* (2013) 33:526–39. doi: 10.1007/s10875-012-9854-1
13. Lee YN, Frugoni F, Dobbs K, Walter JE, Giliani S, Gennery AR, et al. A systematic analysis of recombination activity and genotype-phenotype correlation in human recombination-activating gene 1 deficiency. *J Allergy Clin Immunol.* (2014) 133:1099–108. doi: 10.1016/j.jaci.2013.10.007
14. IJspeert H, Driessen GJ, Moorhouse MJ, Hartwig NG, Wolska-Kusnierz B, Kalwak K, et al. Similar recombination-activating gene (RAG) mutations result in similar immunobiological effects but in different clinical phenotypes. *J Allergy Clin Immunol.* (2014) 133:1124–33. doi: 10.1016/j.jaci.2013.11.028
15. Notarangelo LD, Kim MS, Walter JE, Lee YN. Human RAG mutations: biochemistry and clinical implications. *Nat Rev Immunol.* (2016) 16:234–46. doi: 10.1038/nri.2016.28
16. van Zelm MC, Bartol SJ, Driessen GJ, Mascart F, Reisli I, Franco JL, et al. Human CD19 and CD40L deficiencies impair antibody selection and differentially affect somatic hypermutation. *J Allergy Clin Immunol.* (2014) 134:135–44. doi: 10.1016/j.jaci.2013.11.015
17. van der Velden VH, Flores-Montero J, Perez-Andres M, Martin-Ayuso M, Crespo O, Blanco E, et al. Optimization and testing of dried antibody tube: The EuroFlow LST and PIDOT tubes as examples. *J Immunol Methods.* (2017). doi: 10.1016/j.jim.2017.03.011. [Epub ahead of print].
18. Coulter TI, Chandra A, Bacon CM, Babar J, Curtis J, Screaton N, et al. Clinical spectrum and features of activated phosphoinositide 3-kinase delta syndrome: a large patient cohort study. *J Allergy Clin Immunol.* (2017) 139:597–606 e4. doi: 10.1016/j.jaci.2016.06.021
19. Maecker HT, McCoy JP, Nussenblatt R. Standardizing immunophenotyping for the human immunology project. *Nat Rev Immunol.* (2012) 12:191–200. doi: 10.1038/nri3158
20. Villa A, Sobacchi C, Notarangelo LD, Bozzi F, Abinun M, Abrahamsen TG, et al. V(D)J recombination defects in lymphocytes due to RAG mutations: severe immunodeficiency with a spectrum of clinical presentations. *Blood.* (2001) 97:81–8. doi: 10.1182/blood.V97.1.81
21. Muller SM, Ege M, Pottharst A, Schulz AS, Schwarz K, Friedrich W. Transplacentally acquired maternal T lymphocytes in severe combined immunodeficiency: a study of 121 patients. *Blood.* (2001) 98:1847–51. doi: 10.1182/blood.V98.6.1847
22. Crestani E, Choo S, Frugoni F, Lee YN, Richards S, Smart J, et al. RAG1 reversion mosaicism in a patient with Omenn syndrome. *J Clin Immunol.* (2014) 34:551–4. doi: 10.1007/s10875-014-0051-2
23. Stuchly J, Kanderova V, Vlkova M, Hermanova I, Slamova L, Pelak O, et al. Common variable immunodeficiency patients with a phenotypic profile of immunosenescence present with thrombocytopenia. *Sci Rep.* (2017) 7:39710. doi: 10.1038/srep39710
24. Kalina T, Brdickova N, Glier H, Fernandez P, Bitter M, Flores-Montero J, et al. Frequent issues and lessons learned from EuroFlow QA. *J Immunol Methods.* (2018). doi: 10.1016/j.jim.2018.09.008. [Epub ahead of print].

7

Flow Cytometry for Diagnosis of Primary Immune Deficiencies—A Tertiary Center Experience From North India

Amit Rawat[†], *Kanika Arora*[†], *Jitendra Shandilya, Pandiarajan Vignesh, Deepti Suri, Gurjit Kaur, Rashmi Rikhi, Vibhu Joshi, Jhumki Das, Babu Mathew and Surjit Singh*[*]

Allergy Immunology Unit, Department of Pediatrics, Advanced Pediatrics Center, Post Graduate Institute of Medical Education and Research, Chandigarh, India

***Correspondence:**
Surjit Singh
surjitsinghpgi@rediffmail.com

[†]*These authors share first authorship*

Flow cytometry has emerged as a useful technology that has facilitated our understanding of the human immune system. Primary immune deficiency disorders (PIDDs) are a heterogeneous group of inherited disorders affecting the immune system. More than 350 genes causing various PIDDs have been identified. While the initial suspicion and recognition of PIDDs is clinical, laboratory tools such as flow cytometry and genetic sequencing are essential for confirmation and categorization. Genetic sequencing, however, are prohibitively expensive and not readily available in resource constrained settings. Flow cytometry remains a simple, yet powerful, tool for multi-parametric analysis of cells. While it is confirmatory of diagnosis in certain conditions, in others it helps in narrowing the list of putative genes to be analyzed. The utility of flow cytometry in diagnosis of PIDDs can be divided into four major categories: (a) Enumeration of lymphocyte subsets in peripheral blood. (b) Detection of intracellular signaling molecules, transcription factors, and cytokines. (c) Functional assessment of adaptive and innate immune cells (e.g., T cell function in severe combined immune deficiency and natural killer cell function in familial hemophagocytic lymphohistiocytosis). (d) Evaluation of normal biological processes (e.g., class switching in B cells by B cell immunophenotyping). This review focuses on use of flow cytometry in disease-specific diagnosis of PIDDs in the context of a developing country.

Keywords: flow cytometry, recent advances, clinical applications, immune dysregulation, immune deficiencies, primary immunodefciencies

The term "flow cytometry" refers to evaluation of multiple cell characteristics in a flow system that delivers a single cell suspension at a defined point of measurement (1). Flow cytometry can be used for analysis of intracellular and extracellular proteins, cell sorting, apoptosis, cell proliferation, and quantification of DNA. Utility of flow cytometry in clinical studies was first described by Dr. Louis Kamentsky in the year 1965 (2). Since its first description, there have been major technological advances in the field of flow cytometry, and this technology has revolutionized the field of cell biology.

Flow cytometry is a key investigation for analysis of leucocyte subsets and function and is an essential diagnostic tool in clinical immunology. Primary immune deficiency disorders (PIDDs) are a group of inherited disorders affecting single or multiple components of the immune system, resulting in increased predisposition to infections and immune-dysregulation (3). Flow cytometry is often one of the first investigations to delineate the type of PIDD (4). In our previous review, we highlighted the progress of PIDD research in India and the spectrum of cases with PIDDs at our institute (5). In this review, we discuss the utility of flow cytometry in diagnosis and management of patients with PIDDs in context of a developing country.

SETTING UP OF FLOW CYTOMETRY FACILITY AT OUR CENTER

(a) We have been performing flow cytometry for clinical and research work in PIDDs on a dedicated Beckman Coulter, two-laser, six-color platform (*Navios*) (**Figure 1**). This is a robust and user-friendly instrument but is limited by the number of parameters that can be studied in a single tube.
(b) Majority of samples that we process are obtained from patients who visit our institute and these samples are processed the same day.
(c) Our laboratory is situated in close proximity to the clinical service areas. This facilitates processing of samples and coordination between clinical and laboratory personnel.
(d) However, as we are a designated Center for Advance Research in PIDDs under the Indian Council of Medical Research, we also receive samples from other parts of India (**Figure 1**).
(e) These samples are dispatched by commercial courier and usually reach our laboratory within 48–72 h. All such couriered samples are accompanied by a transport control.
(f) In our experience, these samples do not deteriorate if processed within 48–72 h of having been drawn but we face difficulty during summer months (May–June) when the blood often gets hemolyzed. Assays designed to estimate lymphocyte or neutrophil function (e.g., Dihydrorhodamine 123 assay) are more likely to be jeopardized due to delays in transportation than assays for estimation of cell surface molecules. We also routinely use CD45 as a gating marker and 7-aminoactinomycin D (AAD) to differentiate between live and dead cells. Abnormal results are interpreted in relation to results obtained for travel control.
(g) We usually follow the recommended protocols for processing samples but have made some improvisations based on our experience and keeping in mind cost constraints. We carefully titrate each fresh lot of antibodies and use the antibody concentration with the highest signal-to-noise ratio. This is often much less than the volume recommended by the manufacturer.
(h) All samples are processed with appropriate controls. However, this does add to laboratory costs.
(i) Before acquisition of samples, we run quality control (QC) beads (Flow check beads for Navios) for verification of optical alignment and fluidics stability. This can be checked by calculating coefficient of variation in different detectors. Other set of fluorospheres (Flow set) are also used on a regular basis to standardize light scatter intensity and fluorescent intensity. Stabilized leucocytes with known quantity of surface antigens (Immuno-Trol cells) are used to verify monoclonal antibody performance, sample staining (lysis), and analysis. If coefficient of variation is out of range, we clean the instrument again and rerun the quality control beads. If QC requirements are not met, we withhold processing of samples.
(j) For each lot of antibodies, we perform compensation in a multicolor experiment. This is achieved using cells containing mutually exclusive population of same fluorochromes. Compensation is re-established after any change in hardware, laser alignment, and change in filters or optics.

ROLE OF FLOW CYTOMETRY IN DIAGNOSIS OF COMBINED IMMUNE DEFICIENCY (CID)

Severe Combined Immune Deficiency (SCID)

SCID comprises a group of disorders that predominantly affect T cell development and function. In addition to T cell defects, there may be impaired B cell and/or NK cell development (6).

Immunophenotyping of Lymphocyte Subsets to Classify SCID

A preliminary lymphocyte subset analysis by flow cytometry that includes markers for B lymphocytes (CD19), T lymphocytes (CD3), and natural killer cells (CD56/16) is the first-line investigation for SCID, and it helps in identifying the subtypes of SCID (7–13) (**Table 1, Supplementary Figure 1A**). Isolated CD4 lymphopenia has been described with MHC Class II deficiency (*RFXANK, CIITA, RFXAP*) and hypomorphic *RAG* variants (14). HLA-DR expression by flow cytometry would also be decreased in patients with MHC Class II deficiency. Isolated CD8 lymphopenia with preserved CD4 counts can be seen with *TAP1*, *TAP2*, and *ZAP70* defects (15).

Normal numbers of CD3 counts can be seen in patients with SCID with associated Omenn syndrome (OS) or maternal T cell engraftment. Estimation of naïve T cells (CD45RA+ CD45RO− CD62L+) and memory T cells (CD45RO+CD45RA−CD62L−) in CD4+ and CD8+T lymphocyte populations is helpful in these situations as naïve T cell population is grossly decreased (16) (**Supplementary Figures 1B,C**).

Surface expression of common γ chain (CD132) and interleukin receptor 7α chain (CD127) on monocytes and T lymphocytes, respectively, can also be utilized to characterize X-linked SCID and IL7R deficiency, respectively (17) (**Supplementary Figures 1D,E**).

Functional Assays

Phosphorylation of downstream signal transducer and activator of transcription (STAT) is impaired in cases of defects with *IL2RG* and *JAK3*. Expression of phosphorylated STAT3 or STAT5 in the lymphocytes after stimulation with IL-2 and IL-21 is low in these patients as compared to normal controls (4).

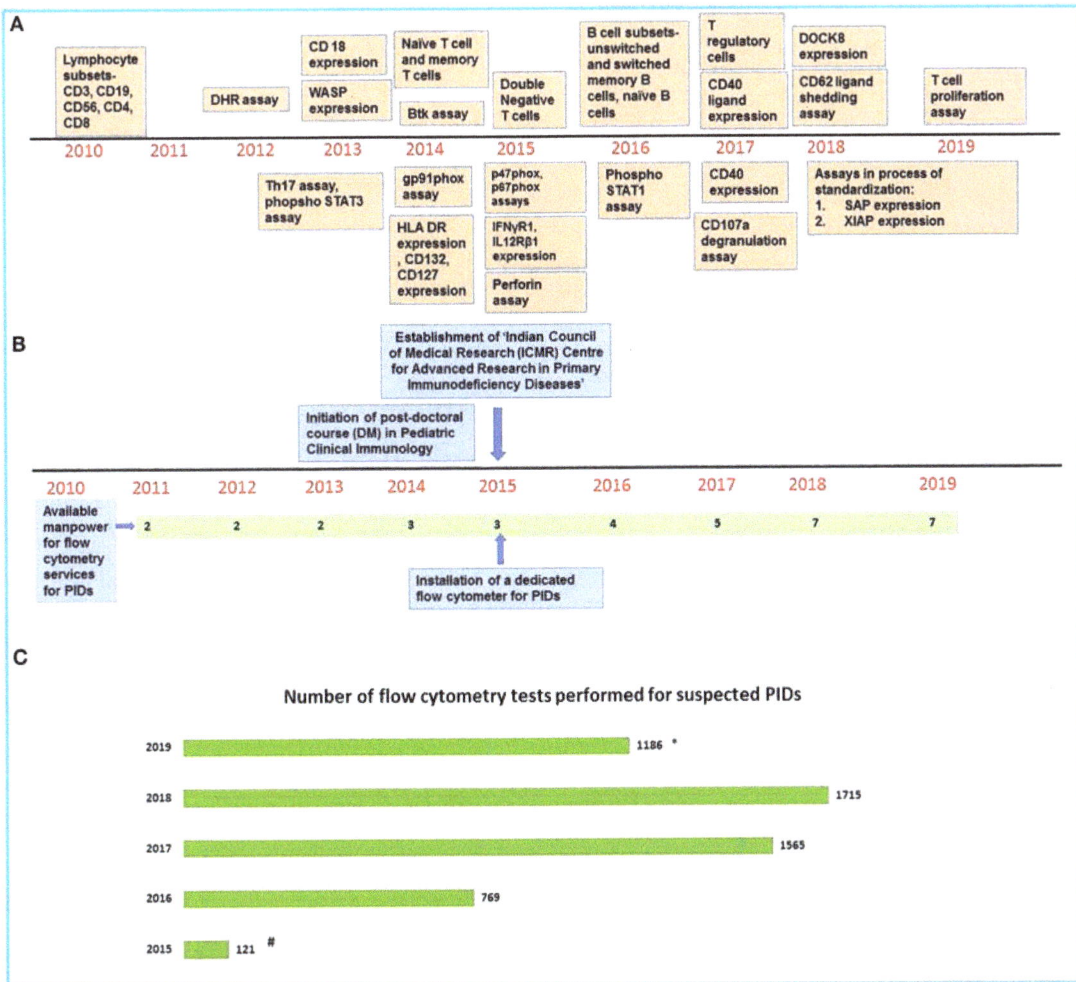

FIGURE 1 | An overview of development of flow cytometry services for PIDs at our center. **(A)** Timeline showing the establishment of flow cytometry tests in the laboratory. **(B)** Timeline showing the increase in manpower and support for the laboratory services. **(C)** Bar graph showing the number of flow cytometry tests for PIDs performed in our laboratory in the last 5 years (#Data available from August 2015 to December 2015/*Data available from January 2019 to July 2019).

Estimation of Lymphocyte Proliferation

Flow cytometry is also used for assessment of T cell proliferation in response to antigens or mitogens using carboxy fluorescein diacetate succinimidyl ester (CFSE) or cell trace dyes that integrate with intracellular proteins of the cell. When T lymphocytes are stimulated with mitogens [e.g., phytohemagglutinin (PHA)] or anti CD3 with CD28, the cells divide and the dye gets apportioned equally between two daughter cells. Patients with SCID show impaired T cell proliferation and decreased response to the dye after stimulation with PHA. Other dyes like Cell Trace Violet and CellTrace Far Red have also been used for lymphocyte proliferation studies (18).

Assessment of Radiosensitive Forms of SCID

Radiosensitivity flow assay is one of the newer techniques that help in functional assessment of patients with radiosensitive forms of SCID (e.g., *DCLRE1C*, *PRKDC*, *LIG4*, *NHEJ1*, and *NBS1*) (19). We have not standardized this in our laboratory yet.

Laboratory Work Flow for SCID at Our Center

In a suspected case of SCID or other CID, we first perform lymphocyte subset analysis using a limited panel of four antibodies, i.e., CD45, CD3, CD19, and CD56. Lymphocytes are gated using SSc vs. CD45 and different subsets are estimated. In patients with SCID with completely absent T cells, we do not assay naïve or memory T cell population. When T cells are present in reduced or normal numbers in a suspected case of SCID or CID, we perform T cell subset analysis using CD3, CD4, CD8, CD45RA, and CD45RO antibodies to estimate the naïve and memory T cells. As we have been getting reasonable results with this antibody cocktail, we have not considered addition of CD62L for processing these samples (20).

HLA-DR estimation on CD3+ T lymphocytes is performed along with naïve and memory T cell estimation in patients with

TABLE 1 | Immunophenotyping in severe combined immune deficiency (SCID) with associated genetic defects.

	Lymphocyte phenotype	Associated genetic defects	Comments
I.	T-B-NK- SCID	*ADA, PNP*	Accumulation of toxic metabolites inhibits DNA synthesis and repair and leads to severe lymphopenia (7).
II.	T-B-NK+ SCID	*RAG1, RAG2, DCLRE1C, LIG4, NHEJ1*	Defects in somatic recombination result in decreased or absent T and B lymphocytes (8).
III.	T-B+NK- SCID	*IL2RG, JAK3*	T-B+NK- SCID results from defects in common gamma chain that is required for normal development of T and NK cells (9). Analysis of surface expression of CD132 may also help in identifying the defect (10).
IV.	T-B+NK+ SCID	*IL7 R*, CD3δ, CD3ε and CD3ζ	Reduced surface expression of CD127 on T cells can help in classifying SCID (11).
V.	Omenn syndrome	*RAG1, RAG2, DCLRE1C, ADA, LIG4, IL2RG, IL7R*, DiGeorge syndrome	Reduced naïve T cells (CD3+45RA+45RO−), elevated memory T cells (CD3+45RA-45RO+), and increased expression of HLA DR on T lymphocytes are noted in Omenn syndrome (12). T cell receptor Vβ repertoire analysis shows skewed Vβ usage indicating oligoclonality (13).

suspected OS. We are not in a position to perform Vβ repertoire analysis in these patients as it is prohibitively expensive.

T cell function is analyzed using CFSE staining. Depending on the immune phenotype and family history we perform expression of IL-2RG on monocytes if the phenotype is T−B+NK− or if there is strong suspicion of X-linked recessive inheritance. Similarly, in patients with T−B+NK+ SCID, we perform IL-7R (CD127) staining. We have erroneously diagnosed IL7R deficiency when CD127 expression was checked on gated lymphocytes and found to be low. This is due to internalization of IL7R during episodes of severe lymphopenia and also due to the fact that if T cells are decreased, gating lymphocytes for IL7R expression is not an appropriate strategy. We have now developed protocols for CD127 expression on CD19+ B lymphocytes.

Clinical Correlate

Flow cytometry also helps in monitoring of engraftment of T cells post-hematopoietic stem cell transplantation in patients with SCID (**Supplementary Figure 2**). We have used flow cytometry for antenatal screening of SCID by measurement of lymphocyte subsets in cord blood samples, especially when amniocentesis or chorionic villous sampling is not possible, and genetic basis of SCID is not available.

DOCK8 Deficiency

DOCK8 defect is an autosomal recessive form of CID characterized clinically by severe cutaneous viral infections such as warts or molluscum contagiosum. Laboratory investigations may reveal eosinophilia and increased serum levels of IgE. Immunological features include low T and B cell numbers, decreased levels of serum IgM, and impaired functional antibody response (21).

DOCK8 is an intracellular protein expressed in myeloid and lymphoid lineages (22). Intracellular staining of DOCK8 in lymphocytes by flow cytometry can be used to recognize patients with *DOCK8* defect and also monitor the expression of DOCK8 in various cell lineages following HSCT in patients with this defect (23).

Laboratory Work Flow for DOCK8 at Our Center

In a suspected case of DOCK8 deficiency, we perform this assay on lymphocytes and neutrophils. As fluorochrome-labeled anti-DOCK8 is presently not available in India, we use a custom-designed antibody labeled with a chosen fluorochrome. This is technically more difficult to standardize.

Hyper-IgM Syndrome

Hyper-IgM syndromes are inherited disorders that mainly affect somatic hypermutation and B cell class switch recombination (24). Serum IgM levels of affected patients may be normal or elevated but IgG and IgA levels are usually decreased.

X-linked Hyper-IgM syndrome occurs due to defect in *CD40L* that encodes for CD40 (CD154) present on activated T cells. The assay is usually performed along with CD69 or CD25 staining of lymphocytes to confirm lymphocyte activation status. Increased expression of CD69 or CD25 along with decreased or absent expression of CD154 on activated lymphocytes is suggestive of CD40L defect (25) (**Supplementary Figure 3**). In our experience, flow cytometry may not give a clue in all patients with CD40L defect. As expression of CD40L can be normal in 5–10% cases, staining with CD40-mulg can be used in these situations. Autosomal recessive hyper-IgM syndrome due to CD40 defect can also be identified by flow cytometry by analyzing expression of CD40 in B cells.

Laboratory Work Flow for Hyper IgM at Our Center

In our center, we study CD40L (CD154) expression by flow cytometry on activated CD4+/CD69+ helper T cells after stimulation with phorbol myristate acetate (PMA) and ionomycin. Percentage expression and median fluorescence intensity of CD40L on activated dual positive CD4+/CD69+ helper T cells is compared with age- and sex-matched healthy controls.

Wiskott-Aldrich Syndrome (WAS)

WAS is an X-linked recessive condition characterized by eczema, thrombocytopenia (with platelets that are characteristically small in size), and CID (26). The *WAS* gene encodes for a 502-amino acid protein (WASp) that contributes to cell motility, actin polymerization, and apoptosis (27). The WASp antibody is directed against WAS protein that is evaluated both on lymphocytes and monocytes.

Flow cytometry plays an important role in detection of WASp through intracellular staining, after fixation and permeabilization of cells (28).

Laboratory Work Flow for WAS at Our Center

In patients with WAS, we perform intracellular staining assay of WAS. We use CD45 and fluorochrome-labeled WAS antibody for this assay. Lymphocytes, monocytes, and neutrophils are gated on CD45 vs. SSc, and expression of WAS protein is checked in each of these leucocyte subsets. The presence or absence of protein is determined by calculating Stain Index (SI) ($\mathbf{SI} = \frac{\textit{Median fluorescence intensity (MFI) of Stained cells}}{\textit{Median Fluorescence Intensity of unstained cells}}$) of controls as well as patient samples and then SI ratio ($\mathbf{SI\ ratio} = \frac{\textit{SI of patient}}{\textit{SI of control}}$) is calculated for each patient. We consider an SI ratio <0.65 on gated lymphocytes to be suggestive of WAS. The SI ratio of patient vs. control remains uniform irrespective of change in MFI, which occurs at each instance when the flow cytometer is recalibrated. We have performed 127 WASp assays from January 2016 to May 2019. In 76 suspected cases, the SI of the test was compared with that of single control/case. Similarly, for 10 cases, the SI of test was compared to the average SI of two controls for each case. Lately, in 41 suspected cases, we have compared the SI of test with an average SI of 3 controls/case. A ratio of 0.65 was determined as a cutoff from these comparisons.

Clinical Correlate

Flow cytometry often provides the first clue in identification of WAS in males being worked up for persistent thrombocytopenia. Normal WASp expression, however, does not rule out WAS as the protein may be non-functional. In such cases, genetic workup is warranted. Flow cytometry can also be used to monitor patients with WAS who have undergone HSCT and also to check for carrier status of females who would typically show a bimodal expression of WASp due to lyonization (**Supplementary Figure 4**).

ROLE OF FLOW CYTOMETRY IN HUMORAL IMMUNE DEFICIENCIES

X-Linked Agammaglobulinemia (XLA)

XLA is an X-linked recessive antibody deficiency due to mutations in the *BTK* gene. Investigations reveal profound hypogammaglobulinemia with decreased or absent peripheral B cells and reduced BTK expression in monocytes on flow cytometry (29). Female carriers of XLA show a bimodal expression of BTK protein (30). In some patients, it becomes necessary to perform genetic analysis and correlate with the BTK flow analysis, as some missense mutations may show near-normal levels of BTK protein expression (31) (**Supplementary Figure 5**).

Laboratory Work Flow for XLA at Our Center

For patients with suspected XLA, we perform CD3/CD19/CD56 lymphocyte subset assay by gating lymphocytes on CD45 vs. SSc. Btk protein expression analysis is carried out on monocytes in patients with low B cell count (<2%). CD14 antibody is used for labeling monocytes for Btk expression. A control sample is always run for comparison. Both percentage and median fluorescence intensity (ΔMFI) are measured in patients and control.

Common Variable Immune Deficiency (CVID)

The term common variable immune deficiency (CVID) refers to a heterogeneous group of diseases defined by low IgG and IgA or IgM deficiency with a decreased antibody response to vaccination (32). Unlike XLA, patients with CVID usually do not have decreased number of B cells. However, most patients with CVID have an abnormal B cell differentiation and reduced memory B cells (33). Memory B cell subsets that are commonly assayed in CVID include class-switched memory B cells (CD19+CD27+IgM−IgD−), marginal zone-like B cells (CD19+CD27+IgM+IgD+), plasmablasts (CD19+CD20−IgM-$CD38^{hi}$CD27+), transitional B cells (CD19+CD27−$CD24^{hi}CD38^{hi}IgM^{hi}$CD10+), and CD21− and CD21+ B cells (34). These can be evaluated by flow cytometry (**Supplementary Figure 6**).

A large number of monogenic defects have been described in patients with CVID. These include defects in *CD19*, *CD81*, *CR2*, *MS4A1*, *ICOS*, *CTLA4*, *LRBA*, *NFKB1*, *NFKB2*, *TNFRSF13C*, *PIK3CD*, and *PIK3R1* (35). However, more than 80% of patients with CVID do not appear to have any monogenic basis for their disease (36). Expression of CD19, CD81, CD21, CD20, ICOS, and BAFF-R can be estimated by flow cytometry. ICOS is detected on activated T cells and BAFF-R is detected on B cells. Cytotoxic T lymphocyte-associated protein 4 (CTLA-4) is a costimulatory molecule. It is expressed on activated T cells and binds to CD28 on B cells. CTLA-4 is essential for functioning of regulatory T cells (37). CTLA-4 expression on flow cytometry is studied on mitogen-stimulated CD4+ T lymphocytes (38). Intracellular expression of Lipopolysaccharide Responsive Beige-like Anchor Protein (LRBA) can be assessed by flow cytometry in monocytes, T cells, and NK cells.

Laboratory Work Flow for CVID at Our Center

We perform B cell immunophenotyping for naïve, switched, and unswitched B lymphocytes in patients with suspected CVID using CD19, CD27, sIgD, and sIgM antibodies. We do not routinely estimate transitional B cells or CD21 low B cells, although this would be useful in defining distinct subsets of CVID patients.

Clinical Correlate

Secondary hypogammaglobulinemia can occur due to drugs or loss of immunoglobulin in conditions such as nephrotic syndrome and protein losing enteropathy. Clinicians often face a dilemma when patients with autoimmune disorders who are receiving steroids turn out to have a low IgG level. This can be a manifestation of CVID or may represent secondary hypogammaglobulinemia due to glucocorticoids. Identification of reduced switch memory B cell patients with low IgA concentration has been reported to be useful in differentiating CVID from secondary hypogammaglobulinemia due to glucocorticoids (39).

ROLE OF FLOW CYTOMETRY IN DISEASES WITH IMMUNE DYSREGULATION

Hemophagocytic Lymphohistiocytosis (HLH)

HLH is a life-threatening disorder due to excessive activation of macrophages and cytotoxic lymphocytes resulting in a cytokine storm. HLH is composed of two major subtypes: primary HLH due to genetic defects and secondary HLH that is associated with an underlying predisposing condition such as an infection, malignancy, or rheumatologic disease (40). Primary HLH results from genetic defects affecting function of NK and cytotoxic CD8+T cells. The most common genetic defect identified is *PRF1* that encodes for perforin, a cytolytic enzyme released by NK cells or CD8+ T cells for killing of intracellular pathogens. Defects in *UNC13D*, *STXBP2*, and *STX11* (41–43) that are involved in cytotoxic lymphocyte degranulation also lead to primary HLH. Flow cytometry helps in measurement of perforin expression and evaluation of CD107a degranulation in NK and CD8+ T cells (44, 45) (**Supplementary Figure 7**). Other defects like Chédiak–Higashi syndrome, Griscelli syndrome Type 2, and Hermansky-Pudlak syndrome Type 2 also have defective degranulation. X-linked lymphoproliferative (XLP) syndrome is a rare disorder characterized by profound hypogammaglobulinemia, Epstein–Barr virus (EBV)-induced lymphoproliferation, and fatal hemophagocytosis. Patients with XLP1 have a defect in the SH2 domain of a SLAM-associated protein (SAP). XLP2 is due to a defect in *XIAP*, which is an X-linked inhibitor of apoptosis gene. Expression of both XIAP and SAP can be detected by intracellular staining on flow cytometry (46) (**Supplementary Table 1**).

Laboratory Work Flow for HLH at Our Center

In patients with suspected HLH, we carry out perforin expression by flow cytometry on CD56+ NK cells after intracellular staining. When NK cells are markedly reduced, we estimate the perforin expression on cytotoxic T cells (CD3+CD8+). If perforin expression is found to be normal, granule release assay (CD107a) is performed on PBMCs by stimulating the cells with PMA and ionomycin and Golgi stop (monensin). We also perform CD107a assay in patients with Chédiak–Higashi syndrome and Griscelli Type 2 syndrome.

Autoimmune Lymphoproliferative Syndrome (ALPS)

ALPS is characterized by lymphoproliferation, multilineage cytopenias, and an increased risk of B cell lymphoma (47). Patients with ALPS usually have defects in FAS and FASL that mediate apoptosis of lymphocytes. Defective apoptosis of developing lymphocytes in thymus results in an increase of double-negative T cells (CD3+TCRαβ+CD4–CD8–) (48) (**Supplementary Figure 8**). Annexin-V^+/propidium iodide (PI2) staining helps in detecting reduced apoptosis in this disorder (49).

Laboratory Work Flow for ALPS at Our Center

We estimate double-negative T (DNT) cells in patients with suspected ALPS using CD3, TCRαβ, CD4, and CD8 antibodies. CD4 and CD8 antibodies are tagged with the same fluorochrome. Percentage of DNTs >1.5% of all lymphocytes or 2.5% of CD3+ T lymphocytes is considered abnormal.

Immune Dysregulation, Polyendocrinopathy, Enteropathy X-Linked (IPEX) Syndrome

IPEX syndrome is a rare x-linked recessive monogenic autoimmune disorder resulting from a mutation in the gene *FOXP3*. Patients present with eczematous dermatitis, enteropathy, and an endocrinopathy (usually diabetes mellitus or hypothyroidism) (50). Most patients with this disorder have reduced CD4+CD25+CD127^{low} Treg or CD4+CD25+FOXP3+ cells. Normal numbers of CD4+CD25+CD127^{low} cells are found in case of hypomorphic *FOXP3* mutation (51). CD25 deficiency is an autosomal recessive defect that has similar clinical manifestations to that of IPEX syndrome. CD25 deficiency is caused by pathogenic variants in the *IL2RA* gene that codes for the α subunit (CD25) of IL2 receptor complex. IL2 α chain with β (CD122) and γ (CD132) subunits forms the high-affinity IL2 receptor. CD25 is present on the surface of T regulatory cells that help maintaining immune homeostasis (52).

Laboratory Work Flow for IPEX Syndrome at Our Center

We analyze T regulatory cells by surface staining with CD4+CD25+CD127+ or by analysis of intracellular FOXP3 expression in suspected cases of IPEX syndrome.

ROLE OF FLOW CYTOMETRY IN PHAGOCYTIC DEFECTS

Chronic Granulomatous Disease (CGD)

CGD results from a dysfunctional NADPH oxidase activity leading to defective oxidative burst in neutrophils (53). The NADPH oxidase complex has six subunits—two cell-membrane-bound proteins (gp91phox and p22phox, encoded by *CYBB* and *CYBA* genes) and four cytosolic components (p47phox, p67phox, p40phox, and cybc1 encoded by *NCF1*, *NCF2*, *NCF4*, and *CYBC1* genes) (54, 55). Patients with CGD have reduced or absent NADPH oxidase activity leading to reduced or no conversion of DHR into fluorescent rhodamine (56) (**Supplementary Figure 9**).

The ΔMFI is markedly decreased in patients with CGD. Further, flow cytometry analysis for NADPH oxidase components may be performed by surface staining of gp91phox for X-linked CGD and intracellular staining for cytoplasmic component p47phox and p67phox in patients with autosomal forms of CGD. In x-linked carriers of CGD, the DHR histogram depicts a pathognomonic double peak pattern due to lyonization (57) (**Supplementary Figure 10**). The DHR assay can also be performed on cord blood for screening of antenatal cases. The laboratory workflow for CGD at our center is summarized in **Supplementary Figure 11**.

Leukocyte Adhesion Defect

Leukocyte adhesion defect is characterized clinically by recurrent bacterial infections with little or no pus formation. Children usually present with omphalitis and delayed separation of umbilical cord. There are three types of LAD:

LAD I: It is an autosomal recessive disorder caused by reduced functioning or expression of CD18, the β subunit of leukocyte β2 integrins. It is caused by mutation in the *ITGB2* (integrin b2, CD18) that encodes for β2 integrin (58). Reduced or absent expression of CD18 or CD11 in neutrophils in LAD1 can be detected by flow cytometry (**Supplementary Figure 12**).

LAD II: Patients with LAD II have abnormalities in fucosylation of cell-surface glycoprotein. Reduced or absent expression of CD15 on neutrophils is characteristic of LADII.

LAD III: Patients with LAD III present with recurrent infections, increased bleeding tendency, and leucocytosis. LAD III deficiency can be detected by *FERMT3* gene sequencing. Neutrophil adherence and chemotaxis are significantly decreased in these patients (59). We currently do not perform neutrophil chemotaxis assay at our laboratory.

Laboratory Work Up of LAD at Our Center

In suspected cases of LAD deficiency, we assess CD18, CD11a, CD11b, and CD11c expression on gated neutrophils.

ROLE OF FLOW CYTOMETRY IN DIAGNOSIS OF OTHER IMMUNE DEFICIENCY SYNDROMES

STAT3 Loss of Function

Autosomal dominant hyper IgE syndrome (HIES) results from a loss of function mutation in STAT3. STAT3 defect impairs the downstream Th17 pathway and this explains the increased frequency of infections with extracellular organisms such as *Staphylococcus aureus* and *Candida albicans* (60). Th17 lymphocyte number and pSTAT3 expression (upon IL-6 stimulation) is reduced in patients with *STAT3* defect.

Clinical Correlate

Clinical presentation of patients with infantile eczema can, at times, be similar to that of HIES. In such situations, the National Institutes of Health (NIH) score can be useful in differentiating the two conditions (61). Flow-cytometry-based assessment of Th17 and pSTAT3 also helps in resolving the clinical dilemma. Patients with STAT3 defect usually have a decreased Th17 number and reduced pSTAT3 expression.

Laboratory Work Flow of HIES at Our Center

In our center, we perform Th17 cell analysis and also study the pSTAT3 expression on peripheral blood mononuclear cells (PBMCs) after stimulation with PMA and ionomycin or IL-6.

ROLE OF FLOW CYTOMETRY IN DIAGNOSIS OF INNATE IMMUNITY

Mendelian Susceptibility to Mycobacterial Disease (MSMD)

Patients with MSMD have a defect in the IFN-γ/IL-12 pathway and are prone to infections with *Mycobacterium* and *Salmonella* spp. (62). Genetic defects that have been shown to result in MSMD include *IFNGR1*, *IFNGR2*, *IL-12RB1*, and *STAT1* (63). Flow cytometry helps in detection of IL-12RB1 on mitogen-stimulated T cells and both subunits of IFN-γ receptor (IFNGR1 and IFNGR2). In autosomal recessive IFN-γR1 deficiency, there is a reduced expression of IFN-γR1 (64). However, in partial autosomal dominant IFNγR1 defect, IFNGR1 is overexpressed due to impaired recycling of the receptor (65). Intracellular staining of STAT1 after stimulation with recombinant IFN-γ may help in assessment of function of IFNγR1 and IFNγR2 (66). Similarly, function of IL-12Rβ1 can be assessed by measuring phosphorylated STAT4 (pSTAT4) in lymphocytes following stimulation with IL-12 (67) (**Supplementary Figure 13**).

Laboratory Work Flow of MSMD at Our Center

In a suspected case of MSMD, we perform IFN-γR1 and IL12Rβ1 assay using flow cytometry. The IFN-γR1 assay is carried out by surface staining using anti-human CD119. Lymphocytes, monocytes, and neutrophils are gated using SSc vs. FSc, and the percentage of IFN-γR1-positive cells is estimated along with the median fluorescence intensity. In patients with complete or partial IFNγR1 deficiency, the expression is reduced. However, in patients with partial dominant IFNγR1 defect, the expression may be paradoxically increased compared to control. Percentage of CD212 is analyzed on CD3-positive cells after stimulation of PBMCs with PHA for 3 days. A significantly reduced SI is a pointer toward IL12Rβ1 defect.

USE OF FLOW CYTOMETRY IN DIAGNOSIS OF IRAK4 AND MYD88 DEFICIENCY

Interleukin-1 receptor-associated kinase (IRAK4) plays an important part in Toll-like receptor and IL-1 receptor signaling. Ligand binding leads to trigger of adapter protein myeloid differentiation primary response 88 (MyD88) that augments the downstream signal induction (68). Mutation in *MYD88* or *IRAK4* impairs TLR signaling pathway. Shedding of CD62L from the surface of granulocytes occurs if the TLR signaling pathway is intact. In case of defect in MYD88 and IRAK-4, CD62L shedding is impaired and this can be assessed with the help of flow cytometry after stimulation of granulocytes with lipopolysaccharide (TLR4 ligand) (**Supplementary Table 2**).

Laboratory Work Flow for MyD88/IRAK4 Deficiency at Our Center

In our laboratory, we stimulate neutrophils with PMA or LPS [such as LPS (TLR4 agonist)] and then stain these with anti-human CD62L. Patients with MyD88, IRAK4, and NEMO do not shed CD62L on stimulated neutrophils. A control sample is always necessary for this assay. We do not have facilities to see the cytokine measurements (TNF α) after stimulation with LPS.

FLOW CYTOMETRY ASSAYS THAT ARE PLANNED TO BE DEVELOPED IN OUR LABORATORY

Activated PI3 Kinase Delta Syndrome (APDS)

Patients with APDS syndrome may harbor heterozygous gain-of-function mutation in *PIK3CD* (APDS1) or loss-of-function mutations in *PIK3R1* (APDS2), resulting in an enhanced PI3K and downstream Akt/mTOR signaling. Premature immunosenescence and immune exhaustion involving T cells leads to an increased predisposition to infection and autoimmunity. T cell immunosenescence is associated with telomere-dependent replicative senescence of cells, which is measured by cell surface expression of CD57 (69). Senescent (CD8+CD57+) T lymphocytes accumulate in the enlarged lymph nodes (70). Flow cytometry can also be used in analysis of enhanced phosphorylation of AKT in CD3 and CD19 cells.

Ataxia Telangiectasia

Ataxia telangiectasia (AT) is a neurodegenerative disorder characterized by conjunctival telangiectasia, radiosensitivity, cerebellar ataxia, immunological defects, and increased susceptibility to malignancy (71).

It is characterized by mutation in the *ATM* gene encoding a protein that assists in cell cycle arrest of damaged cells, recombination, apoptosis, and DNA repair. The earliest event at the double-strand break is phosphorylation of H2AX (histone) protein; measurement of γ-H2AX protein can be carried out by irradiating the cells and staining the cells with γ-H2AX antibody. Levels of γ-H2AX protein are found to be lower in patients with AT as compared to normal control, thereby making it a good diagnostic test for patients with AT (72).

CONCLUSION

Flow cytometry plays a major role in diagnosis and classification of PIDDs and is often used as a first-line investigation. Expression of several surface and intracellular proteins can be reliably assessed and quantified using multicolor flow cytometry. It is also the preferred technique for studying cell signaling pathways and cell–cell interactions and for assaying lymphocyte proliferation. Recent advances in flow cytometry techniques would further facilitate the workup of patients with PIDDs.

AUTHOR CONTRIBUTIONS

AR, KA, JS, PV, SS, and DS drafted the manuscript. AR, KA, JS, RR, GK, VJ, JD, and BM performed the laboratory investigations. SS, AR, and PV reviewed and finalized the manuscript.

ACKNOWLEDGMENTS

The authors thankfully acknowledge the Indian Council of Medical Research and Department of Health Research, Ministry of Health and Family Welfare, Government of India, New Delhi, for support towards the Center for Advanced Research in Primary Immune Deficiency Disorders at Advanced Pediatrics Center, Post Graduate Institute of Medical Education and Research, Chandigarh, India (vide Grant No. GIA/48/2014-DHR). Support provided by the Foundation for Primary Immunodeficiency Diseases (FPID), USA, is also gratefully acknowledged.

SUPPLEMENTARY MATERIAL

Supplementary Figure 1 | (A) Lymphocyte subset analysis depicting normal lymphocyte proportions of lymphocytes in healthy control; Absent T lymphocytes and reduced NK cells in a case of T–B+NK– SCID; Reduced T lymphocytes, normal NK, and relative increase in proportion of B lymphocytes representing T–B+NK+ SCID; Absent T and B lymphocytes with increased proportion of NK cells representing T–B–NK+ SCID; Severe lymphopenia with reduced T, B, and NK cells (T–B–NK– SCID) in an infant with ADA deficiency; Lymphocytes were gated on CD45 vs. SSc and different subsets were estimated on gated lymphocytes. **(B)** Decreased total naïve T lymphocytes (CD3+CD45RA+CD45RO–), naïve helper T cells (CD3+CD4+CD45RA+CD45RO–) and naïve cytotoxic T cells (CD3+CD8+CD45RA+CD45RO–) in a case of SCID; CD3+ T cells were gated on CD3 vs. SSc and CD45RA was observed on CD3, CD4, and CD8 cells. **(C)** Increased expression of HLA DR on T lymphocytes in a patient with Omenn syndrome. **(D)** Reduced expression of CD127 on gated lymphocytes in a case T–B+NK+ SCID due to mutation in IL-7R. **(E)** Reduced expression of CD132 (common γ chain) on neutrophils, monocytes, and lymphocytes in a case of T–B+NK– SCID due to mutation in *IL2RG*.

Supplementary Figure 2 | Lymphocyte subset analysis in a patient with T-B-NK+ SCID **(A)** Pre-transplant; **(B–E)** After hematopoietic stem cell transplantation. Lymphocytes were gated on CD45 vs. SSc and further subsets were analyzed on gated lymphocytes.

Supplementary Figure 3 | Decreased expression of CD40L on activated T Lymphocytes (CD4+CD69+) in response to stimulation with PMA and ionomycin. PBMCs were gated on FSc vs. SSc and activated T lymphocytes were analyzed on the gated PBMCs.

Supplementary Figure 4 | Expression of Wiskott–Aldrich Syndrome protein (WASp) in **(A)** a healthy control; **(B)** a patient with WAS; **(C)** after hematopoietic stem cell transplantation in patient depicted in **(B)**; Lymphocytes were gated on FSc vs. SSc.

Supplementary Figure 5 | (A) Absent B lymphocytes and **(B)** absent Btk protein expression on gated monocytes in a patient with XLA.

Supplementary Figure 6 | B cell phenotyping showing decreased class switched B lymphocytes and reduced switched memory B lymphocytes in a case of CD40 deficiency. **(A)** Control **(B)** Patient. Lymphocytes were gated on FSc. vs SSc, further B lymphocytes were gated on CD19+ to analyze the B cell subsets.

Supplementary Figure 7 | Evaluation for hemophagocytic lymphohistiocytosis. **(A)** Reduced perforin expression on CD56+NK cells in a patient with HLH; lymphocytes were gated on FSc vs. SSc graph. Further, the CD56+ cells are analyzed on gated lymphocytes. **(B)** PBMCs stimulated with PMA and ionomycin and stained with CD107a show reduced expression in a patient. PBMCs were gated on FSc vs. SSc followed by CD56+ NK cells from the gated PBMCs.

Supplementary Figure 8 | Increase in double-negative T cells (TCR αβ+, CD3+, CD4–, CD8–) in a patient with ALPS (FASL mutation). Lymphocytes were gated on CD45 vs. SSc graph and further DNTs were seen on CD4 CD8 vs. TCR-αβ dot plot.

Supplementary Figure 9 | Dihydrorhodamine assay for chronic granulomatous disease: **(A)** Normal shift of fluorescence peak in a control. **(B)** No shift in a patient with CGD. **(C)** Bimodal expression in a female carrier of X-linked CGD. Neutrophils were gated on FSc vs. SSc plot and oxidative burst was evaluated on gated neutrophils.

Supplementary Figure 10 | Flow cytometry analysis of b558 expression. **(A)** Normal expression in a control. **(B)** Patient with X-linked CGD. **(C)** Dual peaks in a carrier female. Neutrophils were gated on FSc vs. SSc plot and b558 was evaluated on gated neutrophils.

Supplementary Figure 11 | Laboratory workflow for patients with chronic granulomatous disease (CGD) diagnosed at our center. *DHR/gp91phox expression in the mother is performed only in cases of males with CGD.

Supplementary Figure 12 | Absent expression of CD18 on gated neutrophils in a patient with LAD-1. Neutrophils were gated on FSc vs. SSc plot.

Supplementary Figure 13 | (A) Decreased expression of IL12Rβ1 after stimulation of PBMCs with PHA; PBMCs were gated on FSc vs. SSc followed by CD3+ T cells from the gated PBMCs. **(B)** Increased expression of IFNγR1 expression on gated neutrophils in a patient with partial dominant IFNγR1 defect. Neutrophils, monocytes, and lymphocytes were gated on FSc vs. SSc plot.

Supplementary Table 1 | Flow cytometry-based tests for diseases of immune dysregulation.

Supplementary Table 2 | Flow cytometry-based tests for defects in intrinsic and innate immunity.

REFERENCES

1. Adan A, Alizada G, Kiraz Y, Baran Y, Nalbant A. Flow cytometry: basic principles and applications. *Crit Rev Biotechnol.* (2017) 37:163–76. doi: 10.3109/07388551.2015.1128876
2. Kamentsky LA, Melamed MR, Derman H. Spectrophotometer: new instrument for ultrarapid cell analysis. *Science.* (1965) 150:630–1. doi: 10.1126/science.150.3696.630
3. Bonilla FA, Khan DA, Ballas ZK, Chinen J, Frank MM, Hsu JT, et al. Practice parameter for the diagnosis and management of primary immunodeficiency. *J Allergy Clin Immunol.* (2015) 136:1186–205.e1–78. doi: 10.1016/j.jaci.2015.04.049
4. Kanegane H, Hoshino A, Okano T, Yasumi T, Wada T, Takada H, et al. Flow cytometry-based diagnosis of primary immunodeficiency diseases. *Allergol Int.* (2018) 67:43–54. doi: 10.1016/j.alit.2017.06.003
5. Jindal AK, Pilania RK, Rawat A, Singh S. Primary immunodeficiency disorders in India—A situational review. *Front Immunol.* (2017) 8:714. doi: 10.3389/fimmu.2017.00714
6. Illoh OC. Current applications of flow cytometry in the diagnosis of primary immunodeficiency diseases. *Arch Pathol Lab Med.* (2004) 128:23–31. doi: 10.1043/1543-2165(2004)128<23:CAOFCI>2.0.CO;2
7. Fischer A. Severe combined immunodeficiencies (SCID). *Clin Exp Immunol.* (2000) 122:143–9. doi: 10.1046/j.1365-2249.2000.01359.x
8. Gaspar HB. Current topic: severe combined immunodeficiency—molecular pathogenesis and diagnosis. *Arch Dis Child.* (2001) 84:169–73. doi: 10.1136/adc.84.2.169
9. Asao H, Okuyama C, Kumaki S, Ishii N, Tsuchiya S, Foster D, et al. Cutting edge: the common gamma-chain is an indispensable subunit of the IL-21 receptor complex. *J Immunol.* (2001) 167:1–5. doi: 10.4049/jimmunol.167.1.1
10. Kuijpers TW, van Leeuwen EMM, Barendregt BH, Klarenbeek P, aan de Kerk DJ, Baars PA, et al. A reversion of an IL2RG mutation in combined immunodeficiency providing competitive advantage to the majority of CD8+ T cells. *Haematologica.* (2013) 98:1030–8. doi: 10.3324/haematol.2012.077511
11. Viprakasit V, Monteerarat Y, Piboonpocanun O, Sanpakit K, Chinchang W, Tachavanich K, et al. Identification of a novel IL7RA mutation (444_450insA) caused marked reduction in CD127 expression from a cohort molecular analysis of severe combined immunodeficiency (T–, B+, NK+ SCID) in Thailand. *Blood.* (2006) 108:1247.
12. Rosenzweig SD, Fleisher TA. Laboratory evaluation for T-cell dysfunction. *J Allergy Clin Immunol.* (2013) 131:622–3.e4. doi: 10.1016/j.jaci.2012.11.018
13. Pilch H, Höhn H, Freitag K, Neukirch C, Necker A, Haddad P, et al. Improved assessment of T-cell receptor (TCR) VB repertoire in clinical specimens: combination of TCR-CDR3 spectratyping with flow cytometry-based TCR VB frequency analysis. *Clin Diagn Lab Immunol.* (2002) 9:257–66. doi: 10.1128/CDLI.9.2.257-266.2002
14. Hanna S, Etzioni A. MHC class I and II deficiencies. *J Allergy Clin Immunol.* (2014) 134:269–75. doi: 10.1016/j.jaci.2014.06.001
15. Gadola SD, Moins-Teisserenc HT, Trowsdale J, Gross WL, Cerundolo V. TAP deficiency syndrome. *Clin Exp Immunol.* (2000) 121:173–8. doi: 10.1046/j.1365-2249.2000.01264.x
16. Knight V. The utility of flow cytometry for the diagnosis of primary immunodeficiencies. *Int J Lab Hematol.* (2019) 41:63–72. doi: 10.1111/ijlh.13010
17. Oliveira JB, Notarangelo LD, Fleisher TA. Applications of flow cytometry for the study of primary immune deficiencies. *Curr Opin Allergy Clin Immunol.* (2008) 6:499–509. doi: 10.1097/ACI.0b013e328312c790
18. Tario JD Jr, Conway AN, Muirhead KA, Wallace PK. Monitoring cell proliferation by dye dilution: considerations for probe selection. *Methods Mol Biol.* (2018) 1678:249–99. doi: 10.1007/978-1-4939-7346-0_12
19. Cowan M, Gennery A. Radiation-sensitive severe combined immunodeficiency: the arguments for and against conditioning prior to hematopoietic cell transplantation—What to do? *J Allergy Clin Immunol.* (2015) 136:1178–85. doi: 10.1016/j.jaci.2015.04.027
20. Aluri J, Desai M, Gupta M, Dalvi A, Terance A, Rosenzweig SD, et al. Clinical, immunological, and molecular findings in 57 patients with severe combined immunodeficiency (SCID) from India. *Front Immunol.* (2019) 10:23. doi: 10.3389/fimmu.2019.00023
21. Aydin SE, Kilic SS, Aytekin C, Kumar A, Porras O, Kainulainen L, et al. DOCK8 deficiency: clinical and immunological phenotype and treatment options—A review of 136 patients. *J Clin Immunol.* (2015) 35:189–98. doi: 10.1007/s10875-014-0126-0
22. Su HC. DOCK8 (Dedicator of cytokinesis 8) deficiency. *Curr Opin Allergy Clin Immunol.* (2010) 10:515–20. doi: 10.1097/ACI.0b013e32833fd718
23. Pai S-Y, de Boer H, Massaad MJ, Chatila TA, Keles S, Jabara HH, et al. Flow cytometry diagnosis of dedicator of cytokinesis 8 (DOCK8) deficiency. *J Allergy Clin Immunol.* (2014) 134:221–3. doi: 10.1016/j.jaci.2014.02.023
24. Gulino AV, Notarangelo LD. Hyper IgM syndromes. *Curr Opin Rheumatol.* (2003) 15:422–9. doi: 10.1097/00002281-200307000-00009
25. Freyer DR, Gowans LK, Warzynski M, Lee W-I. Flow cytometric diagnosis of X-linked hyper-IgM syndrome: application of an accurate and convenient procedure. *J Pediatr Hematol Oncol.* (2004) 26:363–70. doi: 10.1097/00043426-200406000-00006
26. Notarangelo LD, Miao CH, Ochs HD. Wiskott–Aldrich syndrome. *Curr Opin Hematol.* (2008) 15:30–6. doi: 10.1097/MOH.0b013e3282f30448
27. Rivers E, Thrasher AJ. Wiskott-Aldrich syndrome protein: emerging mechanisms in immunity. *Eur J Immunol.* (2017) 47:1857–66. doi: 10.1002/eji.201646715
28. Delmonte OM, Fleisher TA. Flow cytometry: surface markers and beyond. *J Allergy Clin Immunol.* (2019) 143:528–37. doi: 10.1016/j.jaci.2018.08.011
29. Conley ME, Cooper MD. Genetic basis of abnormal B cell development. *Curr Opin Immunol.* (1998) 10:399–406. doi: 10.1016/S0952-7915(98)80112-X

30. Takada H, Kanegane H, Nomura A, Yamamoto K, Ihara K, Takahashi Y, et al. Female agammaglobulinemia due to the Bruton tyrosine kinase deficiency caused by extremely skewed X-chromosome inactivation. *Blood.* (2004) 103:185–7. doi: 10.1182/blood-2003-06-1964
31. Teimourian S, Nasseri S, Pouladi N, Yeganeh M, Aghamohammadi A. Genotype–phenotype correlation in Bruton's tyrosine kinase deficiency. *J Pediatr Hematol Oncol.* (2008) 30:679–83. doi: 10.1097/MPH.0b013e318180bb45
32. Cunningham-Rundles C. The many faces of common variable immunodeficiency. *Hematology Am Soc Hematol Educ Program.* (2012) 2012:301–5. doi: 10.1182/asheducation-2012.1.301
33. Saikia B, Gupta S. Common variable immunodeficiency. *Indian J Pediatr.* (2016) 83:338–44. doi: 10.1007/s12098-016-2038-x
34. Abraham RS, Aubert G. Flow cytometry, a versatile tool for diagnosis and monitoring of primary immunodeficiencies. *Clin Vaccine Immunol.* (2016) 23:254–71. doi: 10.1128/CVI.00001-16
35. Bogaert DJA, Dullaers M, Lambrecht BN, Vermaelen KY, De Baere E, Haerynck F. Genes associated with common variable immunodeficiency: one diagnosis to rule them all? *J Med Genet.* (2016) 53:575–90. doi: 10.1136/jmedgenet-2015-103690
36. van Schouwenburg P, IJspeert H, Pico-Knijnenburg I, Dalm V, van Hagen PM, van Zessen D, et al. Identification of CVID patients with defects in immune repertoire formation or specification. *Front Immunol.* (2018) 9:2545. doi: 10.3389/fimmu.2018.02545
37. Verma N, Burns SO, Walker LSK, Sansom DM. Immune deficiency and autoimmunity in patients with CTLA-4 (CD152) mutations. *Clin Exp Immunol.* (2017) 190:1–7. doi: 10.1111/cei.12997
38. Lo B, Zhang K, Lu W, Zheng L, Zhang Q, Kanellopoulou C, et al. Autoimmune disease. Patients with LRBA deficiency show CTLA4 loss and immune dysregulation responsive to abatacept therapy. *Science.* (2015) 349:436–40. doi: 10.1126/science.aaa1663
39. Wirsum C, Glaser C, Gutenberger S, Keller B, Unger S, Voll RE, et al. Secondary antibody deficiency in glucocorticoid therapy clearly differs from primary antibody deficiency. *J Clin Immunol.* (2016) 36:406–12. doi: 10.1007/s10875-016-0264-7
40. Al-Samkari H, Berliner N. Hemophagocytic lymphohistiocytosis. *Annu Rev Pathol.* (2018) 13:27–49. doi: 10.1146/annurev-pathol-020117-043625
41. Feldmann J, Callebaut I, Raposo G, Certain S, Bacq D, Dumont C, et al. Munc13-4 is essential for cytolytic granules fusion and is mutated in a form of familial hemophagocytic lymphohistiocytosis (FHL3). *Cell.* (2003) 115:461–73. doi: 10.1016/S0092-8674(03)00855-9
42. zurStadt U, Rohr J, Seifert W, Koch F, Grieve S, Pagel J, et al. Familial hemophagocytic lymphohistiocytosis type 5 (FHL-5) is caused by mutations in Munc18-2 and impaired binding to syntaxin 11. *Am J Hum Genet.* (2009) 85:482–92. doi: 10.1016/j.ajhg.2009.09.005
43. zurStadt U, Schmidt S, Kasper B, Beutel K, Diler AS, Henter J-I, et al. Linkage of familial hemophagocytic lymphohistiocytosis (FHL) type-4 to chromosome 6q24 and identification of mutations in syntaxin 11. *Hum Mol Genet.* (2005) 14:827–34. doi: 10.1093/hmg/ddi076
44. Alter G, Malenfant JM, Altfeld M. CD107a as a functional marker for the identification of natural killer cell activity. *J Immunol Methods.* (2004) 294:15–22. doi: 10.1016/j.jim.2004.08.008
45. Kogawa K, Lee SM, Villanueva J, Marmer D, Sumegi J, Filipovich AH. Perforin expression in cytotoxic lymphocytes from patients with hemophagocytic lymphohistiocytosis and their family members. *Blood.* (2002) 99:61–6. doi: 10.1182/blood.V99.1.61
46. Gifford CE, Weingartner E, Villanueva J, Johnson J, Zhang K, Filipovich AH, et al. Clinical flow cytometric screening of SAP and XIAP expression accurately identifies patients with *SH2D1A* and *XIAP/BIRC4* mutations: accuracy of SAP and XIAP flow cytometric screening. *Cytometry B Clin Cytom.* (2014) 86:263–71. doi: 10.1002/cyto.b.21166
47. Shah S, Wu E, Rao VK. Autoimmune lymphoproliferative syndrome: an update and review of the literature. *Curr Allergy Asthma Rep.* (2014) 14:462. doi: 10.1007/s11882-014-0462-4
48. Rieux-Laucat F, Magerus-Chatinet A. Autoimmune lymphoproliferative syndrome: a multifactorial disorder. *Haematologica.* (2010) 95:1805–7. doi: 10.3324/haematol.2010.030395
49. Lopatin U, Yao X, Williams RK, Bleesing JJ, Dale JK, Wong D, et al. Increases in circulating and lymphoid tissue interleukin-10 in autoimmune lymphoproliferative syndrome are associated with disease expression. *Blood.* (2001) 97:3161–70. doi: 10.1182/blood.V97.10.3161
50. Torgerson TR, Ochs HD. Immune dysregulation, polyendocrinopathy, enteropathy, X-linked: forkhead box protein 3 mutations and lack of regulatory T cells. *J Allergy Clin Immunol.* (2007) 120:744–50. doi: 10.1016/j.jaci.2007.08.044
51. Otsubo K, Kanegane H, Kamachi Y, Kobayashi I, Tsuge I, Imaizumi M, et al. Identification of FOXP3-negative regulatory T-like (CD4+CD25+CD127low) cells in patients with immune dysregulation, polyendocrinopathy, enteropathy, X-linked syndrome. *Clin Immunol.* (2011) 141:111–20. doi: 10.1016/j.clim.2011.06.006
52. Vignoli M, Ciullini Mannurita S, Fioravanti A, Tumino M, Grassi A, Guariso G, et al. CD25 deficiency: a new conformational mutation prevents the receptor expression on cell surface. *Clin Immunol.* (2019) 201:15–9. doi: 10.1016/j.clim.2019.02.003
53. Rawat A, Bhattad S, Singh S. Chronic granulomatous disease. *Indian J Pediatr.* (2016) 83:345–53. doi: 10.1007/s12098-016-2040-3
54. Roos D. Chronic granulomatous disease. *Br Med Bull.* (2016) 118:50–63. doi: 10.1093/bmb/ldw009
55. Arnadottir GA, Norddahl GL, Gudmundsdottir S, Agustsdottir AB, Sigurdsson S, Jensson BO, et al. A homozygous loss-of-function mutation leading to CYBC1 deficiency causes chronic granulomatous disease. *Nat Commun.* (2018) 9:4447. doi: 10.1038/s41467-018-06964-x
56. Vowells SJ, Sekhsaria S, Malech HL, Shalit M, Fleisher TA. Flow cytometric analysis of the granulocyte respiratory burst: a comparison study of fluorescent probes. *J Immunol Methods.* (1995) 178:89–97. doi: 10.1016/0022-1759(94)00247-T
57. Marciano BE, Zerbe CS, Falcone EL, Ding L, DeRavin SS, Daub J, et al. X-linked carriers of chronic granulomatous disease: illness, lyonization, and stability. *J Allergy Clin Immunol.* (2018) 141:365–71. doi: 10.1016/j.jaci.2017.04.035
58. Hanna S, Etzioni A. Leukocyte adhesion deficiencies: leukocyte adhesion deficiencies. *Ann N Y Acad Sci.* (2012) 1250:50–5. doi: 10.1111/j.1749-6632.2011.06389.x
59. Moser M, Bauer M, Schmid S, Ruppert R, Schmidt S, Sixt M, et al. Kindlin-3 is required for beta2 integrin-mediated leukocyte adhesion to endothelial cells. *Nat Med.* (2009) 15:300–5. doi: 10.1038/nm.1921
60. Freeman AF, Holland SM. The hyper IgE syndromes. *Immunol Allergy Clin North Am.* (2008) 28:277–viii. doi: 10.1016/j.iac.2008.01.005
61. Grimbacher B, Schäffer AA, Holland SM, Davis J, Gallin JI, Malech HL, et al. Genetic linkage of hyper-IgE syndrome to chromosome 4. *Am J Hum Genet.* (1999) 65:735–44. doi: 10.1086/302547
62. de Beaucoudrey L, Samarina A, Bustamante J, Cobat A, Boisson-Dupuis S, Feinberg J, et al. Revisiting human IL-12Rβ1 deficiency. *Medicine.* (2010) 89:381–402. doi: 10.1097/MD.0b013e3181fdd832
63. Bustamante J, Boisson-Dupuis S, Abel L, Casanova J-L. Mendelian susceptibility to mycobacterial disease: genetic, immunological, and clinical features of inborn errors of IFN-γ immunity. *Semin Immunol.* (2014) 26:454–70. doi: 10.1016/j.smim.2014.09.008
64. Sologuren I, Boisson-Dupuis S, Pestano J, Vincent QB, Fernández-Pérez L, Chapgier A, et al. Partial recessive IFN-γR1 deficiency: genetic, immunological and clinical features of 14 patients from 11 kindreds. *Hum Mol Genet.* (2011) 20:1509–23. doi: 10.1093/hmg/ddr029
65. Jouanguy E, Lamhamedi-Cherradi S, Lammas D, Dorman SE, Fondanèche M-C, Dupuis S, et al. A human IFNGR1 small deletion hotspot associated with dominant susceptibility to mycobacterial infection. *Nat Genet.* (1999) 21:370–8. doi: 10.1038/7701
66. Fleisher TA, Dorman SE, Anderson JA, Vail M, Brown MR, Holland SM. Detection of intracellular phosphorylated STAT-1 by Flow Cytometry. *Clin Immunol.* (1999) 90:425–30. doi: 10.1006/clim.1998.4654
67. Uzel G, Frucht DM, Fleisher TA, Holland SM. Detection of intracellular phosphorylated STAT-4 by flow cytometry. *Clin Immunol.* (2001) 100:270–6. doi: 10.1006/clim.2001.5078
68. Vidya MK, Kumar VG, Sejian V, Bagath M, Krishnan G, Bhatta R. Toll-like receptors: significance, ligands, signaling pathways,

and functions in mammals. *Int Rev Immunol.* (2018) 37:20–36. doi: 10.1080/08830185.2017.1380200

69. CuraDaball P, Ventura Ferreira MS, Ammann S, Klemann C, Lorenz MR, Warthorst U, et al. CD57 identifies T cells with functional senescence before terminal differentiation and relative telomere shortening in patients with activated PI3 kinase delta syndrome. *Immunol Cell Biol.* (2018) 96:1060–71. doi: 10.1111/imcb.12169
70. Coulter TI, Chandra A, Bacon CM, Babar J, Curtis J, Screaton N, et al. Clinical spectrum and features of activated phosphoinositide 3-kinase δ syndrome: a large patient cohort study. *J Allergy Clin Immunol.* (2017) 139:597–606.e4. doi: 10.1016/j.jaci.2016.06.021
71. Rothblum-Oviatt C, Wright J, Lefton-Greif MA, McGrath-Morrow SA, Crawford TO, Lederman HM. Ataxia telangiectasia: a review. *Orphanet J Rare Dis.* (2016) 11:159. doi: 10.1186/s13023-016-0543-7
72. Porcedda P, Turinetto V, Brusco A, Cavalieri S, Lantelme E, Orlando L, et al. A rapid flow cytometry test based on histone H2AX phosphorylation for the sensitive and specific diagnosis of ataxia telangiectasia. *Cytometry A.* (2008) 73A:508–16. doi: 10.1002/cyto.a.20566

8

Flow Cytometric Determination of Actin Polymerization in Peripheral Blood Leukocytes Effectively Discriminate Patients with Homozygous Mutation in ARPC1B from Asymptomatic Carriers and Normal Controls

Andreja N. Kopitar[1], *Gašper Markelj*[2], *Miha Oražem*[3], *Štefan Blazina*[2], *Tadej Avčin*[2,4], *Alojz Ihan*[1] *and Maruša Debeljak*[5*]

[1] *Faculty of Medicine, Institute of Microbiology and Immunology, University of Ljubljana, Ljubljana, Slovenia,* [2] *Department of Allergology, Rheumatology and Clinical Immunology, University Children's Hospital, University Medical Center Ljubljana, Ljubljana, Slovenia,* [3] *Department of Radiation Oncology, Institute of Oncology Ljubljana, Ljubljana, Slovenia,* [4] *Department of Pediatrics, Faculty of Medicine, University of Ljubljana, Ljubljana, Slovenia,* [5] *Unit for Special Laboratory Diagnostics, University Children's Hospital, University Medical Center Ljubljana, Ljubljana, Slovenia*

Correspondence:
Maruša Debeljak
marusa.debeljak@kclj.si

Actin nucleators initiate formation of actin filaments. Among them, the Arp2/3 complex has the ability to form branched actin networks. This complex is regulated by members of the Wiscott-Aldrich syndrome protein (WASp) family. Polymerization of actin filaments can be evaluated through flow cytometry by fluorescent phalloidin staining before and after stimulation with N-formyl-methionyl-leucyl-phenylalanine (fMLP). We identified a missense mutation in the gene ARPC1B (Arp2/3 activator subunit) resulting in defective actin polymerization in four patients (three of them were related). All patients (1 male, 3 female) developed microthrombocytopenia, cellular immune deficiency, eczema, various autoimmune manifestations, recurrent skin abscesses and elevated IgE antibodies. Besides four patients with homozygous mutation in ARPC1B, we also identified six heterozygous carriers without clinical disease (3 males, 3 females) within the same family. We developed a functional test to evaluate Arp2/3 complex function, which consists of flow cytometric detection of intracellular polymerized actin after *in vitro* fMLP stimulation of leukocytes. Median fluorescence intensities of FITC-phalloidin stained actin were measured in monocytes, neutrophils and lymphocytes of patients, carriers, and healthy control subjects. We detected non-efficient actin polymerization in monocytes and neutrophils of homozygous patients compared to carriers or the healthy subjects. In monocytes, the increase in median fluorescence intensities was significantly lower in patients compared to carriers (104 vs. 213%; $p < 0.01$) and healthy controls (104 vs. 289%; $p < 0.01$). Similarly, the increase in median fluorescence intensities in neutrophils was significantly increased in the group with carriers (208%; $p < 0.01$) and healthy controls (238%; $p < 0.01$) and significantly decreased in the patient's group (94%). Our functional fMLP/phalloidin test can therefore be used as a practical tool to separate symptomatic patients from asymptomatic mutation associated to actin polymerization.

Keywords: ARPC1B deficiency, Arp2/3, actin polymerization, flow cytometry, functional test, peripheral blood leukocytes

INTRODUCTION

Polymerization of actin plays an important role in many immune functions like proliferation and differentiation of immune cells, migration, intercellular and intracellular signaling and activation of both, innate and adaptive immune responses. Dynamic rearrangement of cell shape relies on rapid assembly and disassembly of filamentous actin (1). To initiate actin assembly during such processes, cells generate free barbed ends that act as templates for polymerization by uncapping or severing existing filaments or by nucleating from monomers *de novo* (2). The microfilamentous cytoskeleton is a highly dynamic network that is made of actin and numerous actin-associated proteins (3). Polymerization is initiated by three classes of actin nucleators, the actin related protein 2/actin related protein 3 (Arp2/3) complex, the formin family, and the more recently identified Spire, cordon-bleu, and leiomodin family (1). They promote nucleation, in response to specific upstream signals such as integrin activation, T-cell and B-cell receptor ligation and chemokine stimulation (4). Each class of nucleators has a distinct mechanism for initiating actin polymerization (1). The first major actin nucleator to be discovered was the Arp2/3 complex, which is composed of evolutionarily-conserved subunits including the actin-related proteins Arp2 and Arp3 and five additional subunits ARPC1–5 (5). Arp2/3 complex is a macromolecular machine that nucleates branched actin filaments in response to cellular signals. Wiskott-Aldrich syndrome proteins (WASp) family regulates the nucleation activity of Arp2/3 complex, providing a way for cells to assemble branched actin filament networks (6). Rho-family GTPases like Cdc42 and Rac2 are involved in regulation of actin polymerization by directly interacting with WASp (7).

Control of actin dynamics is essential to many cellular processes, including motility, vesicle trafficking, and cell division. The Arp2/3 complex nucleates new (daughter) filaments on the sides of existing (mother) filaments in response to activating stimulus from the WASp family [reviewed in Smith et al. (8)]. Dynamic associations of Arp2/3 complex with mother filament and WASp is temporally coordinated to initiation daughter filament growth which is necessary to perform a variety of cellular functions including motility (9). Phalloidin has been widely used for studying actin polymerization in biochemical assays and in fluorescent microscopy (10). It is a small toxic molecule produced by the poisonous mushrooms *Amanita phalloides*. Phalloidin stabilizes actin structures and therefore prevents the depolymerization of the actin polymers, resulting in cytotoxicity (11).

Over 300 genes have been causally linked to monogenic forms of primary immunodeficiency disorder (PID), including a number that are associated with actin polymerization are mostly due to genetic defects in such regulatory proteins. Known cytoskeleton-associated PIDs present either as combined or severe combined immunodeficiencies or as phagocyte disorders (4).

Our study focused on ARPC1B deficiency, a recently described PID (12, 13). Disease is characterized by recurrent infections, hypersensitivity, autoimmunity and increased risk of malignancies. Majority of the patients have increased bleeding tendency due to thrombocytopenia and platelet disfunction. Recurrent infections are both bacterial and viral most commonly in the respiratory tract, skin and gastrointestinal tract. Hypersensitivity features include eczema, food allergies, and asthma. Predominant autoimmune features are skin vasculitis and inflammatory bowel disease. Disease clinically resembles with loss-of-function mutations in WAS gene (13, 14).

The aim of our study was to introduce a rapid, very specific and simple functional test to evaluate impaired actin polymerization in patients with mutation in ARPC1B. Intracellularly polymerized actin was measured by flow cytometry with fluorescent phalloidin before and after *in vitro* fMLP stimulation of leukocytes.

METHODS

Patients/Study Design

In the period from November 2016 to December 2018, we evaluated patients that were initially identified as having Wiskott-Aldrich like syndrome (thrombocytopenia, eczema, variable degree of immunodeficiency), but later ARPC1 mutation were identified. Four patients with homozygous ARPC1B mutation (1 male, 3 females), 6 heterozygous carriers without clinical disease (3 males, 3 females) within the same family and twelve healthy subjects (without ARPC1B mutation) were included in the study. Clinical and immunological parameters of the patients are summarized in **Tables 1**, **2**.

Genetic Tests

We extracted genomic DNA from whole blood EDTA samples of four patients and their relatives (siblings, parents, grandparents) according to established laboratory protocols using FlexiGene DNA isolation kit (Qiagen, Germany). We performed whole exome sequencing of an index patient in collaboration with Eurofins Genomics (Ebersberg, Germany) using Ion AmpliSeq Exome kit for whole exome enrichment preparation and Ion

TABLE 1 | Clinical parameters of the patients with ARPC1B mutation at the first evaluation.

Patient	Age	Infections	Allergy	Autoimmunity	Malignancy	Other
P1	27 year	Recurrent bonchiolitis and pneumonias, recurrent skin abscesses	eczema, Food, pollen and mites allergy	Enterocolitis, Small vessels vasculitis, Autoimmune thrombocytopenia, panniculitis	/	Stunted growth
P2	24 year	Prolonged pneumonias, Gastroenteritis, Candida esophagitis, Chronic warts - Epidermodysplasia verruciformis	Eczema, Food allergy	Enterocolitis, Pernicous anemia	Metaplasia in gastric mucosa, bowel adenoma *in situ*	Stunted growth
P3	30 year	Recurrent pneumonias, lung abscesses, Gastroenteritis, Recurrent skin abscess, chronic leg ulceration, Gastroenteritis, Genital condyloma and severe warts	Eczema, Food, mites, animal epithelia allergy, Allergic asthma	Enterocolitis, Small vessels vasculitis	Cervical intraepithelial neoplasia grade 2	Stunted growth
P4	16 months	/	Mild eczema	Evans syndrome	/	/

TABLE 2 | Immunological parameters of the patients with mutations in ARPC1B at the first evaluation.

Patient	IgE	IgG	IgA	IgM	CD3	CD19	CD4	CD8	NK	T cell prolif. (PHA)	T cell prolif. (CD3+CD28)
	IE/L	g/L			10^9 cells/L					%	%
NV1	0–100	7.0–16.0	0.7–5.0	0.4–2.8	0.7–1.9	0.1–0.4	0.4–1.3	0.2–0.7	0.04–0.2	29–57	50–85
P1	1746↑	13.4	0.98	2.52	0.626↓	0.562↑	0.305↓	0.498	0.369	15↓	52
P2	932↑	11.3	4.7	0.85	0.967	0.521↑	0.459	0.546	0.468	22↓	70
P3	716↑	13.6	6.3↑	0.6	1.006	0.542↑	0.730	0.126↓	0.066↓	33	66
NV2	0-60	4.7-12.0	0.14-0.91	0.4-1.5	2.2-5.5	0.9-2.5	1.1-3.6	0.5-1.8	0.1-1.1	29-57	50-85
P4	<19	12.4↑	2.21↑	1.33	1.551↓	2.066	1.024↓	0.408↓	0.777	38	77

Immunoglobulin classes were measured in serum. The concentration of IgE is in IE/L, and IgG, IgA, IgM in g/L. The concentration of lymphocytes subpopulations are presented as $\times 10^9$ cells/L, the proliferation of T lymphocytes after stimulation with PHA or CD3 and CD28 in percentage of proliferating cells. CD3, T lymphocytes; CD19, B lymphocytes; CD4, helper T cells; CD8, cytotoxic T cells; NK, Natural killer cells; PHA, phytohaemagglutinin; anti-CD3, anti-CD28 – monoclonal antibodies, P, patients, NV1, normal values for adults, NV2, normal values for 16 month. An arrow indicates deviation from normal values (15, 16).

PI™ Sequencing 200 Kit v3 together with Ion Proton Sequencer (Life Technologies, USA) to perform whole exon sequencing. We analyzed genetic variants with coverage >15x with Variant Studio 2.2 software (Illumina). Since pathogenic mutations leading to WAS-like are likely rare in unaffected populations, we filtered out all variants identified from the latest draft of the 1000 Genomes Project and dbSNP build 132. The search tool for the retrieval of interacting genes/proteins (STRING, http://string-db.org/) was used to construct protein-protein interactions, which are involved downstream and upstream of the WASP protein, and could be involved in defective actin reorganization, cell trafficking and synapse formation. We directed and focused the analysis on actin reorganization defects using the panel of genes (*ACTR2, ACTR3, ARPC1A, ARPC1B, ARPC2, ARPC3, ARPC4, ARPC5, ARPC5L, BTK, FYN, GRB2, NCK1, PSTPIP, WIPF1*). We excluded from further analysis all variants exceeding the threshold value for known variant minor allele frequency at 1%. We used the autosomal recessive inheritance model to further reduce the number of potential causative variants. We confirmed the identified candidate variant and its family segregation by a targeted Sanger sequencing run on ABI Genetic Analyzer 3500 (Applied Biosystems, USA) using custom oligonucleotides and BigDye Terminator v3.1 sequencing kit (Applied Biosystems, USA). We analyzed the potential deleterious effect of identified genetic variant with several *in silico* prediction tools: SIFT (Sorting Intolerant from Tolerant; http://sift.bii.a-star.edu.sg), Polyphen2 (http://genetics.bwh.harvard.edu/pph2/), CADD score (http://cadd.gs.washington.edu/score) and Mutation taster (http://www.mutationtaster.org/).

Functional fMLP/Phalloidin Test

The actin polymerization was determined by a flow cytometric assay. Fifty microliter of citrated whole blood was incubated for 20 s with or without 10 μl of N-formyl-methionyl-leucyl-phenylalanine (fMLP) (final concentration 0.83×10^{-3}M).

The stimulation time with fMLP was selected among different incubation times; 10, 20, 30, 40, 50, 60, 120, and 180 s as optimized for cell viability and phalloidin mean fluorescence intensity (MFI). Thereafter cells were fixed with 50 μL 4% formaldehyde and incubated for 25 min at room temperature. Red blood cells were lysed with 2 mL BD FACSTM Lysing Solution (BD Biosciences, San Jose, CA, USA) for 10 min, centrifuged (5 min, 450 g) and resuspended in 100 μl PBS containing 1% BSA. Cells were then stained with 10 μL CD14 PE (cat. No. 345785; clone MφP9) and 10 μL CD45 PerCP-Cy5.5 (cat. No. 332784: clone 2D1) monoclonal antibodies (Becton Dickinson, CA, USA) and incubated in the dark for another 15 min. Cells were then permeabilized with 1 mL BD Perm/WashTM buffer (BD Biosciences), centrifuged and intracellularly stained with 5 μL of 1,5 μM FITC-phalloidin, final concentration 150 nM (Sigma-Aldrich, USA). The optimal dilution of phalloidin was determined by titration. Following 60 min incubation in dark at 4°C, the sample was washed twice with 1 mL of PBS containing 1% BSA before analysis by flow cytometry within 30 min. Samples were evaluated by a BD FACS Canto I or II cytometer (BD Biosciences, CA, USA), using DIVA software (BD Biosciences, San Diego, USA). At least 10,000 cells were acquired. The data analysis was performed using FlowJo version 10.1 software (TreeStar, Ashland, USA). The cells were gated into monocytes, neutrophils and lymphocytes according to CD45-PerCP Cy5.5 and CD14-PE distribution (**Figure 2**). The gates were checked by backgating on scatter plots. The FITC-phalloidin fluorescence on monocytes, neutrophils and lymphocytes was displayed on histograms. Patient samples were always measured in duplicates. Normalization was performed by setting the fluorescence intensity of unstimulated samples to 100%. Increase in MFI in the fMLP stimulated samples was calculated as $\frac{\textit{stimulated sample*100}}{\textit{unstimulated sample}}$.

Apoptotic and viable cells we distinguished by 7-AAD vs. annexin V-APC (both from BD Pharmingen) staining. Aggregated doublet cells were excluded from analysis.

Morphological Assay for Actin Polymerization

Mononuclear cells were isolated on a Ficoll–Hypaque gradient. Distribution of F-actin was evaluated in cells fixed with 4% formaldehyde, centrifuged on slides and air dried. After washing with PBS, cells were stained with 100 μL 5M FITC-phalloidin. Labeled samples were again washed in PBS and mounted using VECTASHIELD® mounting medium with DAPI. Slides were examined at 400-or 1,000-fold magnification on a DMRB Leica fluorescence microscope.

Burst Test

The quantitative determination of leukocyte oxidative burst was performed in heparinized whole blood according to instructions of the manufacturer (Glycotope Biotechnology GmbH, Heidelberg, Germany). Briefly, 100 μL of whole blood were stimulated with unlabelled opsonized bacteria (*Escherichia coli*) as a particular stimulator, protein kinase C ligand phorbol 12-myristate 13-acetate (PMA) as a strong stimulus, or fMLP as low stimulant. This stimulations induce monocytes and granulocytes to produce reactive oxygen metabolites. Radical formation was measured at 37°C by conversion of dihydrorhodamine 123 to the fluorescent rhodamine 123. A sample without stimulus served as negative background control. The reaction was stopped by addition of lysing solution, which also removed erythrocytes. After a washing step, DNA staining was performed to exclude aggregation artifacts. Cells were analyzed by flow cytometry (FACSCanto; Becton Dickinson), using DIVA software (Becton Dickinson) for data acquisition and analysis, and the results were expressed as MFI plotted on histograms (17).

Phagocytosis Test

To determinate the phagocytosis of neutrophil granulocytes and monocytes the cells were ingesting FITC-labeled opsonized *E. coli* according to instructions of the manufacturer. We used PHAGOTEST kit from Glycotope Biotechnology GmbH. Briefly, heparinized whole blood was incubated with bacteria at 37°C, a negative control sample remains on ice. The phagocytosis was stopped by placing the samples on ice and adding quenching solution, which discrimination between attachment and internalization of bacteria. Erythrocytes were lysed and DNA staining solution was added just before measurement. Cells were analyzed on FACSCanto flow cytometer, using DIVA software (Becton Dickinson). The percentage of cells, which ingested the FITC labeled *E. coli*, was determinate using the gate on negative control sample on FITC fluorescence histogram.

Statistical Analysis

Increase in median fluorescent intensity was analyzed with independent two-tailed Student's t-test. Statistics were presented as mean of the results ± standard error of the mean (SEM). $P < 0.05$ were considered statistically significant. Whenever two or more replicate samples where measured on the same day for the same donor, we used the calculated average value of the measurements.

RESULTS

Patients

All patients and carriers came from the north-east Slovenian Roma community. Three patients presented in neonatal period with eczema, thrombocytopenia and bloody diarrhea. Later they developed recurrent bacterial infections of lung and skin, therapy resistant inflammatory bowel disease, allergic reactions and other various autoimmune features (AI vasculitis, AI thrombocytopenia, and pernicious anemia). Forth patient presented with mild excema and autoimmune hemolytic anemia and thrombocytopenia (Evans syndrome) at 7 months. They had decreased IgM and elevated IgA and IgE antibodies, a mild cellular immune deficiency, slightly decreased phagocytic assays. Clinical characteristics of the patients with mutations in ARPC1B are summarized in **Table 1**.

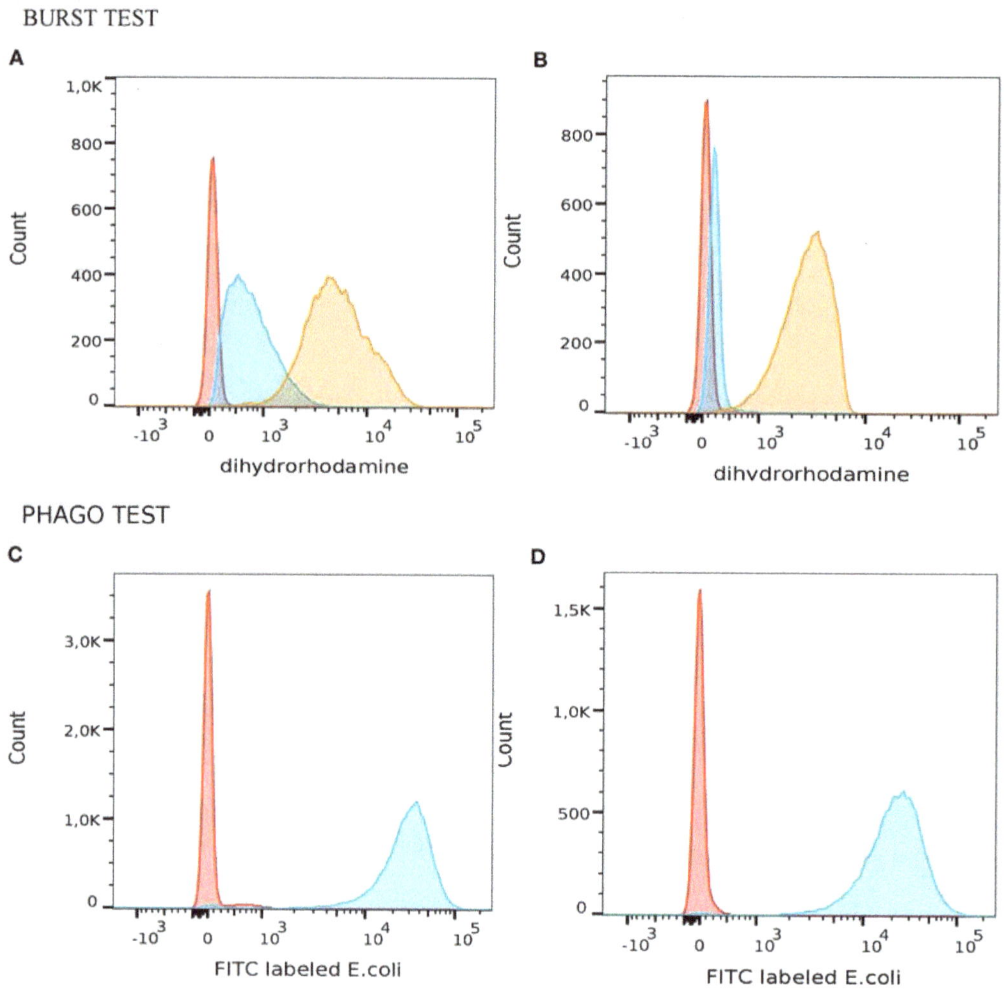

FIGURE 1 | Measurement of oxidative burst and phagocitosis in granulocytes with PHAGOBURST^{TM} test (Glycotope Biotechnology GmbH, Heidelberg, Germany) by flow cytometer. A representative example of functional granulocyte activity which produced different amount of reactive oxidants in patient with mutation in ARPC1B **(A)** and healthy control **(B)**. Red – unstimulated granulocytes; blue – fMLP stimulated granulocytes; orange – PMA stimulated granulocytes. Different phagocytic activity of granulocytes from patients with mutation in ARPC1B **(C)** and healty control **(D)** after phagocytosis of *E. coli* (blue histogram) and negative control (red histogram).

Genetic Studies

Whole exome sequencing identified a mutation in ARPC1B gene (Arp2/3 activator), resulting in defective actin polymerization.

A novel mutation fits in an autosomal recessive model of inheritance. In ARPC1B gene which codes for p41protein in ARP2/3 complex the homozygous substitution c.265A>C was found. It changes amino acid threonine at position 89 into proline (p.Thr89Pro). We predicted the mutation pathogenicity using several *in silico* programs: SIFT (deleterious 0.01), Polyphen2 (possibly_damaging 0.903), CADD score (25.5) and Mutation taster (disease causing 0.999). We cite nomenclature according to the HGVS guidelines (www.hgvs.org/mutnomen). Sequence variants were checked using the Mutalyzer program (http://www.LOVD.nl/mutalyzer). The variant was confirmed with Sanger sequencing. Variant is not present in dbSNP or ExAC database (Exome Aggregattion Consortium: http://exac.broadinstitute.org/). Another three patients were also homozygous for the c.265A>C substitution.

Family segregation analysis was performed in several family members. Parents of all patients are heterozygous carriers of the mutation and have not developed clinical signs of the disease.

All patients with mutation in ARPC1B had slightly decreased phagocytosis and normal oxidative burst after stimulation of monocytes and granulocytes with opsonized *E. coli* or PMA. However, we observed increased respiratory burst in neutrophils after mild stimulation with fMLP in average 67% (**Figure 1**).

Functional fMLP/Phalloidin Test

Median fluorescence intensities of FITC-phalloidin stained actin in monocytes, lymphocytes, and neutrophils were measured by flow cytometry. The data was normalized to percentage of increase in MFI, to compensate for variation in fluorescence intensity between different days. This calculation is described in the methods. The increase of MFI in FITC-phalloidin stained actin was measured on leukocytes populations from patients, carriers, and healthy controls (**Figure 2**). In monocytes, increase

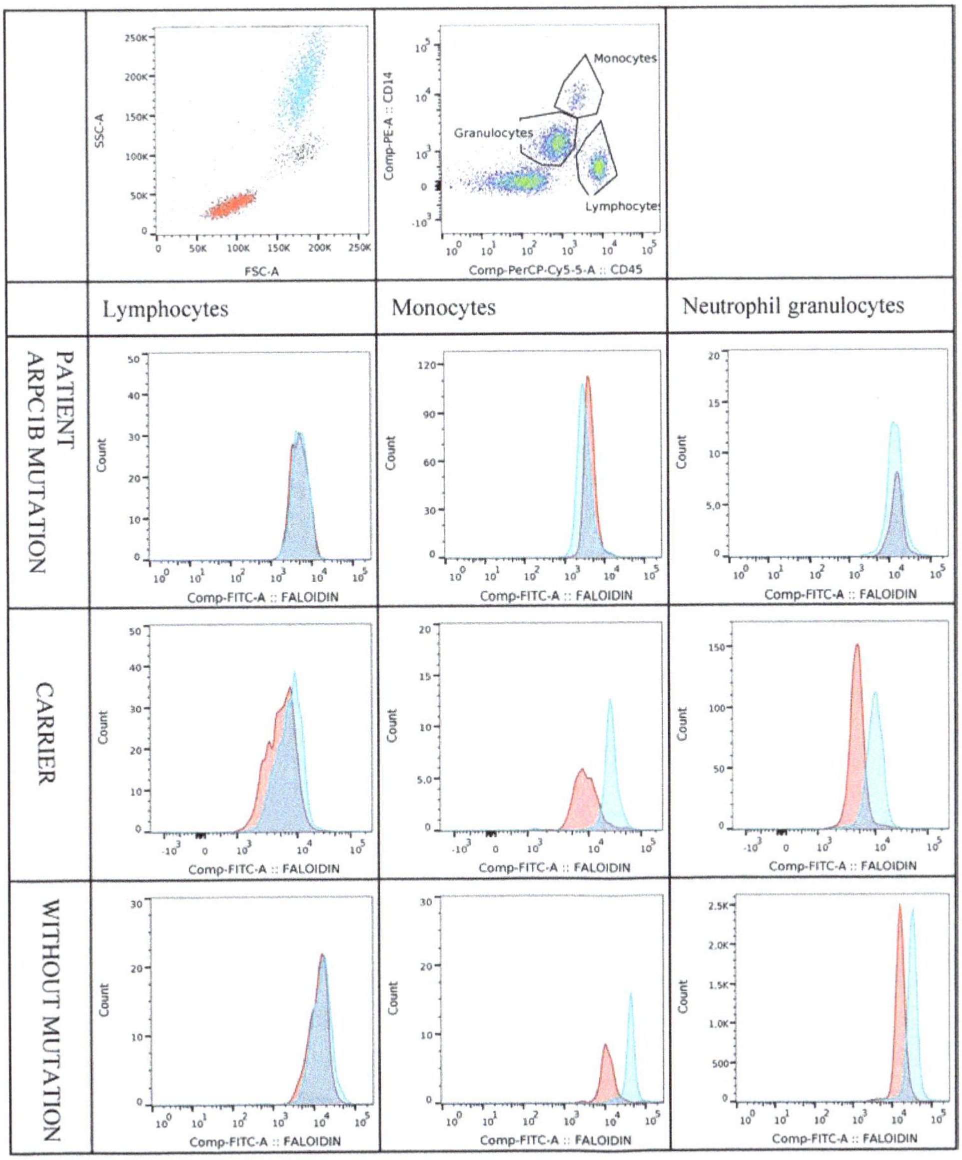

FIGURE 2 | Figure shows an example of multicolour staining and flow cytometry analysis of FITC-phalloidin staining. In the representative pseudocolor plot, leukocytes are separated according to CD45 vs. CD14 staining and gated on lymphocytes, monocytes and neutrophil granulocytes. Histograms show the staining profile of intracellular actin in unstimulated (red) and fMLP stimulated samples (blue). A shift in FITC-phalloidin intensity is easily seen in the histogram overlays. The first three histograms show FITC-phalloidin expression on gated lymphocytes, monocytes or neutrophil granulocytes for patient with mutation in ARPC1B. The second and the third row of histograms shows examples of carrier and healthy control.

in MFI in patients was significantly lower than in carriers ($p = 0.02$) or healthy subjects ($p \leq 0.01$). In lymphocytes, increase in MFI in patients was not statistically significantly lower than in heterozygotic carries ($p = 0.101$) or healthy controls ($p = 0.108$). The most significant differences were observed in neutrophils. In the group with carriers and healthy subjects without ARPC1B mutation, the MFI showed a statistically significant increase ($p \leq 0.01$) while in the patient's group there was a significant decrease ($p \leq 0.01$) (**Figure 3**). Average MFI with or without fMLP stimulation as well as increases in MFI for all three groups are shown in **Table 3**. Morphological and fluorescence images of fMLP activated and non-activated patient's and healthy subject's phalloidin-marked cells are depicted in **Figure 4**.

DISCUSSION

Phalloidin is widely used in studies of actin filament assembly, including analysis of branch formation by Arp2/3 complex. This cyclic peptide binds and stabilizes actin filaments (18). However, the flow cytometry measurement of phalloidin on monocytes and neutrophils in patients with deficiencies in actin polymerization has not yet been considered. Here we have shown that FITC-phalloidin is simple and rapid functional test that can evaluate the last stage of actin polymerization. We identified a missense mutation in the gene ARPC1B resulting in defective actin polymerization in four patients. ARPC1B is prominently expressed in blood/immune cells and is one of two isoforms Arp2/3, which is required for actin filament branching. Thus, ARPC1B deficiency in humans results in defective Arp2/3 actin filament branching that is associated with multisystem disease including platelet abnormalities, cutaneous vasculitis, eosinophilia and predisposition to inflammatory diseases (19). ARPC1B deficiency has a similar multisystem pathogenesis as a lack of expression of WASp, which is also involved in migration and pseudopod formation (20). Mutations in genes that encode actin regulatory proteins in immune cells, give rise to a distinct subset of PIDs. Defects in actin cytoskeleton affect nearly every stage of the immune response: proliferation of hematopoietic cells in the bone marrow, migration, trans-migration through the endothelium to the sight of infection, dramatic shape change needed to phagocytose invading pathogens, presentation of antigens, and the intimate cellular interactions needed for direct cell to cell signaling (1). Immune cells like many other motile cells make 3D actin-filled pseudopodie and navigate through complex environment at speeds of 20 μm/min (20).

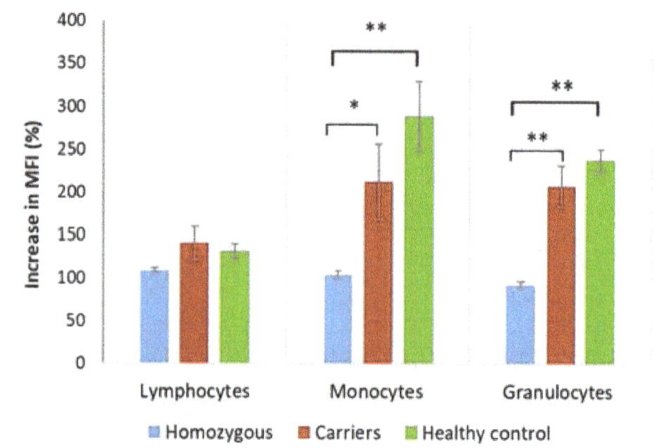

FIGURE 3 | Actin polymerization in patients, carriers and healthy controls. Graphical presentation of mean increase in mean fluorescent intensity (MFI) ± standard error of the mean (SEM) on lymphocytes, monocytes and neutrophil granulocytes. The percentages of increase in fluorescent intensity are presented by setting the fluorescence intensity of unstimulated samples to 100% as described by the equation $\frac{\textit{stimulated sample*100}}{\textit{unstimulated sample}}$. Increase in median fluorescent intensity was analyzed with independent two-tailed Student's *t*-test. Significant differences (*$p \leq 0.05$; **$p \leq 0.01$) between homozygous, carriers and healthy controls are shown.

Neutrophils respond to chemotactic stimuli, such as fMLP by increasing the nucleation and polymerization of actin filaments. They respond to a gradient of chemoattractant by extending actin-rich pseudopodia preferentially in the direction of the highest concentration of chemotactic molecules. The response to fMLP occur very rapidly, within 5 to 30 s they begin to extend

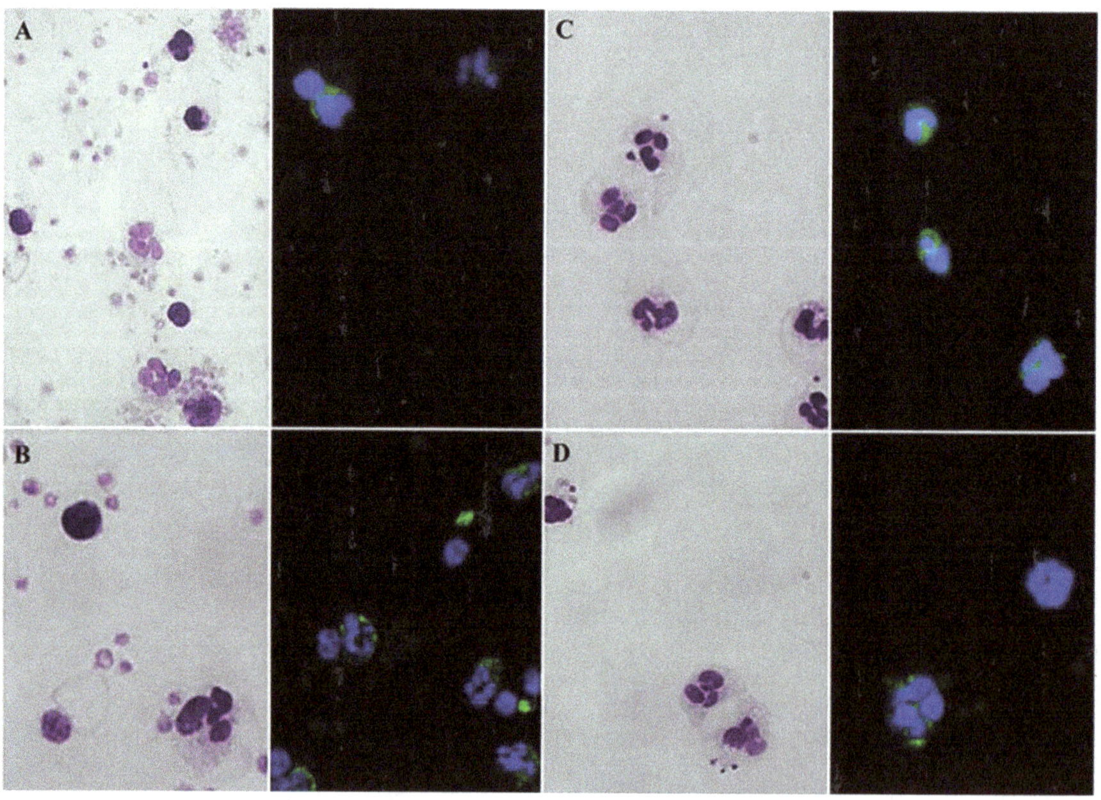

FIGURE 4 | Giemsa stained blood smears and fluorescent microscopy images of FITC-phalloidin stained cells. **(A)** Smears of non-stimulated blood specimen of a healthy subject. **(B)** fMLP-stimulated blood cells of a healthy subject. **(C)** Non-stimulated patient's blood cells. **(D)** fMLP-stimulated patient's blood cells.

TABLE 3 | Average median fluorescence intensity (MFI) of neutrophils and monocytes before and after 20 s stimulation with fMLP in three different groups–homozygous (patients), carriers, and healthy subjects without mutation in ARPC1B.

	Average MFI FITC-phalloidin stained actin		
	Without stimulation	**With stimulation**	**Increase in MFI**
Monocytes			
Homozygous ($n = 4$)	17,382 ± 2,665	17,334 ± 2,113	104 ± 5%
Carriers ($n = 6$)	22,809 ± 7,655	33784 ± 5,684	213 ± 44%
Without mutation ($n = 12$)	26,710 ± 7,050	58,280 ± 14,269	289 ± 41%
Neutrophils			
Homozygous ($n = 4$)	4,791 ± 430	4,497 ± 477	94 ± 4%
Carriers ($n = 6$)	6,570 ± 279	13,405 ± 561	208 ± 24%
Without mutation ($n = 12$)	12,701 ± 3,120	31,975 ± 9,503	238 ± 13%
Lymphocytes			
Homozygous ($n = 4$)	5,993 ± 404	6,478 ± 380	109 ± 3%
Carriers ($n = 6$)	7,432 ± 1,858	9,226 ± 1,589	141 ± 19%
Without mutation ($n = 12$)	12,611 ± 2,484	15,290 ± 2,672	131 ± 9%

The results are presented as the mean with the standard error of the mean (SEM).

their surface toward the gradient of chemoattractant (21). A few minutes later, neutrophils develop a polarized shape with formation of contracted tail in the rear and F-actin-rich ruffles at the front. Actin acts as the engine that drives neutrophil motility. The cellular amount of polymerized actin can be determined by assessing the content of fluorescent phalloidin, which binds to F-actin in a 1:1 ratio more tightly than to G-actin and, at saturation, the amount of phalloidin bound is a measure of the amount of F-actin present (22). This can be observed with a fluorescence microscope or measured with a flow cytometer (3). Phagocytic cells have very rapid changes in actin polymerization, which is needed for detection and migration toward pathogens, and destroy their targets. According to our results, they are the most appropriate to measure fluorescence intensity of intracellular actin stained with FITC-phalloidin in patients with defect of actin polymerization (**Figure 3**). Significant difference in fluorescence intensity between patients with mutation in ARPC1B, carriers and healthy controls indicates that the content of polymerized actin in activated monocytes is indeed lower in patients. The same holds for neutrophils, where the observed decrease in actin content below basal levels can be attributed to fMLP-activation induced damage of cells **Table 3**.

In ARPC1B homozygous patients, we observed increased respiratory burst in neutrophils after mild stimulation with fMLP. Three of our patients with ARPC1B mutation had developed problems with recurrent infection. This could have an effect on the increased oxidative burst after fMLP stimulation, which was not observed in normal blood neutrophils (**Figure 1B**). It is known that priming of fMLP receptor with cytokines (e.g., TNF-α) facilitates stronger oxidative burst, which in turn has detrimental effect on these oxidizing granulocytes (23, 24). Since higher than normal values of oxidizing granulocytes were also found in PHAGOBURST^{TM} test (**Figure 1**), we believe the paradoxical decrease in actin content in neutrophils after stimulation can be explained by the mechanism mentioned above. Therefore, activation of cytokine-primed fMLP receptors triggers prominent oxidative burst in granulocytes. Oxidizing cells are consequently damaged in this process, which leads to the release of actin, resulting in lower fluorescence intensity detection (25). The neutrophil and macrophage abnormalities caused by defective actin polymerization might explain increase frequency of bacterial infections.

WASp and Arp2/3 function has been reported to have crucial role in the formation of immunological synapse between dendritic cells (DC) and lymphocytes (26). In WAS patient's, for example, DC uptake of soluble antigen is normal, but phagocytosis and presentation of particulate antigens is impaired (27). Bouma et al. hypothesized that reduced proliferation of lymphocytes is due to impaired antigen presentation and reduced IL-12 release from the DC (28). On the other hand, poor DC migration after antigen uptake may lead to maturation of DCs before they reach lymph nodes, with ectopic cytokine and chemokine release likely to recruit other immune cells that may contribute to inflammatory processes such as eczema (1). All our patients had eczema and all but the younger one had elevated levels of total IgE which is characteristic for WAS and ARPC1B immunodeficiency. However, the youngest patient had increased levels of food-specific IgE. All patients had thrombocytopenia and developed autoimmune diseases.

On lymphocytes, we did not observe significant differences in actin polymerization between homozygotes, asymptomatic heterozygote and healthy controls. The actin polymerization is not as extensive in lymphocytes compare to more motile monocytes and neutrophils. In our group of patients, we have observed mild cellular deficiency (**Table 2**), which coincides with previous reports (12). A major defect in T cells with abnormal actin polymerization is their altered immunological synapses formation and reduced chemotaxis. This can lead to defective response to CD3 and antigens in some cases (14). However, *in vitro* T-cell proliferation in response to combination of anti-CD3 and anti-CD28, cytokines (IL-15, IL-2) and mitogens was in largely normal (12). In our patients, the response to anti-CD3 and anti-CD28 was normal, but response to mitogen phytohaemagglutinin (PHA) was reduced in two related patients. T lymphocytes successfully participated in immunoglobulin isotype switching, because all patients had increased IgG and IgA levels during the course of their disease. Until now, 14 patients with ARPC1B deficiency have been reported in addition to our four patients, and they all had increased–immunoglobulin E (12, 14, 19).

In summary, by measuring actin polymerization on neutrophils and monocytes with a functional fMLP/phalloidin test, we have efficiently distinguished between symptomatic homozygous patients with mutation in ARPC1B, asymptomatic heterozygous carriers and healthy controls. The mutation of Arp2/3 activator subunit (ARPC1B) resulted in defective polymerization of actin. In blood leukocytes, we have observed the biggest differences in increase of median fluorescence intensity on neutrophils and monocytes. Flow cytometry assays may represent a very useful and rapid tool to detect mutation in ARPC1B that leads to impaired actin polymerization. In the future, it would be very interesting to see if similar differences can be observed also in other primary immunodeficiencies due to abnormalities of actin cytoskeleton, for example Wiskott-Aldrich syndrome.

AUTHOR CONTRIBUTIONS

AK, MO, and MD performed the experiments and analyzed the data. AK, AI, and MD wrote the paper. All of the authors revised the manuscript, approved the final version submitted for publication and contributed to the conception and design of the study.

ACKNOWLEDGMENTS

The authors wish to thank Maja Zabel, Katka Pohar, and Jasmina Livk for assistance in the laboratory and Claudio Vallan for helpful discussions. This work was partially supported by the Slovenian Research Agency grant P3-0083, grant L7-8274, grant P3-0343 and by the University Medical Center Ljubljana research grant 20180093.

REFERENCES

1. Moulding DA, Record J, Malinova D, Thrasher AJ. Actin cytoskeletal defects in immunodeficiency. *Immunol Rev.* (2013) 256:282–99. doi: 10.1111/imr.12114
2. Campellone KG, Welch MD. A nucleator arms race: cellular control of actin assembly. *Nat Rev Mol Cell Biol.* (2010) 11:237–51. doi: 10.1038/nrm2867
3. Torres M, Coates TD. Function of the cytoskeleton in human neutrophils and methods for evaluation. *J Immunol Methods.* (1999) 232:89–109.
4. Burns SO, Zarafov A, Thrasher AJ. Primary immunodeficiencies due to abnormalities of the actin cytoskeleton. *Curr Opin Hematol.* (2017) 24:16–22. doi: 10.1097/moh.0000000000000296
5. Firat-Karalar EN, Welch MD. New mechanisms and functions of actin nucleation. *Curr Opin Cell Biol.* (2011) 23:4–13. doi: 10.1016/j.ceb.2010.10.007
6. Luan Q, Zelter A, MacCoss MJ, Davis TN, Nolen BJ. Identification of Wiskott-Aldrich syndrome protein (WASP) binding sites on the branched actin filament nucleator Arp2/3 complex. *Proc Natl Acad Sci USA.* (2018) 115:E1409–e18. doi: 10.1073/pnas.1716622115
7. Spiering D, Hodgson L. Dynamics of the Rho-family small GTPases in actin regulation and motility. *Cell Adh Migr.* (2011) 5:170–80. doi: 10.4161/cam.5.2.14403
8. Pollard TD., Cooper JA. Actin, a central player in cell shape and movement. *Science.* (2009) 326:1208–12. doi: 10.1126/science.1175862
9. Smith BA, Padrick SB, Doolittle LK, Daugherty-Clarke K, Correa IR Jr, Xu MQ, et al. Three-color single molecule imaging shows WASP detachment from Arp2/3 complex triggers actin filament branch formation. *eLife.* (2013) 2:e01008. doi: 10.7554/eLife.01008
10. Kakley MR, Velle KB, Fritz-Laylin LK. Relative quantitation of polymerized actin in suspension cells by flow cytometry. *Bio Protoc.* (2018) 8:3094. doi: 10.21769/BioProtoc.3094
11. Vandekerckhove J, Deboben A, Nassal M, Wieland T. The phalloidin binding site of F-actin. *EMBO J.* (1985) 4:2815–8.
12. Volpi S, Cicalese MP, Tuijnenburg P, Tool ATJ, Cuadrado E, Ahanchian H, et al. A combined immunodeficiency with severe infections, inflammation and allergy caused by ARPC1B deficiency. *J Allergy Clin Immunol.* (2019) 143:2296–9 doi: 10.1016/j.jaci.2019.02.003
13. Kuijpers TW, Tool ATJ, van der Bijl I, de Boer M, van Houdt M, de Cuyper IM, et al. Combined immunodeficiency with severe inflammation and allergy caused by ARPC1B deficiency. *J Allergy Clin Immunol.* (2017) 140:273–7.e10. doi: 10.1016/j.jaci.2016.09.061
14. Brigida I, Zoccolillo M, Cicalese MP, Pfajfer L, Barzaghi F, Scala S, et al. T-cell defects in patients with ARPC1B germline mutations account for combined immunodeficiency. *Blood.* (2018) 132:2362–74. doi: 10.1182/blood-2018-07-863431
15. Comans-Bitter WM, de Groot R, van den Beemd R, Neijens HJ, Hop WC, Groeneveld K, et al. Immunophenotyping of blood lymphocytes in childhood. Reference values for lymphocyte subpopulations. *J Pediatr.* (1997) 130:388–93.
16. Lothar T. Immunoglobulins (Ig). In: Lothar T, editor. *Clinical Laboratory Diagnostics.* Frankfurt: TH Books Verlagsgesellschaft (1998). p. 667–81.
17. Lun A, Schmitt M, Renz H. Phagocytosis and oxidative burst: reference values for flow cytometric assays independent of age. *Clin Chem.* (2000) 46:1836–9.
18. Mahaffy RE, Pollard TD. Influence of phalloidin on the formation of actin filament branches by Arp2/3 complex. *Biochemistry.* (2008) 47:6460–7. doi: 10.1021/bi702484h
19. Kahr WH, Pluthero FG, Elkadri A, Warner N, Drobac M, Chen CH, et al. Loss of the Arp2/3 complex component ARPC1B causes platelet abnormalities and predisposes to inflammatory disease. *Nat Commun.* (2017) 8:14816. doi: 10.1038/ncomms14816
20. Fritz-Laylin LK, Lord SJ, Mullins RD. WASP and SCAR are evolutionarily conserved in actin-filled pseudopod-based motility. *J Cell Biol.* (2017) 216:1673–88. doi: 10.1083/jcb.201701074
21. Weiner OD, Servant G, Welch MD, Mitchison TJ, Sedat JW, Bourne HR. Spatial control of actin polymerization during neutrophil chemotaxis. *Nat Cell Biol.* (1999) 1:75–81. doi: 10.1038/10042
22. Carulli G, Mattii L, Azzara A, Brizzi S, Galimberti S, Zucca A, et al. Actin polymerization in neutrophils from donors of peripheral blood stem cells: divergent effects of glycosylated and nonglycosylated recombinant human granulocyte colony-stimulating factor. *Am J Hematol.* (2006) 81:318–23. doi: 10.1002/ajh.20604
23. Marasco WA, Phan SH, Krutzsch H, Showell HJ, Feltner DE, Nairn R, et al. Purification and identification of formyl-methionyl-leucyl-phenylalanine as the major peptide neutrophil chemotactic factor produced by *Escherichia coli. J Biol Chem.* (1984) 259:5430–9.
24. Elbim C, Chollet-Martin S, Bailly S, Hakim J, Gougerot-Pocidalo MA. Priming of polymorphonuclear neutrophils by tumor necrosis factor alpha in whole

blood: identification of two polymorphonuclear neutrophil subpopulations in response to formyl-peptides. *Blood.* (1993) 82:633–40.

25. Menegazzi R, Cramer R, Patriarca P, Scheurich P, Dri P. Evidence that tumor necrosis factor alpha (TNF)-induced activation of neutrophil respiratory burst on biologic surfaces is mediated by the p55 TNF receptor. *Blood.* (1994) 84:287–93.
26. Malinova D, Fritzsche M, Nowosad CR, Armer H, Munro PM, Blundell MP, et al. WASp-dependent actin cytoskeleton stability at the dendritic cell immunological synapse is required for extensive, functional T cell contacts. *J Leukoc Biol.* (2016) 99:699–710. doi: 10.1189/jlb.2A0215-050RR
27. Westerberg L, Wallin RP, Greicius G, Ljunggren HG, Severinson E. Efficient antigen presentation of soluble, but not particulate, antigen in the absence of Wiskott-Aldrich syndrome protein. *Immunology.* (2003) 109:384–91. doi: 10.1046/j.1365-2567.2003.01668.x
28. Bouma G, Mendoza-Naranjo A, Blundell MP, de Falco E, Parsley KL, Burns SO, et al. Cytoskeletal remodeling mediated by WASp in dendritic cells is necessary for normal immune synapse formation and T-cell priming. *Blood.* (2011) 118:2492–501. doi: 10.1182/blood-2011-03-340265

9

A Computational Pipeline for the Diagnosis of CVID Patients

Annelies Emmaneel[1,2], Delfien J. Bogaert[3,4], Sofie Van Gassen[1,2], Simon J. Tavernier[3,5,6], Melissa Dullaers[7], Filomeen Haerynck[3,4] and Yvan Saeys[1,2]*

[1] Department of Applied Mathematics, Computer Science and Statistics, Ghent University, Ghent, Belgium, [2] Data Mining and Modeling for Biomedicine, VIB Center for Inflammation Research, Ghent, Belgium, [3] Primary Immunodeficiency Research Lab, Center for Primary Immunodeficiency Ghent, Jeffrey Modell Diagnosis and Research Center, Ghent University Hospital, Ghent, Belgium, [4] Department of Internal Medicine and Pediatrics, Ghent University, Ghent, Belgium, [5] Department of Biomedical Molecular Biology, Ghent University, Ghent, Belgium, [6] Unit of Molecular Signal Transduction in Inflammation, VIB Center for Inflammation Research, Ghent, Belgium, [7] Ablynx, A Sanofi Company, Zwijnaarde, Belgium

***Correspondence:**
Yvan Saeys
yvan.saeys@ugent.be

Common variable immunodeficiency (CVID) is one of the most frequently diagnosed primary antibody deficiencies (PADs), a group of disorders characterized by a decrease in one or more immunoglobulin (sub)classes and/or impaired antibody responses caused by inborn defects in B cells in the absence of other major immune defects. CVID patients suffer from recurrent infections and disease-related, non-infectious, complications such as autoimmune manifestations, lymphoproliferation, and malignancies. A timely diagnosis is essential for optimal follow-up and treatment. However, CVID is by definition a diagnosis of exclusion, thereby covering a heterogeneous patient population and making it difficult to establish a definite diagnosis. To aid the diagnosis of CVID patients, and distinguish them from other PADs, we developed an automated machine learning pipeline which performs automated diagnosis based on flow cytometric immunophenotyping. Using this pipeline, we analyzed the immunophenotypic profile in a pediatric and adult cohort of 28 patients with CVID, 23 patients with idiopathic primary hypogammaglobulinemia, 21 patients with IgG subclass deficiency, six patients with isolated IgA deficiency, one patient with isolated IgM deficiency, and 100 unrelated healthy controls. Flow cytometry analysis is traditionally done by manual identification of the cell populations of interest. Yet, this approach has severe limitations including subjectivity of the manual gating and bias toward known populations. To overcome these limitations, we here propose an automated computational flow cytometry pipeline that successfully distinguishes CVID phenotypes from other PADs and healthy controls. Compared to the traditional, manual analysis, our pipeline is fully automated, performing automated quality control and data pre-processing, automated population identification (gating) and deriving features from these populations to build a machine learning classifier to distinguish CVID from other PADs and healthy controls. This results in a more reproducible flow cytometry analysis, and improves the diagnosis compared to manual analysis: our pipelines achieve on average a balanced accuracy score of 0.93 (±0.07), whereas using the manually extracted populations, an averaged balanced accuracy score of 0.72 (±0.23) is achieved.

Keywords: CVID, flow cytometry, FlowSOM, computational pipeline, PAD

INTRODUCTION

Primary antibody deficiencies (PADs), the largest group of primary immune deficiency disorders, are characterized by markedly reduced serum levels of one or more immunoglobulin isotypes and/or inadequate antibody responses to specific antigens due to genetically determined defects in B cell development and/or function, without major impairments in other parts of the immune system. Common variable immunodeficiency (CVID) is one of the most prevalent PAD disorders, and defined as a marked decrease in serum immunoglobulin (Ig) G with a marked decrease in serum IgM and/or IgA, poor antibody responses to vaccination, and exclusion of secondary or other defined causes of hypogammaglobulinemia (1). As CVID is a diagnosis of exclusion, it encompasses a clinically and immunologically heterogeneous patient population with varying age of onset and severity. CVID patients typically have recurrent infections, mainly of the respiratory, and gastrointestinal tracts. In addition, CVID patients are prone to developing disease-related, non-infectious, complications due to immune dysregulation such as autoimmunity, polyclonal lymphoproliferation, granulomatous manifestations, and malignancy (1–3). Although various abnormalities in B and T cell subsets have been previously reported, the pathophysiological mechanisms of CVID are incompletely understood (1). In recent years, several disease genes for monogenic forms of CVID have been identified, but these only account for 2–10% of patients (4). Timely diagnosis of CVID remains an important challenge in clinical practice, where many other disease possibilities often have to be excluded before a definite diagnosis of CVID can be established (5, 6).

To aid the diagnosis of CVID patients, immunophenotyping by flow cytometry is often performed to obtain an overview of which immune cell populations are affected. Recent advances in multi-parameter flow cytometry allow the measurement of larger marker panels, so that increasingly detailed cell subsets can be identified (7–9).

Currently, flow cytometry data is typically analyzed manually by iteratively selecting cell populations on two-dimensional scatterplots. This manual approach is not only time-consuming, but also researcher-dependent and biased toward expected cell populations. In contrast, automated techniques may facilitate the analysis of larger marker panels by testing countless marker combinations, possibly identifying cell populations that might be indicative of disease status, which may have been overlooked during manual gating (10). In recent years, various computational techniques to analyze flow cytometry data have been developed (11). These techniques automate the different steps in the flow cytometry data analysis pipeline, making data analysis exactly reproducible. For example, pre-processing techniques such as FlowAI (12), and flowClean (13) can be used to perform data quality control. They automatically evaluate scatter and marker values over time and filter out regions that show abnormal behavior. To gain insight into the data structure, various techniques can be applied. Dimensionality reduction techniques such as PCA, t-SNE (14), or UMAP (15) perform dimensionality reduction, and project the high-dimensional cytometry data to a lower-dimensional (often two-dimensional) space, allowing a more comprehensive overview. On the other hand, automated population identification techniques also exist, that aim to group (cluster) similar cells into cell populations with similar phenotypes. To this end, many clustering algorithms have been developed (16), some of which also offer specific visualizations [e.g., FlowSOM (17) and Phenograph (18)]. Here, we develop a novel computational pipeline that combines several of these tools to help distinguish CVID patients from patients with other forms of PADs as well as healthy controls.

MATERIALS AND METHODS

Study Cohort

The study cohort was described earlier in Bogaert et al. (9), in which extensive flow cytometric immunophenotyping was performed in patients with different forms of PADs, including CVID, and several control groups. From this cohort, we have reexamined the flow cytometry data from 28 CVID patients, 23 patients with idiopathic primary hypogammaglobulinemia, 21 patients with IgG subclass deficiency, six patients with isolated IgA deficiency, one patient with isolated IgM deficiency, and 100 healthy controls (HCs). CVID was defined as decreased [from hereon always meaning: at least two standard deviations (SD) below the age-adjusted mean according to the local lab reference values, measured at least twice] IgG, decreased IgA and/or IgM, and poor antibody responses to protein and/or polysaccharide vaccines (1). Idiopathic primary hypogammaglobulinemia was defined as decreased IgG, normal or decreased IgA and/or IgM, and good antibody responses to protein and/or polysaccharide vaccines. IgGSD was defined as decreased IgG2 and/or IgG3, normal total IgG and IgM, normal or decreased IgA, and good or poor antibody responses to protein and/or polysaccharide vaccines. Isolated IgA and IgM deficiencies were defined as an isolated decrease in IgA or IgM, respectively, normal IgG, and good antibody responses to protein and/or polysaccharide vaccines. Each patient was verified to fulfill the appropriate definition before enrollment in the study. Patients with other defined causes of antibody deficiency and/or profound T cell defects, as determined by the ESID registry criteria for CVID (http://esid.org/Working-Parties/Registry/Diagnosis-criteria), were excluded. For the current study, the patients with idiopathic primary hypogammaglobulinemia, IgG subclass deficiency, isolated IgA deficiency and isolated IgM deficiency were combined in one patient group from hereon referred to as "other PADs" ($n = 51$).

Three different marker panels were measured. The first panel focused on identifying the main cell populations in peripheral blood mononuclear cells (PBMCs), the second panel focused on B cell subsets, and the third panel focused on T cell subsets. A detailed overview of the marker panels can be found in **Supplementary Table 1**. The clinical variables gender, age, and diagnosis were collected from the patients' records. The patients were divided into eight age groups to adjust for age-dependent differences in white blood cell subsets [see **Supplementary Table 2**; (9, 19)]. Data were measured over 21 experiment days.

The study was approved by the ethical committee of Ghent University Hospital (2012/593). All reported subjects (or their parents in case of pediatric subjects) provided written informed consent for participation in the study, in accordance with the Helsinki Declaration of 1975.

Computational Pipelines

We automated most steps of cytometry data analysis workflow, including quality control and data preprocessing, automated population detection, feature extraction, and predictive model building using machine learning methods to perform diagnosis. The scripts for the computational pipelines can be found on https://github.com/saeyslab/Computational_Pipeline_CVID.

Preprocessing and Quality Control

The fcs files were read into R, compensated with the compensation matrices determined in the previous study and transformed with the estimate Logicle function of the flowCore package. Cells with unreliable measurements (e.g., out of the detection range) were removed. Quality control was done with the FlowAI (12) package. Only the high quality measurements were selected for further processing. Additionally, only live single cells were used for further analysis, based on the manual pregating of the data.

Alongside the computational analysis, results were compared to the manual analysis performed in the original study [see **Supplementary Figure 1**; (9)]. The cell populations identified for panel 1 included B cells, CD4+ T cells, CD4- T cells, monocytes, natural killer T (NKT) cells, natural killer (NK) cells, basophils, dendritic cells (DCs), plasmacytoid DCs, and conventional DCs. For panel 2 this included IgD+CD27- naive B cells, IgD-CD27+ switched memory B cells (mem B cells), IgD+CD27+ marginal zone-like (MZ-like) B cells, IgD-CD27- B cells, CD24-CD38++ plasmablasts, CD24++CD38++ transitional (trans) B cells, CD21-CD38+ B cells, CD21low B cells, and CD19lowCD138+ plasma cells. The T cell panel 3 populations include CD31+RO-CD4+ T cells, CD31+RO-CD8+ T cells, CD4+ naive T cells, CD4+ effector memory T cells, CD4+ effector memory RA T cells, CD4+ central memory T cells, CD8+ central memory T cells, CD8+ effector memory T cells, CD8+ naive T cells, CD8+ effector memory RA T cells, gamma delta T cells, and regulatory T cells (Treg) cells.

Automated Population Identification and Feature Extraction

Cell populations were identified by FlowSOM, one of the best performing automated gating techniques identified in the benchmark by Weber et al. (16). FlowSOM uses a Self-Organizing Map (SOM) to group similar cells into fine-grained cell types, which are subsequently grouped into metaclusters (coarse-grained cell types) and visualized in a next step using a minimal spanning tree. FlowSOM trees were built separately for each panel with the FlowSOM R package. An aggregated file was created for each panel and contained 3.000.000 cells sampled from all the files for that panel. For panel 1, a FlowSOM model with a 10 × 10 grid and 14 metaclusters was created using the following markers: FSC-A, SSC-A, CD56, CD3, CD123, CD14, CD127, CD4, CD19, HLA-DR, iNKT/CD34, CD16, and CD11c. A FlowSOM model was created for panel 2 using a 10 × 10 grid and 18 metaclusters using the following markers: CD21, CD24, CD27, CD38, CD138, IgA, IgD, IgG, and IgM. The FlowSOM model created for panel 3 was also built with a 10 × 10 grid and 18 metaclusters using the following markers: CCR7, CXCR5, CD45RO, g/dTCR, FoxP3, CD278, CD8, CD31, and CD4. These were compared with the manual gating labels using the purity and F1-measure. Note that the purity is weighted for the number of cells belonging to a cluster.

Purity: $\frac{1}{N} \sum_{m \in M} \max_{d \in D} |m \cap d|$ (M: set of clusters, D: set of classes, N: number of cells)

F1-measure: $2^* \frac{precision \cdot recall}{precision + recall}$ Precision: $\frac{TP}{TP+FP}$ Recall: $\frac{TP}{TP+FN}$

(TP: True positives, FP: False positives, FN: False negatives)

For each panel, the following set of features were extracted to be used as input for the machine learning models in the next step: cell percentages for each file per cluster (percentages_clusters), per metacluster (percentages_metaclusters), and the cell percentages in the clusters compared to their respective metacluster (percentages_clusters_to_metaclusters). The median fluorescence intensities (MFIs) for all markers were also obtained for every cluster (MFI_cluster) and metacluster (MFI_metacluster). Zero-imputation was used for MFI values of clusters without cells. This resulted in a total of 1,696 features for panel 1, 1,162 features for panel 2 and 1,282 features for panel 3, yielding in total 4,140 features that can be used as input variables for the classifiers to perform automated diagnosing.

To eliminate effects linked to the aging of the immune system, a z-score was applied per age group on the extracted features of the clustering methods and on the features determined from the manual gating. The score was based on the mean (μ) and standard deviation (σ) of the healthy controls in each age group. All the individual values (x) for that age group and feature are normalized with the z-score: $Z_{age} = \frac{x_{age} - \mu_{age}}{\sigma_{age}}$

Automated Diagnosing Using Machine Learning

To perform automated diagnosis, we compared a number of machine learning models that aim to predict a patient's disease status from the features obtained from the automated gating. To this end, we explored two different types of classifiers: Random Forests, an ensemble based classifier based on a large combination of randomized decision trees, and Support Vector Machines (SVMs), a linear classifier that makes use of structural risk minimization to stimulate model generalization. Random Forest models were constructed using 500 decision trees, and SVM models were trained with a linear kernel function and C-parameter set to one. For each model type, two versions were trained. The first version formulated the problem as a three-class classification problem, distinguishing between CVID, other PADs and healthy patients. The second model version combined the other PADs and healthy control patients into a joint Non-CVID class vs. the CVID patients.

The full classification models were built with six different datasets consisting of the features extracted from the FlowSOM objects: percentages_clusters, percentages_metaclusters, percentages_clusters_to_metaclusters, Clusters (percentages_clusters + MFI_clusters), Meta_clusters (percentages_metaclusters + MFI_metaclusters), and total (percentages_clusters, percentages_metaclusters + MFI_clusters + MFI_metaclusters + percentages_clusters_to_metaclusters).

Model performance was measured using 21-fold cross-validation, leaving one experiment day out at the time. This ensures that the impact of batch effects on individual experiment days can be estimated accurately. The performance was assessed using the balanced accuracy measure due to the class imbalance for the CVID population compared to the other PAD and healthy control population.

Balanced accuracy: $(\frac{TP}{P} + \frac{TN}{N})/2$ (TP: True positives, P: Positives, TN: True negatives, Negatives)

For each cross-validation run, one experiment day was left out to test generalization performance. Aggregated fcs files were created with the patient's fcs files missing for the left-out experiment day. FlowSOM objects were built for each aggregation file and age-group specific means and standard deviations for applying the z-scores were calculated at this point. Then all the files, including the left-out files, were mapped onto the FlowSOM object to extract their features and apply the z-scoring. Classification models were built with the features belonging to the train data (not the samples belonging to the left-out experiment day) and the test data was then used to predict their corresponding label.

Feature Selection

To get more insight into which features contribute most to model performance, and check whether removing unimportant features had a beneficial effect on classification performance, feature selection was performed. A feature selection method was applied to both the manual gating cell populations and the features derived from FlowSOM and is based on the feature selection step in Van Gassen et al. (20). For the classification models with two classes, Wilcoxon tests were calculated for every feature in the dataset based on the two labels (CVID vs. No-CVID). A Kruskal-Wallis test was performed for every feature if a classification model was built with CVID, other PADs, and HC labels. The *p*-values of these tests were then sorted and used for the feature selection step. The two features with the lowest *p*-values were selected, whereafter new features were iteratively added from the sorted list if the pairwise Pearson correlation between the selected features and the new candidate feature was lower than 0.2. These features were then used to build the classification models described in the previous section.

Classification Models Based on Manual Gating

In the original study, 47 features were extracted from the manual gating to describe the patients' immunophenotype. These values were normalized using the z-score and were also used as features to build the classification models. In the cross-validation step, the features calculated for the patients and healthy controls belonging to one experiment day were iteratively left out of the z-scoring and classification step and used as test data to predict their labels.

RESULTS

We compared the results of the automated pipeline based on automated quality control and population identification with FlowSOM to the results based on the manual gating. In a first step, we aimed to find out whether the population identification by FlowSOM corresponded to the manually gated populations. Subsequently, we evaluated the predictive power of features derived from both automated as well as manually gated populations in combination with machine learning models. Finally, we aimed to identify those features that seem most promising as biomarkers to diagnose CVID from other PADs and healthy controls.

FlowSOM Accurately Identifies the Cell Populations

The FlowSOM tree built for panel 1 coincided well with the manual labels, with an average purity per cluster of 0.94 (**Figure 1**). When grouping the clusters into metaclusters, the average purity was 0.78 and there was a clear correspondence with the manual populations (e.g., metacluster 10 corresponds with B cells). This translates into an F1-measure of 0.96 and is confirmed when looking at two-dimensional scatter plots corresponding with the manual gating strategy in **Supplementary Figure 3**.

For the second panel, the average purity was 0.82 per cluster and 0.73 per metacluster, but the F1 measure only 0.60. This lower number is mainly due to a lower recall, which indicates that not all cells from the manually identified populations are captured together in one metacluster. When we noticed this discrepancy, we compared again the labeling on the tree (**Figure 2**) and the two-dimensional gating (**Supplementary Figure 4**). This inspection revealed that in the manual gating strategy, the cell populations are first determined based on their expression of CD markers and are later subdivided into smaller populations based on Ig expression. In contrast, the FlowSOM tree is largely split up into quadrants of immunoglobulins, and only then further split based on the CD markers.

The average purity per cluster and metacluster was 0.83 and 0.67, respectively, for panel 3 (**Figure 3**). The F-measure for this panel was 0.60. This lower purity and F-measure again indicate that not all the manually identified populations were captured together in one metacluster but the higher purity of the clusters indicates that the cells that are assigned to one cluster mostly belong to the same manually gated population. The purity of the clusters and metaclusters can also be visually inspected on **Supplementary Figure 5**.

The labeling of the clusters and metaclusters of all FlowSOM trees are depicted in **Supplementary Figure 2**.

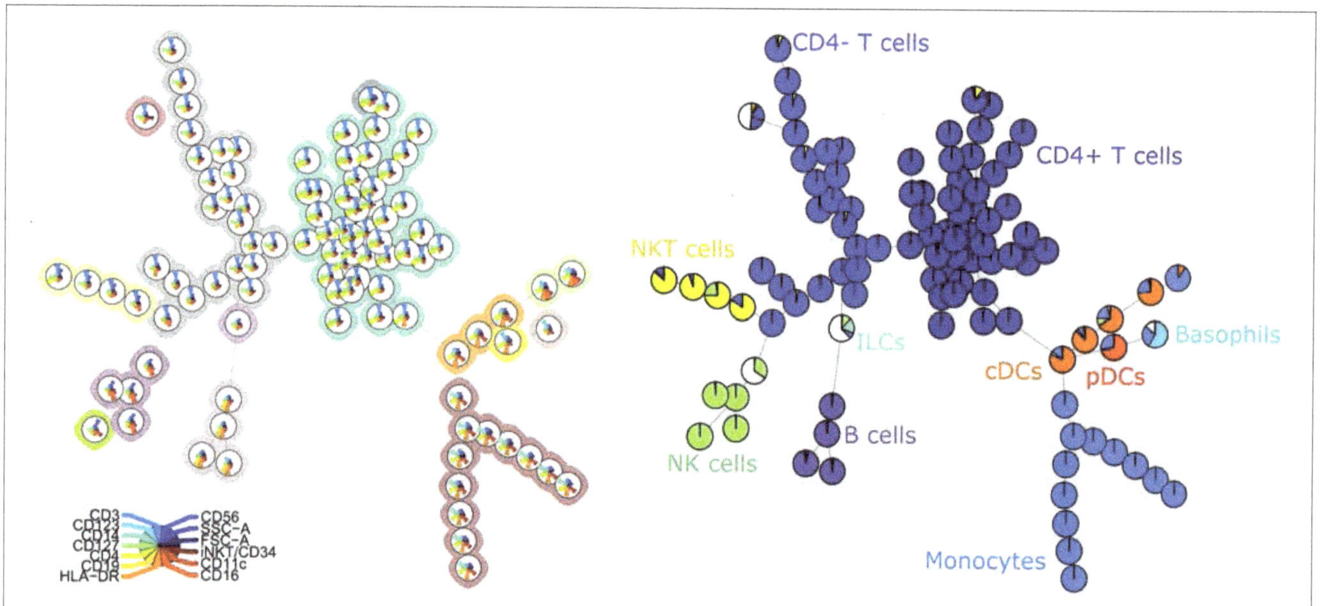

FIGURE 1 | Left: FlowSOM tree for the PBMCs panel 1. The background coloring indicates the metaclustering. **Right:** FlowSOM tree were the cells from Healthy control PIDHC011 were mapped onto the original FlowSOM tree for panel 1. The colors of the nodes correspond to the manually gated labels.

Machine Learning Models Accurately Diagnose CVID

To assess the predictive power of the different classification models, a 21-fold cross-validation was performed for every classification model. The balanced accuracy was calculated in order to determine the predictive power of the extracted cell populations of FlowSOM or the manually extracted cell populations in combination with a classifier (random forest or SVM). An overview is given in **Figure 4**.

Overall, it is clear that the models with FlowSOM derived features are able to obtain higher scores than the pipelines using the features from the manual gating. The average balanced accuracy of all manual gating models for the prediction of the CVID and No-CVID class was 0.63 (±0.10) with feature selection and 0.79 (±0.15) without feature selection while the average balanced accuracy of all FlowSOM models was 0.80 (±0.13) and 0.91 (±0.07) with and without feature selection, respectively. For the three-class models the average accuracies was 0.45 (±0.10) with selection and 0.72 (±0.23) without selection for the manual gating features and 0.81 (±0.16) with selection and 0.93 (±0.0) without selection for the FlowSOM features. Several models only misclassified one patient, obtaining a balanced accuracy of 0.982.

In general, the SVM models gave more accurate results than the random forest classifiers if no feature selection step was used, except for a number of classification models built with the manually selected populations and the models using the FlowSOM metacluster percentages of the individual panels. If a feature selection step was used, all models with an SVM classifier performed worse than the random forests models that were built with the selected features. The decrease is smaller when the FlowSOM cluster MFIs and percentages are used together, or if all FlowSOM features are used for panel 2 or for the three panels combined. Feature selection before training the random forest models resulted most of the times in an equal or less result than the models where no initial feature selection step was performed. When using the features derived from the manually gated populations, feature selection always had a negative impact.

The models where features from panel 2 were used also had an overall better performance than the models based on features from panel 1, and were only slightly better in comparison with the models based on the features of the panels combined. When only the features of panel 3 were used, the performance decreased slightly for the FlowSOM features and greatly when the manually gated populations were used compared to the other two panels. When the information was combined of all three panels, the results generally increased compared to the individual panels. Only panel 2 generated some better results for particular models. The top accuracy was only reached for models built for panel 2 for the two-class model but the overall performance of the models is higher when three classes are classified.

In total, 112 models were built for both the two-class and three-class classification problems and built with either an SVM or random forest classifier, with one of the six different feature sets of FlowSOM or the manually selected populations and with or without a feature selection step. From all the possible two-class classification models, 79 individuals (out of 179) were misclassified at least once and nine patients were misclassified in more than 1/3th of the models (listed in **Table 1**). From all possible three-class classification models, 168 people were misclassified in the three-class classification models from which seven individuals were mislabeled in more than 1/3th of the models. This increase in mistakes between classification problems is due to added misclassifications between healthy controls and other PADs. For four of these ten patients, further

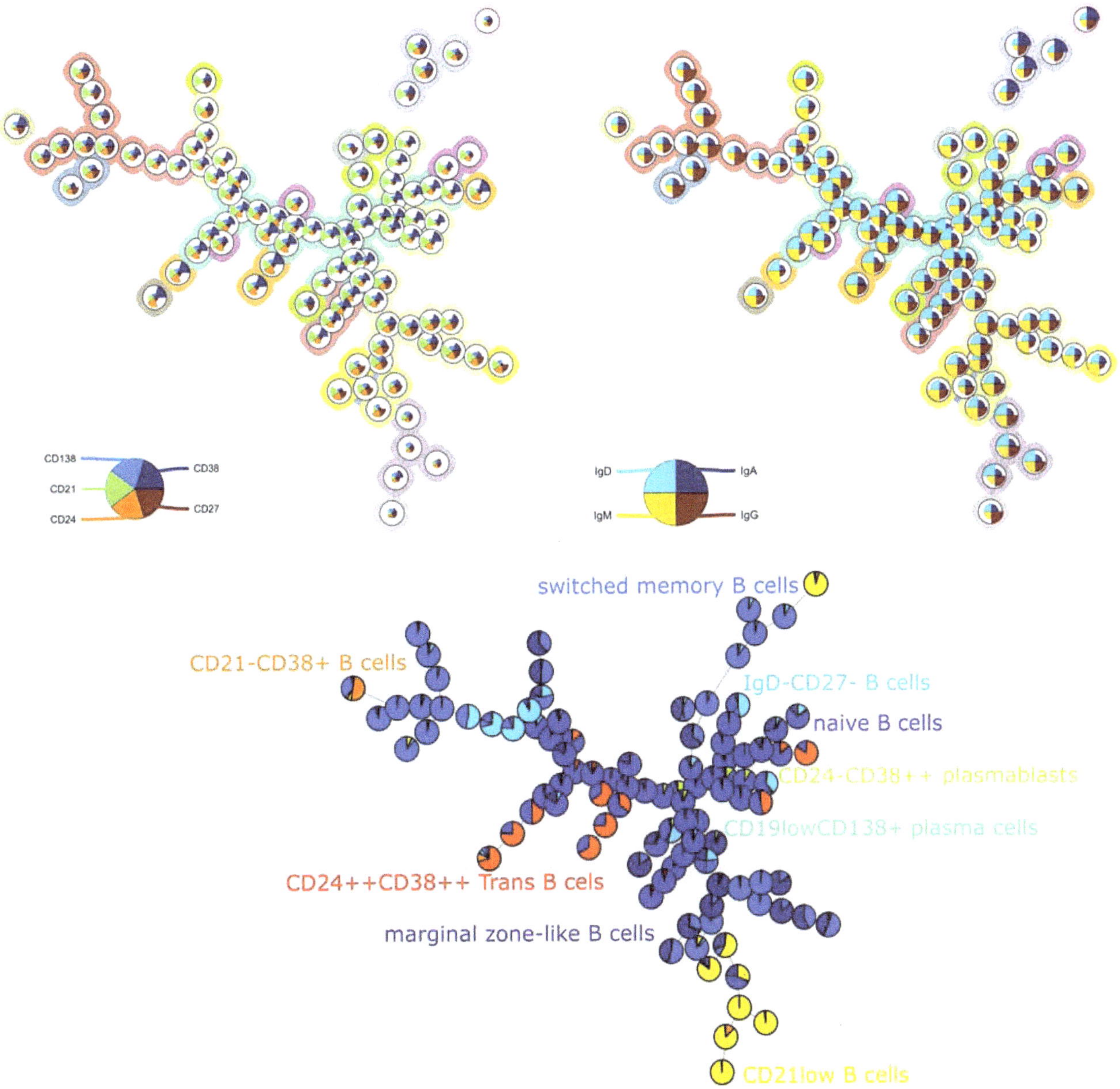

FIGURE 2 | Top left: FlowSOM tree for the B cell subset panel 2 with expressed CD markers displayed. The background coloring indicates the metaclustering. **Top right:** FlowSOM tree with expression of immunoglobulins displayed. **Bottom:** FlowSOM tree where the cells from Healthy control PIDHC011 were mapped onto original FlowSOM tree for panel 2. The colors of the nodes correspond to the manually gated labels.

follow-up with their physician indicated that they might have been misdiagnosed in our database.

Visual Exploration of the Immune State Space Allows for Visual Separation of CVID Patients

To explore the underlying structure of the patient population, dimensionality reduction using t-SNE was performed on the three features with the highest importance scores in the SVM models built on either the manual gating results for the three panels individually or the total feature set extracted from FlowSOM for both panels individually (**Figure 5**). For both models, there is no grouping visible based on age or gender.

Looking at diagnosis, there is a grouping of healthy controls for both the model built on the manual features and for the model built on the FlowSOM features. Most CVID patients also seem to group together for both models with the exception of some. The other PAD patients however seem to be spread across the healthy controls and the CVID patients.

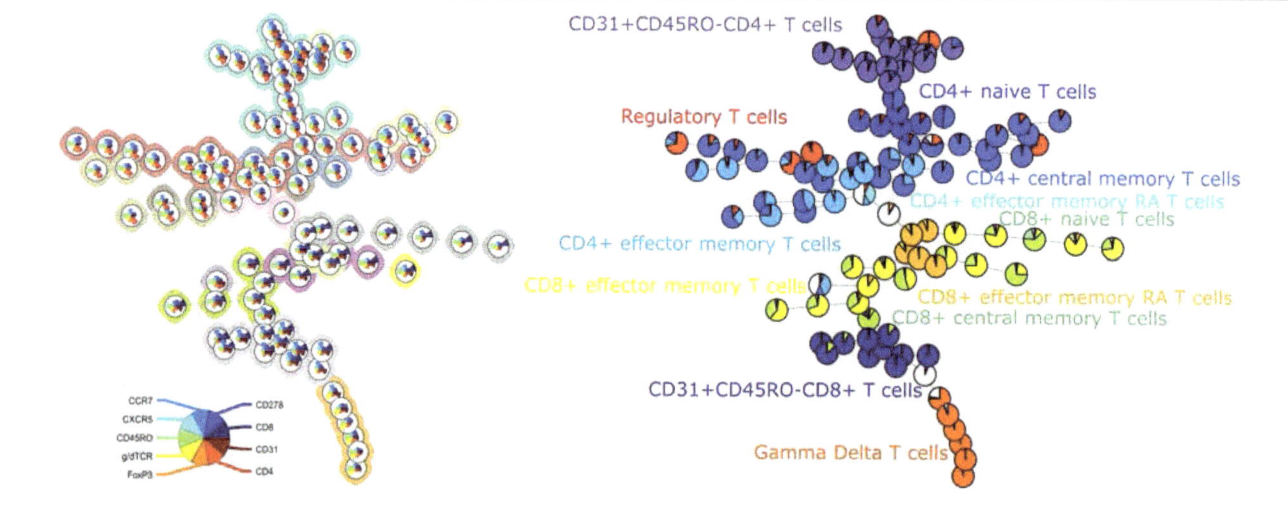

FIGURE 3 | Left: FlowSOM tree for the T cell subset panel 3. The background coloring indicates the metaclustering. **Right**: FlowSOM tree were the cells from Healthy control PIDHC011 were mapped onto the original FlowSOM tree for panel 3. The colors of the nodes correspond to the manually gated labels.

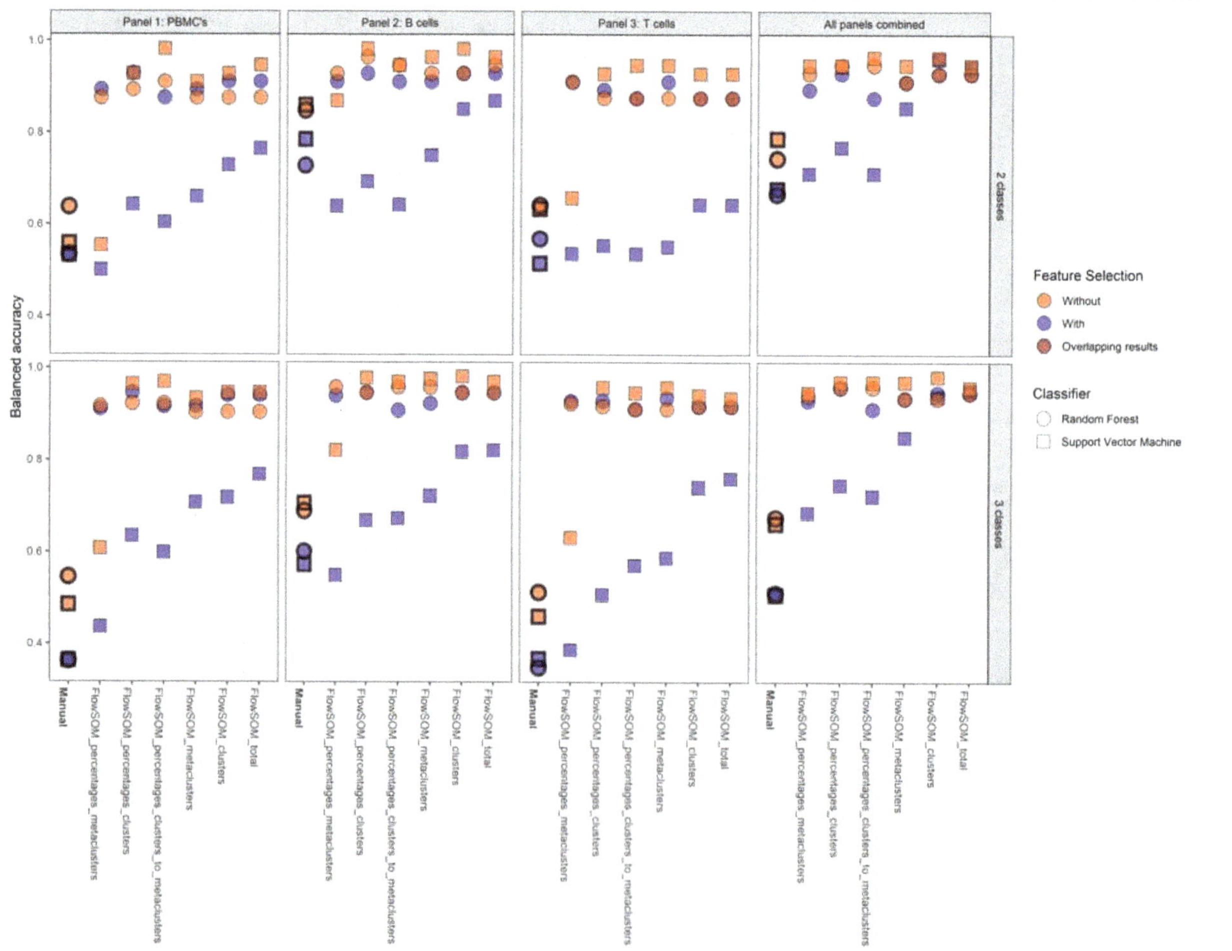

FIGURE 4 | Overview of the balanced accuracy scores of the different classification models (performed with 21-fold cross-validation). Color indicates whether feature selection was applied, shape indicates which classification model was used. Overall, FlowSOM features can clearly improve on features extracted from the manual gating.

TABLE 1 | Overview of the most frequently misclassified patients.

	Nr. misclassifications for two-class classification model	Nr. misclassifications three-class classification model	Remarks
PID030 (CVID)	52	45	No explanation found yet.
PID040 (CVID)	70	73	Syndromic primary immunodeficiency initially presenting with CVID phenotype.
PID041 (CVID)	59	63	Syndromic primary immunodeficiency initially presenting with CVID phenotype. First degree family member of PID040.
PID043 (Other PAD)	0	64	Early loss to follow-up, no information on progression of disease phenotype.
PID053 (CVID)	111	110	No explanation found yet.
PID054 (CVID)	104	100	No explanation found yet. First degree family member of PID053.
PID055 (CVID)	78	70	Presumably secondary CVID after autoimmune—induced subacute liver failure with need of liver transplantation.
PID060 (CVID)	42	35	No explanation found yet.
PID257 (CVID)	38	29	No explanation found yet.
PID285 (CVID)	39	33	No explanation found yet.

All the patients listed in the first column were misclassified by the models in more than 1/3 of the 112 possible model combinations (built with or without a feature selection, with either an SVM or random forest classifier, with one of six different feature sets of FlowSOM or the manually selected populations). The second column depicts the results for all two-class models while the third column shows the results for the three-class models. In the last column, remarks are listed as possible explanations for the frequent misclassification. The red color of a number indicates that that patient was not misclassified in more than 1/3th of the 112 models.

Most Important Features in SVM Classification Identify Relevant Populations for CVID Diagnosis

In order to find populations that could play a role in the identification of CVID patients, importance scores were ranked from the SVM result in the three-class classification models for panels 1-3 individually. These are the same features as in the dimensionality exploration section. The expression of the top three features from the models that were built with all the FlowSOM features (i.e., the MFIs and percentages of clusters and metaclusters and the percentages of clusters compared to the metaclusters) were compared across the three different classes and are visualized in **Figure 6** for the three panels.

For all features of the first panel, an increasing trend is visible of the feature values for the CVID patients. These results indicate an increase in a certain CD4+ T cell population compared to the entire CD4+ T cell population and an increase of CD14 expression on a certain population of cDCs. For the second panel there seems to be a decrease of CD27 expression for a particular switched memory B cell population with IgG, CD24 and CD21 expression. A similar trend is visible for another switched memory B cell population where no immunoglobulins but the same CD markers are expressed. The last feature of panel 2 indicates an increase of a CD21low B cell population in CVID patients compared to the other two classes. Three different types of T cells were selected for panel 3. The first population consists of a specific gamma delta T cell population that appears to have decreased in the other PAD and CVID patients. There seems to be a decrease of the CD4+ naive T cells (CD45RO-CCR7+) in the other PAD patients opposed to the healthy controls but this decrease is not greatly extended to the CVID patients. The last feature indicates an increase in MFI expression of FoxP3 for a certain regulatory T cell population.

Feature Selection Identifies Relevant Population for CVID Diagnosis

Although the feature selection steps did not seem to improve the models, the selected features with the lowest p-values still seem to be relevant in the identification of the CVID patients.

The number of selected FlowSOM features ranged from 2 to 43 features with a median of 13 features while the number of the selected manual populations ranged from 4 to 15 features with a median of seven features.

To inspect these features for the three-class classification problem, Kruskal Wallis tests were performed on all the FlowSOM features. The two features with the lowest p-values and the next feature with the lowest p-value and with a low correlation with the first two features were selected. They all had a value smaller than 1.10–10 and are depicted in **Figure 7**. The features selected for panel 1 indicate an increase of a certain NK cell population compared to the entire NK cell population for the other PAD and CVID patients. For another NK cell population however, there seems to be a decrease in cell counts compared to all immune cells. The difference between the two populations is the expression of CD56. Cluster 89 shows a very low expression of the marker. The final selected feature of panel 1 suggests that for cluster 22, cells (labeled as CD4+ T cells) have a larger cell size due to higher FSC-A values in the other PAD and CVID patients. Upon further inspection, we confirmed that this significant increase was not only the case for cluster 22, but also for the FSC-A MFI of most CD4+ T cell clusters and the metacluster 1 which represents the CD4+ T cells. Unfortunately this could not be confirmed in panel 3 due to altered scattered

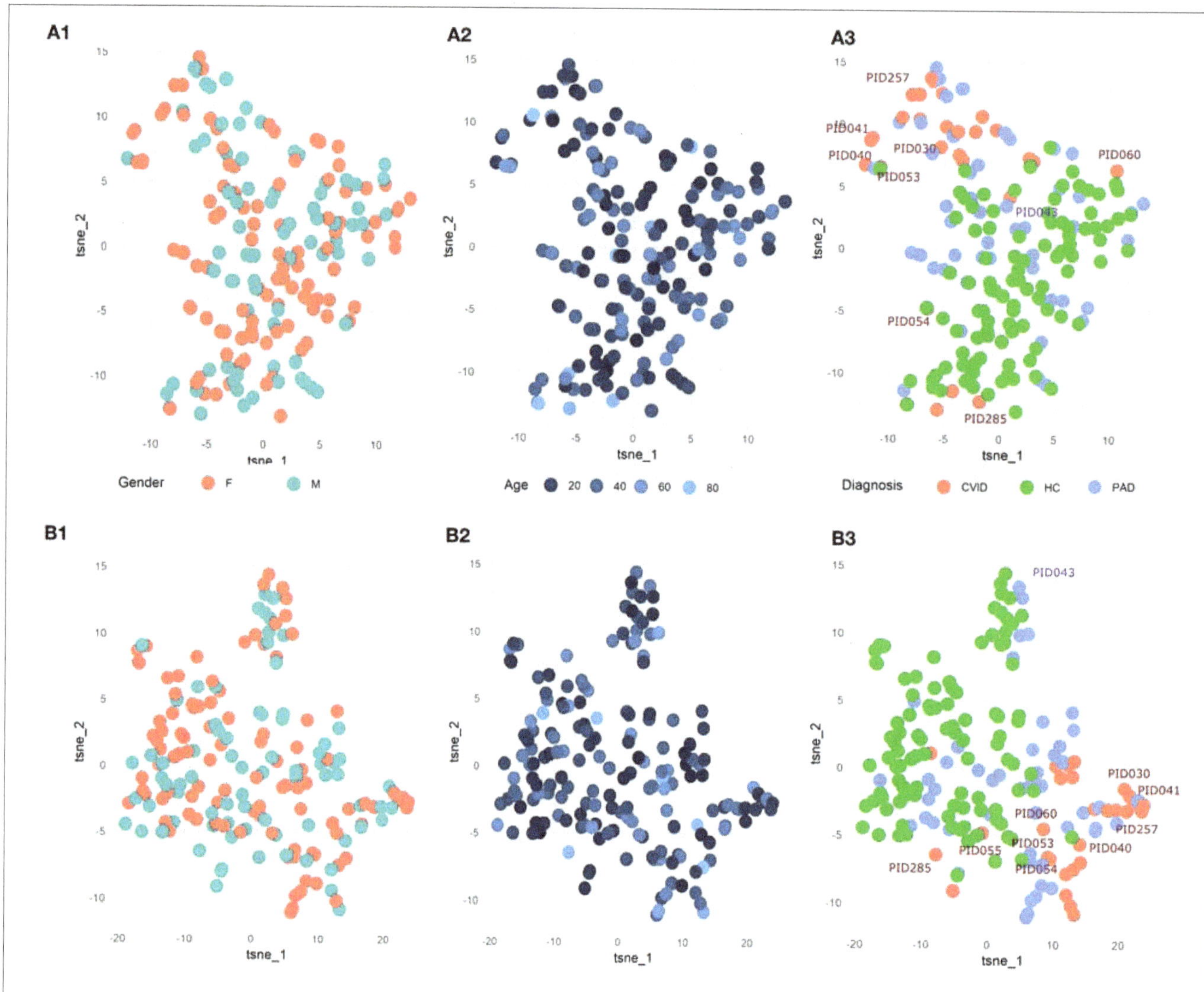

FIGURE 5 | (A1-3) t-SNE result of the patient population with manually gated cell populations of the most important features determined by the SVM model for the three panels individually. **(B1-3)** t-SNE result of the patient population with the total features of FlowSOM of the most important features determined by the SVM model for the three panels individually. The perplexity for both t-SNEs was set to 15. A z-score was applied on the used features first to eliminate age-linked immune changes.

values because of the fixation step necessary for the use of the intracellular marker FoxP3.

For panel 2, a significant decrease is present in two certain switched memory B cell populations, with IgG, CD38, and CD21 expressed, compared to the healthy controls and the other PAD patients. A second switched memory B cell population seems to be increased in CVID patients compared to the other two classes that expresses CD21, IgA, and CD24.

In panel 3, an increase can be found for a certain population of CD8+ effector memory T cells (CD45RO+CCR7-) compared to the other populations in its metacluster in the other PAD patients. This increase toward the healthy controls is also present in the CVID patients but not as pronounced. The MFI however of CCR7 in a certain cluster of regulatory T cells is increased gradually from the healthy controls to the other PADs and the CVID patients. The third important feature of the SVM model is again a cluster to metacluster ratio where a great decrease is noticed in the other PADs compared to the healthy controls and a smaller decrease in the CVID patients of a certain CD31+CD45RO-CD8+ T cell population.

Diagnosis of a New Patient Is Much Faster by Automated Classification Than by Manual Analysis

A big advantage of using automated models during the diagnostic process of patients is that the computational time is much less than the time necessary to manually gate every population in 2D plots. It took our model 2.54 min in total to load the necessary objects to make a prediction, to map the fcs file of a randomly chosen patient on the FlowSOM tree created for panel 1, to extract all possible features (percentages and MFIs), to apply the z-score to these features and to make a prediction with the SVM of a three-class model built on all possible FlowSOM features.

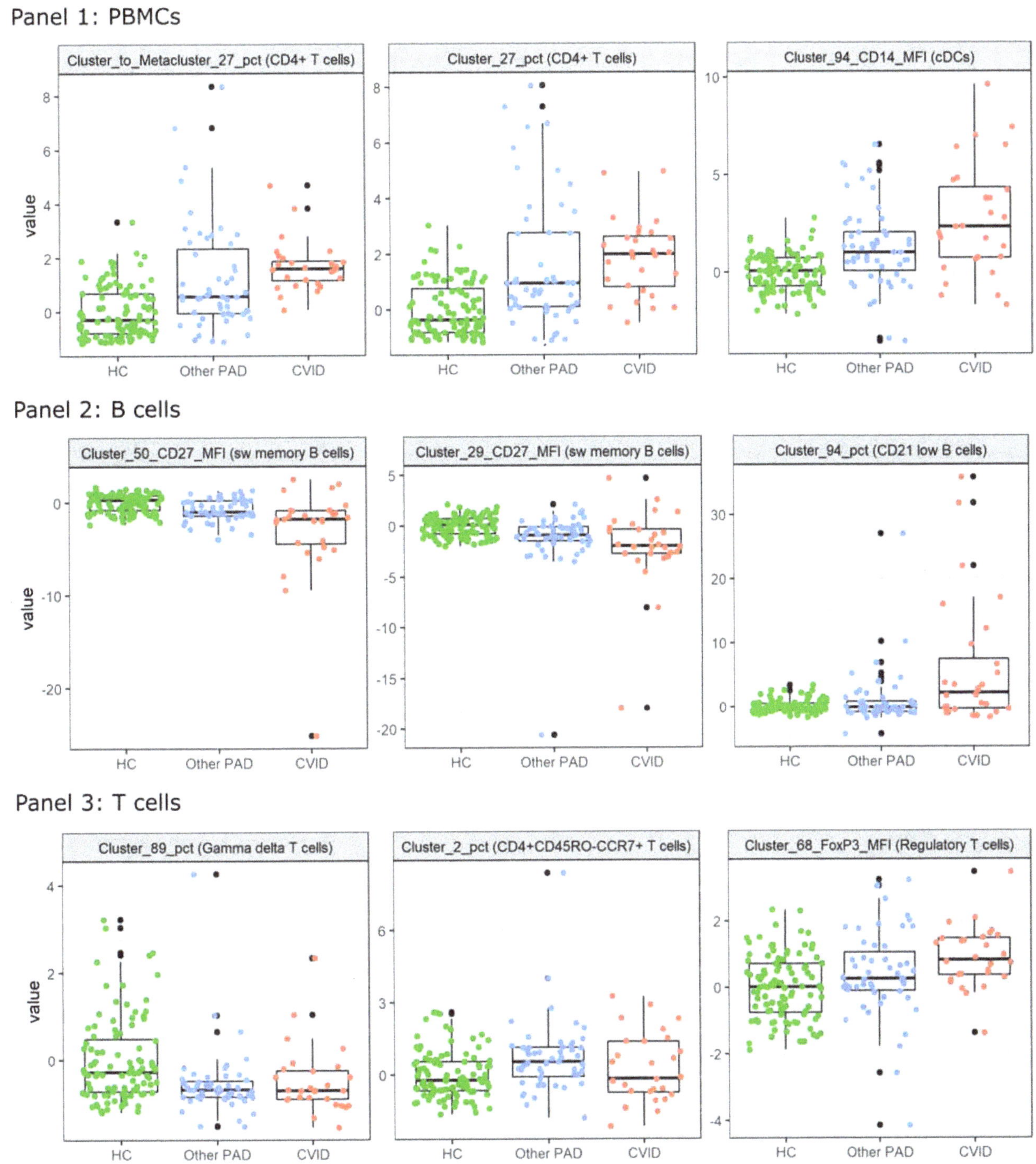

FIGURE 6 | Boxplots calculated for the most important features in the support vector machines built for the three-way classification of all FlowSOM features for either panel 1, 2, or 3. The colored points indicate the values on which the boxplots were built. A z-score was applied on the used features first to eliminate age-linked immune changes.

When the classification would be done with a manual gating strategy it would take at least 15 min to gate the entire manual gating strategy and classify the patient based on the known CVID criteria. The classifier built on these gated populations, as performed in this study, still uses the populations that have to be gated first which occupies most of the work and time. This means that the usage of a full computational model is much faster than performing classification based on manually placed gates.

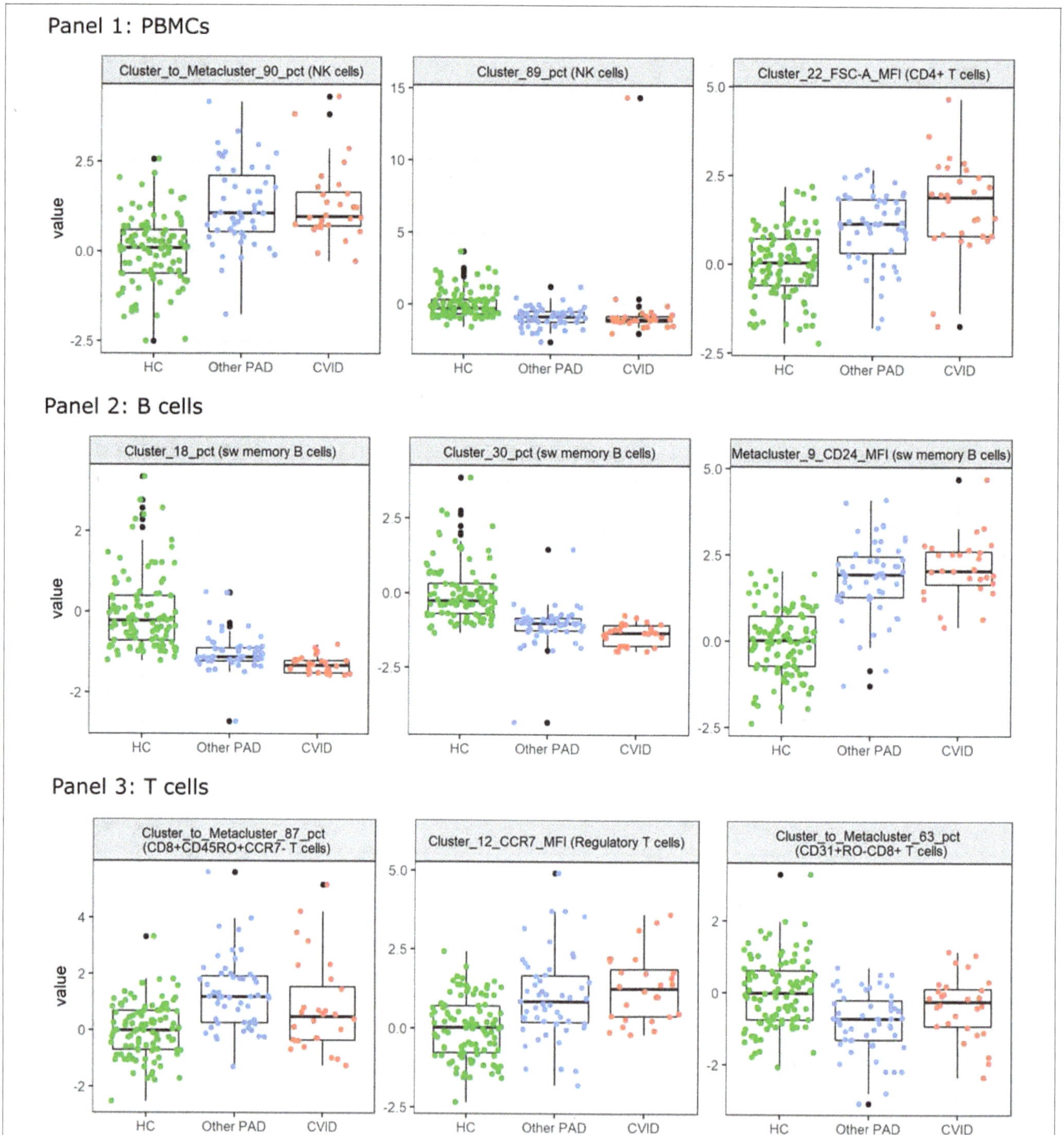

FIGURE 7 | Boxplots calculated for the features selected by the feature selection step in the three-class classification model calculated on all FlowSOM features for either panel 1, 2, or 3. This feature selection step is performed before the classification step in the automated models. The first three features selected with the lowest *p*-value are displayed for both panels. The colored points indicate the values on which the boxplots were built. A z-score was applied on the used features first to eliminate age-linked immune changes.

DISCUSSION

In this study, the efficiency and accuracy of different models built with varying FlowSOM feature sets or manually gated cell populations were compared in their ability to identify CVID patients, patients with other PADs and healthy controls.

Both types of automated techniques can be used to diagnose CVID but models built on FlowSOM features proved to be faster and more accurate than models built on manually gated cell populations. Even when the number of FlowSOM features dropped lower than the total number of manually gated populations due to feature selection, the random forest models still obtained better results than the models built with all manual features.

The FlowSOM models accurately represented the manually gated cell populations and captured more detail allowing for better classification results with either an SVM or a random forest as classifier. This is confirmed by the features extracted from the FlowSOM tree of panel 2. Although the structure of the tree of this panel does not coincide with the manual gating strategy since it first splits up the immunoglobulins instead of the CD markers, the classification results of the extracted features from this tree still managed to obtain better accuracies in predicting the class labels.

The comparison between these classifiers showed that models built with an SVM outperformed the models with a random forest when no feature selection was applied. However, when this selection limited the number of features, the accuracy of the SVM models dropped below the accuracy of the random forest models.

Adding this feature selection step, in order to remove unimportant features, did not increase the accuracy of the models. For the models built on the manually gated populations, this is explained by the limited number of cell populations that were gated. These populations were specifically selected according to commonly used gating guidelines in order to investigate CVID patients, meaning that filtering these cell populations resulted in a loss of information needed to classify the patients correctly. The fact that CVID is an immunologically heterogeneous disease could explain the accuracy drop for all models built on FlowSOM features. This would indicate that there are many differential alterations in the immune system in CVID patients, other PAD patients and healthy controls and that the distinction between these groups cannot be made based on only a few of them. By performing a feature selection step, too much valuable information would be lost. The heterogeneity of the disease is confirmed by the selection of other features that were considered as most important in the classification step for the different models and by selecting other features during the feature selection step than those that were most important in the SVM or random forest models.

Though it did not seem that feature selection added an advantage in increasing accuracy of the predictions, it still gave valuable insights into the CVID phenotype next to the features that were ranked as most important in the SVM classification. Most of these insights are confirmed in the original study of Bogaert et al. (9) where they also noticed a general decrease of switched memory B cell populations, a decrease of switched memory B cells that express IgG and an increase of CD21low B cells in CVID patients, a decrease in CD4+ naïve T cells and a decrease in NK cells in CVID patients and in patients with other PADs. However, two features, concerning CD4+ T cells, seem to contradict results from the original study. The original results showed a decrease of the general CD4+ T cell population while these features indicates an increase for one CD4+ T cell population in CVID patients and in patients with other PADs. Nevertheless, this is merely an indication of only one CD4+ T cell population that seems to be increased as opposed to the entire CD4+ T cell population.

The advantage of using a FlowSOM model allowed for a deeper insight into these results and delivered a more specific marker profile of the cells (i.e., the decreasing szitched memory B cell percentages for clusters 18 and 30 expressed next to IgG also CD38 and CD21). This also allowed for the comparison in MFIs of markers between cell populations which lead to a certain sw memory B cell population that expressed CD21, CD24, and IgA. For this cell population in CVID and other PAD patients, the CD24 expression was increased. Other examples of the specificity of FlowSOM are the features that either showed the increase of FoxP3 for a certain regulatory T cell population in other PAD but mostly in CVID patients and the feature that showed the increase of CCR7 for another regulatory T cell population.

Multiple features highlighted in this study have not yet been discussed in literature. They concern the increase of the FSC-A marker in the CD4+ T cell population in CVID and other PAD patients, the increase of the CD14 markers for a certain conventional dendritic cell population, the increase in CD8+ effector memory T cells and in CD8+CD45RO-CD31+ T cells and the decrease of certain gamma delta T cells in the other PAD and CVID patients.

There are two features that did not seem to be related to the CVID or other PAD phenotypes that indicate a decrease of the CD27 marker for two switched memory B cell populations. This is explained by the mapping of IgD-CD27- cells instead of switched memory B cells on these clusters of the FlowSOM model for the CVID and other PAD patients.

Another important aspect of the classification models concerns the frequently misdiagnosed patients. Although the best model could predict almost all CVID patients, mistakes were still made. It was shown that these mistakes could be valid and that the follow-up of these patients can give valuable insights into the model. It seemed that two misclassified patients were wrongly diagnosed and that secondary complications have a marked influence on the classification of the patients. However, most of these patients with secondary complications are still correctly diagnosed in the best performing models.

The final conclusion of this study tells us that the use of a classification model built on FlowSOM features would be a quick, accurate and useful tool in the diagnosis of patients with CVID. This, however, should still be confirmed in a larger cohort with a more generalized marker panel in order to integrate the classification models in the daily diagnostic procedures.

AUTHOR CONTRIBUTIONS

AE, DB, SV, FH, ST, and YS all contributed to writing the manuscript. AE generated the results of the manuscript under supervision of SV and YS. DB and MD set up the original study and provided the manually gated labels and all fcs files and clinical information for this study. FH, ST, and DB explained the biology of the disease and linked the outcome of the computational models to the clinical phenotypes of the patients.

FUNDING

SV was supported by an FWO postdoctoral research grant (Research Foundation - Flanders). YS and SV were ISAC Marylou Ingram Scholars. FH was funded by University Research Grant (BOF-University Ghent) and Centre for Primary Immune deficiency Ghent was funded by Jeffrey Modell Foundation. ST was funded by Bijzonder onderzoeksfonds. This project has received funding within the Grand Challenges Program of VIB. This VIB Program received support from the Flemish Government under the Management Agreement 2017–2021 (VR 2016 2312 Doc.1521/4).

SUPPLEMENTARY MATERIAL

Supplementary Figure 1 | Manual gating strategies. The manual gated strategies used to determine the manually selected cell populations is depicted in the figure for panel 1, panel 2, and panel 3.

Supplementary Figure 2 | Overview of clustering and meta-clustering labels of FLowSOM trees. Cluster- and meta-clusterlabels were created by building the FlowSOM models for the three panels. These clusterlabels (left) and meta-clusterlabels (right) are used for labeling in the feature extraction step. **(A)** FlowSOM model created for the panel 1 with focus on Peripheral Blood Mononuclear cells. **(B)** FlowSOM model created for the panel 2 with focus on B cell subsets. **(C)** FlowSOM model created for the panel 3 with focus on T cell subsets.

Supplementary Figure 3 | Comparison of metaclusters with manual gating panel 1. The manual gated plots are depicted on the first row for PIDHC011 and correspond to the same marker combinations visualized in **Supplementary Figure 1**. The following rows visualize 2D scatterplots of the same marker combinations of the manual gates in the first row for each metacluster. 100,000 cells were randomly sampled from the FlowSOM tree from panel 1. The background cells are colored black while those of the selected metacluster are plotted in color.

Supplementary Figure 4 | Comparison of metaclusters with manual gating panel 2. The manual gated plots are depicted on the first row for PIDHC011 and correspond to the same marker combinations visualized in **Supplementary Figure 1**. The following rows visualize 2D scatterplots of the same marker combinations of the manual gates in the first row for each metacluster. 100,000 cells were randomly sampled from the FlowSOM tree from panel 2. The background cells are colored black while those of the selected metacluster are plotted in color.

Supplementary Figure 5 | Comparison of metaclusters with manual gating panel 3. The manual gated plots are depicted on the first row for PIDHC011 and correspond to the same marker combinations visualized in **Supplementary Figure 1**. The following rows visualize 2D scatterplots of the same marker combinations of the manual gates in the first row for each metacluster. 100,000 cells were randomly sampled from the FlowSOM tree from panel 1. The background cells are colored black while those of the selected metacluster are plotted in color.

REFERENCES

1. Bonilla FA, Barlan I, Chapel H, Costa-Carvalho BT, Cunningham-Rundles C, de la Morena MT, et al. International consensus document (ICON): common variable immunodeficiency disorders. *J Aller Clin Immunol Pract.* (2016) 4:38–59. doi: 10.1016/j.jaip.2015.07.025
2. Durandy A, Kracker S, Fischer A. Primary antibody deficiencies. *Nat Rev Immunol.* (2013) 13:519–33. doi: 10.1038/nri3466
3. Gathmann B, Mahlaoui N, Gérard L, Oksenhendler E, Warnatz K, et al. Clinical picture and treatment of 2,212 patients with common variable immunodeficiency. *J Aller Clin Immunol.* (2014) 134:116–26. doi: 10.1016/j.jaci.2013.12.1077
4. Bogaert DJ, Dullaers M, Lambrecht BN, Vermaelen KY, De Baere E, Haerynck F. Genes associated with common variable immunodeficiency: one diagnosis to rule them all? *J Med Genet.* (2016) 53:575–90. doi: 10.1136/jmedgenet-2015-103690
5. Conley ME, Notarangelo LD, Etzioni A. Diagnostic criteria for primary immunodeficiencies. *Clin Immunol.* (1999) 93:190–7. doi: 10.1006/clim.1999.4799
6. Chapel H. Common variable immunodeficiency disorders (CVID) — diagnoses of exclusion, especially combined immune defects. *J Aller Clin Immunol.* (2016) 4:1158–9. doi: 10.1016/j.jaip.2016.09.006
7. Stuchlý J, Kanderová V, Vlková M, Hermanová I, Slámová L, Pelák O, et al. Common variable immunodeficiency patients with a phenotypic profile of immunosenescence present with thrombocytopenia. *Sci Rep.* (2017) 7:39710. doi: 10.1038/srep39710
8. Warnatz K, Schlesier M. Flowcytometric phenotyping of common variable immunodeficiency. *Cytometr B Clin Cytometr.* (2008) 74:261–71. doi: 10.1002/cyto.b.20432
9. Bogaert DJ, De Bruyne M, Debacker V, Depuydt P, De Preter K, Bonroy C, et al. The immunophenotypic fingerprint of patients with primary antibody deficiencies is partially present in their asymptomatic first-degree relatives. *Haematologica.* (2017) 102:192–202. doi: 10.3324/haematol.2016.149112
10. Kvistborg P, Gouttefangeas C, Aghaeepour N, Cazaly A, Chattopadhyay PK, Chan C, et al. Thinking outside the gate: single-cell assessments in multiple dimensions. *Immunity.* (2015) 42:591–2. doi: 10.1016/j.immuni.2015.04.006
11. Saeys Y, Van Gassen S, Lambrecht BN. Computational flow cytometry: helping to make sense of high-dimensional immunology data. *Nat Rev Immunol.* (2016) 16:449–62. doi: 10.1038/nri.2016.56
12. Monaco G, Chen H, Poidinger M, Chen J, de Magalhães JP, Larbi A. flowAI: automatic and interactive anomaly discerning tools for flow cytometry data. *Bioinformatics.* (2016) 32:2473–80. doi: 10.1093/bioinformatics/btw191
13. Fletez-Brant K, Špidlen J, Brinkman RR, Roederer M, Chattopadhyay PK. flowClean: Automated identification and removal of fluorescence

anomalies in flow cytometry data. *Cytomet A J Int Soc Analyt Cytol.* (2016) 89:461–71. doi: 10.1002/cyto.a.22837

14. Van der Maaten L, Hinton G. Visualizing data using t-SNE. *J Mach Learn Res JMLR.* (2008) 9:2579–605.
15. McInnes L, Healy J, Saul N, Großberger L. UMAP: uniform manifold approximation and projection. *J Open Source Softw.* (2018) 3:861. doi: 10.21105/joss.00861
16. Weber LM, Robinson MD. Comparison of clustering methods for high-dimensional single-cell flow and mass cytometry data. *Cytometry Part A.* (2016) 89:1084–96. doi: 10.1002/cyto.a.23030
17. Van Gassen S, Callebaut B, Van Helden MJ, Lambrecht BN, Demeester P, Dhaene T, et al. FlowSOM: using self-organizing maps for visualization and interpretation of cytometry data. *Cytomet A J Int Soc Analyt Cytol.* (2015) 87:636–45. doi: 10.1002/cyto.a.22625
18. Levine JH, Simonds EF, Bendall SC, Davis KL, El-Amir AD, Tadmor MD, et al. Data-driven phenotypic dissection of AML reveals progenitor-like cells that correlate with prognosis. *Cell.* (2015) 162:184–97. doi: 10.1016/j.cell.2015.05.047
19. Castelo-Branco C, Soveral I. The immune system and aging: a review. *Gynecol Endocrinol.* (2014) 3016-22. doi: 10.3109/09513590.2013.852531
20. Van Gassen S, Vens C, Dhaene T, Lambrecht BN, Saeys Y. FloReMi: flow density survival regression using minimal feature redundancy. *Cytometr A J Int Soc Analyt Cytol.* (2016) 89:22–9. doi: 10.1002/cyto.a.22734

10

Flow Cytometry Contributions for the Diagnosis and Immunopathological Characterization of Primary Immunodeficiency Diseases with Immune Dysregulation

Otavio Cabral-Marques[1], Lena F. Schimke[2], Edgar Borges de Oliveira Jr.[3], Nadia El Khawanky[4,5], Rodrigo Nalio Ramos[6], Basel K. Al-Ramadi[7], Gesmar Rodrigues Silva Segundo[8], Hans D. Ochs[9] and Antonio Condino-Neto[1]*

[1] Department of Immunology, Institute of Biomedical Sciences, University of São Paulo, São Paulo, Brazil, [2] Department of Rheumatology and Clinical Immunology, Faculty of Medicine, Center for Chronic Immunodeficiency (CCI), Medical Center-University of Freiburg, University of Freiburg, Freiburg im Breisgau, Germany, [3] Immunogenic Inc., São Paulo, Brazil, [4] Department of Hematology, Oncology and Stem Cell Transplantation, Freiburg University Medical Center, Freiburg im Breisgau, Germany, [5] Precision Medicine Theme, The South Australian Health and Medical Research Institute (SAHMRI), Adelaide, SA, Australia, [6] INSERM U932, SiRIC Translational Immunotherapy Team, Institut Curie, Paris Sciences et Lettres Research University, Paris, France, [7] Department of Medical Microbiology and Immunology, College of Medicine and Health Sciences, UAE University, Al Ain, United Arab Emirates, [8] Department of Pediatrics, Federal University of Uberlandia Medical School, Uberlândia, Brazil, [9] Department of Pediatrics, University of Washington School of Medicine, and Seattle Children's Research Institute, Seattle, WA, United States

***Correspondence:**
Otavio Cabral-Marques
otavio.cmarques@gmail.com

Almost 70 years after establishing the concept of primary immunodeficiency disorders (PIDs), more than 320 monogenic inborn errors of immunity have been identified thanks to the remarkable contribution of high-throughput genetic screening in the last decade. Approximately 40 of these PIDs present with autoimmune or auto-inflammatory symptoms as the primary clinical manifestation instead of infections. These PIDs are now recognized as diseases of immune dysregulation. Loss-of function mutations in genes such as *FOXP3, CD25, LRBA, IL-10, IL10RA, and IL10RB,* as well as heterozygous gain-of-function mutations in *JAK1* and *STAT3* have been reported as causative of these disorders. Identifying these syndromes has considerably contributed to expanding our knowledge on the mechanisms of immune regulation and tolerance. Although whole exome and whole genome sequencing have been extremely useful in identifying novel causative genes underlying new phenotypes, these approaches are time-consuming and expensive. Patients with monogenic syndromes associated with autoimmunity require faster diagnostic tools to delineate therapeutic strategies and avoid organ damage. Since these PIDs present with severe life-threatening phenotypes, the need for a precise diagnosis in order to initiate appropriate patient management is necessary. More traditional approaches such as flow cytometry are therefore a valid option. Here, we review the application of flow cytometry and discuss the relevance of this powerful technique in diagnosing patients with PIDs presenting with immune dysregulation. In addition, flow cytometry represents a fast, robust, and sensitive approach that efficiently uncovers new immunopathological mechanisms underlying monogenic PIDs.

Keywords: flow cytometry, diagnosis, primary immunodeficiency diseases, immune dysregulation, mutation

INTRODUCTION

An effective immune response is required for defending the host from infections as well as playing a fundamental role in physiological homeostasis (1–9). In this context, the investigation of inborn errors of immunity leading to primary immunodeficiency diseases (PIDs) has considerably expanded our understanding of how the immune system works to eliminate infections while avoiding autoimmune diseases (10–17). The first PID was identified in 1952 by Ogden Bruton who reported a male patient with agammaglobulinemia who suffered from recurrent bacterial infections (18). By 2003, mutations in approximately 100 genes were found to cause molecularly defined PIDs (19). The introduction of next-generation sequencing (NGS) (e.g., whole exome sequencing or WES; whole genome sequencing or WGS) led to the discovery of ~120 new genes by 2015 (20–23). The most recent International Union of Immunological Societies (IUIS) report lists more than 320 monogenic causes of PID (24).

The longitudinal observation and molecular evaluation of PID patients revealed that the phenotype of PID patients comprises not only the susceptibility to bacterial, fungal, and viral infections diseases, but also autoinflammatory and autoimmune disorders as well as an increased incidence of malignancies (15, 16, 25–28). The group of PIDs associated with inflammation and autoimmunity has been recognized by the IUIS Phenotypic Classification Committee for PIDs as "diseases of immune dysregulation" (24). The prototype for this group is the syndrome of Immune Dysregulation, Polyendocrinopathy, Enteropathy, X-linked (IPEX) (29) caused by mutations in the Forkhead Box P3 (*FOXP3*) gene that results in the defective development of $CD4^{+}CD25^{+}$ regulatory T cells (Tregs). To date, mutations in some 40 genes have been identified that can present with symptoms of immune dysregulation [**Figure 1**; (24)]. Patients suspected to have one of these disorders require a rapid and precise diagnosis for prognostic and therapeutic considerations.

Although WES and WGS are powerful tools that have improved the genetic characterization of patients with undefined PIDs, these are laborious, time-consuming, and expensive tests. Flow cytometry, which is readily available in most laboratories, represents a useful low cost and rapid technology for the

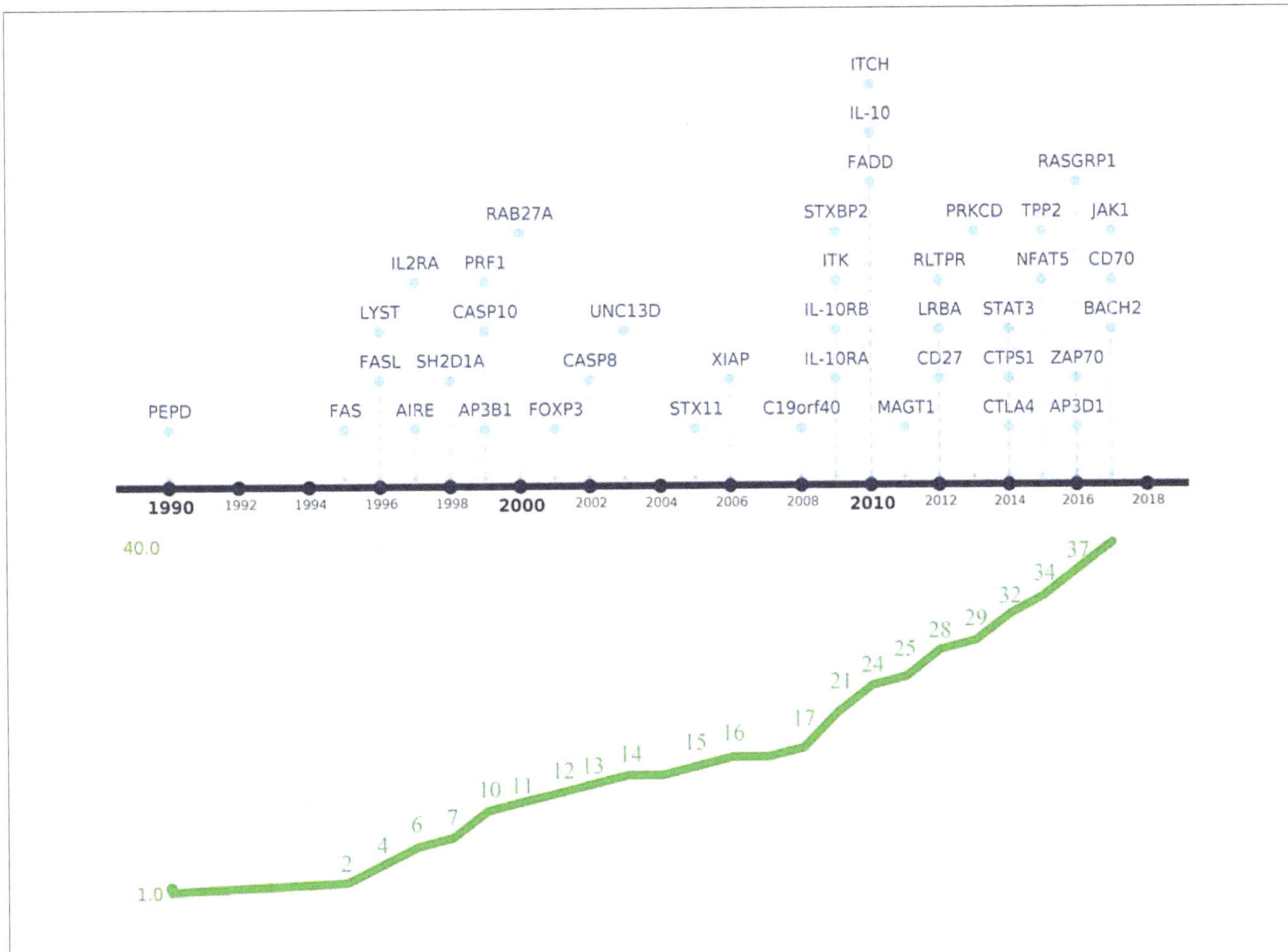

FIGURE 1 | Timeline depicting the discovery of genetic defects that cause PIDs associated with immune dysregulation. Genes are shown above the timeline by year of first reported mutation. The graphic below the timeline shows the cumulative increase of PIDs with immune dysregulation that were genetically characterized. The Y-axis represents the 40 genes associated with diseases of immune dysregulation that were discovered between 1990 and 2017 when the last IUIS phenotypic classification for PIDs was published (shown in the X-axis). The image was created using Time.Graphics (30).

investigation of PIDs, including patients with symptoms of immune dysregulation. This tool can identify not only the abnormal expression of extra- and intracellular molecules but can also be used to assess functional responses of specific subpopulations of lymphocytes. Flow cytometry-based assays have the advantage of being more quantitative, widely available and relatively easier to perform in a diagnostic laboratory setting compared with other techniques such as western blot analysis, fluorescent and confocal microscopy.

The advantage of using flow cytometry for the diagnosis of PIDs, in general, has been extensively discussed (31–36). Here, we review the progress made in using flow cytometry for the diagnosis of PIDs associated with immune dysregulation and its contributions for a better understanding of disease immunopathology. Although the genetic dissection of several PIDs have provided relevant insights into molecular pathways associated with host defense and immune tolerance (24, 37–43), we discuss here only the inborn errors of immunity presented by the last IUIS phenotypic classification for PIDs in 2017 (44).

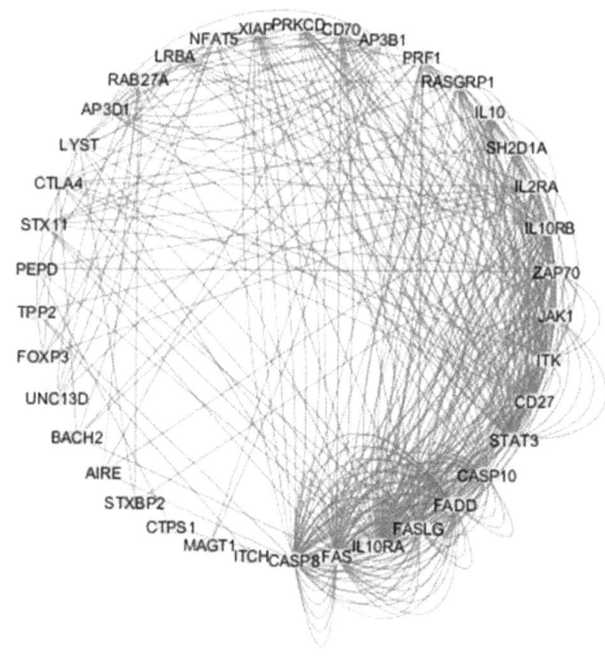

FIGURE 2 | Network of 40 genes that cause PIDs associated with immune dysregulation. The interactive circular graph illustrates the connections (e.g., physical interaction, common signaling pathways, co-localization.) between the causative genes and was developed using the GeneMANIA Cytoscape plugin (47). The genes were provided as a query and are represented by the blue nodes while their connections are represented by the gray lines. Related genes are closer together in the network and have more connecting lines among them.

Flow Cytometry for Diseases of Immune Dysregulation

Since the first attempt by Cooper et al. to provide a classification for PIDs in 1973 (45), the number of PIDs have exponentially increased as most recently summarized by the IUIS Inborn Errors of Immunity Committee classification [**Figure 1** (24)]. The first PIDs with features of immune dysregulation appeared in the IUIS Phenotypic Classification for Primary Immunodeficiencies in 1999 (Wiskott-Aldrich syndrome, PNP deficiency, selective IgA deficiency, early complement component deficiencies, and ALPS) (46). In subsequent reports, increased numbers of PIDs with features of immune dysregulation were reported, currently comprising a total of 40 monogenic diseases of immune dysregulation (**Figure 2**), divided into two main groups labeled "Hemophagocytic Lymphohistiocytosis (HLH) & Epstein-Barr virus (EBV) susceptibility" and "Syndromes with Autoimmunity and Others" (**Figure 3**). We use this classification throughout this article. The genes causing these disorders are listed in **Figure 4** (HLH and EBV susceptibility) and **Figure 7** (syndromes with autoimmunity).

With a few exceptions, the flow cytometry contributions for the characterization of diseases of immune dysregulation are discussed below and summarized in **Tables 1**, **2**. We have not included the Fanconi anemia-associated protein 24 (FAAP24) (91) and Itch E3 ubiquitin ligase (ITCH) (92) deficiencies, which are molecules that play a critical role in DNA repair (91, 93) and the negative regulation of T cell activation (92, 94). There are only single reports (91, 92) of these deficiencies and flow cytometry methods for the characterization of their immunopathological mechanisms are not available. This is also the case for prolidase D (*PEPD*) deficiency (95), which has been associated with the development of systemic lupus erythematosus (SLE) (96), and zeta chain of T cell receptor-associated protein kinase 70 (ZAP-70) (97) and nuclear factor of activated T cells 5 (NFAT5) deficiencies (98). Only two ZAP-70-deficient siblings have been reported with combined hypomorphic and activation mutations, and flow cytometry was only used to analyze T cell activation by measuring CD69 expression on activated T cells. Only a single patient with NFAT5 deficiency was reported, for whom flow cytometry was used mainly for immunophenotyping and cell death analysis (98).

Flow Cytometry Guidelines

Before reviewing the contribution of flow cytometry to the characterization of PIDs with immune dysregulation, we emphasize that in order to perform molecular characterization of inborn errors of immunity in diagnostic laboratories, one needs to become familiar with the flow cytometry guidelines and parameters, which have been previously reported (31, 99–104) They were discussed in detail with focus on technical flow cytometry aspects. For example, flow cytometry parameters of general importance are the determination and validation of flow cytometry positive controls (e.g., fluorescence compensation controls as well as resting and activation controls in the case of inducible molecules), the establishment of appropriate cutoffs (e.g., by defining the 10th percentile of normal controls as a center-specific lower limit of normal), and avoiding misinterpretation of results due to inter-laboratory variability, specificity, and sensitivity, particularly in patients with low peripheral blood lymphocyte counts. Another important issue is

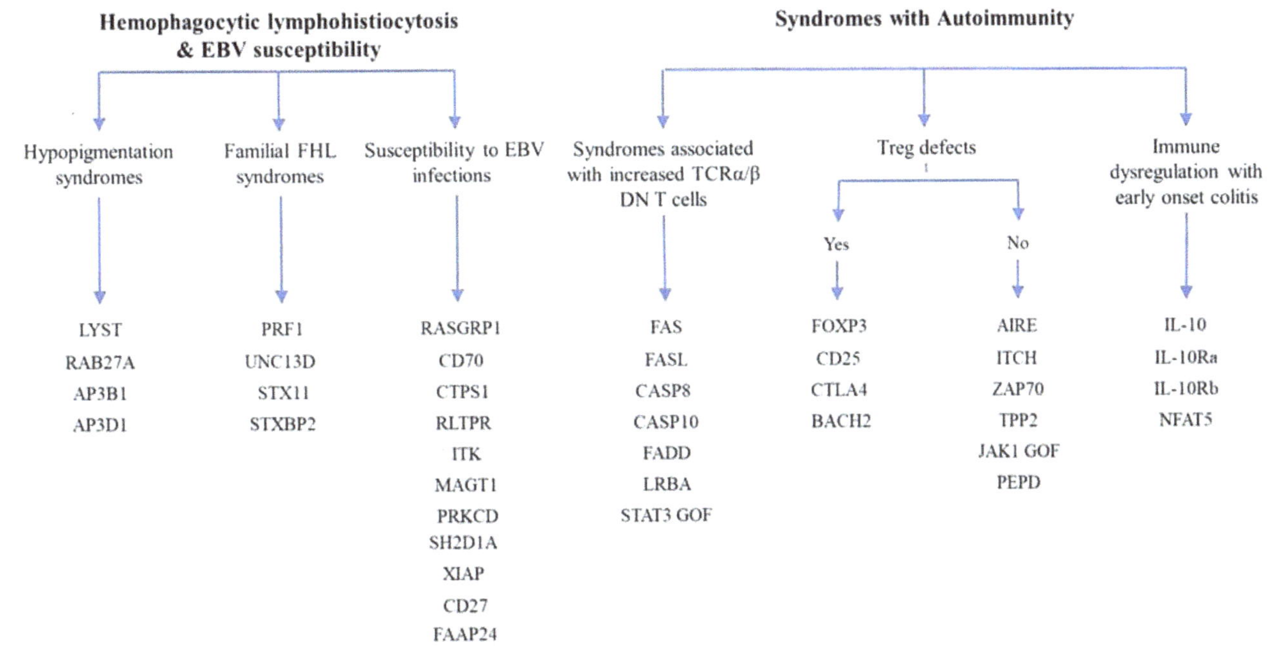

FIGURE 3 | Diagram of the 40 genes that cause PIDs associated with immune dysregulation. The genes are classified according the 2017 IUIS phenotypic classification for PIDs (24).

that some functional assays have a time frame (normally within 24 h after venous puncture) within the test must be performed, due to changes in cell viability or the activation of affected cell pathways during blood shipment. Thus, it is important to obtain blood from healthy controls at the same time of patient sampling and ship them together for flow cytometry screening tests (49, 105). In cases that the cells obtained from the same-day healthy control show results outside the normal range, i.e., not expressing or overexpressing a specific molecule, which is used as experimental readout such as in degranulation assays (49), the shipment and test have to be repeated. Altogether, the above mentioned factors as well as other experimental procedures such as correct definition of instrument setup and evaluation of cell viability prior to the experiment are of major importance for the proper execution of diagnostic flow cytometry. Importantly, following the initial flow cytometry screening tests, there is a significant amount of work to be performed by functional validation studies (e.g., by combining site-directed mutagenesis combined with flow cytometric assays) when identifying new molecular defects.

HEMOPHAGOCYTIC LYMPHOHISTIOCYTOSIS AND EBV SUSCEPTIBILITY

HLH is a hyper-inflammatory syndrome directly linked to abnormalities in cytotoxicity as a result of defective degranulation. This syndrome is characterized by prolonged fever and massive hepatosplenomegaly associated with laboratory findings such as cytopenia, hypertriglyceridemia, hypofibrinogenemia, and NK cells and cytotoxic ($CD8^+$) T lymphocytes (CTLs) exhibiting reduced cytotoxicity (24, 106). Clinical and immunological features of FHL syndromes have previously been reviewed in detail (107, 108). Natural killer (NK) and cytotoxic T cells from these patients show an impaired capacity to control viral infections. The unique curative therapy for HLH is hematopoietic stem cell transplantation (HSCT) (109–111).

Several different genetic disorders are associated with an HLH phenotype and are classified as HLH with hypopigmentation or without hypopigmentation (familial hemophagocytic lymphohistiocytosis syndromes or FHL). Secondary HLH, generally seen in older children and adults without a known genetic defect, are triggered by viral infections such as EBV (most commonly), cytomegalovirus, and herpes simplex virus, or by hematologic malignancies, rheumatologic conditions, or tuberculosis (112). The 19 causative genes associated with the HLH and EBV susceptibility group are summarized in **Figure 4** as well as a summarized guideline is shown in **Figure 5**, which describes the flow cytometric assays required to diagnose patients with syndromes that present with autoimmunity.

Hypopigmentation Syndromes

Four different inborn errors of immunity causing HLH with hypopigmentation/albinism have been described: Chediak-Higashi syndrome, genetically characterized by mutations in the lysosomal trafficking regulator (*LYST*) gene (50, 51); Griscelli syndrome type 2 due to mutations in Ras-Related Protein Rab-27A (*RAB27A*) (52); and Hermansky-Pudlak syndrome type 2

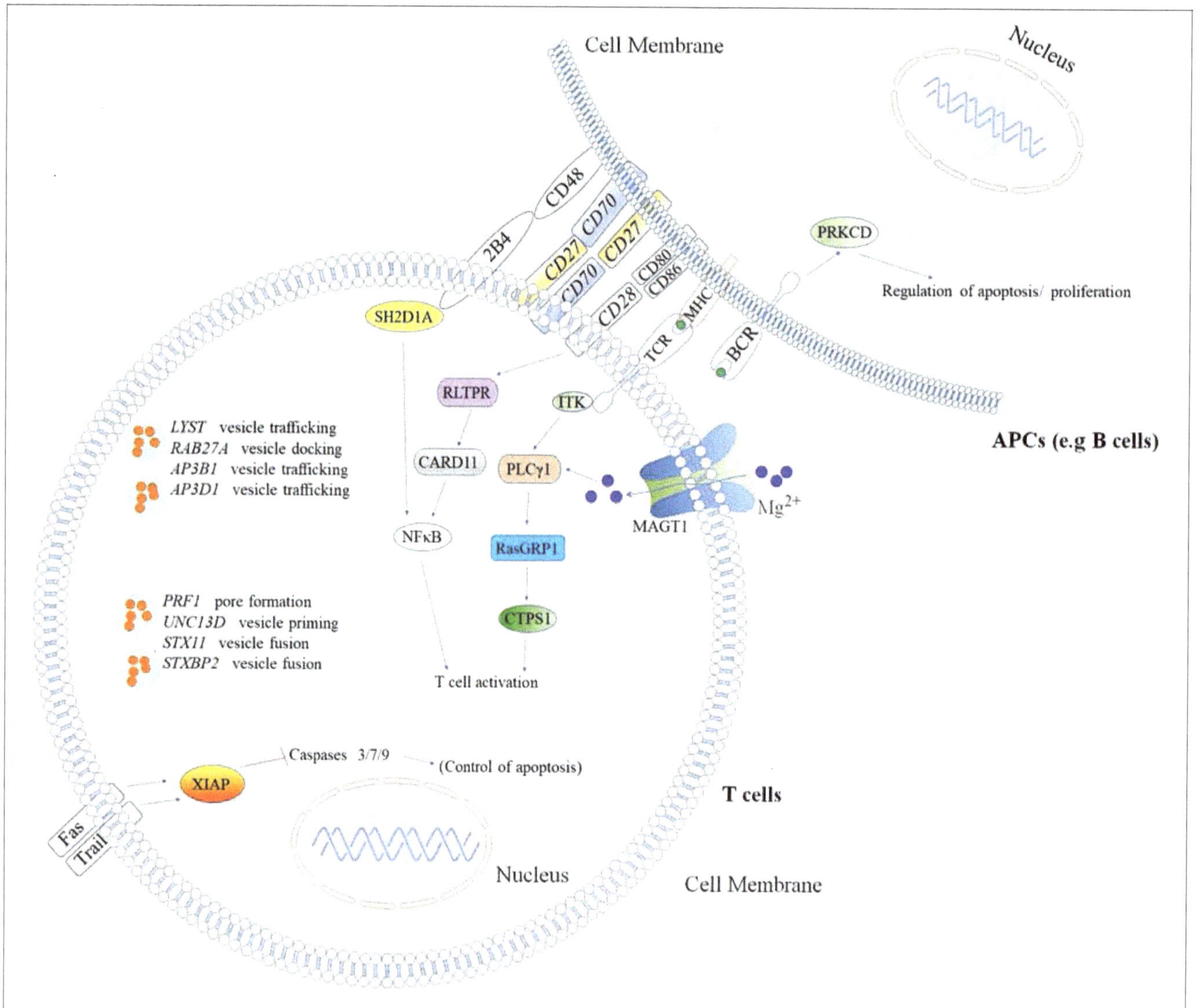

FIGURE 4 | Inborn errors of immunity that cause increased susceptibility to Hemophagocytic Lymphohistiocytosis (HLH) & Epstein–Barr virus (EBV)*. Illustration of mutated genes associated with HLH and increased susceptibility to EBV are shown with colored backgrounds. To allow a better comprehension of signaling pathways involved, other molecules (Fas, Trail, MHC, NFκB, 2BA, CD48, CD28, CD80, CD86, and BCR) not associated with HLH and EBV susceptibility are shown in the white background. *Named according to the 2017 IUIS phenotypic classification for PIDs (24). The illustration was constructed using Motifolio Drawing Toolkits (48).

and type 10 caused by mutations in the adaptor related protein complex 3 beta 1 (*AP3B1*) (53) and adaptor related protein complex 3 delta 1 (*AP3D1*) (54), respectively. These diseases generally manifest as hypopigmentation, immunodeficiency, neutropenia, or decreased NK and cytotoxic T cell activity, and bleeding tendency. However, a few cases of patients with Griscelli syndrome type 2 with biallelic mutations in *RAB27A* have been reported with normal pigmentation (113).

Interestingly, the overlapping clinical features shown by inborn errors of immunity causing HLH with hypopigmentation/albinism might be explained by defects in the molecular machinery responsible for the biogenesis and transport of secretory lysosome-related organelles in different cell types (54). These physiologic processes are essential for production and secretion of perforin and granzyme by NK cells and cytotoxic CD8^{+} T lymphocytes (54, 55), as well as secretion of melanin by melanosomes (114, 115) and release of small molecules by δ granules from platelets during blood vessel damage, which facilitates platelet adhesion and activation during coagulation (114).

Since there is no specific flow cytometry approach established to detect the expression of LYST, RAB27A, AP3B1, or AP3D1, the differential diagnosis of these syndromes, based on flow cytometry, is not possible and thus the diagnosis relies on biochemical and molecular criteria (50, 109, 116). A few specific features differentiate these disorders, such as the presence of large inclusions (lysosome) in white blood cells from patients with Chediak Higashi syndrome (49, 50, 116), specific hair shaft

TABLE 1 | Summary of flow cytometry contributions for the immunopathological characterization of Hemophagocytic Lymphohistiocytosis (HLH) and Epstein–Barr virus (EBV) susceptibility.

HLH and EBV susceptibility	Flow cytometric (FC) application and immunopathological mechanisms identified	Genetic defect (References)	Inheritance
Hypopigmentation Syndromes			
Chediak Higashi sd	Reduced degranulation based on the surface up-regulation of CD107a (49) in Natural killer (NK) cells and cytotoxic T lymphocytes (CTLs)	*LYST* (50, 51)	AR
Griscelli sd type 2	Reduced degranulation based on the surface up-regulation of CD107a (49) in NK and CTLs	*RAB27A* (52)	AR
Hermansky-Pudlak sd type 2	Reduced degranulation based on the surface up-regulation of CD107a (49) in NK and CTLs	*AP3B1* (53)	AR
Hermansky-Pudlak sd, type 10	Reduced degranulation based on the surface up-regulation of CD107a (49) in NK and CTLs	*AP3D1* (54)	AR
Familial HLH			
Perforin deficiency (FHL2)	Perforin expression in NK cells and CTLs Normal CD107a expression in NK and CTLs	*PRF1* (55)	AR
UNC13D or Munc13-4 deficiency (FHL3)	Munc13-4 expression in NK cells, CTLs, and platelets.	*UNC13D* (56)	AR
Syntaxin 11 deficiency (FHL4)	STX11 expression not available by FC (no antibody validated). Reduced CD107a expression in NK and CTLs	*STX11* (57)	AR
STXBP2 or Munc18-2 deficiency (FHL5)	STXBP2 expression by FC not available (no antibody validated). Reduced CD107a expression in NK and CTLs	STXBP2 (58)	AR
Susceptibility to EBV infections			
RASGRP1 deficiency	Reduced cell proliferation using fluorescent cell staining dye; impaired T cell activation by measuring CD69 expression; defective CTPS1 expression; reduced intracellular expression of active caspase 3; reduced T cell apoptosis using annexin V/propidium iodide staining, all in response to CD3/TCR activation	RASGRP1 (59–63)	AR
CD70 deficiency	CD70 expression on phytohaemagglutinin (PHA)-stimulated T cells; binding of a CD27-Fc fusion protein on T cells	CD70 (64)	AR
CTPS1 deficiency	Defective cell proliferation using fluorescent cell staining dye	CTPS1 (65)	AR
RLTPR deficiency	RLTPR expression in adaptive (B and T lymphocytes) and innate (monocytes and dendritic cells) immune cells. Reduced phospho-nuclear factor (NF)-κB P65-(pS259) expression and inhibitor (I)κBα degradation in CD4$^+$ and CD8$^+$, specifically after CD28 co-stimulation; CD107a expression after K562 stimulation	RLTPR or CARMIL2 (66)	
ITK deficiency	ITK expression by FC not available (no antibody validated). Reduced T cell receptor (TCR)-mediated calcium flux; absence of Natural Killer T (NKT) cells determined as TCR Vβ11 and TCR Vα24 double-positive cells	ITK (67)	AR
MAGT1 deficiency	MAGT1 expression by FC not available (no antibody validated). Reduced CD69 expression in CD4$^+$ T cells after anti-CD3 stimulation. Low CD31$^+$ cells in the naïve (CD27$^+$, CD45RO$^-$) CD4$^+$ T cell population. Impaired Mg influx using Mg2$^+$-specific fluorescent probe MagFluo4. Reduced NKG2D expression in NK cells and CTLs	MAGT1 (68)	XL
PRKCD deficiency	Increased B cell proliferation after anti-IgM stimulation; resistance to PMA-induced cell death; low CD27 expression on B cells	PRKCD (69–71)	AR
XLP1	SH2D1A expression, low numbers of circulating NKT cells (Vα24TCR+/Vβ11TCR+). Impaired apoptosis.	SH2D1A (72)	XL
XLP2	XIAP expression, low numbers of circulating NKT cells (Vα24TCR+/Vβ11TCR+). Enhanced apoptosis	XIAP (73)	XL
CD27 deficiency	CD27 expression on B cells	CD27 (74)	AR

Diseases are classified as reported by the 2017 IUIS phenotypic classification for PIDs (24). AP3B1, Adaptor Related Protein Complex 3 Beta 1; AP3D1, Adaptor Related Protein Complex 3 Delta 1; AR, Autosomal recessive; CD27, Cluster of Differentiation 27; CD70, Cluster of Differentiation 70; CTPS1, Cytidine triphosphate synthase 1; FHL, familial hemophagocytic lymphohistiocytosis; ITK, IL2 Inducible T Cell Kinase; LYST, Lysosomal Trafficking Regulator; MAGT1, Magnesium Transporter 1; PRF1, Perforin 1; PRKCD, Protein Kinase C Delta; RAB27A, Ras-Related Protein Rab-27A; RASGRP1, RAS guanyl-releasing protein 1; RLTPR, RGD motif, leucine rich repeats, tropomodulin domain and proline-rich containing; sd, syndrome; SH2D1A, SH2 Domain Containing 1A; STX11, Syntaxin 11; STXBP2, Syntaxin Binding Protein 2; UNC13D, Protein unc-13 homolog D; XL, X-linked; XIAP, X-linked inhibitor of apoptosis protein.

anomalies, and the detection of a platelet storage pool deficiency characteristic of Hermansky-Pudlak syndrome (54). However, flow cytometry has been used successfully as a screening tool for primary (i.e., genetic) degranulation defects. The approach relies on measuring the up-regulation of CD107a on NK cells (with/without K562 stimulation) (49) and cytotoxic T lymphocytes (with/without anti-CD3 stimulation) (54). CD107a is a lysosomal protein that co-localizes with perforin and granzyme in cytolytic granules (117, 118) and is expressed on the cell surface upon activation-induced degranulation following the engagement of T cell receptor (TCR) and NK cell activating receptors (119, 120). This assay has been performed in parallel with a cytotoxicity assay using K562 or P815 target cells to functionally confirm the degranulation defect suggested by a reduced CD107a expression following 48 h with phytohemagglutinin (PHA)/IL-2 or anti-CD3/anti-CD28

TABLE 2 | Summary of flow cytometry contributions for the immunopathological characterization of Syndromes with autoimmunity.

Syndromes with autoimmunity	Flow cytometric (FC) application and immunopathological mechanisms identified	Genetic defect (References)	Inheritance
Syndromes associated with increased TCRα/β DN T cells			
ALPS-FAS	FAS expression, reduced T cell apoptosis	*TNFRSF6* (75)	AD/AR
ALPS-FASLG	FASL expression, reduced T cell apoptosis	*TNFSF6* (76)	AD/AR
ALPS-Caspase8	Reduced T cell apoptosis	*CASP8* (77)	AR
ALPS-Caspase 10	Reduced T cell apoptosis	*CASP10* (78)	AD
FADD deficiency	Reduced T cell apoptosis	*FADD* (79)	AR
LRBA deficiency	Reduced T regulatory (T reg) cells, low CTLA4 and Helios; Increased B cell apoptosis and low levels of IgG^+/IgA^+ $CD27^+$ switched-memory B cells; reduced B proliferative capacity, and impaired activation (using CD138 staining)	LRBA (80)	AR
STAT3 gain-of-function (GOF) mutation	Delayed de-phosphorylation of STAT3; diminished STAT5 and STAT1 phosphorylation; which is in line with the role in the negative regulation of several STATs162. High levels of Th17 cells; reduced $FOXP3^+CD25^+$ Treg population; decreased FASL-induced apoptosis	STAT3 (81)	AD
Defective regulatory T cells			
IPEX	Decreased or absent FOXP3 expression by $CD4^+CD25^+$ regulatory T cells	FOXP3 (82)	XL
CD25 deficiency	Impaired CD25 expression; defective proliferative responses following anti-CD3 or PH; defective NK cell maturation increased (CD56brightCD16hi and reduced CD56dimCD16hi NK cells in peripheral blood); increased degranulation by elevated CD107a expression and higher perforin and granzyme B expression in NK cells;	CD25 or IL2RA (83)	AR
CTLA4 haploinsufficiency	CTLA4 expression, trafficking, binding to its ligand, and CTLA4-mediated trans-endocytosis	CTLA4 (84)	AD
BACH2 deficiency	Reduced BACH2 expression in T and B lymphocytes, decreased FOXP3 expression by $CD4^+CD25^+$ regulatory T cells, reduced total and class-switched memory B cells, increased T-bet expression	BACH2 (85)	AD
Normal regulatory T cell function			
APECED	Expression of IL-17A, IL-17F, and IL-22 by PBMCs. AIRE expression by FC is not available (no antibody validated)	AIRE (86)	AR
Tripeptidyl-Peptidase II deficiency	Lymphocytes expressing high levels of major histocompatibility complex (MHC) class I molecules, a predominant T $CD8^+CD27^-CD28^-CD127^-$ phenotype; increased percentage of IFN-γ and IL-17 positive T cells; high expression of T-bet and perforin. Defective proliferation lymphoproliferation and increased susceptibility to apoptosis; increased levels of CD21low B cells	TPP2 (87)	AR
JAK1 GOF	Increased JAK1, STAT1, and STAT3 phosphorylation	JAK1 (88)	AD
Immune dysregulation with early onset Colitis			
IL-10 deficiency	No FC assay available. Normal STAT3 phosphorylation in response to IL-10	IL-10(89)	AR
IL-10RA deficiency	IL-10RA expression; defective STAT3 phosphorylation in response to IL-10. Normal STAT3 phosphorylation in response to IL-23	IL-10Ra (90)	AR
IL-10RB deficiency	IL-10RB expression; defective STAT3 phosphorylation in response to IL-10. Normal STAT3 phosphorylation in response to IL-23	IL-10Rb (90)	AR

Diseases are classified as reported by the 2017 IUIS phenotypic classification for PIDs (24). AD, Autosomal dominant; ALPS-FAS, Autoimmune lymphoproliferative syndrome-Fas cell surface death receptor; ALPS-FASLG, Autoimmune lymphoproliferative syndrome FAS ligand gene; APECED, Autoimmune polyendocrinopathy candidiasis ectodermal dystrophy; AR, Autosomal recessive; BACH2, BTB Domain And CNC Homolog 2; CASP8, cysteine-aspartic acid protease 8;CASP10, cysteine-aspartic acid protease 10; CD25 or IL2RA, Interleukin 2 Receptor A; CTLA4, cytotoxic T-lymphocyte-associated Protein 4; DN, double negative; FADD, Fas Associated Via Death Domain; IL-10, Interleukin-10; IL-10Ra, Interleukin-10 Receptor alpha; IL-10Rb, Interleukin-10 Receptor beta; IPEX, Immune dysregulation; polyendocrinopathy; enteropathy; XL, X-linked; JAK1, Janus Kinase 1; LRBA, LPS Responsive Beige-Like Anchor Protein; NFAT5, Nuclear Factor Of Activated T Cells 5; STAT3, signal transducer and activator of transcription 3; TPP2, Tripeptidyl Peptidase 2.

beads stimulation (49, 109, 112, 121). This degranulation assay allows the differentiation between primary and secondary HLH. The latter express CD107a normally upon cell activation (49). Furthermore, as elegantly reported by Bryceson et al. (49), the analysis of CD107a expression by flow cytometry has the advantage of being a sensitive assay even when patients receive immunosuppressive therapy or have very low numbers of T/NK cells. Detailed methodological information about the detection of T and NK cell degranulation by flow cytometry can be found elsewhere (36, 122).

Familial Hemophagocytic Lymphohistiocytosis (FHL) Syndromes

FHL is a life-threatening autosomal-recessive inherited hyperinflammatory syndrome that usually develops within the first 2 years of age (56). FHL syndromes are caused by mutations in *perforin-1* (*PRF1*), designated as FLH2, accounting for 30–50% of known cases (105, 108), or proteins involved in perforin secretion: protein unc-13 homolog D (*UNC13D*) (56), Syntaxin-11 (*STX11*) (57), and Syntaxin Binding Protein 2 (*STXBP2*)

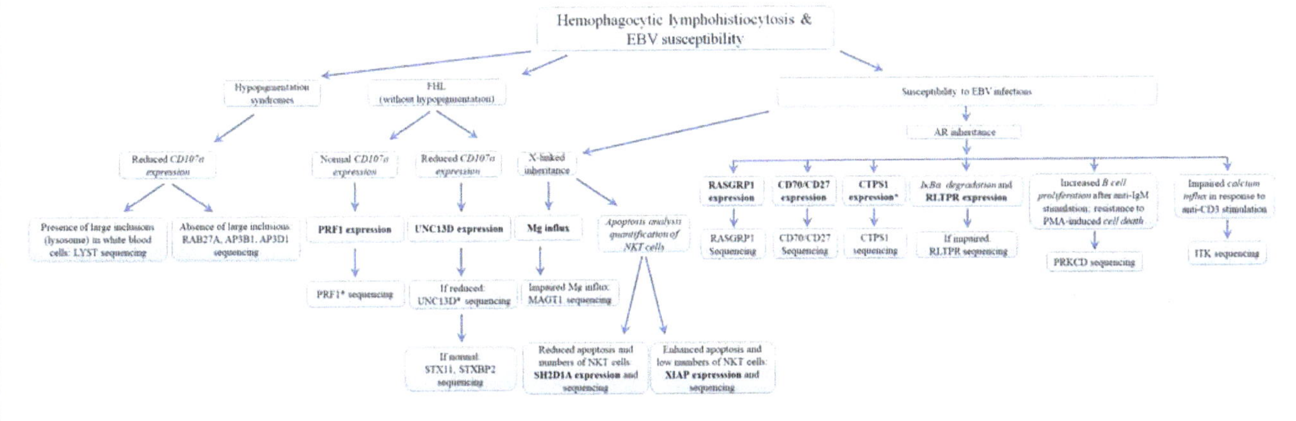

FIGURE 5 | Flowchart depicting the immunophenotypic analysis used to define the molecular genetic defects of patients with hemophagocytic lymphohistiocytosis & EBV susceptibility, with flow cytometry. In those cases with normal protein by flow cytometry, if there is a strong clinical indication for a specific immune dysregulation disease, it is recommended to perform gene sequencing to exclude missense mutations that do not impair protein expression. While it has been estimated that PRF1 deficiency accounts for 30–60% of known FHL cases and UNC13D deficiency for up to 20% of FHL cases, the frequency for most of the other immune dysregulation syndromes remains unknown. *Flow cytometry assay validated in HepG2 cells, but remains to be tested with cells from PID patients. Bold and italic texts are disease-specific and non-disease specific flow cytometry tests, respectively.

(58), known as FHL3, FHL4, and FHL5, respectively. The gene responsible for FHL1 has not yet been identified (107).

Defective perforin expression by NK cells ($CD3^-CD56^+CD16^+$) and cytotoxic T lymphocytes ($CD3^+CD8^+$) can be detected by flow cytometry and has been used as a screening approach for FHL2 (34). Likewise, patients with UNC13D deficiency, which accounts for up to 20% of FHL cases, can be identified by decreased UNC13D expression using flow cytometry. Usually, UNC13D expression is assessed on NK cells and T lymphocytes. Since patients with UNC13D deficiency frequently present with significantly reduced leukocyte counts (pancytopenia), UNC13D expression can instead be analyzed on platelets ($CD41a^+$) (34, 105, 123), since platelets express UNC13D more abundantly than peripheral blood leukocytes (105).

There is no specific or commercially available antibody for flow cytometry to screen patients with STX11 and STXBP2 deficiencies. Therefore, these two deficiencies have been identified indirectly by measuring CD107a expression, or by the exclusion of defective PRF1 and UNC13D expression. While cells from patients with FHL3-5 present reduced CD107a expression on the surface of NK cells and CTLs, CD107a expression is normal in subjects with PRF-1 deficiency (49, 58, 123). This phenomenon is explained by the fact that perforin constitutes part of the lytic granule content, but in contrast to UNC13D, STX11, and STXBP2, it is not essential for the transport of secretory lysosome-related organelles (55, 58, 106, 107, 124, 125).

Susceptibility to EBV Infection

More than 90% of the global population are EBV-seropositive, with the majority being asymptomatic or manifesting a self-limiting disease (126). Patients with inborn errors of immunity that result in susceptibility to EBV may develop severe or fatal mononucleosis, B cell lymphoma, lymphoproliferative disease, or HLH (67, 127–129). Mutations in at least 11 genes (four of them with *EBV-associated HLH*) are known to cause increased susceptibility to EBV (24), demonstrating the non-redundant role of signaling pathways that generate EBV-specific immunity, and the pivotal role of continuous immune surveillance to ensure virus-host homeostasis (129, 130). The signaling pathways and outcomes involved in the immunopathogenesis of severe EBV infections (129) are summarized in **Figure 4**.

Notably, T cell proliferation by patients with susceptibility to EBV can be reduced, normal or even increased (**Table 3**); however, some subjects belonging to the same PID subgroup may display variable proliferation results where some patients with CTPS1 (65, 131) and CD27 (74, 134) deficiencies have reduced T cell proliferation and others do not. Moreover, the abnormal proliferative responses might be stimulus dependent. For instance, patients with ITK deficiency may demonstrate reduced T cell proliferation in response to CD3/CD28 stimulation, but normal proliferation in response to PHA stimulation (132). Therefore, in addition to be a non-specific assay to screen different PIDs, the analysis of T cell proliferation from patients with susceptibility to EBV needs to be carefully scrutinized as a screening flow cytometry tool to direct the definitive diagnosis of these PIDs.

RASGRP1 Deficiency

RAS guanyl-releasing protein 1 (*RASGRP1*) is a guanine nucleotide exchange factor and activator of the RAS-MAPK pathway initiated by diacylglycerol following TCR signaling (129). Mutations in RASGRP1 have been found in patients with a combined immunodeficiency (a ALPS-like disease) (59) presenting with recurrent respiratory infections in association with EBV-induced lymphoproliferative disease, chronic lymphadenopathy, hepatosplenomegaly, autoimmune hemolytic anemia, and immune thrombocytopenia (59–63). In addition to its availability as a screening tool to establish the diagnosis of RASGRP1 deficiency (59), flow cytometry has been

TABLE 3 | T cell proliferation response of PIDs with susceptibility to EBV.

	Susceptibility to EBV									
Deficiency	RASGRP1	CD70	CTPS1	RLTPR	ITK	MAGT1	PRKCD	XLP1	XIAP	CD27
T cell proliferation	Reduced	Reduced	Reduced	Reduced	Reduced	Reduced	Normal	Increased	Reduced	Reduced
References	(60)	(64)	(65, 131)	(66)	(132)	(68)	(70)	(133)	(73)	(74, 134)

widely applied to evaluate functional defects resulting from RASGRP1 mutations. For instance, this approach can be used to detect reduced T cell expansion by a cell proliferation kit (e.g., CellTrace), impaired T cell activation by CD69 staining, and markedly reduced phosphorylation of ERK. Diminished intracellular expression of active caspase 3 in lymphocytes associated with reduced apoptosis using annexin V (AV) and propidium iodide (PI) staining has been observed (59–61).

CD70/CD27 Deficiencies

Disorders of T cell co-signaling pathways such as those caused by deficiencies in CD40L, SAP, OX40, or CD70/CD27 highlight the critical role of co-stimulation for host defense (135–137). Patients with mutations affecting the co-stimulatory molecules CD70 and CD27 (**Figure 4**), which are expressed on the surface of T, B and NK cells (138–140) present with similar clinical phenotypes. These patients exhibit impaired effector $CD8^+$ T cell generation, hypogammaglobulinemia, lack of memory B cells, and reduced cytolytic and proliferative responses of T cells resulting in chronic EBV infections (EBV-associated lymphoproliferation, EBV-associated HLH, and B cell lymphoma). Additionally, affected patients might develop severe forms of other viral infections including influenza, herpesviruses (e.g., varicella-zoster virus), and cytomegalovirus (CMV) (64, 74, 134, 141–143). Cell-surface expression of both CD70 and CD27 are assessed by flow cytometry using specific monoclonal antibodies. Similar to other combined deficiencies, it is possible that a mutated non-functional protein is expressed on the cell surface (144, 145) in which case it is possible to analyse the ability of a CD27Fc fusion protein that binds to CD70, by flow cytometry (64).

RLTPR Deficiency

The RLTPR (RGD motif, leucine-rich repeats, tropomodulin domain, and proline-rich containing) is a scaffold protein that bridges CD28 located on the cell-surface to the cytosolic adaptor called Caspase Recruitment Domain Family Member 11 (CARD11), enabling proper activation of the TCR-induced NF-κB signaling pathway (146, 147). Although human CD28 deficiency has not yet been characterized, RLTPR deficiency was recently reported as an autosomal recessive combined immunodeficiency highlighting the critical role of the CD28 pathway for T- and B-cell activation (66). RLTPR-deficient patients present with low numbers of memory $CD4^+$ T cells, reduced numbers of T helper (Th)1, Th17, and T follicular helper cells, as well as reduced memory B cells, and show poor antibody responses to vaccines (67, 148). RLTPR deficiency causes susceptibility to a variety of pathogens, including bacteria, fungi, and viruses (e.g., EBV). RLTPR expression can be detected by flow cytometry in adaptive (B and T lymphocytes) and innate (monocytes and dendritic cells) immune cells. Moreover, NF-κB signaling defects (149, 150) in $CD4^+$ and $CD8^+$ T cells from patients with RLTPR mutations have been characterized by flow cytometry, primarily manifested by reduced NF-κB P65 phosphorylation and IκBα degradation following anti-CD28 stimulation (66). In this context, there is a debatable paradigm that CD28 co-stimulation is not necessary for the activation of memory T cells. In agreement, flow cytometric analysis of T cell proliferation has shown that the lack of RLTPR only impairs the proliferation of naïve, but not memory T cells (66). Flow cytometric analysis also points out a critical role of RLTPR in NK cells, since their degranulation capacity is impaired after K562 stimulation, depicted by reduced CD107a expression (151).

CTPS1 Deficiency

The cytidine nucleotide triphosphate synthase 1 (*CTPS1*) is a molecule involved in DNA synthesis in lymphocytes (152) and therefore plays a central role in lymphocyte proliferation (65, 131). Loss-of-function homozygous mutations in CTPS1 cause a combined immunodeficiency characterized by the impaired capacity of activated T and B cells to proliferate in response to antigen receptor-mediated activation (65). CTPS1-deficient patients are susceptible to life-threatening bacterial and viral infections, including those caused by EBV (e.g., EBV-related B-cell non-Hodgkin lymphoma). Flow cytometry has only been used to evaluate T lymphocyte proliferation in response to an anti-CD3 antibody or anti-CD3/CD28 coated beads, as well as B cells in response to anti-BCR plus CpG, which were found to be defective (65). However, patients with normal lymphoproliferative response have also been reported (131). There is no anti-CTPS1 fluorochrome-conjugated antibody commercially available. Therefore, CTPS1 expression is analyzed by western blot (65). CTPS1 expression by flow cytometry has been validated in HepG2 cells through incubation of primary unconjugated antibody followed by a dye-conjugated secondary antibody staining (153). This staining strategy represents a potential approach to screen patients with CTPS1 deficiency by flow cytometry.

ITK Deficiency

Mutations in the IL-2-inducible T cell kinase (ITK) causes a life-threatening syndrome of immune dysregulation and therapy-resistant EBV-associated lymphoproliferative disease (154–156). ITK is a signaling molecule located proximal to the TCR (**Figure 4**). ITK is expressed in thymocytes and peripheral T cells, regulating the thresholds of TCR signaling and specific development of $CD8^+$ T cells (131). Flow cytometry analysis has shown that ITK deficient patients exhibit a reduced TCR-mediated calcium flux in T cells (67) and an absence of NKT cells as determined by the lack of TCR Vβ11 and TCR Vα24 double-positive cells (156).

MAGT1 Deficiency

In addition to its essential role as a co-factor for nucleic acids and metabolic enzymes (157, 158), a critical role of magnesium ion (Mg^{2+}) in immune responses has been demonstrated by disease-causing mutations in the magnesium transporter 1 gene (*MAGT1*). Li et al. (68) reported Mg^{2+} as an intracellular second messenger following TCR activation in patients with an X-linked inborn error of immunity characterized by $CD4^+$ T cell lymphopenia, severe chronic viral infections (e.g., EBV infection associated with lymphoproliferative disease or lymphoma), and defective T lymphocyte activation. Flow cytometry was used by the authors to characterize several immunological defects, but not the expression of MAGT1, which was investigated by Western blots. A reduced CD69 expression by $CD4^+$ T cells after anti-CD3 stimulation was identified, while the response to phorbol 12-myristate 13-acetate (PMA) plus Ionomycin was normal, thus suggesting a specific defective TCR signaling that was confirmed by impaired NF-κB and NFAT nuclear translocation using confocal microscopy. Reduced levels of naïve $CD4^+$ T cells ($CD27^+$, $CD45RO^-$) expressing CD31, a cell surface marker of naive TREC-rich T cells, suggest a diminished thymic output (159–161). Kinetic analysis by flow cytometry also revealed abrogation of TCR-induced Mg^{2+} influx, which can be detected by the Mg^{2+}-specific fluorescent probe, MagFluo4 (68). Another immunologic feature of the disease is the impaired cytotoxic function of NK and $CD8^+$ T cells. Chaigne-Delalande et al. (162) elegantly demonstrated that decreased intracellular free Mg^{2+} causes impaired expression of the natural killer activating receptor NKG2D in NK and $CD8^+$ T cells, impairing cytolytic responses against EBV.

PRKCD Deficiency

Protein kinase C delta (PKCδ) (69–71, 163) belongs to a family of at least 11 serine/threonine kinase members involved in several pathological conditions (164, 165). Mutations in this gene cause a monogenic disease that presents either as SLE-like disease or as autoimmune lymphoproliferative syndrome (ALPS)-like disorder. PKCδ deficiency is associated with uncontrolled lymphoproliferation and chronic EBV infection. Immunologically, human PKCδ deficiency results in a B cell disorder characterized by B cell resistance to apoptosis, B cell hyperproliferation, increased production of autoantibodies, and decreased numbers of memory B cells (69–71, 163). A similar phenotype has been identified in PKCδ knockout mice (166–168), demonstrating the essential role of PKCδ in B cell tolerance. Flow cytometry applications to investigate this disease are designed to demonstrate increased B cell proliferation after anti-IgM stimulation, resistance to PMA-induced cell death (70), and the almost absence of CD27 expression on B cells (69), i.e., absence of memory cells.

X-Linked Lymphoproliferative Syndromes

X-linked lymphoproliferative syndrome (XLP) is a PID that presents with severe or fatal EBV infection, acquired hypogammaglobulinemia, malignant lymphoma, and HLH (72, 169). Most XLP cases are due to mutations in the SH2 domain protein 1A (*SH2D1A*) gene (XLP type 1), which encodes the signaling lymphocytic activation molecule (SLAM)-associated protein (SAP) (72). SAP is an adapter molecule that controls several signaling pathways involved in lymphocyte activation, proliferation, cytotoxicity, and also promotion of apoptosis [**Figure 4**; (170–172)]. The defect in antibody production exhibited by SH2D1A-deficient patients probably arise from impaired $CD4^+$ T cell interaction with B cells rather than an intrinsic B cell failure (169, 173).

Mutations in the gene encoding the X-linked inhibitor of apoptosis (*XIAP*), which inhibits caspase-3,−7, and−9 by direct binding (174), are responsible for XLP type 2 syndrome (73).The clinical phenotype and the disease pathogenesis have been reviewed and compared in detail elsewhere (129, 172, 175, 176). Flow cytometry can be used to evaluate apoptosis, in order to distinguish both XLP forms. Due to the distinct physiological roles of SH2D1A and XIAP, enhanced apoptosis of T lymphocytes is observed in patients with XIAP-deficiency, while the absence of SAP in SH2D1A deficiency is consistently associated with impaired cell apoptosis (133, 170, 172). This might explain why cytopenia is common in XIAP but not in SH2D1A deficiency (129). The EBV-associated immune dysregulation in XIAP deficiency might, in part, be due to the combination of an intrinsic exacerbated proliferation of immune cells plus the incapacity to respond to EBV. The lymphoproliferative disease reported in SH2D1A deficiency seems to be more the consequence of extrinsic and constant stimulation induced by EBV that cannot be properly controlled. For both XLP forms, flow cytometry to test intracellular testing for SAP and XIAP protein expression is available [**Figure 6**; (34)]. In addition, flow cytometric testing has demonstrated that the absence of SAP or XIAP proteins results in reduced numbers of circulating NKT ($V\alpha24TCR^+/V\beta11TCR^+$) cells (73).

SYNDROMES WITH AUTOIMMUNITY

The second major group of diseases of immune dysregulation named "Syndromes with Autoimmunity and Others," is subdivided based on the increased percentage of $CD4^-CD8^-TCR\alpha/\beta$ (double negative [DN] T cells), on Treg defects, and the development of colitis (24). The 21 disease-causing genes belonging to this group are represented in **Figure 7** as well as a summarized guideline (**Figure 8**) which describes the flow cytometric assays required to diagnose patients with syndromes that include autoimmunity.

Syndromes Associated With an Increased Percentage of $CD4^-CD8^-TCR\alpha/\beta$ Cells

Autoimmune Lymphoproliferative Syndromes (ALPS)

TCRα/β DN T cells are useful biomarkers, frequently elevated in children with autoimmune lymphoproliferative syndromes

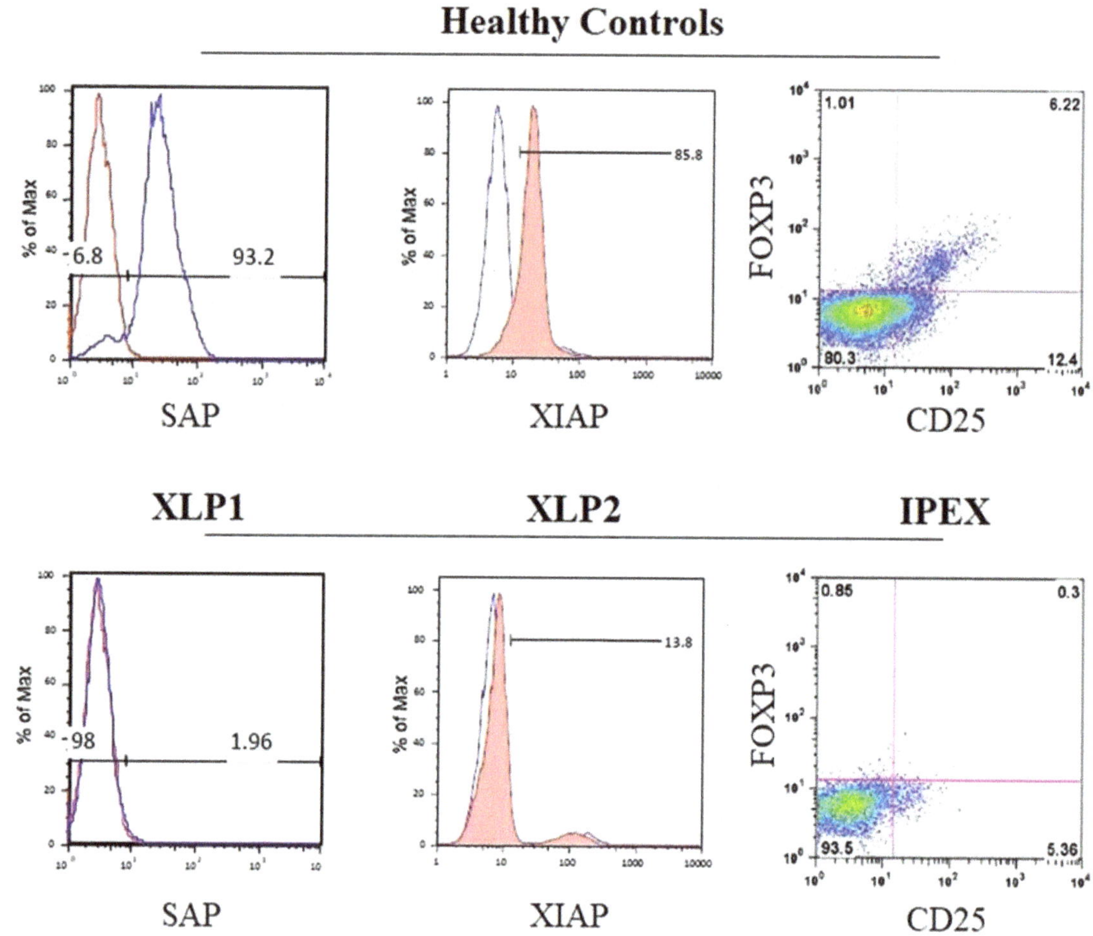

FIGURE 6 | Disease-specific flow cytometry tests for PIDs with immune dysregulation. The histograms show the normal expression of SAP and XIAP from healthy control lymphocytes (upper panels) compared with the absent expression of SAP and XIAP in lymphocytes from patients with X-linked lymphoproliferative syndrome type 1 (XLP1) and XLP2 (lower panels), respectively. The dot plot exhibits the absence of nuclear forkhead box P3 (FOXP3) expression in $CD4^{+}CD25^{+}$ regulatory T cells from patient PBMCs with immune dysregulation, polyendocrinopathy, enteropathy, X-linked inheritance syndrome (IPEX) (bottom right panel) compared with healthy control PBMCs (top right panel).

(ALPS) (179). The immunological functions of these cells have been reviewed in detail elsewhere (180). However, their precise role in the pathogenesis of autoimmune diseases is not well understood (179). ALPS is caused by mutations in five different genes: *FAS, FASL, FADD, CASP8, and CASP10.* The interaction between Fas (CD95) and Fas ligand or FasL (CD178), both expressed by activated T lymphocytes (the former also present on other cell types), triggers the formation of a death-inducing signaling complex (181, 182). This process involves the recruitment of Fas-associated death domain (FADD), cysteine-aspartic acid protease 8 (*CASP8*), and *CASP10*, initiating a cascade of signaling events that result in apoptotic cell death (183). This process regulates lymphocyte life span and promotes the elimination of autoreactive lymphocytes (**Figure 7**). The syndromes caused by mutations in these five genes have been classified by the National Institutes of Health (NIH) (177) as ALPS-FAS cell surface death receptor (the most frequent) (75), ALPS-FASL (76), ALPS-Caspase 8 (77), ALPS-Caspase 10 (78), and the FADD-deficiency (79). These disorders generally present as lymphadenopathy, splenomegaly, and autoimmune manifestations such as autoimmune hemolytic anemia, and severe recurrent thrombocytopenia (75–79, 184). Laboratory findings also include polyclonal hypergammaglobulinaemia, T lymphocyte apoptosis defect, and increased percentages of TCRα/β DN T cells (177).

Flow cytometry analysis demonstrates defective T cell apoptosis in response to anti-Fas antibody, recombinant FasL, or after phytohaemagglutinin (PHA)-/IL-2 stimulation by using FasT Kill assays or AV/PI or 7-AAD-staining. The technique of detecting increased percentages of TCRα/β DN T cells within peripheral blood mononuclear cells (PBMCs) is well established (76, 185, 186). Moreover, protein expression of FAS (187) and FASL (186) (both after T-cell blast generation by PHA plus IL-2) by flow cytometry is available to investigate ALPS-FAS and ALPS-FASL, respectively. Although the other ALPS forms (due to FADD (79), CASP8, or CASP10 deficiency) have not yet been studied by flow cytometry due to the unavailability of specific fluorescent conjugated antibodies, mutations in the FAS

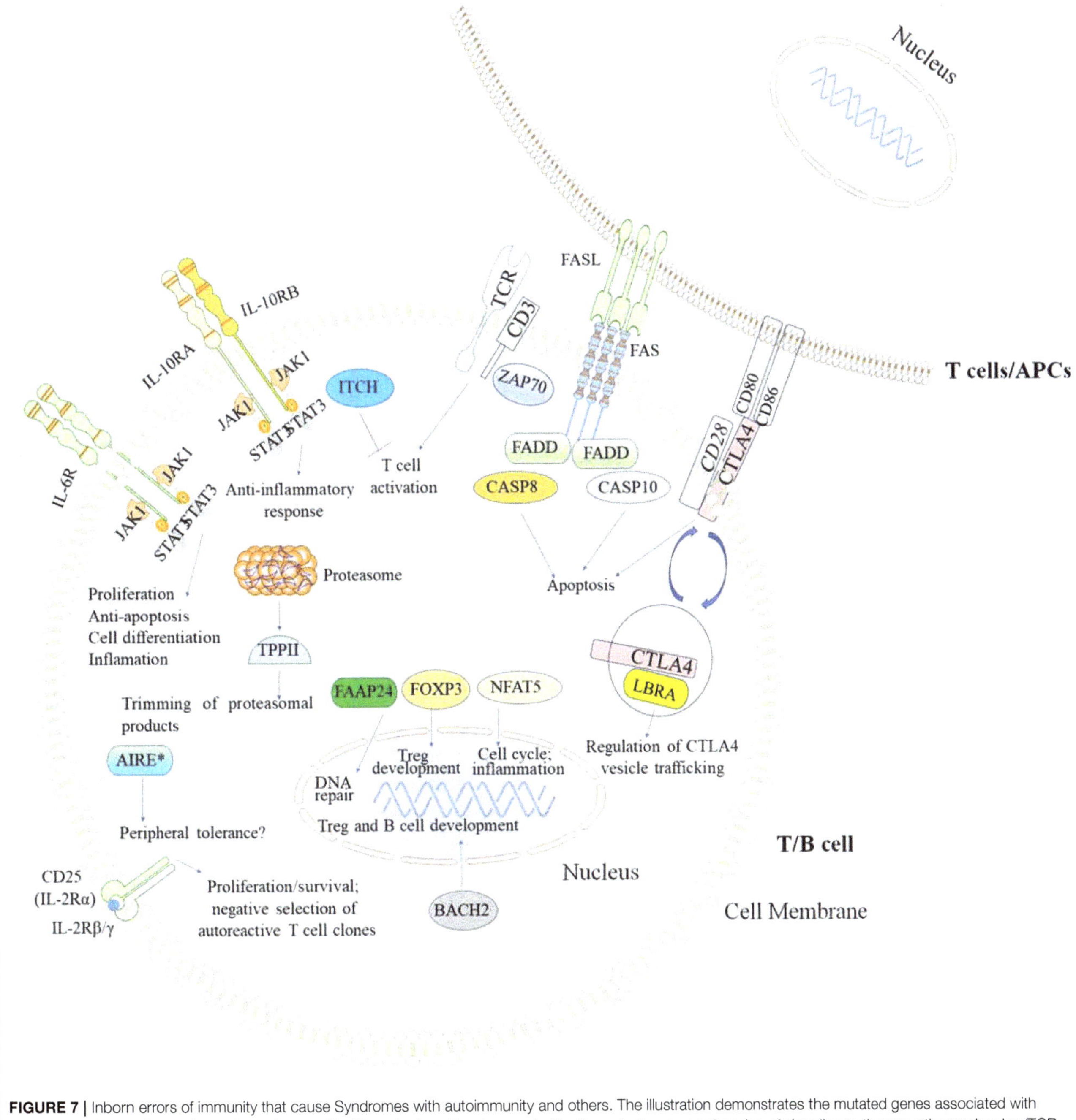

FIGURE 7 | Inborn errors of immunity that cause Syndromes with autoimmunity and others. The illustration demonstrates the mutated genes associated with syndromes with autoimmunity, and are shown with different colored backgrounds. To allow a better comprehension of signaling pathways, other molecules (TCR, CD3, CD28, CD80, and CD86) not associated with syndromes associated with autoimmunity are shown in white background. Nomenclature as designated by the 2017 IUIS phenotypic classification of PIDs (24). The illustration was constructed using Motifolio Drawing Toolkits (48).

receptor is the most frequent disease form of ALPS found in ~70% of genetically defined ALPS (177, 178) thereby making flow cytometry an essential screening tool for patients suspected to have ALPS.

STAT3 Gain-of-function Mutations

While heterozygous germline inactivating mutations in the signal transducer and activator of transcription 3 (STAT3) with dominant negative effect cause autosomal dominant hyper IgE syndrome (188), heterozygous gain-of-function (GOF) mutations in STAT3 result in an ALPS-like phenotype (81). Patients can develop early-onset poly-autoimmunity (e.g., type 1 diabetes), autoimmune hypothyroidism, enteropathy, pulmonary disease, cytopenias, arthritis, short stature, myelodysplastic syndrome, aplastic anemia, and lymphocytic leukemia (81, 189, 190). Increased percentages of TCRαβ^{+}-DN

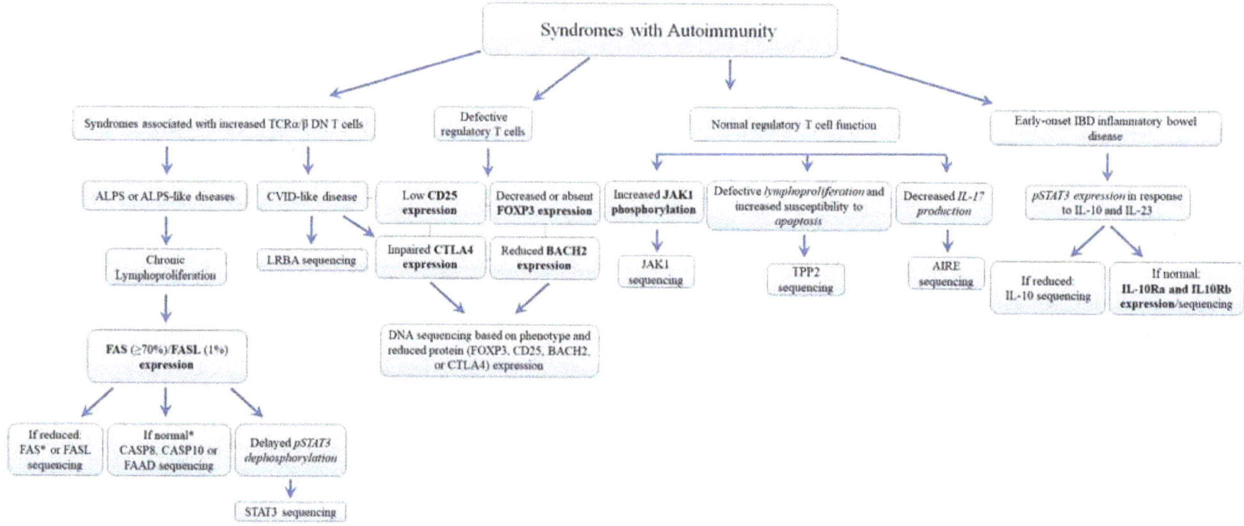

FIGURE 8 | Flowchart depicting the recommended immunophenotypic analysis used to define the molecular genetic defects of patients with immunodeficiency syndromes with Autoimmunity. In those cases with normal protein by flow cytometry, if there is a strong clinical indication for a specific immune dysregulation disease, it is recommended to perform gene sequencing to exclude missense mutations that do not impair protein expression. It is estimated that mutations in the FAS receptor are the most frequent pathology of ALPS (≅70% of genetically defined ALPS) (177, 178). However, the frequency of other immune dysregulation syndromes remains unknown. Bold and italic texts are disease-specific and non-disease specific flow cytometry tests, respectively.

T cells are occasionally identified (189). So far, STAT3 GOF mutations have been shown to enhance transcriptional activity and delay dephosphorylation of STAT3, without inducing constitutive phosphorylation as shown by flow cytometry studies. In agreement with the involvement of STAT3 in the inhibition of Tregs (191, 192) and enhancement of Th17 cell differentiation (193), flow cytometry has also shown increased Th17 levels while the FOXP3$^+$CD25$^+$ Treg population is reduced and the expression of CD25 (IL2RA) is decreased in patients with STAT3 GOF mutations (189). Due to its activity as a repressor of FAS-FASL activity, decreased FASL-induced apoptosis has been observed (190).

LRBA Deficiency

Mutations in the lipopolysaccharide responsive beige-like anchor protein (*LRBA*) gene cause a common variable immunodeficiency (CVID)-like disease with predominant antibody deficiency (hypogammaglobulinemia) and autoimmunity (e.g., autoimmune hemolytic anemia as well as atrophic gastritis with autoantibodies against intrinsic factor, autoimmune enteropathy, hypothyroidism, myasthenia gravis, polyarthritis), and inflammatory bowel disease (80, 194, 195). The phenotype of LRBA deficiency has been well-characterized elsewhere (196). LRBA is highly expressed in immune cells such as T and B cells (80). The application of flow cytometry to screen patients with LRBA deficiency has been recently developed (197) as well as its application to evaluate several immunopathological mechanisms of this disease. More than 70% of the LRBA-deficient patients have reduced levels of Tregs (196) (CD4$^+$CD25$^+$FOXP3$^+$), which may be related to the low surface expression of cytotoxic T lymphocyte–associated antigen 4 (CTLA4 or CD152) (198). CTLA4 is a cell surface molecule required for the proper suppressive function of Tregs (199–201). The reduced CTLA4 levels can be explained by the fact that LRBA is a regulator of CTLA4 vesicle trafficking [**Figure 5**; (197)]. Increased percentages of TCRα/β DN T cells have been found in up to 50% of LRBA-deficient patients (196). Several other defects associated with LRBA deficiency have been identified by flow cytometry (80). Among them are increased B cell apoptosis, low levels of IgG$^+$IgA$^+$CD27$^+$ switched-memory B cells, reduced B cell proliferation, and impaired activation (as measured by CD138 expression).

Defective Regulatory T Cells

The next two subgroups of Syndromes with Autoimmunity are based on the presence or absence of Treg defects (24). Tregs play a central role in peripheral immune tolerance, which controls the response of mature B and T cells that egressed from the primary lymphoid organs (202–204). Several autoimmune diseases have demonstrated the essential role of Tregs (202, 205), whose development is orchestrated by the transcription factor FOXP3.

Immune Dysregulation Due to Abnormal Tregs

IPEX

The immune dysregulation, polyendocrinopathy, enteropathy, X-linked syndrome (IPEX) is caused by loss of function mutations in the *FOXP3* gene (82). Clinical, immunological, and molecular features of IPEX syndrome have recently been characterized in a large cohort of patients (206). Flow cytometry of CD4$^+$FOXP3$^+$CD25$^+$ cells is well established to screen patients suspected to have IPEX who normally have low or absent nuclear FOXP3 expression in Tregs [**Figure 6**; (34)]. However, patients with missense mutations in *FOXP3* may present with normal protein expression and are not suitable for flow analysis. The identification of *FOXP3* mutations is essential to differentiate patients with IPEX from those with IPEX-like syndromes caused by mutations in other immune regulatory genes (e.g., *LRBA*, *CTLA4*, and CD25) (83, 206).

CD25 deficiency

Although CD25-deficient patients display normal percentage of $FOXP3^+$ cells, mutations in the *CD25* gene, which encodes the high-affinity subunit IL-2 receptor alpha chain (IL-12RA) of the tripartite receptor for IL-2 (83), causes an IPEX-like syndrome. This observation is explained by the fact that CD25, which can be detected by flow cytometry, is required for the production of the immunoregulatory cytokine IL-10 by Tregs (207). This suggests that CD25 is required for the function but not the survival of Tregs (207). $CD4^+$ lymphocytes are decreased in numbers, and the proliferative response following stimulation with anti-CD3, PHA, or other mitogens is diminished (208). In addition, CD25 deficiency decreases apoptosis in the thymus, impairing negative selection of autoreactive T cell clones, resulting in inflammation in multiple organs (208).

Flow cytometry has also defined a role of CD25 in NK cell maturation and function, as suggested by the accumulation of $CD56^{bright}CD16^{high}$ and reduced frequency of $CD56^{dim}CD16^{hi}$ NK cell in the peripheral blood as well as the expression of higher amounts of perforin and granzyme B. Increased degranulation (by increased CD107a expression) while reduced IFN-γ production by NK cells has also been reported (209).

CTLA4 deficiency

Mutations in the inhibitory receptor *CTLA4*, which acts to terminate the proliferation of activated T cells, have recently been recognized as a monogenic cause of CVID (210, 211). Therefore, for diagnostic assays of CTLA4, LRBA, and BACH2, defects in these molecules need to be evaluated in parallel (**Figure 7**; see section BACH2 Deficiency). CTLA4 is also constitutively expressed by Tregs and functions as a key checkpoint molecule for immune tolerance (211, 212). Details of CTLA4 biology and immunophenotyping of CTLA4 haploinsufficiency have recently been reviewed (213, 214). Briefly, CTLA4 competes effectively with CD28 because of higher affinity for binding to the costimulatory molecules CD80 and CD86, which are expressed on the surface of antigen-presenting cells (215). Patients with CTLA4 haploinsufficiency develop a T cell hyperproliferative syndrome resulting in lymphocytic infiltration of multiple organs (e.g., brain, gastrointestinal, and lung), autoimmune thrombocytopenia, hemolytic anemia, and other cytopenias, as well as hypogammaglobulinemia (84, 210), and increased susceptibility for cancer (216). Decreased CTLA4 expression can be demonstrated by flow cytometry. This tool is also useful to assess the effect of different mutations on CTLA4 function, which would normally require complex assays. For instance, flow cytometry can be used to demonstrate that CTLA4 loses its ability to interact with its natural ligands (CD80 and CD86), to traffic from the intracellular compartment to the cell membrane, and to inhibit T cell activation by physical removal of CD80/CD86 by CTLA4-mediated trans-endocytosis (211, 217, 218).

BACH2 deficiency

The gene encoding the BTB and CNC homology 1, basic leucine zipper transcription factor 2 (BACH2) is involved in the maturation of T and B lymphocytes. BACH2 is required for class switch recombination (CSR), somatic hypermutation (SHM) of immunoglobulin genes, and generation of regulatory T cells (219, 220). BACH2 haploinsufficiency has recently been associated with CVID and lymphocytic colitis. Low BACH2 protein expression in $CD4^+$, $CD8^+$ T and B lymphocytes can be demonstrated by flow cytometry, together with significantly decreased numbers of $Foxp3^+$ Treg cells, increased Th1 cells, reduced $CD19^+CD27^+$ memory, and low IgG class-switched $CD27^+IgG^+$ B cells (85).

Normal Treg Function

APECED

The discovery that mutations in the autoimmune regulator (*AIRE*) gene cause the autoimmune-polyendocrinopathy-candidiasis-ectodermal-dystrophy (APECED) syndrome (221) provided the novel concept that a monogenic defect can cause a systemic human autoimmune disease (86). The endocrinopathies presented by APECED patients are characterized by hypoparathyroidism, hypothyroidism, adrenal failure, gonadal failure, and autoimmune hepatitis. The ectodermal dystrophies comprise vitiligo, alopecia, keratopathy, and dystrophy of dental enamel, nails, and tympanic membranes (86, 222).

AIRE mediates central T cell tolerance by promoting the expression of thousands of tissue-specific self-antigens by medullary thymic epithelial cells (mTEC), leading to the deletion of T cells with strongly self-reactive TCR (223). Extrathymic AIRE expression has recently been reported in response to antigen and interleukin 2 stimulation in human peripheral blood cells such as $CD4^+$ T cells, suggesting a role of AIRE in mature lymphocytes (224). However, there is no flow cytometry assay available to analyze AIRE expression in peripheral blood lymphocytes. To explore the expression of AIRE in $CD4^+$ T cells to screen patients with APECED could improve the precise diagnosis of this disease, once the screening is currently based on the presence of the classical triad of CMC, hypoparathyroidism and adrenal insufficiency (Addison's disease) (225).

Tripeptidyl-peptidase II deficiency

Tripeptidyl peptidase II (TPPII) is a cytosolic peptidase that works downstream of proteasomes in cytosolic proteolysis by trimming proteasomal degradation products [**Figure 7**; (226)]. TPPII modulates several cellular processes, including antigen presentation by major histocompatibility complex (MHC) I molecules, T cell proliferation, and survival (87, 227). Among others, patients with TPPII deficiency develop autoimmune manifestations (e.g., immune hemolytic anemia, immune thrombocytopenia, and other cytopenias), and they are susceptible to viral infections such as CMV and severe chickenpox (87).

Although not used to assess TPPII expression in lymphocytes for establishing the diagnosis of TPPII deficiency, flow cytometry has been broadly employed to immunophenotypes and characterize lymphocyte function in affected patients. Lymphocytes from TPPII-deficient patients express higher levels of HLA class I molecules, present a skewed T-effector memory phenotype, and have a predominant $CD8^{+}CD27^{-}CD28^{-}CD127^{-}$ phenotype (87), which has been associated with enhanced effector functions and increased percentages of IFN-γ- and IL-17- positive T cells, as well as high levels of T-bet and perforin expression. Defective lymphoproliferation and increased susceptibility to apoptosis were also characterized by flow cytometry using Carboxyfluorescein succinimidyl ester (CFSE) and AV/PI. Furthermore, the patients showed increased levels of $CD21^{low}$ cells, an autoreactive B cell population often associated with CVID and autoimmune diseases. $CD21^{low}$ B cells are thought to have undergone activation and proliferation *in vivo* while exhibiting defective proliferation in response to B cell receptor stimulation (228, 229).

JAK1 gain-of function

The janus kinase 1 (JAK1) plays a central role in cytokine (e.g., interferon-α, IFN-γ, IL-6) signaling by phosphorylating STAT proteins (e.g., STAT1, STAT2, and STAT3). STAT proteins translocate to the nucleus and activate the transcription of many genes involved in immune responses (230). A family with a JAK1 germline GOF mutation that causes a systemic immune dysregulatory disease has recently been reported. Affected patients present with severe atopic dermatitis, profound eosinophilia, and autoimmune thyroid disease. A phospho-flow cytometry assay was able to demonstrate increased JAK1 and STAT1 phosphorylation at baseline and following IFN-α stimulation as well as enhanced IL-6-induced STAT3 phosphorylation (88).

Challenges to evaluating Treg function by flow cytometry

Due to their relevant pathophysiological role in the maintenance of immune homeostasis, we briefly reflect on the challenges associated with evaluating Treg number and function by flow cytometry. Distinct markers have been used to characterize human $CD4^{+}$ regulatory T cells since their first *ex-vivo* characterization in 2001 (231–233). The stable expression of the transcription factor FOXP3 represents one of the hallmarks of Tregs in both human and mice (234) and has been used to evaluate Tregs by flow cytometry, not only in PIDs with immune dysregulation but also other human diseases, including cancer (235) and diabetes (236). However, the functional characterization of human Tregs by flow cytometry still represents a challenge due to several factors; (I) FOXP3 can also be transiently expressed by activated $CD4^{+}$ T cells (237, 238); (II) FOXP3 evaluation requires the permeabilization of the nucleus membrane thereby impeding the possibility of FACS-sorting; (III) Circulating Tregs represent a very low frequency of the blood composition (representing 10% of the $CD4^{+}$ T cell compartment) and therefore a large number of PBMCs are required for adequate analysis. (IV) Classic Treg definition requires the *ex-vivo* evaluation of their suppressive capability.

Phenotypically, the evaluation of Tregs goes beyond the expression of FOXP3 in $CD4^{+}$ T cells, requiring the combination of distinct surface markers. In order to detect the high expression of the alpha chain of the IL-2 receptor (CD25) (232, 233), flow cytometric panels have shown that Treg cells exhibit low expression of both CD45RA (239) and IL-7 alpha receptor (CD127) (240, 241). Recent works have also shown that Tregs from tissues might express high levels of activation markers such as the coinhibitory receptor T cell Ig and ITIM domain (TIGIT) (242), the inducible T-cell co-stimulator (ICOS) (243), and the ectonucleotidase CD39 (244–246), which could be used for further *ex-vivo* isolation and characterization.

Another challenge for the laboratorial evaluation of Tregs consist of the low frequency of these cells in peripheral blood, which limits adequate functional assessment of these cells. To overcome this limitation, *in vitro* strategies for Treg expansion may include an initial cell enrichment step by selecting T cells, phenotypically characterized by $CD4^{+}CD25^{high}CD127^{low}$ expression, that will subsequently be subjected to cell culture in the presence of IL-2, rapamycin or TCR-stimulation (e.g., anti-CD3 or APCs) (247–249). These strategies may be considered to achieve the number of cells required for screening or classical suppression assays using cells from patients with PIDs and immune dysregulation. In this context, Tregs are co-cultured and proliferated with conventional $CD4^{+}$ T cells or $CD8^{+}$ T cells under polyclonal stimulation followed by assessing suppression of proliferation with fluorescent-labeling methods. The ratios of Tregs to target cells, duration of co-culture and readout need to be adapted to each set of assays, considering variation of donors, cell viability and the sensitivity of the suppression method (250).

Immune Dysregulation With Early Onset Colitis

IL-10, IL-10Ra, and IL-10Rb Deficiencies

Interleukin 10 (*IL-10*) is an important anti-inflammatory cytokine produced by cells like APCs. Early-onset (within the first months of life) of severe inflammatory bowel disease (EO-IBD), i.e., Crohn's disease and ulcerative colitis (UC), can be caused by IL-10 and IL10- receptor deficiencies (89, 90, 251). The expression of both IL-10 receptor alpha (IL-*10RA*) and IL-10 receptor beta (*IL10RB*) can be assessed by flow cytometry (90). Of note, IL-10 binds to its receptor, leading to the activation of the JAK1-STAT3 pathway [**Figure 9A**; (252)]. Normal or defective IL-10-induced phosphorylation of STAT3 in T cells has been evaluated by flow cytometry to distinguish patients with EO-IBD due to IL-10 or IL-10R deficiencies (**Figure 9B**). Recombinant IL-6 or IL-23 are used in parallel with IL-10 as stimuli to distinguish the specificity of IL-10 or IL10R deficiencies.

CONCLUSION AND FUTURE PERSPECTIVES

Since the identification of the specific mutation is the definitive approach for a specific molecular diagnosis, flow cytometry represents an extremely useful and versatile tool to effectively and rapidly evaluate patients with PIDs at relatively low costs (32–35). Of note, most of the other PIDs associated with immune

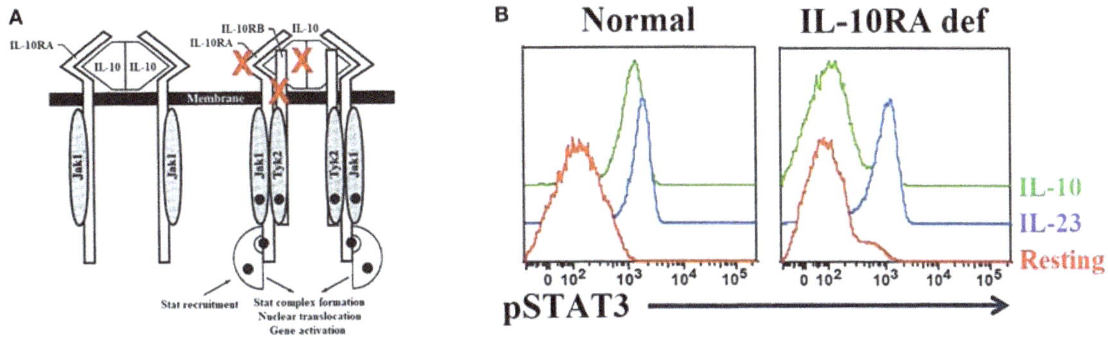

FIGURE 9 | IL-10 and IL-10 receptor deficiencies and the relevant role of flow cytometry analysis for precise diagnosis. **(A)** The interaction between IL-10 and its receptor (left side) as well as the downstream signaling events (right side) are exhibited. The red X highlights the IL-10 and IL-10 receptors (IL-10RA/B) that if mutated cause immune dysregulation with early onset colitis. **(B)** Flow cytometric histograms from a healthy control and an IL-10RA deficient patient, in resting or after IL-23 or IL-10 stimulation, illustrating the importance of flow cytometric application for functional assessment of inborn errors of immunity.

dysregulation (**Figure 3**) seem to be rare diseases. This current landscape is also influenced by the fact that, while some diseases have been described earlier (e.g., mutations in *FAS*, *FASL*, and *LYST*) (75, 184) and investigated in more detail, the molecular defects that cause most PIDs with immune dysregulation have only recently been discovered (**Figure 1**). However, we can confidently estimate that *PRF1 deficiency* accounts for 30–50%, and UNC13D deficiency for up to 20% of all FHL cases (34, 105, 108, 123), and mutations in the FAS receptor are the most frequent cause of ALPS [~70% of genetically defined ALPS (177, 178)]. The incidence of several other PIDs with immune dysregulation remains to be determined when additional patients are discovered. While more than 250 patients with Chediak-Higashi syndrome due to LYST deficiency were described 13 years ago (**?**), other PIDs we included in this review have been reported only in the last decade and we expect that only a small proportion of these patients have been discovered to date. The establishment of more laboratories capable of molecularly characterizing PIDs with immune dysregulation syndromes throughout the world, including developing countries, will be essential in advancing this new field of immunology. This will allow us to elucidate which defects are indeed rare or common.

Since these syndromes are rare, there is not a high request of specialized assays (e.g., FAS/FASL expression) when compared to other less specialized laboratory tests (e.g., complete blood count and quantitative immunoglobulins determination). Consequently, while the former assays are routinely only performed in PID research centers (often in state universities), which are supported by research grants, less specialized examinations are broadly available in most laboratories. We hope that improving the diagnoses of previously described and newly discovered PIDs with immune dysregulation will encourage governments and other funding sources to promote the establishment of new PID specialized laboratories in underserved geographic areas such as developing countries, where the true incidence of PIDs with immune dysregulation remains to be determined.

Finally, beyond its utility as a screening tool for patients with symptoms of immune dysregulation, flow cytometry has helped to characterize novel immunopathological mechanisms of several recently reported new PIDs. However, new flow cytometric technologies such as time-of-flight mass cytometry (CyTOF) (253) have not yet been applied for characterizing the immunopathology of immune dysregulation syndromes. Equally, flow cytometry is not currently applied in the context of systems immunology studies (254, 255) to better understand the immunopathology of diseases of immune dysregulation. For instance, traditional flow cytometry can be used to validate the findings obtained from combinatorial techniques such as CyTOF with high-throughput sequencing of mRNA (RNA-seq) or mass spectrometry, and uncovering systemic immunology defects (256, 257). Systems immunology will provide a more comprehensive understanding of the role of specific molecules across immune cells, potentially revealing novel therapeutic targets for patients with diseases of immune dysregulation.

AUTHOR CONTRIBUTIONS

OC-M: acquisition of data, wrote the manuscript, edited the manuscript, and proof reading. LS, NE, RR, and GS: wrote the manuscript. EO: figure configuration and wrote the manuscript. BA-R: wrote the manuscript, proof reading, and edited the manuscript. HO and AC-N: proof reading, wrote, and edited the manuscript.

ACKNOWLEDGMENTS

HO is supported by a grant of the Jeffrey Modell Foundation.

REFERENCES

1. Matzinger P. The danger model: a renewed sense of self. *Science.* (2002) 296:301–5. doi: 10.1126/science.1071059
2. Cabral-Marques O, Marques A, Giil LM, De Vito R, Rademacher J, Günther J, et al. GPCR-specific autoantibody signatures are associated with physiological and pathological immune homeostasis. *Nat Commun.* (2018) 9:5224. doi: 10.1038/s41467-018-07598-9
3. Kotas MEE, Medzhitov R. Homeostasis, inflammation, and disease susceptibility. *Cell.* (2015) 160:816–27. doi: 10.1016/j.cell.2015.02.010
4. Immunity in the tissues. *Nat Immunol.* (2013) 14:977. doi: 10.1038/ni.2722
5. Qu F, Guilak F, Mauck RL. Cell migration: implications for repair and regeneration in joint disease. *Nat Rev Rheumatol.* (2019) 15:167–79. doi: 10.1038/s41584-018-0151-0
6. Bednarski JJ, Sleckman BP. At the intersection of DNA damage and immune responses. *Nat Rev Immunol.* (2019) 19:231–42. doi: 10.1038/s41577-019-0135-6
7. Schmidt RE, Grimbacher B, Witte T. Autoimmunity and primary immunodeficiency: two sides of the same coin? *Nat Rev Rheumatol.* (2018) 14:7–18. doi: 10.1038/nrrheum.2017.198
8. Cabral-Marques O, Riemekasten G. Functional autoantibodies targeting G protein-coupled receptors in rheumatic diseases. *Nat Rev Rheumatol.* (2017) 13:648–56. doi: 10.1038/nrrheum.2017.134
9. Cabral-Marques O, Carvalho-Marques AH, Schimke LF, Heidecke H, Riemekasten G. Loss of balance in normal GPCR-mediated cell trafficking. *Front Biosci.* (2019) 24:18–34. doi: 10.2741/4707
10. Sánchez-Ramón S, Bermúdez A, González-Granado LI, Rodríguez-Gallego C, Sastre A, Soler-Palacín P, et al. Primary and Secondary Immunodeficiency Diseases in Oncohaematology: Warning Signs, Diagnosis, and Management. *Front Immunol.* (2019) 10:586.
11. Israel L, Wang Y, Bulek K, Della Mina E, Zhang Z, Pedergnana V, et al. Human adaptive immunity rescues an inborn error of innate immunity. *Cell.* (2017) 168:789–800.e10. doi: 10.1016/j.cell.2017.01.039
12. Meyts I, Bosch B, Bolze A, Boisson B, Itan Y, Belkadi A, et al. Exome and genome sequencing for inborn errors of immunity. *J Allergy Clin Immunol.* (2016) 138:957–69. doi: 10.1016/j.jaci.2016.08.003
13. Casanova J-L, Abel L. Genetic dissection of immunity to mycobacteria: the human model. *Annu Rev Immunol.* (2002) 20:581–620. doi: 10.1146/annurev.immunol.20.081501.125851
14. Casanova J-L. Human genetic basis of interindividual variability in the course of infection. *Proc Natl Acad Sci USA.* (2015) 112:201521644. doi: 10.1073/pnas.1521644112
15. Casanova J-L, Abel L. Inborn errors of immunity to infection: the rule rather than the exception. *J Exp Med.* (2005) 202:197–201. doi: 10.1084/jem.20050854
16. Casanova J-L. Severe infectious diseases of childhood as monogenic inborn errors of immunity. *Proc Natl Acad Sci USA.* (2015) 112:201521651. doi: 10.1073/pnas.1521651112
17. Casanova J-L, Abel L. Human genetics of infectious diseases: a unified theory. *EMBO J.* (2007) 26:915–22. doi: 10.1038/sj.emboj.7601558
18. Bruton OC. Agammaglobulinemia. *Pediatrics.* (1952) 9:722–8.
19. Notarangelo L, Casanova JL, Fischer A, Puck J, Rosen F, Seger R, Geha R. Primary immunodeficiency diseases: an update. *J Allergy Clin Immunol.* (2004) 114:677–87. doi: 10.1016/j.jaci.2004.06.044
20. Picard C, Al-Herz W, Bousfiha A, Casanova J-LL, Chatila T, Conley ME, et al. Primary immunodeficiency diseases: an update on the classification from the international union of immunological societies expert committee for primary immunodeficiency 2015. *J Clin Immunol.* (2015) 35:696–726. doi: 10.1007/s10875-015-0201-1
21. Chinen J, Notarangelo LD, Shearer WT, Turvey SE, Durandy A, Fischer A, et al. Advances in basic and clinical immunology in 2014. *J Allergy Clin Immunol.* (2015) 135:1132–41. doi: 10.1016/j.jaci.2015.02.037
22. Greil J, Rausch T, Giese T, Bandapalli OR, Daniel V, Bekeredjian-Ding I, et al. Whole-exome sequencing links caspase recruitment domain 11 (CARD11) inactivation to severe combined immunodeficiency. *J Allergy Clin Immunol.* (2013) 131:1376–83.e3. doi: 10.1016/j.jaci.2013.02.012
23. Itan Y, Casanova J-L. Novel primary immunodeficiency candidate genes predicted by the human gene connectome. *Front Immunol.* (2015) 6:142. doi: 10.3389/fimmu.2015.00142
24. Bousfiha A, Jeddane L, Picard C, Ailal F, Bobby Gaspar H, Al-Herz W, et al. The 2017 IUIS phenotypic classification for primary immunodeficiencies. *J Clin Immunol.* (2018) 38:129–43. doi: 10.1007/s10875-017-0465-8
25. Parvaneh N, Casanova J-L, Notarangelo LD, Conley ME. Primary immunodeficiencies: a rapidly evolving story. *J Allergy Clin Immunol.* (2013) 131:314–23. doi: 10.1016/j.jaci.2012.11.051
26. Tangye SG. Genetic cause of immune dysregulation one gene or two? *J Clin Invest.* (2016) 126:4065–7. doi: 10.1172/JCI90831
27. Alcaïs A, Quintana-Murci L, Thaler DS, Schurr E, Abel L, Casanova J-L. Life-threatening infectious diseases of childhood: single-gene inborn errors of immunity? *Ann NY Acad Sci.* (2010) 1214:18–33. doi: 10.1111/j.1749-6632.2010.05834.x
28. Meyts I, Casanova J-L. A human inborn error connects the α's. *Nat Immunol.* (2016) 17:472–4. doi: 10.1038/ni.3420
29. Torgerson TR. Genetic disorders of immune tolerance: the flip side of immune deficiency where autoimmunity trumps infection. *Blood.* (2017) 130.
30. *Free Online Timeline Maker.* Available online at: https://time.graphics/ (accessed August 13, 2019).
31. van der Burg M, Kalina T, Perez-Andres M, Vlkova M, Lopez-Granados E, Blanco E, et al. The EuroFlow PID orientation tube for flow cytometric diagnostic screening of primary immunodeficiencies of the lymphoid system. *Front Immunol.* (2019) 10:246. doi: 10.3389/fimmu.2019.00246
32. Oliveira JB, Notarangelo LD, Fleisher TA. Applications of flow cytometry for the study of primary immune deficiencies. *Curr Opin Allergy Clin Immunol.* (2008) 8:499–509. doi: 10.1097/ACI.0b013e328312c790
33. Abraham RS, Aubert G. Flow cytometry, a versatile tool for diagnosis and monitoring of primary immunodeficiencies. *Clin Vaccine Immunol.* (2016) 23:254–71. doi: 10.1128/CVI.00001-16
34. Kanegane H, Hoshino A, Okano T, Yasumi T, Wada T, Takada H, Okada S, et al. Flow cytometry-based diagnosis of primary immunodeficiency diseases. *Allergol Int.* (2018) 67:43–54. doi: 10.1016/j.alit.2017.06.003
35. Takashima T, Okamura M, Yeh T, Okano T, Yamashita M, Tanaka K, et al. Multicolor flow cytometry for the diagnosis of primary immunodeficiency diseases. *J Clin Immunol.* (2017) 37:486–95. doi: 10.1007/s10875-017-0405-7
36. Chiang SCC, Bleesing JJ, Marsh RA. Current flow cytometric assays for the screening and diagnosis of primary HLH. *Front Immunol.* (2019) 10:1740. doi: 10.3389/fimmu.2019.01740
37. Massaad MJ, Zhou J, Tsuchimoto D, Chou J, Jabara H, Janssen E, et al. Deficiency of base excision repair enzyme NEIL3 drives increased predisposition to autoimmunity. *J Clin Invest.* (2016) 126:4219–36. doi: 10.1172/JCI85647
38. Janssen E, Morbach H, Ullas S, Bannock JM, Massad C, Menard L, et al. Dedicator of cytokinesis 8–deficient patients have a breakdown in peripheral B-cell tolerance and defective regulatory T cells. *J Allergy Clin Immunol.* (2014) 134:1365–74. doi: 10.1016/j.jaci.2014.07.042
39. Issac JM, Mohamed YA, Bashir GH, Al-Sbiei A, Conca W, Khan TA, et al. Induction of hypergammaglobulinemia and autoantibodies by Salmonella infection in MyD88-deficient mice. *Front Immunol.* (2018) 9:1384. doi: 10.3389/fimmu.2018.01384
40. Romberg N, Al Moussawi K, Nelson-Williams C, Stiegler AL, Loring E, Choi M, et al. Mutation of NLRC4 causes a syndrome of enterocolitis and autoinflammation. *Nat Genet.* (2014) 46:1135–9. doi: 10.1038/ng.3066
41. Sauer AV, Morbach H, Brigida I, Ng Y-S, Aiuti A, Meffre E. Defective B cell tolerance in adenosine deaminase deficiency is corrected by gene therapy. *J Clin Invest.* (2012) 122:2141–52. doi: 10.1172/JCI61788
42. Ombrello MJ, Remmers EF, Sun G, Freeman AF, Datta S, Torabi-Parizi P, et al. Cold urticaria, immunodeficiency, and autoimmunity related to PLCG2 deletions. *N Engl J Med.* (2012) 366:330–8. doi: 10.1056/NEJMoa1102140
43. Isnardi I, Ng Y-S, Srdanovic I, Motaghedi R, Rudchenko S, von Bernuth H, et al. IRAK-4- and MyD88-dependent pathways are essential for the removal of developing autoreactive B cells in humans. *Immunity.* (2008) 29:746–57. doi: 10.1016/j.immuni.2008.09.015

44. Du Y, Yan L, Wang J, Zhan W, Song K, Han X, et al. β1-Adrenoceptor autoantibodies from DCM patients enhance the proliferation of T lymphocytes through the β1-AR/cAMP/PKA and p38 MAPK pathways. *PLoS ONE.* (2012) 7:e52911. doi: 10.1371/journal.pone.0052911
45. Cooper MD, Faulk WP, Fudenberg HH, Good RA, Hitzig W, Kunkel H, et al. Classification of primary immunodeficiencies. *N Engl J Med.* (1973) 288:966–7. doi: 10.1056/NEJM197305032881814
46. Primary Immunodeficiency Diseases Report of an IUIS Scientific Committee. *Clin Exp Immunol.* (1999) 118:1–28.
47. Montojo J, Zuberi K, Rodriguez H, Kazi F, Wright G, Donaldson SL, et al. GeneMANIA Cytoscape plugin: fast gene function predictions on the desktop. *Bioinformatics.* (2010) 26:2927–8. doi: 10.1093/bioinformatics/btq562
48. *Motifolio: Scientific illustration Toolkits for Presentations and Publications.* Available online at: www.motifolio.com
49. Bryceson YT, Pende D, Maul-Pavicic A, Gilmour KC, Ufheil H, Vraetz T, et al. A prospective evaluation of degranulation assays in the rapid diagnosis of familial hemophagocytic syndromes. *Blood.* (2012) 119:2754–63. doi: 10.1182/blood-2011-08-374199
50. Nagle DL, Karim MA, Woolf EA, Holmgren L, Bork P, Misumi DJ, et al. Identification and mutation analysis of the complete gene for Chediak–Higashi syndrome. *Nat Genet.* (1996) 14:307–11. doi: 10.1038/ng1196-307
51. Barbosa MDFS, Nguyen QA, Tchernev VT, Ashley JA, Detter JC, Blaydes SM, et al. Identification of the homologous beige and Chediak–Higashi syndrome genes. *Nature.* (1996) 382:262–5. doi: 10.1038/382262a0
52. Ménasché G, Pastural E, Feldmann J, Certain S, Ersoy F, Dupuis S, et al. Mutations in RAB27A cause Griscelli syndrome associated with haemophagocytic syndrome. *Nat Genet.* (2000) 25:173–6. doi: 10.1038/76024
53. Dell'Angelica EC, Shotelersuk V, Aguilar RC, Gahl WA, Bonifacino JS. Altered trafficking of lysosomal proteins in Hermansky-Pudlak syndrome due to mutations in the beta 3A subunit of the AP-3 adaptor. *Mol Cell.* (1999) 3:11–21. doi: 10.1016/S1097-2765(00)80170-7
54. Ammann S, Schulz A, Krageloh-Mann I, Dieckmann NMG, Niethammer K, Fuchs S, et al. Mutations in AP3D1 associated with immunodeficiency and seizures define a new type of Hermansky-Pudlak syndrome. *Blood.* (2016) 127:997–1006. doi: 10.1182/blood-2015-09-671636
55. Stepp SE, Dufourcq-Lagelouse R, Le Deist F, Bhawan S, Certain S, Mathew PA, et al. Perforin gene defects in familial hemophagocytic lymphohistiocytosis. *Science.* (1999) 286:1957–9. doi: 10.1126/science.286.5446.1957
56. Allen M, De Fusco C, Legrand F, Clementi R, Conter V, Danesino C, et al. Familial hemophagocytic lymphohistiocytosis: how late can the onset be? *Haematologica.* (2001) 86:499–503.
57. zur Stadt U, Schmidt S, Kasper B, Beutel K, Diler AS, Henter J-I, et al. Linkage of familial hemophagocytic lymphohistiocytosis (FHL) type-4 to chromosome 6q24 and identification of mutations in syntaxin 11. *Hum Mol Genet.* (2005) 14:827–34. doi: 10.1093/hmg/ddi076
58. Côte M, Ménager MM, Burgess A, Mahlaoui N, Picard C, Schaffner C, et al. Munc18-2 deficiency causes familial hemophagocytic lymphohistiocytosis type 5 and impairs cytotoxic granule exocytosis in patient NK cells. *J Clin Invest.* (2009) 119:3765–73. doi: 10.1172/JCI40732
59. Mao H, Yang W, Latour S, Yang J, Winter S, Zheng J, et al. RASGRP1 mutation in autoimmune lymphoproliferative syndrome-like disease. *J Allergy Clin Immunol.* (2018) 142:595–604.e16. doi: 10.1016/j.jaci.2017.10.026
60. Salzer E, Cagdas D, Hons M, Mace EM, Garncarz W, Petronczki ÖY, et al. RASGRP1 deficiency causes immunodeficiency with impaired cytoskeletal dynamics. *Nat Immunol.* (2016) 17:1352–60. doi: 10.1038/ni.3575
61. Winter S, Martin E, Boutboul D, Lenoir C, Boudjemaa S, Petit A, et al. Loss of RASGRP1 in humans impairs T-cell expansion leading to Epstein-Barr virus susceptibility. *EMBO Mol Med.* (2018) 10:188–99. doi: 10.15252/emmm.201708292
62. Platt CD, Fried AJ, Hoyos-Bachiloglu R, Usmani GN, Schmidt B, et al. Combined immunodeficiency with EBV positive B cell lymphoma and epidermodysplasia verruciformis due to a novel homozygous mutation in RASGRP1. *Clin Immunol.* (2017) 183:142–4. doi: 10.1016/j.clim.2017.08.007
63. Somekh I, Marquardt B, Liu Y, Rohlfs M, Hollizeck S, Karakukcu M, et al. Novel mutations in RASGRP1 are associated with immunodeficiency, immune dysregulation, and EBV-induced lymphoma. *J Clin Immunol.* (2018) 38:699–710. doi: 10.1007/s10875-018-0533-8
64. Izawa K, Martin E, Soudais C, Bruneau J, Boutboul D, Rodriguez R, et al. Inherited CD70 deficiency in humans reveals a critical role for the CD70-CD27 pathway in immunity to Epstein-Barr virus infection. *J Exp Med.* (2017) 214:73–89. doi: 10.1084/jem.20160784
65. Martin E, Palmic N, Sanquer S, Lenoir C, Hauck F, Mongellaz C, et al. CTP synthase 1 deficiency in humans reveals its central role in lymphocyte proliferation. *Nature.* (2014) 510:288–92. doi: 10.1038/nature13386
66. Wang Y, Ma CS, Ling Y, Bousfiha A, Camcioglu Y, Jacquot S, et al. Dual T cell- and B cell-intrinsic deficiency in humans with biallelic RLTPR mutations. *J Exp Med.* (2016) 213:2413–35. doi: 10.1084/jem.20160576
67. Linka RM, Risse SL, Bienemann K, Werner M, Linka Y, Krux F, et al. Loss-of-function mutations within the IL-2 inducible kinase ITK in patients with EBV-associated lymphoproliferative diseases. *Leukemia.* (2012) 26:963–71. doi: 10.1038/leu.2011.371
68. Li F-Y, Chaigne-Delalande B, Kanellopoulou C, Davis JC, Matthews HF, Douek DC, et al. Second messenger role for $Mg2^{+}$ revealed by human T-cell immunodeficiency. *Nature.* (2011) 475:471–6. doi: 10.1038/nature10246
69. Salzer E, Santos-Valente E, Klaver S, Ban SA, Emminger W, Prengemann NK, et al. B-cell deficiency and severe autoimmunity caused by deficiency of protein kinase C δ. *Blood.* (2013) 121:3112–6. doi: 10.1182/blood-2012-10-460741
70. Kuehn HS, Niemela JE, Rangel-Santos A, Zhang M, Pittaluga S, Stoddard JL, et al. Loss-of-function of the protein kinase C δ(PKCδ) causes a B-cell lymphoproliferative syndrome in humans. *Blood.* (2013) 121:3117–25. doi: 10.1182/blood-2012-12-469544
71. Belot A, Kasher PR, Trotter EW, Foray A-P, Debaud A-L, Rice GI, et al. Protein kinase cδ deficiency causes mendelian systemic lupus erythematosus with B cell-defective apoptosis and hyperproliferation. *Arthritis Rheum.* (2013) 65:2161–71. doi: 10.1002/art.38008
72. Coffey AJ, Brooksbank RA, Brandau O, Oohashi T, Howell GR, Bye JM, et al. Host response to EBV infection in X-linked lymphoproliferative disease results from mutations in an SH2-domain encoding gene. *Nat Genet.* (1998) 20:129–35. doi: 10.1038/2424
73. Rigaud S, Fondanèche M-C, Lambert N, Pasquier B, Mateo V, Soulas P, et al. XIAP deficiency in humans causes an X-linked lymphoproliferative syndrome. *Nature.* (2006) 444:110–4. doi: 10.1038/nature05257
74. van Montfrans JM, Hoepelman AIM, Otto S, van Gijn M, van de Corput L, de Weger RA, et al. CD27 deficiency is associated with combined immunodeficiency and persistent symptomatic EBV viremia. *J Allergy Clin Immunol.* (2012) 129:787–793.e6. doi: 10.1016/j.jaci.2011.11.013
75. Rieux-Laucat F, Le Deist F, Hivroz C, Roberts I, Debatin K, Fischer A, et al. Mutations in Fas associated with human lymphoproliferative syndrome and autoimmunity. *Science.* (1995) 268:1347–9. doi: 10.1126/science.7539157
76. Wu J, Wilson J, He J, Xiang L, Schur PH, Mountz JD. Fas ligand mutation in a patient with systemic lupus erythematosus and lymphoproliferative disease. *J Clin Invest.* (1996) 98:1107–13. doi: 10.1172/JCI118892
77. Chun HJ, Zheng L, Ahmad M, Wang J, Speirs CK, Siegel RM, et al. Pleiotropic defects in lymphocyte activation caused by caspase-8 mutations lead to human immunodeficiency. *Nature.* (2002) 419:395–9. doi: 10.1038/nature01063
78. Wang J, Zheng L, Lobito A, Chan FK-M, Dale J, Sneller M, et al. Inherited human caspase 10 mutations underlie defective lymphocyte and dendritic cell apoptosis in autoimmune lymphoproliferative syndrome type II. *Cell.* (1999) 98:47–58. doi: 10.1016/S0092-8674(00)80605-4
79. Bolze A, Byun M, McDonald D, Morgan NV, Abhyankar A, Premkumar L, et al. Whole-exome-sequencing-based discovery of human FADD deficiency. *Am J Hum Genet.* (2010) 87:873–81. doi: 10.1016/j.ajhg.2010.10.028
80. Lopez-Herrera G, Tampella G, Pan-Hammarström Q, Herholz P, Trujillo-Vargas CM, Phadwal K, et al. Deleterious mutations in LRBA are associated with a syndrome of immune deficiency and autoimmunity. *Am J Hum Genet.* (2012) 90:986–1001. doi: 10.1016/j.ajhg.2012.04.015
81. Flanagan SE, Haapaniemi E, Russell MA, Caswell R, Allen HL, De Franco E, et al. Activating germline mutations in STAT3 cause early-onset multi-organ autoimmune disease. *Nat Genet.* (2014) 46:812–4. doi: 10.1038/ng.3040

82. Bennett CL, Christie J, Ramsdell F, Brunkow ME, Ferguson PJ, Whitesell L, et al. The immune dysregulation, polyendocrinopathy, enteropathy, X-linked syndrome (IPEX) is caused by mutations of FOXP3. *Nat Genet.* (2001) 27:20–1. doi: 10.1038/83713
83. Sharfe N, Dadi HK, Shahar M, Roifman CM. Human immune disorder arising from mutation of the α chain of the interleukin-2 receptor. *Proc Natl Acad Sci USA.* (1997) 94:3168–71. doi: 10.1073/pnas.94.7.3168
84. Kuehn HS, Ouyang W, Lo B, Deenick EK, Niemela JE, Avery DT, et al. Immune dysregulation in human subjects with heterozygous germline mutations in CTLA4. *Science.* (2014) 345:1623–7. doi: 10.1126/science.1255904
85. Afzali B, Grönholm J, Vandrovcova J, O'Brien C, Sun H-W, Vanderleyden I, et al. BACH2 immunodeficiency illustrates an association between super-enhancers and haploinsufficiency. *Nat Immunol.* (2017) 18:813–23. doi: 10.1038/ni.3753
86. Aaltonen J, Björses P, Perheentupa J, Horelli-Kuitunen N, Palotie A, Peltonen L, et al. An autoimmune disease, APECED, caused by mutations in a novel gene featuring two PHD-type zinc-finger domains. *Nat Genet.* (1997) 17:399–403. doi: 10.1038/ng1297-399
87. Stepensky P, Rensing-Ehl A, Gather R, Revel-Vilk S, Fischer U, Nabhani S, et al. Early-onset Evans syndrome, immunodeficiency, and premature immunosenescence associated with tripeptidyl-peptidase II deficiency. *Blood.* (2015) 125:753–61. doi: 10.1182/blood-2014-08-593202
88. Del Bel KL, Ragotte RJ, Saferali A, Lee S, Vercauteren SM, Mostafavi SA, Schreiber RA, et al. JAK1 gain-of-function causes an autosomal dominant immune dysregulatory and hypereosinophilic syndrome. *J Allergy Clin Immunol.* (2017) 139:2016–20.e5. doi: 10.1016/j.jaci.2016.12.957
89. Glocker E-O, Kotlarz D, Klein C, Shah N, Grimbacher B. IL-10 and IL-10 receptor defects in humans. *Ann NY Acad Sci.* (2011) 1246:102–7. doi: 10.1111/j.1749-6632.2011.06339.x
90. Glocker E-O, Kotlarz D, Boztug K, Gertz EM, Schäffer AA, Noyan F, et al. Inflammatory bowel disease and mutations affecting the interleukin-10 receptor. *N Engl J Med.* (2009) 361:2033–45. doi: 10.1056/NEJMoa0907206
91. Collis SJ, Ciccia A, Deans AJ, Horejší Z, Martin JS, Maslen SL, et al. FANCM and FAAP24 function in ATR-mediated checkpoint signaling independently of the fanconi anemia core complex. *Mol Cell.* (2008) 32:313–24. doi: 10.1016/j.molcel.2008.10.014
92. Lohr NJ, Molleston JP, Strauss KA, Torres-Martinez W, Sherman EA, Squires RH, et al. Human ITCH E3 ubiquitin ligase deficiency causes syndromic multisystem autoimmune disease. *Am J Hum Genet.* (2010) 86:447–53. doi: 10.1016/j.ajhg.2010.01.028
93. Ciccia A, Ling C, Coulthard R, Yan Z, Xue Y, Meetei AR, et al. Identification of FAAP24, a fanconi anemia core complex protein that interacts with FANCM. *Mol Cell.* (2007) 25:331–43. doi: 10.1016/j.molcel.2007.01.003
94. Mueller DL. E3 ubiquitin ligases as T cell anergy factors. *Nat Immunol.* (2004) 5:883–90. doi: 10.1038/ni1106
95. Tanoue A, Endo F, Kitano A, Matsuda I. A single nucleotide change in the prolidase gene in fibroblasts from two patients with polypeptide positive prolidase deficiency. Expression of the mutant enzyme in NIH 3T3 cells. *J Clin Invest.* (1990) 86:351–5. doi: 10.1172/JCI114708
96. Shrinath M, Walter JH, Haeney M, Couriel JM, Lewis MA, Herrick AL. Prolidase deficiency and systemic lupus erythematosus. *Arch Dis Child.* (1997) 76:441–4. doi: 10.1136/adc.76.5.441
97. Chan AY, Punwani D, Kadlecek TA, Cowan MJ, Olson JL, Mathes EF, et al. A novel human autoimmune syndrome caused by combined hypomorphic and activating mutations in ZAP-70. *J Exp Med.* (2016) 213:155–65. doi: 10.1084/jem.20150888
98. Boland BS, Widjaja CE, Banno A, Zhang B, Kim SH, Stoven S, et al. Immunodeficiency and autoimmune enterocolopathy linked to NFAT5 haploinsufficiency. (2015) 194:2551–60. doi: 10.4049/jimmunol.1401463
99. Cady FM, Morice WG. Flow cytometric assessment of T-cell chronic lymphoproliferative disorders. *Clin Lab Med.* (2007) 27:513–32. doi: 10.1016/j.cll.2007.05.004
100. Maecker HT, Trotter J. Flow cytometry controls, instrument setup, and the determination of positivity. *Cytometry A.* (2006) 69:1037–42. doi: 10.1002/cyto.a.20333
101. Cossarizza A, Chang H-D, Radbruch A, Akdis M, Andrä I, Annunziato F, et al. Guidelines for the use of flow cytometry and cell sorting in immunological studies. *Eur J Immunol.* (2017) 47:1584–797. doi: 10.1002/eji.201646632
102. Richardson AM, Moyer AM, Hasadsri L, Abraham RS. Diagnostic tools for inborn errors of human immunity (primary immunodeficiencies and immune dysregulatory diseases). *Curr Allergy Asthma Rep.* (2018) 18:19. doi: 10.1007/s11882-018-0770-1
103. Kalina T, Lundsten K, Engel P. Relevance of antibody validation for flow cytometry. *Cytom Part A.* (2019). doi: 10.1002/cyto.a.23895. [Epub ahead of print].
104. Kalina T. Reproducibility of flow cytometry through standardization: opportunities and challenges. *Cytometry A.* (2019). doi: 10.1002/cyto.a.23901. [Epub ahead of print].
105. Murata Y, Yasumi T, Shirakawa R, Izawa K, Sakai H, Abe J, et al. Rapid diagnosis of FHL3 by flow cytometric detection of intraplatelet Munc13-4 protein. *Blood.* (2011) 118:1225–30. doi: 10.1182/blood-2011-01-329540
106. Kogawa K, Lee SM, Villanueva J, Marmer D, Sumegi J, Filipovich AH. Perforin expression in cytotoxic lymphocytes from patients with hemophagocytic lymphohistiocytosis and their family members. *Blood.* (2002) 99:61–6. doi: 10.1182/blood.V99.1.61
107. Sieni E, Cetica V, Hackmann Y, Coniglio ML, Da Ros M, Ciambotti B, et al. Familial hemophagocytic lymphohistiocytosis: when rare diseases shed light on immune system functioning. *Front Immunol.* (2014) 5:167. doi: 10.3389/fimmu.2014.00167
108. Voskoboinik I, Smyth MJ, Trapani JA. Perforin-mediated target-cell death and immune homeostasis. *Nat Rev Immunol.* (2006) 6:940–52. doi: 10.1038/nri1983
109. Lozano ML, Rivera J, Sánchez-Guiu I, Vicente V. Towards the targeted management of Chediak-Higashi syndrome. *Orphanet J Rare Dis.* (2014) 9:132. doi: 10.1186/s13023-014-0132-6
110. Griscelli C, Durandy A, Guy-Grand D, Daguillard F, Herzog C, Prunieras M. A syndrome associating partial albinism and immunodeficiency. *Am J Med.* (1978) 65:691–702. doi: 10.1016/0002-9343(78)90858-6
111. Jordan MB, Filipovich AH. Hematopoietic cell transplantation for hemophagocytic lymphohistiocytosis: a journey of a thousand miles begins with a single (big) step. *Bone Marrow Transplant.* (2008) 42:433–7. doi: 10.1038/bmt.2008.232
112. Cairo MS, Vandeven C, Toy C, Tischler D, Sender L. Fluorescent cytometric analysis of polymorphonuclear leukocytes in Chediak-Higashi Syndrome: diminished C3bi receptor expression (OKM1) with normal granular cell density. *Pediatr Res.* (1988) 24:673–6. doi: 10.1203/00006450-198812000-00004
113. Cetica V, Hackmann Y, Grieve S, Sieni E, Ciambotti B, Coniglio ML, et al. Patients with Griscelli syndrome and normal pigmentation identify RAB27A mutations that selectively disrupt MUNC13-4 binding. *J Allergy Clin Immunol.* (2015) 135:1310–8.e1. doi: 10.1016/j.jaci.2014.08.039
114. Marks MS, Seabra MC. The melanosome: membrane dynamics in black and white. *Nat Rev Mol Cell Biol.* (2001) 2:738–48. doi: 10.1038/35096009
115. Stinchcombe J, Bossi G, Griffiths GM. Linking albinism and immunity: the secrets of secretory lysosomes. *Science.* (2004) 305:55–9. doi: 10.1126/science.1095291
116. Kaplan J, De Domenico I, Ward DM. Chediak-Higashi syndrome. *Curr Opin Hematol.* (2008) 15:22–9. doi: 10.1097/MOH.0b013e3282f2bcce
117. Bryceson YT, March ME, Barber DF, Ljunggren H-G, Long EO. Cytolytic granule polarization and degranulation controlled by different receptors in resting NK cells. *J Exp Med.* (2005) 202:1001–12. doi: 10.1084/jem.20051143
118. Peters PJ, Borst J, Oorschot V, Fukuda M, Krähenbühl O, Tschopp J, et al. Cytotoxic T lymphocyte granules are secretory lysosomes, containing both perforin and granzymes. *J Exp Med.* (1991) 173:1099–109. doi: 10.1084/jem.173.5.1099
119. Betts MR, Brenchley JM, Price DA, De Rosa SC, Douek DC, Roederer M, et al. Sensitive and viable identification of antigen-specific CD8+ T cells by a flow cytometric assay for degranulation. *J Immunol Methods.* (2003) 281:65–78. doi: 10.1016/S0022-1759(03)00265-5
120. Alter G, Malenfant JM, Altfeld M. CD107a as a functional marker for the identification of natural killer cell activity. *J Immunol Methods.* (2004) 294:15–22. doi: 10.1016/j.jim.2004.08.008
121. Jessen B, Bode SFN, Ammann S, Chakravorty S, Davies G, Diestelhorst J, et al. The risk of hemophagocytic lymphohistiocytosis

in Hermansky-Pudlak syndrome type 2. *Blood.* (2013) 121:2943–51. doi: 10.1182/blood-2012-10-463166

122. Betts MR, Koup RA. Detection of T-cell degranulation: CD107a and b. *Methods Cell Biol.* (2004) 75:497–512. doi: 10.1016/S0091-679X(04)75020-7
123. Shibata H, Yasumi T, Shimodera S, Hiejima E, Izawa K, Kawai T, et al. Human CTL-based functional analysis shows the reliability of a munc13-4 protein expression assay for FHL3 diagnosis. *Blood.* (2018) 131:2016–25. doi: 10.1182/blood-2017-10-812503
124. Marcenaro S, Gallo F, Martini S, Santoro A, Griffiths GM, Aricó M, et al. Analysis of natural killer-cell function in familial hemophagocytic lymphohistiocytosis (FHL): defective CD107a surface expression heralds Munc13-4 defect and discriminates between genetic subtypes of the disease. *Blood.* (2006) 108:2316–23. doi: 10.1182/blood-2006-04-015693
125. Feldmann J, Callebaut I, Raposo G, Certain S, Bacq D, Dumont C, et al. Munc13-4 is essential for cytolytic granules fusion and is mutated in a form of familial hemophagocytic lymphohistiocytosis (FHL3). *Cell.* (2003) 115:461–73. doi: 10.1016/S0092-8674(03)00855-9
126. Daschkey S, Bienemann K, Schuster V, Kreth HW, Linka RM, Hönscheid A, et al. Fatal lymphoproliferative disease in two siblings lacking functional FAAP24. *J Clin Immunol.* (2016) 36:684–92. doi: 10.1007/s10875-016-0317-y
127. Ovadia A, Dalal I. Epstein–Barr virus infection in primary immunodeficiency. *LymphoSign J.* (2018) 5:65–85. doi: 10.14785/lymphosign-2018-0011
128. Worth AJJ, Houldcroft CJ, Booth C. Severe Epstein-Barr virus infection in primary immunodeficiency and the normal host. *Br J Haematol.* (2016) 175:559–76. doi: 10.1111/bjh.14339
129. Tangye SG, Palendira U, Edwards ESJ. Human immunity against EBV—lessons from the clinic. *J Exp Med.* (2017) 214:269–83. doi: 10.1084/jem.20161846
130. Taylor GS, Long HM, Brooks JM, Rickinson AB, Hislop AD. The immunology of Epstein-Barr virus-induced disease. *Annu Rev Immunol.* (2015) 33:787–821. doi: 10.1146/annurev-immunol-032414-112326
131. Trück J, Kelly DF, Taylor JM, Kienzler AK, Lester T, Seller A, et al. Variable phenotype and discrete alterations of immune phenotypes in CTP synthase 1 deficiency: report of 2 siblings. *J Allergy Clin Immunol.* (2016) 138:1722–5.e6. doi: 10.1016/j.jaci.2016.04.059
132. Serwas NK, Cagdas D, Ban SA, Bienemann K, Salzer E, Tezcan I, et al. Identification of ITK deficiency as a novel genetic cause of idiopathic CD4+ T-cell lymphopenia. *Blood.* (2014) 124:655–7. doi: 10.1182/blood-2014-03-564930
133. Nichols KE, Harkin DP, Levitz S, Krainer M, Kolquist KA, Genovese C, et al. Inactivating mutations in an SH2 domain-encoding gene in X-linked lymphoproliferative syndrome. *Proc Natl Acad Sci USA.* (1998) 95:13765–70. doi: 10.1073/pnas.95.23.13765
134. Alkhairy OK, Perez-Becker R, Driessen GJ, Abolhassani H, van Montfrans J, Borte S, et al. Novel mutations in TNFRSF7/CD27: clinical, immunologic, and genetic characterization of human CD27 deficiency. *J Allergy Clin Immunol.* (2015) 136:703–712.e10. doi: 10.1016/j.jaci.2015.02.022
135. França TT, Barreiros LA, al-Ramadi BK, Ochs HD, Cabral-Marques O, Condino-Neto A. CD40 ligand deficiency: treatment strategies and novel therapeutic perspectives. *Expert Rev Clin Immunol.* (2019) 15:529–40. doi: 10.1080/1744666X.2019.1573674
136. Cabral-Marques O, França TT, Al-Sbiei A, Schimke LF, Khan TA, Feriotti C, et al. CD40 ligand deficiency causes functional defects of peripheral neutrophils that are improved by exogenous IFN-γ. *J Allergy Clin Immunol.* (2018) 142:1571–88. doi: 10.1016/j.jaci.2018.02.026
137. Fischer A. Recent advances in understanding the pathophysiology of primary T cell immunodeficiencies. *Trends Mol Med.* (2015) 21:408–16. doi: 10.1016/j.molmed.2015.04.002
138. Grommé M, Uytdehaag FG, Janssen H, Calafat J, van Binnendijk RS, Kenter MJ, et al. Recycling MHC class I molecules and endosomal peptide loading. *Proc Natl Acad Sci USA.* (1999) 96:10326–31. doi: 10.1073/pnas.96.18.10326
139. Kobata T, Jacquot S, Kozlowski S, Agematsu K, Schlossman SF, Morimoto C. CD27-CD70 interactions regulate B-cell activation by T cells. *Proc Natl Acad Sci USA.* (1995) 92:11249–53. doi: 10.1073/pnas.92.24.11249
140. Keller AM, Groothuis TA, Veraar EAM, Marsman M, de Buy Wenniger LM, Janssen H, et al. Costimulatory ligand CD70 is delivered to the immunological synapse by shared intracellular trafficking with MHC class II molecules. *Proc Natl Acad Sci USA.* (2007) 104:5989–94. doi: 10.1073/pnas.0700946104
141. Munitic I, Kuka M, Allam A, Scoville JP, Ashwell JD. CD70 deficiency impairs effector CD8 T cell generation and viral clearance but is dispensable for the recall response to lymphocytic choriomeningitis virus. *J Immunol.* (2013) 190:1169–79. doi: 10.4049/jimmunol.1202353
142. Abolhassani H, Edwards ESJ, Ikinciogullari A, Jing H, Borte S, Buggert M, et al. Combined immunodeficiency and Epstein-Barr virus-induced B cell malignancy in humans with inherited CD70 deficiency. *J Exp Med.* (2017) 214:91–106. doi: 10.1084/jem.20160849
143. Salzer E, Daschkey S, Choo S, Gombert M, Santos-Valente E, Ginzel S, et al. Combined immunodeficiency with life-threatening EBV-associated lymphoproliferative disorder in patients lacking functional CD27. *Haematologica.* (2013) 98:473–8. doi: 10.3324/haematol.2012.068791
144. Seyama K, Nonoyama S, Gangsaas I, Hollenbaugh D, Pabst HF, Aruffo A, et al. Mutations of the CD40 ligand gene and its effect on CD40 ligand expression in patients with X-linked hyper IgM syndrome. *Blood.* (1998) 92:2421–34. doi: 10.1182/blood.V92.7.2421
145. Cabral-Marques O, Klaver S, Schimke LF, Ascendino EH, Khan TA, Pereira PVS, et al. First report of the hyper-IgM syndrome registry of the latin american society for immunodeficiencies: novel mutations, unique infections, and outcomes. *J Clin Immunol.* (2014) 34:146–56. doi: 10.1007/s10875-013-9980-4
146. Roncagalli R, Cucchetti M, Jarmuzynski N, Grégoire C, Bergot E, Audebert S, et al. The scaffolding function of the RLTPR protein explains its essential role for CD28 co-stimulation in mouse and human T cells. *J Exp Med.* (2016) 213:2437–57. doi: 10.1084/jem.20160579
147. Schober T, Magg T, Laschinger M, Fröhlich T, Rohlfs M, Liu Y, Puchalka J, et al. Rltpr is a central scaffold protein regulating human TCR co-signaling and cytoskeletal dynamics. *Blood.* (2016) 128:131. doi: 10.1182/blood.V128.22.131.131
148. Alazami AM, Al-Helale M, Alhissi S, Al-Saud B, Alajlan H, Monies D, et al. Novel CARMIL2 mutations in patients with variable clinical dermatitis, infections, and combined immunodeficiency. *Front Immunol.* (2018) 9:203. doi: 10.3389/fimmu.2018.00203
149. Schimke LF, Rieber N, Rylaarsdam S, Cabral-Marques O, Hubbard N, Puel A, et al. A novel gain-of-function IKBA mutation underlies ectodermal dysplasia with immunodeficiency and polyendocrinopathy. *J Clin Immunol.* (2013) 33:1088–99. doi: 10.1007/s10875-013-9906-1
150. Khan TA, Schimke LF, Amaral EP, Ishfaq M, Barbosa Bonfim CC, Rahman H, et al. Interferon-gamma reduces the proliferation of M. tuberculosis within macrophages from a patient with a novel hypomorphic NEMO mutation. *Pediatr Blood Cancer.* (2016) 63:1863–6. doi: 10.1002/pbc.26098
151. Schober T, Magg T, Laschinger M, Rohlfs M, Linhares ND, Puchalka J, et al. A human immunodeficiency syndrome caused by mutations in CARMIL2. *Nat Commun.* (2017) 8:14209. doi: 10.1038/ncomms14209
152. van den Berg AA, van Lenthe H, Kipp JB, de Korte D, van Kuilenburg AB, van Gennip AH. Cytidine triphosphate (CTP) synthetase activity during cell cycle progression in normal and malignant T-lymphocytic cells. *Eur J Cancer.* (1995) 31A:108–12. doi: 10.1016/0959-8049(94)00442-8
153. Proteintech. *CTP Synthase Antibody.* Available online at: https://www.ptglab.com/Products/CTPS-Antibody-15914-1-AP.htm (accessed June 14, 2019).
154. Atherly LO, Lucas JA, Felices M, Yin CC, Reiner SL, Berg LJ. The Tec family tyrosine kinases Itk and Rlk regulate the development of conventional CD8+ T cells. *Immunity.* (2006) 25:79–91. doi: 10.1016/j.immuni.2006.05.012
155. Ghosh S, Drexler I, Bhatia S, Adler H, Gennery AR, Borkhardt A. Interleukin-2-inducible T-cell kinase deficiency-new patients, new insight? *Front Immunol.* (2018) 9:979. doi: 10.3389/fimmu.2018.00979
156. Huck K, Feyen O, Niehues T, Rüschendorf F, Hübner N, Laws H-J, et al. Girls homozygous for an IL-2-inducible T cell kinase mutation that leads to protein deficiency develop fatal EBV-associated lymphoproliferation. *J Clin Invest.* (2009) 119:1350–8. doi: 10.1172/JCI37901
157. Yang W, Lee JY, Nowotny M. Making and breaking nucleic acids: two-$Mg2^{+}$-ion catalysis and substrate specificity. *Mol Cell.* (2006) 22:5–13. doi: 10.1016/j.molcel.2006.03.013
158. Cowan JA. Structural and catalytic chemistry of magnesium-dependent enzymes. *Biometals.* (2002) 15:225–35. doi: 10.1023/A:1016022730880

159. Junge S, Kloeckener-Gruissem B, Zufferey R, Keisker A, Salgo B, Fauchere J-C, et al. Correlation between recent thymic emigrants and CD31+ (PECAM-1) CD4+ T cells in normal individuals during aging and in lymphopenic children. *Eur J Immunol.* (2007) 37:3270–80. doi: 10.1002/eji.200636976
160. Douek DC, McFarland RD, Keiser PH, Gage EA, Massey JM, Haynes BF, et al. Changes in thymic function with age and during the treatment of HIV infection. *Nature.* (1998) 396:690–5. doi: 10.1038/25374
161. Kohler S, Wagner U, Pierer M, Kimmig S, Oppmann B, Möwes B, et al. Post-thymic *in vivo* proliferation of naive CD4+ T cells constrains the TCR repertoire in healthy human adults. *Eur J Immunol.* (2005) 35:1987–94. doi: 10.1002/eji.200526181
162. Chaigne-Delalande B, Li F-Y, O'Connor GM, Lukacs MJ, Jiang P, Zheng L, et al. $Mg2^{+}$ regulates cytotoxic functions of NK and CD8 T cells in chronic EBV infection through NKG2D. *Science.* (2013) 341:186–91. doi: 10.1126/science.1240094
163. Lei L, Muhammad S, Al-Obaidi M, Sebire N, Cheng IL, Eleftheriou D, et al. Successful use of ofatumumab in two cases of early-onset juvenile SLE with thrombocytopenia caused by a mutation in protein kinase C δ. *Pediatr Rheumatol.* (2018) 16:61. doi: 10.1186/s12969-018-0278-1
164. Altman A, Kong K-F. Protein kinase C enzymes in the hematopoietic and immune systems. *Annu Rev Immunol.* (2016) 34:511–38. doi: 10.1146/annurev-immunol-041015-055347
165. Spitaler M, Cantrell DA. Protein kinase C and beyond. *Nat Immunol.* (2004) 5:785–90. doi: 10.1038/ni1097
166. Mecklenbräuker I, Saijo K, Zheng N-Y, Leitges M, Tarakhovsky A. Protein kinase Cδ controls self-antigen-induced B-cell tolerance. *Nature.* (2002) 416:860–5. doi: 10.1038/416860a
167. Miyamoto A, Nakayama K, Imaki H, Hirose S, Jiang Y, Abe M, et al. Increased proliferation of B cells and auto-immunity in mice lacking protein kinase Cδ. *Nature.* (2002) 416:865–9. doi: 10.1038/416865a
168. Salzer E, Santos-Valente E, Keller B, Warnatz K, Boztug K. Protein kinase C δ: a gatekeeper of immune homeostasis. *J Clin Immunol.* (2016) 36:631–40. doi: 10.1007/s10875-016-0323-0
169. Booth C, Gilmour KC, Veys P, Gennery AR, Slatter MA, Chapel H, et al. X-linked lymphoproliferative disease due to SAP/SH2D1A deficiency: a multicenter study on the manifestations, management and outcome of the disease. *Blood.* (2011) 117:53–62. doi: 10.1182/blood-2010-06-284935
170. Nagy N, Matskova L, Kis LL, Hellman U, Klein G, Klein E. The proapoptotic function of SAP provides a clue to the clinical picture of X-linked lymphoproliferative disease. *Proc Natl Acad Sci USA.* (2009) 106:11966–71. doi: 10.1073/pnas.0905691106
171. Nagy N, Matskova L, Hellman U, Klein G, Klein E. The apoptosis modulating role of SAP (SLAM associated protein) contributes to the symptomatology of the X linked lymphoproliferative disease. *Cell Cycle.* (2009) 8:3086–90. doi: 10.4161/cc.8.19.9636
172. Pachlopnik Schmid J, Canioni D, Moshous D, Touzot F, Mahlaoui N, Hauck F, et al. Clinical similarities and differences of patients with X-linked lymphoproliferative syndrome type 1 (XLP-1/SAP deficiency) versus type 2 (XLP-2/XIAP deficiency). *Blood.* (2011) 117:1522–9. doi: 10.1182/blood-2010-07-298372
173. Ma CS, Hare NJ, Nichols KE, Dupré L, Andolfi G, Roncarolo M-G, et al. Impaired humoral immunity in X-linked lymphoproliferative disease is associated with defective IL-10 production by CD4+ T cells. *J Clin Invest.* (2005) 115:1049–59. doi: 10.1172/JCI200523139
174. Salvesen GS, Duckett CS. IAP proteins: blocking the road to death's door. *Nat Rev Mol Cell Biol.* (2002) 3:401–10. doi: 10.1038/nrm830
175. Ma CS, Nichols KE, Tangye SG. Regulation of cellular and humoral immune responses by the SLAM and SAP families of molecules. *Annu Rev Immunol.* (2007) 25:337–79. doi: 10.1146/annurev.immunol.25.022106.141651
176. Nichols KE, Ma CS, Cannons JL, Schwartzberg PL, Tangye SG. Molecular and cellular pathogenesis of X-linked lymphoproliferative disease. *Immunol Rev.* (2005) 203:180–99. doi: 10.1111/j.0105-2896.2005.00230.x
177. Oliveira JB, Bleesing JJ, Dianzani U, Fleisher TA, Jaffe ES, Lenardo MJ, et al. Revised diagnostic criteria and classification for the autoimmune lymphoproliferative syndrome (ALPS): report from the 2009 NIH International Workshop. *Blood.* (2010) 116:e35–40. doi: 10.1182/blood-2010-04-280347
178. Bride K, Teachey D. Autoimmune lymphoproliferative syndrome: more than a FAScinating disease. *F1000Research.* (2017) 6:1928. doi: 10.12688/f1000research.11545.1
179. Tarbox JA, Keppel MP, Topcagic N, Mackin C, Ben Abdallah M, Baszis KW, et al. Elevated double negative T cells in pediatric autoimmunity. *J Clin Immunol.* (2014) 34:594–9. doi: 10.1007/s10875-014-0038-z
180. Hillhouse EE, Lesage S. A comprehensive review of the phenotype and function of antigen-specific immunoregulatory double negative T cells. *J Autoimmun.* (2013) 40:58–65. doi: 10.1016/j.jaut.2012.07.010
181. Alderson MR, Tough TW, Davis-Smith T, Braddy S, Falk B, Schooley KA, et al. Fas ligand mediates activation-induced cell death in human T lymphocytes. *J Exp Med.* (1995) 181:71–7. doi: 10.1084/jem.181.1.71
182. Dhein J, Walczak H, Bäumler C, Debatin K-M, Krammer PH. Autocrine T-cell suicide mediated by APO-1/(Fas/CD95). *Nature.* (1995) 373:438–41. doi: 10.1038/373438a0
183. Krueger A, Fas SC, Baumann S, Krammer PH. The role of CD95 in the regulation of peripheral T-cell apoptosis. *Immunol Rev.* (2003) 193:58–69. doi: 10.1034/j.1600-065X.2003.00047.x
184. Le Deist F, Emile J-F, Rieux-Laucat F, Benkerrou M, Roberts I, Brousse N, et al. Clinical, immunological, and pathological consequences of Fas-deficient conditions. *Lancet.* (1996) 348:719–23. doi: 10.1016/S0140-6736(96)02293-3
185. Lo B, Ramaswamy M, Davis J, Price S, Rao VK, Siegel RM, et al. A rapid *ex vivo* clinical diagnostic assay for fas receptor-induced T lymphocyte apoptosis. *J Clin Immunol.* (2013) 33:479–88. doi: 10.1007/s10875-012-9811-z
186. Nabhani S, Ginzel S, Miskin H, Revel-Vilk S, Harlev D, Fleckenstein B, et al. Deregulation of Fas ligand expression as a novel cause of autoimmune lymphoproliferative syndrome-like disease. *Haematologica.* (2015) 100:1189–98. doi: 10.3324/haematol.2014.114967
187. Kuehn HS, Caminha I, Niemela JE, Rao VK, Davis J, Fleisher TA, et al. FAS haploinsufficiency is a common disease mechanism in the human autoimmune lymphoproliferative syndrome. *J Immunol.* (2011) 186:6035–43. doi: 10.4049/jimmunol.1100021
188. Holland SM, DeLeo FR, Elloumi HZ, Hsu AP, Uzel G, Brodsky N, et al. STAT3 mutations in the Hyper-IgE syndrome. *N Engl J Med.* (2007) 357:1608–19. doi: 10.1056/NEJMoa073687
189. Milner JD, Vogel TP, Forbes L, Ma CA, Stray-Pedersen A, Niemela JE, et al. Early-onset lymphoproliferation and autoimmunity caused by germline STAT3 gain-of-function mutations. *Blood.* (2015) 125:591–9. doi: 10.1182/blood-2014-09-602763
190. Nabhani S, Schipp C, Miskin H, Levin C, Postovsky S, Dujovny T, et al. STAT3 gain-of-function mutations associated with autoimmune lymphoproliferative syndrome like disease deregulate lymphocyte apoptosis and can be targeted by BH3 mimetic compounds. *Clin Immunol.* (2017) 181:32–42. doi: 10.1016/j.clim.2017.05.021
191. Laurence A, Amarnath S, Mariotti J, Kim YC, Foley J, Eckhaus M, et al. STAT3 transcription factor promotes instability of nTreg cells and limits generation of iTreg cells during acute murine graft-versus-host disease. *Immunity.* (2012) 37:209–22. doi: 10.1016/j.immuni.2012.05.027
192. Huber M, Steinwald V, Guralnik A, Brustle A, Kleemann P, Rosenplanter C, et al. IL-27 inhibits the development of regulatory T cells via STAT3. *Int Immunol.* (2008) 20:223–34. doi: 10.1093/intimm/dxm139
193. Milner JD, Brenchley JM, Laurence A, Freeman AF, Hill BJ, Elias KM, et al. Impaired TH17 cell differentiation in subjects with autosomal dominant hyper-IgE syndrome. *Nature.* (2008) 452:773–6. doi: 10.1038/nature06764
194. Soler-Palacín P, Garcia-Prat M, Martín-Nalda A, Franco-Jarava C, Rivière JG, Plaja A, et al. LRBA deficiency in a patient with a novel homozygous mutation due to chromosome 4 segmental uniparental isodisomy. *Front Immunol.* (2018) 9:2397. doi: 10.3389/fimmu.2018.02397
195. Lévy E, Stolzenberg M-C, Bruneau J, Breton S, Neven B, Sauvion S, et al. LRBA deficiency with autoimmunity and early onset chronic erosive polyarthritis. *Clin Immunol.* (2016) 168:88–93. doi: 10.1016/j.clim.2016.03.006
196. Gámez-Díaz L, August D, Stepensky P, Revel-Vilk S, Seidel MG, Noriko M, et al. The extended phenotype of LPS-responsive beige-like anchor

protein (LRBA) deficiency. *J Allergy Clin Immunol.* (2016) 137:223–30. doi: 10.1016/j.jaci.2015.09.025

197. Lo B, Zhang K, Lu W, Zheng L, Zhang Q, Kanellopoulou C, et al. Patients with LRBA deficiency show CTLA4 loss and immune dysregulation responsive to abatacept therapy. *Science.* (2015) 349:436–40. doi: 10.1126/science.aaa1663
198. Charbonnier L-M, Janssen E, Chou J, Ohsumi TK, Keles S, Hsu JT, Massaad MJ, et al. Regulatory T-cell deficiency and immune dysregulation, polyendocrinopathy, enteropathy, X-linked-like disorder caused by loss-of-function mutations in LRBA. *J Allergy Clin Immunol.* (2015) 135:217–227.e9. doi: 10.1016/j.jaci.2014.10.019
199. Sebastian M, Lopez-Ocasio M, Metidji A, Rieder SA, Shevach EM, Thornton AM. Helios controls a limited subset of regulatory T cell functions. *J Immunol.* (2016) 196:144–55. doi: 10.4049/jimmunol.1501704
200. Thornton AM, Korty PE, Tran DQ, Wohlfert EA, Murray PE, Belkaid Y, et al. Expression of Helios, an Ikaros transcription factor family member, differentiates thymic-derived from peripherally induced Foxp3 + T regulatory cells. *J Immunol.* (2010) 184:3433–41. doi: 10.4049/jimmunol.0904028
201. Jain N, Nguyen H, Chambers C, Kang J. Dual function of CTLA-4 in regulatory T cells and conventional T cells to prevent multiorgan autoimmunity. *Proc Natl Acad Sci USA.* (2010) 107:1524–8. doi: 10.1073/pnas.0910341107
202. Montgomery RA, Tatapudi VS, Leffell MS, Zachary AA. HLA in transplantation. *Nat Rev Nephrol.* (2018) 14:558–70. doi: 10.1038/s41581-018-0039-x
203. Serra P, Santamaria P. Antigen-specific therapeutic approaches for autoimmunity. *Nat Biotechnol.* (2019) 37:238–51. doi: 10.1038/s41587-019-0015-4
204. Anderson MS, Su MA. AIRE expands: new roles in immune tolerance and beyond. *Nat Rev Immunol.* (2016) 16:247–58. doi: 10.1038/nri.2016.9
205. Charbonnier L-M, Wang S, Georgiev P, Sefik E, Chatila TA. Control of peripheral tolerance by regulatory T cell–intrinsic Notch signaling. *Nat Immunol.* (2015) 16:1162–73. doi: 10.1038/ni.3288
206. Gambineri E, Ciullini Mannurita S, Hagin D, Vignoli M, Anover-Sombke S, DeBoer S, et al. Clinical, immunological, and molecular heterogeneity of 173 patients with the phenotype of immune dysregulation, polyendocrinopathy, enteropathy, x-linked (IPEX) syndrome. *Front Immunol.* (2018) 9:2411. doi: 10.3389/fimmu.2018.02411
207. Caudy AA, Reddy ST, Chatila T, Atkinson JP, Verbsky JW. CD25 deficiency causes an immune dysregulation, polyendocrinopathy, enteropathy, X-linked–like syndrome, and defective IL-10 expression from CD4 lymphocytes. *J Allergy Clin Immunol.* (2007) 119:482–7. doi: 10.1016/j.jaci.2006.10.007
208. Roifman CM. Human IL-2 receptor α chain deficiency. *Pediatr Res.* (2000) 48:6–11. doi: 10.1203/00006450-200007000-00004
209. Caldirola MS, Rodríguez Broggi MG, Gaillard MI, Bezrodnik L, Zwirner NW. Primary immunodeficiencies unravel the role of IL-2/CD25/STAT5b in human natural killer cell maturation. *Front Immunol.* (2018) 9:1429. doi: 10.3389/fimmu.2018.01429
210. Schubert D, Bode C, Kenefeck R, Hou TZ, Wing JB, Kennedy A, et al. Autosomal dominant immune dysregulation syndrome in humans with CTLA4 mutations. *Nat Med.* (2014) 20:1410–6. doi: 10.1038/nm.3746
211. Zheng Hou T, Verma N, Wanders J, Kennedy A, Soskic B, Janman D, et al. Identifying functional defects in patients with immune dysregulation due to LRBA and CTLA-4 mutations. *Regul Artic Immunobiol.* (2017) 129:1458–68. doi: 10.1182/blood-2016-10-745174
212. Friedline RH, Brown DS, Nguyen H, Kornfeld H, Lee J, Zhang Y, et al. CD4+ regulatory T cells require CTLA-4 for the maintenance of systemic tolerance. *J Exp Med.* (2009) 206:421–34. doi: 10.1084/jem.20081811
213. Mitsuiki N, Schwab C, Grimbacher B. What did we learn from CTLA-4 insufficiency on the human immune system? *Immunol Rev.* (2019) 287:33–49. doi: 10.1111/imr.12721
214. Schwab C, Gabrysch A, Olbrich P, Patiño V, Warnatz K, Wolff D, et al. Phenotype, penetrance, and treatment of 133 cytotoxic T-lymphocyte antigen 4–insufficient subjects. *J Allergy Clin Immunol.* (2018) 142:1932–46. doi: 10.1016/j.jaci.2018.02.055
215. Greene JL, Leytze GM, Emswiler J, Peach R, Bajorath J, Cosand W, et al. Covalent dimerization of CD28/CTLA-4 and oligomerization of CD80/CD86 regulate T cell costimulatory interactions. *J Biol Chem.* (1996) 271:26762–71. doi: 10.1074/jbc.271.43.26762
216. Egg D, Schwab C, Gabrysch A, Arkwright PD, Cheesman E, Giulino-Roth L, et al. Increased risk for malignancies in 131 affected CTLA4 mutation carriers. *Front Immunol.* (2018) 9:2012. doi: 10.3389/fimmu.2018.02012
217. Zeissig S, Petersen B-S, Tomczak M, Melum E, Huc-Claustre E, Dougan SK, et al. Early-onset Crohn's disease and autoimmunity associated with a variant in CTLA-4. *Gut.* (2015) 64:1889–97. doi: 10.1136/gutjnl-2014-308541
218. Qureshi OS, Zheng Y, Nakamura K, Attridge K, Manzotti C, Schmidt EM, et al. Trans-endocytosis of CD80 and CD86: a molecular basis for the cell-extrinsic function of CTLA-4. *Science.* (2011) 332:600–3. doi: 10.1126/science.1202947
219. Muto A, Tashiro S, Nakajima O, Hoshino H, Takahashi S, Sakoda E, et al. The transcriptional programme of antibody class switching involves the repressor Bach2. *Nature.* (2004) 429:566–71. doi: 10.1038/nature02596
220. Roychoudhuri R, Hirahara K, Mousavi K, Clever D, Klebanoff CA, Bonelli M, et al. BACH2 represses effector programs to stabilize Treg-mediated immune homeostasis. *Nature.* (2013) 498:506–10. doi: 10.1038/nature12199
221. Heino M, Peterson P, Kudoh J, Shimizu N, Antonarakis SE, Scott HS, et al. APECED mutations in the autoimmune regulator (AIRE) gene. *Hum Mutat.* (2001) 18:205–11. doi: 10.1002/humu.1176
222. Ahonen P, Myllärniemi S, Sipilä I, Perheentupa J. Clinical variation of autoimmune polyendocrinopathy–candidiasis–ectodermal dystrophy (APECED) in a series of 68 patients. *N Engl J Med.* (1990) 322:1829–36. doi: 10.1056/NEJM199006283222601
223. Klein L, Kyewski B, Allen PM, Hogquist KA. Positive and negative selection of the T cell repertoire: what thymocytes see (and don't see). *Nat Rev Immunol.* (2014) 14:377–91. doi: 10.1038/nri3667
224. Nagafuchi S, Katsuta H, Koyanagi-Katsuta R, Yamasaki S, Inoue Y, Shimoda K, et al. Autoimmune regulator (AIRE) gene is expressed in human activated CD4+ T-cells and regulated by mitogen-activated protein kinase pathway. *Microbiol Immunol.* (2006) 50:979–87. doi: 10.1111/j.1348-0421.2006.tb03876.x
225. Constantine GM, Lionakis MS. Lessons from primary immunodeficiencies: autoimmune regulator and autoimmune polyendocrinopathy-candidiasis-ectodermal dystrophy. *Immunol Rev.* (2019) 287:103–20. doi: 10.1111/imr.12714
226. Geier E, Pfeifer G, Wilm M, Lucchiari-Hartz M, Baumeister W, Eichmann K, et al. A giant protease with potential to substitute for some functions of the proteasome. *Science.* (1999) 283:978–81. doi: 10.1126/science.283.5404.978
227. Reits E, Neijssen J, Herberts C, Benckhuijsen W, Janssen L, Drijfhout JW, et al. A major role for TPPII in trimming proteasomal degradation products for MHC class I antigen presentation. *Immunity.* (2004) 20:495–506. doi: 10.1016/S1074-7613(04)00074-3
228. Rakhmanov M, Keller B, Gutenberger S, Foerster C, Hoenig M, Driessen G, et al. Circulating CD21low B cells in common variable immunodeficiency resemble tissue homing, innate-like B cells. *Proc Natl Acad Sci USA.* (2009) 106:13451–6. doi: 10.1073/pnas.0901984106
229. Moir S, Ho J, Malaspina A, Wang W, DiPoto AC, O'Shea MA, et al. Evidence for HIV-associated B cell exhaustion in a dysfunctional memory B cell compartment in HIV-infected viremic individuals. *J Exp Med.* (2008) 205:1797–805. doi: 10.1084/jem.20072683
230. Khodarev NN, Roizman B, Weichselbaum RR. Molecular pathways: interferon/stat1 pathway: role in the tumor resistance to genotoxic stress and aggressive growth. *Clin Cancer Res.* (2012) 18:3015–21. doi: 10.1158/1078-0432.CCR-11-3225
231. Levings MK, Sangregorio R, Roncarolo MG. Human cd25(+)cd4(+) t regulatory cells suppress naive and memory T cell proliferation and can be expanded *in vitro* without loss of function. *J Exp Med.* (2001) 193:1295–302. doi: 10.1084/jem.193.11.1295
232. Jonuleit H, Schmitt E, Stassen M, Tuettenberg A, Knop J, Enk AH. Identification and functional characterization of human CD4(+)CD25(+) T cells with regulatory properties isolated from peripheral blood. *J Exp Med.* (2001) 193:1285–94. doi: 10.1084/jem.193.11.1285

233. Dieckmann D, Plottner H, Berchtold S, Berger T, Schuler G. *Ex vivo* isolation and characterization of CD4(+)CD25(+) T cells with regulatory properties from human blood. *J Exp Med.* (2001) 193:1303–10. doi: 10.1084/jem.193.11.1303
234. Rudensky AY. Regulatory T cells and Foxp3. *Immunol Rev.* (2011) 241:260–8. doi: 10.1111/j.1600-065X.2011.01018.x
235. Gobert M, Treilleux I, Bendriss-Vermare N, Bachelot T, Goddard-Leon S, Arfi V, et al. Regulatory T cells recruited through CCL22/CCR4 are selectively activated in lymphoid infiltrates surrounding primary breast tumors and lead to an adverse clinical outcome. *Cancer Res.* (2009) 69:2000–9. doi: 10.1158/0008-5472.CAN-08-2360
236. Putnam AL, Brusko TM, Lee MR, Liu W, Szot GL, Ghosh T, et al. Expansion of human regulatory T-cells from patients with type 1 diabetes. *Diabetes.* (2009) 58:652–62. doi: 10.2337/db08-1168
237. Gavin MA, Torgerson TR, Houston E, DeRoos P, Ho WY, Stray-Pedersen A, et al. Single-cell analysis of normal and FOXP3-mutant human T cells: FOXP3 expression without regulatory T cell development. *Proc Natl Acad Sci USA.* (2006) 103:6659–64. doi: 10.1073/pnas.0509484103
238. Wang J, Ioan-Facsinay A, van der Voort EIH, Huizinga TWJ, Toes REM. Transient expression of FOXP3 in human activated nonregulatory CD4+ T cells. *Eur J Immunol.* (2007) 37:129–38. doi: 10.1002/eji.200636435
239. Miyara M, Yoshioka Y, Kitoh A, Shima T, Wing K, Niwa A, et al. Functional delineation and differentiation dynamics of human CD4+ T cells expressing the FoxP3 transcription factor. *Immunity.* (2009) 30:899–911. doi: 10.1016/j.immuni.2009.03.019
240. Liu W, Putnam AL, Xu-Yu Z, Szot GL, Lee MR, Zhu S, et al. CD127 expression inversely correlates with FoxP3 and suppressive function of human CD4+ T reg cells. *J Exp Med.* (2006) 203:1701–11. doi: 10.1084/jem.20060772
241. Seddiki N, Santner-Nanan B, Martinson J, Zaunders J, Sasson S, Landay A, et al. Expression of interleukin (IL)-2 and IL-7 receptors discriminates between human regulatory and activated T cells. *J Exp Med.* (2006) 203:1693–700. doi: 10.1084/jem.20060468
242. Fuhrman CA, Yeh W-I, Seay HR, Saikumar Lakshmi P, Chopra G, Zhang L, et al. Divergent phenotypes of human regulatory T cells expressing the receptors TIGIT and CD226. *J Immunol.* (2015) 195:145–55. doi: 10.4049/jimmunol.1402381
243. Landuyt AE, Klocke BJ, Colvin TB, Schoeb TR, Maynard CL. Cutting edge: ICOS-deficient regulatory T cells display normal induction of IL-10 but readily downregulate expression of Foxp3. *J Immunol.* (2019) 202:1039–44. doi: 10.4049/jimmunol.1801266
244. Borsellino G, Kleinewietfeld M, Di Mitri D, Sternjak A, Diamantini A, Giometto R, et al. Expression of ectonucleotidase CD39 by Foxp3+ Treg cells: hydrolysis of extracellular ATP and immune suppression. *Blood.* (2007) 110:1225–32. doi: 10.1182/blood-2006-12-064527
245. Gourdin N, Bossennec M, Rodriguez C, Vigano S, Machon C, Jandus C, et al. Autocrine adenosine regulates tumor polyfunctional CD73+CD4+ effector T cells devoid of immune checkpoints. *Cancer Res.* (2018) 78:3604–18. doi: 10.1158/0008-5472.CAN-17-2405
246. Álvarez-Sánchez N, Cruz-Chamorro I, Díaz-Sánchez M, Lardone PJ, Guerrero JM, Carrillo-Vico A. Peripheral CD39-expressing T regulatory cells are increased and associated with relapsing-remitting multiple sclerosis in relapsing patients. *Sci Rep.* (2019) 9:2302. doi: 10.1038/s41598-019-38897-w
247. Hippen KL, Merkel SC, Schirm DK, Sieben CM, Sumstad D, Kadidlo DM, et al. Massive *ex vivo* expansion of human natural regulatory T cells (T(regs)) with minimal loss of *in vivo* functional activity. *Sci Transl Med.* (2011) 3:83ra41. doi: 10.1126/scitranslmed.3001809
248. Jin X, Lu Y, Zhao Y, Yi S. Large-scale *in vitro* expansion of human regulatory T cells with potent xenoantigen-specific suppression. *Cytotechnology.* (2016) 68:935–45. doi: 10.1007/s10616-015-9845-1
249. Battaglia M, Stabilini A, Migliavacca B, Horejs-Hoeck J, Kaupper T, Roncarolo M-G. Rapamycin promotes expansion of functional $CD4^{+}$ CD25 $^{+}$ FOXP3 $^{+}$ regulatory T cells of both healthy subjects and type 1 diabetic patients. *J Immunol.* (2006) 177:8338–47. doi: 10.4049/jimmunol.177.12.8338
250. McMurchy AN, Levings MK. Suppression assays with human T regulatory cells: a technical guide. *Eur J Immunol.* (2012) 42:27–34. doi: 10.1002/eji.201141651
251. Engelhardt KR, Shah N, Faizura-Yeop I, Kocacik Uygun DF, Frede N, Muise AM, et al. Clinical outcome in IL-10- and IL-10 receptor–deficient patients with or without hematopoietic stem cell transplantation. *J Allergy Clin Immunol.* (2013) 131:825–30.e9. doi: 10.1016/j.jaci.2012.09.025
252. Begue B, Verdier J, Rieux-Laucat F, Goulet O, Morali A, Canioni D, et al. Defective IL10 signaling defining a subgroup of patients with inflammatory bowel disease. *Am J Gastroenterol.* (2011) 106:1544–55. doi: 10.1038/ajg.2011.112
253. O'Donnell EA, Ernst DN, Hingorani R. Multiparameter flow cytometry: advances in high resolution analysis. *Immune Netw.* (2013) 13:43–54. doi: 10.4110/in.2013.13.2.43
254. Villani A-C, Sarkizova S, Hacohen N. Systems immunology: learning the rules of the immune system. *Annu Rev Immunol.* (2018) 36:813–42. doi: 10.1146/annurev-immunol-042617-053035
255. Davis MM, Tato CM, Furman D. Systems immunology: just getting started. *Nat Immunol.* (2017) 18:725–32. doi: 10.1038/ni.3768
256. Choi J, Fernandez R, Maecker HT, Butte MJ. Systems biology approach to uncover signaling defects in primary immunodeficiency diseases. *J Immunol.* (2016) 196(1 Suppl.):209.7.
257. Choi J, Fernandez R, Maecker HT, Butte MJ. Systems approach to uncover signaling networks in primary immunodeficiency diseases. *J Allergy Clin Immunol.* (2017) 140:881–4.e8. doi: 10.1016/j.jaci.2017.03.025

11

Impaired STAT3-Dependent Upregulation of IL2Rα in B Cells of a Patient with a STAT1 Gain-of-Function Mutation

Menno C. van Zelm [1,2,3], Julian J. Bosco [2,3], Pei M. Aui [1,3], Samuel De Jong [1,3], Fiona Hore-Lacy [2,3], Robyn E. O'Hehir [2,3], Robert G. Stirling [2,3] and Paul U. Cameron [3,4,5]**

[1] Department of Immunology and Pathology, Central Clinical School, Monash University, Melbourne, VIC, Australia, [2] Allergy, Asthma and Clinical Immunology Service, Department of Respiratory, Allergy and Clinical Immunology (Research), Central Clinical School, Monash University, The Alfred Hospital, Melbourne, VIC, Australia, [3] The Jeffrey Modell Diagnostic and Research Centre for Primary Immunodeficiencies in Melbourne, Melbourne, VIC, Australia, [4] Department of Infectious Diseases, Alfred Hospital and Monash University, Melbourne, VIC, Australia, [5] The Peter Doherty Institute for Infection and Immunity, University of Melbourne and Royal Melbourne Hospital, Melbourne, VIC, Australia

***Correspondence:**
Menno C. van Zelm
menno.vanzelm@monash.edu
Paul U. Cameron
paul.cameron@unimelb.edu.au

Heterozygous *STAT1* gain-of-function (GOF) mutations form the most common genetic cause of chronic mucocutaneous candidiasis (CMC). In such patients, increased STAT1 function leads to impaired STAT3-dependent activation of IL-17A and IL-17F in T cells, thereby causing impaired Th17 responses to *Candida*. In spite of the critical role of STAT3 in IL-21 signaling in B cells, nearly all STAT1 GOF patients have normal or high serum IgG. We here present a 44 year-old male with childhood onset of CMC and antibody deficiency since early adulthood. Sequence analysis of *STAT1* revealed a heterozygous missense mutation in the coiled-coil domain (p.D168E), which resulted in increased STAT1 phosphorylation of B-cells activated with IFNα and IFNγ. IL-21 induced STAT3 phosphorylation and nuclear localization were normal, but resulted in impaired upregulation of IL2Rα. This newly identified B-cell intrinsic impairment of STAT3 function could underlie the progressive development of hypogammaglobulinemia. Considering the high risk of bronchiectasis and irreversible organ damage, this case illustrates the need for monitoring of IgG levels and/or function in adult patients with STAT1 GOF mutations.

Keywords: chronic mucocutaneous candidiasis, hypogammaglobulinemia, STAT1, gain-of-function, STAT3, IL2Rα

BACKGROUND

Chronic mucocutaneous candidiasis (CMC) is a persistent or recurrent infection by *Candida* and typically affects the nails, skin, oral, and genital mucosae. In recent years, many cases have been shown to result from primary immunodeficiencies (PIDs) with impaired helper-T(h)17 cell immunity (1). This can be due to inhibitory autoantibodies against Th17 cytokines in patients with autosomal recessive (AR) polyendocrine syndrome type I (APS-1), or alternatively, inherited mutations that impair development and function of Th17 cells. Heterozygous *STAT1* gain-of-function (GOF) mutations form the most common genetic cause of CMC with mutations found in more than 50% of patients (2–4). These mutations are typically found in exons 7-14 which encode the coiled-coil and DNA-binding domains. As a result, increased STAT1 phosphorylation occurs upon stimulation of immune cells with STAT1-activating cytokines, such as interferon (IFN)α and IFNγ. Importantly, increased STAT1 signaling reciprocally inhibits STAT3-dependent cytokine production, which include IL-17A and IL-17F in T cells. Thus, STAT1 GOF predisposes to impaired Th17 responses to *Candida* (2, 4).

Patients with *STAT1* GOF mutations often present with additional bacterial and viral complications. Furthermore, autoimmunity/autoinflammatory disease has been observed in 37% of patients in a large cohort study ($n = 274$), and several patients have been shown to develop solid tumors (3). Effects on B-cells and humoral immunity are variable. 19% of 209 patients carried reduced total B cell numbers and 49% of the 53 patients examined had reduced memory B cell numbers. In addition, up to 23% of patients have impaired antibody responses to vaccinations with protein antigens, although only 3% have hypogammaglobulinemia (3, 5). As STAT3 is critical for IL21-dependent signaling in T-cell dependent B-cell responses, it is possible that STAT1 GOF mutations affect antibody responses and humoral immunity by inadvertent repression of STAT3-mediated transcription. We here identify a defect in STAT3-dependent upregulation of IL2Rα (CD25) in B cells of a patient with STAT1 GOF.

METHODS

Ethics

Diagnostic work-up of blood and laboratory research studies including genetics of the patient were carried out with approval of Human Research Ethics committee of The Alfred Hospital (Study 109/15) and obtained after written informed consent. In addition, the patient has consented to publication of the case report. Data from healthy controls were collected after written consent was obtained and with approval of the human ethics committee of Monash University (Study 2016-0289). All studies were performed in accordance with the Declaration of Helsinki.

Flowcytometric Immunophenotyping and *in vitro* Cell Stimulation

Patient and control subjects were included over a time period of 3 years. Standardized sample preparation, antibody staining, and flow cytometer instrument settings were used to ensure consistency in flow cytometry (6). In short, absolute counts of CD3+, CD4+ and CD8+ T cells, CD19+ B cells, and CD16+/CD56+ natural killer cells were obtained with a diagnostic lyse-no-wash protocol by using commercial Trucount tubes (BD Biosciences, San Jose, CA). For detailed 11-color flow cytometry, red blood cells were lysed with NH_4Cl before incubation of 1–2 million nucleated cells for 15 min at room temperature in a total volume of 100 μL. After preparation, cells were measured on 4-laser flow cytometer (LSRII or LSRFortessa, BD Biosciences) by using standardized settings (6). Data were analyzed with FACSDiva (V8.0; BD Biosciences) and FlowJo software (v10) Naive and memory B-cells, and CD4+ T-cell subsets were defined as previously described (7).

Immortalization of patient's and control B cells with EBV derived from supernatant of the B95–8 cell line was performed as described previously (8). The EBV LCL were stimulated *in vitro* for 30 min with IFNα (10,000 U/ml; pbl assay science), IFN-γ (10,000 U/ml; Peprotech), or IL-21 (50 ng/ml; Lonza). Subsequently, the cells were stained with CD20-BV605 (clone 2H7; BioLegend) and Fixable Viability Stain 700 (BD Biosciences) prior to fixation, permeabilization, and staining with STAT1(pY701)-AF67 (clone 4a) and STAT3(pY705)-PE (clone 4/P-STAT3) according to manufacturer's instructions (BD Biosciences). Following acquisition on a 4-laser LSRII (BD Biosciences), live single cells that were positive for CD20 expression were analyzed for intracellular pSTAT1 and pSTAT3 expression (FlowJo v10). In addition, nuclear localization of pSTAT3 following 30 min IL-21 stimulation was determined in EBV LCL from the patient and from a healthy control using an imaging flow cytometer (Imagestream^X MKII; Amnis/Millennium Science, Mulgrave, VIC, Australia) equipped with four lasers (405, 488, 642, and 785 nm). Images (60x) were obtained from >1,000 cells per condition and similarity scores were derived for pSTAT3 and the nucleus (stained with Vybrant™ DyeCycle™ Violet; Thermo Scientific). Similarity scores for surface CD20 (BV605) and the nucleus were derived as negative control.

Sequence Analysis of STAT1

Following genomic DNA isolation from post-Ficoll granulocytes (GenElute Mammalian Genomic DNA Miniprep Kit, Sigma-Aldrich, St Louis, Mo), exons 7-14 of the *STAT1* gene were PCR-amplified using previously published primers (9), and sequenced by the Micromon facility of Monash University on an Applied Biosystems 3730s DNA Analyzer (Thermo Fisher). Obtained sequences were aligned with the reference sequence from Ensembl using CLC Main Workbench 7 software.

Molecular Analysis of Ig Gene Rearrangements

RNA was isolated from post-Ficoll mononuclear cells of the patient with a GenElute mammalian RNA kit (Sigma-Aldrich) and reverse transcribed to cDNA with random primers (Invitrogen Life technologies). Rearranged IgG and IgA transcripts were amplified in a multiplex PCR approach using 4 different *IGHV*-family leader forward primers in combination with an *IGHG*-consensus or *IGHA*-consensus reverse primer (10, 11). PCR products were cloned into a pGEMT easy vector (Promega, Madison WI), amplified by colony PCR, and sequenced as above. Sequences were analyzed using the IMGT database (http://www.imgt.org/IMGT_vquest/vquest) to assign the *IGHV*, *IGHD*, and *IGHJ* genes and alleles, and to identify somatic hypermutations (SHM). Of each unique clone, the position and frequency of mutations were determined within the entire *IGHV* gene (FR1-CDR1-FR2-CDR2-FR3). SHM were determined as variations on the best matched V-gene and represented as the percentage of mutations of the total sequenced V-gene nucleotides. The IgG and IgA receptor subclasses were determined using the *IGH* reference sequence (NG_001019). All results of the patient were compared with previously generated data sets of controls (12).

CASE PRESENTATION

Clinical History

We here present a 44 year-old male with a history of CMC treated since early childhood with azole antifungal agents. The patient is the second of three children from non-consanguineous parents. He has developed resistance to antifungal drugs including nystatin, fluconazole, and partially to voriconazole to which he had an allergic drug reaction of troublesome and persistent photodermatitis. He is currently controlled on posaconazole and amphotericin lozenges.

The CMC has been associated with the development of esophageal strictures requiring repeated dilation. At the age of 39 years this procedure was complicated by esophageal rupture and mediastinitis requiring a prolonged ICU admission. The esophageal rupture was treated surgically but subsequent investigations for recurrent stenosis led to diagnosis of esophageal cancer at age 40. He underwent esophageal resection a year later with clear surgical margins, followed by adjuvant chemotherapy which was truncated because of severe mucositis. Radiotherapy was commenced for this cancer due to poor prognosis in young age.

Shortly after diagnosis with esophageal cancer, the patient was started on G-CSF therapy (2 times 300 μg per week) for almost 2 years (Dec 2014–July 2016). As the patient reported increased discomfort following discontinuation, G-CSF therapy was re-started a year later at age 43 years and is still current.

During early adulthood, the patient developed progressive hypogammaglobulinemia (**Table 1**) with poor vaccine responses and commenced IVIG replacement at age 35. In spite of adequate trough IgG with monthly IVIG, he continues to suffer from recurrent lower respiratory tract infections requiring antibiotics and has been hospitalized on at least 4 occasions with bacterial infections, including salmonella gastroenteritis. He has required periodic courses of IV caspafungin for candida partially resistant to azoles.

TABLE 1 | Immunological data.

Laboratory measurement	Patient 35 year	Patient 42 year	Normal range*
SERUM IG LEVELS (g/L)			
IgG	**3.4**	–	7.0–15.5
IgG1	**1.8**	–	3.8–9.3
IgG2	**1.8**	–	2.4–7.0
IgG3	0.3	–	0.22–1.76
IgG4	0.1	–	0.04–0.86
IgA	1.6	–	0.76–3.9
IgM	**0.3**	–	0.45–2.3
LYMPHOCYTE SUBSETS (CELLS/μl BLOOD)			
B cells	**51**	103	76–608
Transitional	–	0.9	0.4–29
Naive mature	–	87	31–398
IgD+ memory	–	7.1	3.4–79
IgD- memory	–	**2.4**	12–114
T cells	1,248	1,013	773–2,757
CD8	576	475	243–950
CD4	624	409	307–1,600
Tfh (CD45RA-CXCR5+)	–	26	16–175
Th17 (CD45RA-CCR6-CCR4+CXCR3-)	–	**7.4**	11–98

For cell subsets: 5–95% of adult controls; B cells, n = 44; T cells, n = 34. Values below normal range are depicted in bold font.

Identification of a Heterozygous Gain-of-Function Mutation in *STAT1*

Given the severity of the CMC and the antibody deficiency, more detailed immunological work-up was performed in the context of a research study. Detailed flowcytometric immunophenotyping of the patient's B- and T-cells revealed a severe reduction in CD27+ memory B cells and low circulating numbers of Th17 cells at age 42 years following discontinuation of G-CSF therapy (**Table 1**). As the patient did not have typical clinical associations of APS-1, a *STAT1* GOF mutation was considered and genetic analysis of *STAT1* exons 7-14 was performed on DNA of the patient. Sanger sequencing revealed a heterozygous variant in exon 7 (c.504T>A) resulting in a missense mutation in the coiled-coil domain (p.D168E) (**Figure 1A**). The same mutation has been previously described in a 5 year old female patient, but was not functionally addressed (3). To examine the effects of the mutation, we studied phosphorylation of STAT1 in EBV-immortalized B-lymphocytes of the patient. Thirty minutes after stimulation with either IFNα or IFNγ, the patient's cells showed increased levels of pSTAT1 confirming a GOF phenotype as a result of the D168E missense mutation (**Figure 1B**).

T-Helper and T-Follicular Helper Cell Subsets

Given that the patient reported beneficial effects of G-CSF treatment, we retrospectively analyzed immune cells prior-to and during the treatment period. Extensive follow-up of total leukocyte and neutrophil count showed a general increase in numbers during therapy (**Figure 2A**). Three stored PBMC samples were available for detailed T-cell immunophenotyping, and reporting of relative frequencies of Th17 and Tfh cells. Th17 cell frequencies were within the normal range on only 1 occasion under G-CSF therapy, whereas Tfh cell frequencies were not below the normal range (**Figure 2B**). Hence, G-CSF therapy was associated with normalization of Th17 cells on at least one occasion.

STAT3 Signaling Defect in B Cells

To gain more insight into the nature of the hypogammaglobulinemia and reduced memory B cells in the patient, we first quantified SHM in IgG transcripts from blood B cells. Overall, SHM levels were normal. However, IgG3 transcripts of the patient contained negligible SHM, in contrast to IgG1 and IgG2 (**Figure 3A**). Further analysis of the IgG transcripts demonstrated a predominant usage of IgG3 compared to IgG2 (**Figure 3B**).

T-cell dependent B-cell responses critically depend on IL-21R signaling via STAT3. As STAT1 GOF mutations can

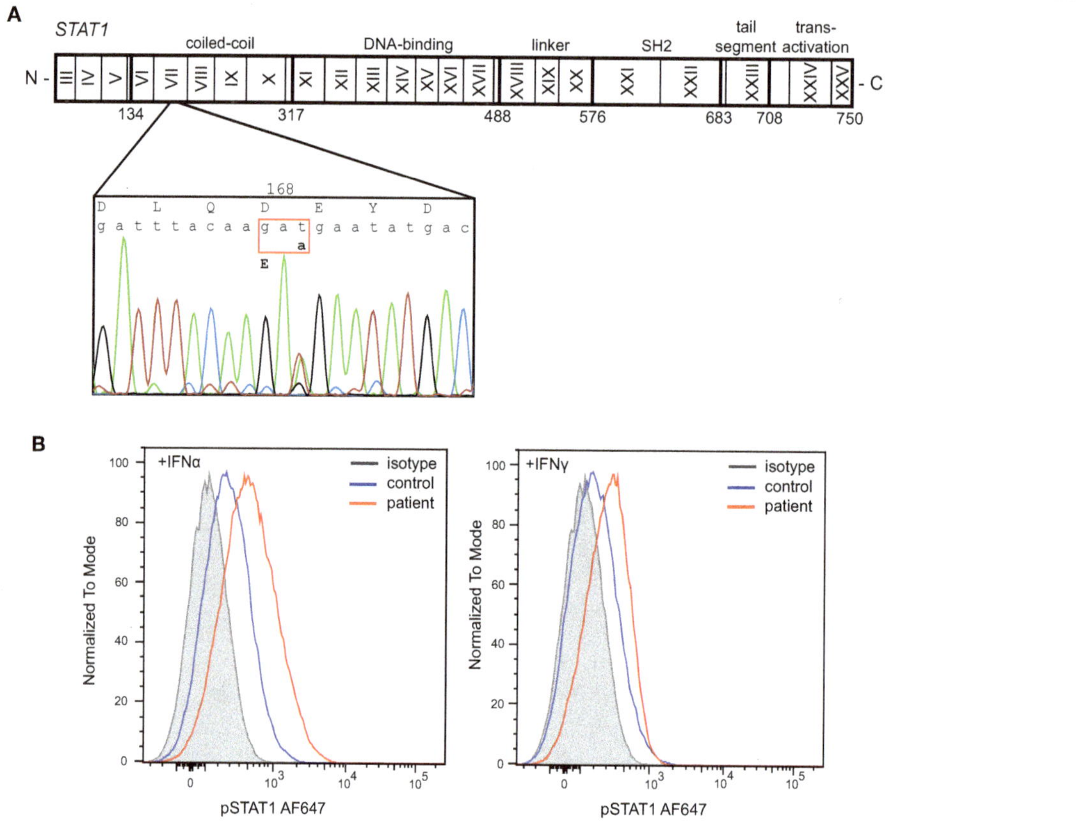

FIGURE 1 | Identification of a heterozygous mutation in STAT1 leading to a gain of function. **(A)** Sanger sequencing revealed a heterozygous c.504T>A mutation in exon 7 resulting in a missense mutation in the coiled-coil domain (p.D168E). **(B)** Increased phosphorylation of STAT1 following *in vitro* stimulation of patient's EBV-LCL with IFNα and IFNγ.

inhibit STAT3 activity, we here questioned whether the patient's B cells had intrinsically impaired STAT3 responsiveness. Indeed, in EBV-immortalized B cells from the patient, IL-21 stimulation normally induced STAT3 phosphorylation (**Figure 3C**). Moreover, nuclear localization studies with imaging flowcytometry revealed normal nuclear localization of pSTAT3 after IL-21 stimulation as well (**Figure 3D**). Therefore, we next evaluated functional STAT3 signaling by evaluation of expression of CD25, the IL2Rα chain, which is a direct target of STAT3 in B cells (13). Following 24 h incubation with IL-21, EBV-LCL from a healthy control upregulated CD25 surface expression (**Figure 3E**). In contrast, EBV-LCL from the patient had lower levels of CD25 expression. These findings are consistent with previous finding that STAT3 activity was inhibited by STAT1 GOF at the target gene activation level, but not upstream of that (14).

DISCUSSION

We here report a patient with STAT1 GOF and adult-onset antibody deficiency in the context of reduced total and memory B cells and impaired SHM and class switching to IgG2. Despite the known inhibition of STAT3 function due to STAT1 GOF, this has not been extensively addressed in previous studies. In contrast to the highly penetrant defects in Th17 function, the impact of *STAT1* GOF mutations on B-cell function and antibody responses is variable among reported patients (3). In B cells from our patient, we confirmed that following stimulation with IL-21, STAT3 phosphorylation and nuclear localization were not affected, but that activation of expression of the target gene encoding CD25 (IL-2Rα) was impaired. Hence, these B-cells will not be optimally sensitized to the stimulatory effects of IL-2 (13), and subject to suboptimal humoral immune responses.

Using *in vitro* functional analysis, we showed that the heterozygous *STAT1* D168E mutation in our patient had a dominant GOF effect on STAT1 phosphorylation. The increased amount of pSTAT1 protein following activation is generally assumed to be the result of a larger fraction of the mutant STAT1 being phosphorylated. However, as we were unable to measure total STAT1 protein, it remains possible that the mutant STAT1 is expressed at a higher level than the wild type, providing more total protein to be phosphorylated upon activation.

The same D168E mutation has been identified previously in a 5 year-old from Moroccan descent (patient 167 from kindred 111), but was not functionally assessed (3). The Moroccan girl did not present with hypogammaglobulinemia (IgG, 15.86 g/L),

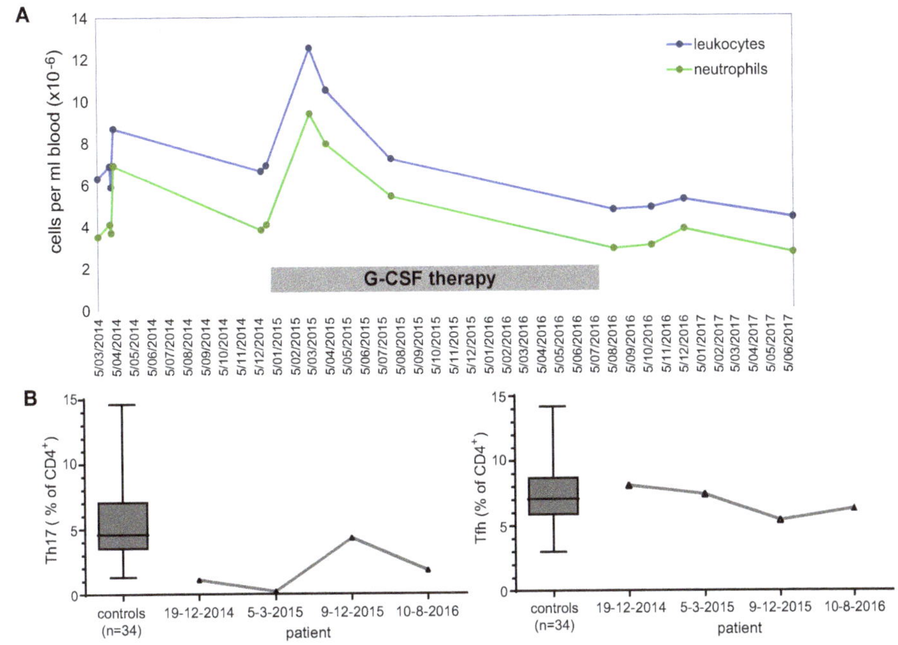

FIGURE 2 | Immunological effects of immunotherapy with G-CSF. **(A)** Longitudinal measurements of blood leukocyte and neutrophil cell counts over a 3 year interval. **(B)** Frequencies of Th17 and Tfh cell subsets within total CD4 T cells prior to, during (2 timepoints; 2015) and after discontinuation of G-CSF therapy.

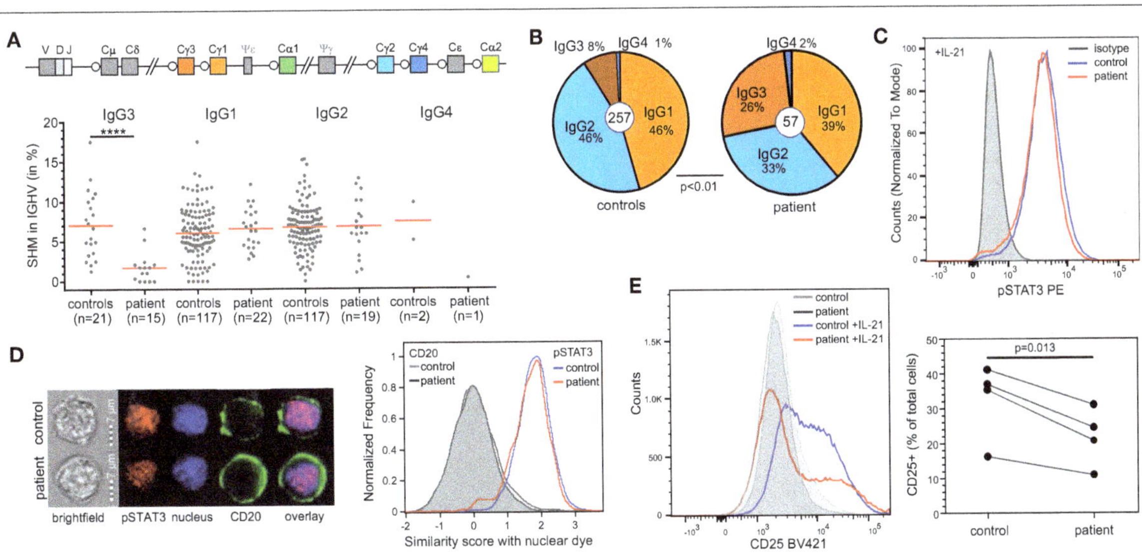

FIGURE 3 | B-cell defects in STAT1 GOF. **(A)** Somatic hypermutation levels in IgG subclass transcripts of the patient and controls. **(B)** Relative distributions of IgG subclasses of unique transcripts. **(C)** STAT3 phosphorylation in EBV-LCL upon stimulation with IL-21. **(D)** Nuclear localization of pSTAT3 in EBV-LCL following stimulation with IL-21 as determined with the AMNIS ImageStream. Example images are shown on the left, and the collated events as overlays for nuclear localization scores on the right. **(E)** CD25 (IL2Rα) expression on EBV-LCL following stimulation with IL-21. Overlays are shown for one experiment to illustrate on the left and the combined data from 4 independent experiments on the right. Statistics: Paired *t*-test.

nor did our patient before early adulthood. It is therefore possible that patients with STAT1 GOF mutations are susceptible for a progressive decline in serum IgG levels and consequent antibody deficiency. This decline in antibody responses could be the accumulated effect of Tfh cell defects and the B-cell intrinsic defect to respond to IL-21. As shown by our *in vitro* data, this potentially mimics STAT3 LOF mutations with impaired activation of STAT3 target genes (13).

In this patient the STAT1 GOF may have directly contributed to the development of esophageal cancer. Early onset cancers were present in 6% of patients in the large series (3), and suggest that immunological abnormalities including Th17 and B cell function may also be associated with risk for malignancies.

Prior to the genetic diagnosis of STAT1 GOF, the patient was started on experimental G-CSF treatment based on the well-described anti candida function of this cytokine, as well as indications in the literature of a beneficial effect of adjunctive immunotherapy for the treatment of disseminated candidiasis (15). G-CSF therapy in our patient did increase Th17 cell frequencies, but did not resolve the candidiasis. The latter is in line with a recent report of an impaired capacity for killing of *C. albicans* by G-CSF recruited neutrophils (16). Moreover, it was previously reported that Th17 responses in STAT1 GOF patients were not restored by G-CSF immunotherapy (17). We here show a partial effect of G-CSF resulting in a clinical benefit. Increasing evidence is accumulating that Jak inhibitors are successful in resolving candidiasis in STAT1 GOF patients (18–20), but this is not entirely risk-free (21). Unfortunately, we have not yet been able to obtain compassionate access to Jak inhibitors for our patient, and as he does not experience adverse effects of G-CSF therapy this therapy is still continued.

CONCLUDING REMARKS

We describe a B-cell intrinsic impairment of STAT3 function in a patient with a STAT1 GOF mutation and progressive development of hypogammaglobulinemia. Currently, a minority of the reported patients with STAT1 GOF mutations suffer from hypogammaglobulinemia with a larger proportion showing impaired responses to vaccination (3). Considering the high risk of bronchiectasis and irreversible organ damage (22, 23), this case illustrates the need for monitoring of IgG levels and/or function in adult patients with STAT1 GOF mutations.

AUTHOR CONTRIBUTIONS

MvZ, JB, and PC designed and wrote the manuscript. PA and SDJ performed experiments. FH-L, RO, and RS contributed to essential discussion of the paper. All authors critically read and commented on manuscript drafts and approved of the final version.

FUNDING

This work was supported by The Jeffrey Modell Foundation, and by a National Health and Medical Research Council Senior Research Fellowship (GNT1117687) to MvZ.

ACKNOWLEDGMENTS

We gratefully acknowledge technical support from Dr. Geza Paukovic and Steven Lim (AMREP Flow Cytometry Core Facility), and the support of Dr. Raffi Gugasyan and Mr. Jasper (Burnet Institute) with imaging flowcytometry. We thank Dr. Anne Puel (Paris, France) for sharing unpublished data.

REFERENCES

1. Puel A, Cypowyj S, Marodi L, Abel L, Picard C, Casanova JL. Inborn errors of human IL-17 immunity underlie chronic mucocutaneous candidiasis. *Curr Opin Allergy Clin Immunol.* (2012) 12:616–22. doi: 10.1097/ACI.0b013e328358cc0b
2. Liu L, Okada S, Kong XF, Kreins AY, Cypowyj S, Abhyankar A, et al. Gain-of-function human STAT1 mutations impair IL-17 immunity and underlie chronic mucocutaneous candidiasis. *J Exp Med.* (2011) 208:1635–48. doi: 10.1084/jem.20110958
3. Toubiana J, Okada S, Hiller J, Oleastro M, Lagos Gomez M, Aldave Becerra JC, et al. Heterozygous STAT1 gain-of-function mutations underlie an unexpectedly broad clinical phenotype. *Blood.* (2016) 127:3154–64. doi: 10.1182/blood-2015-11-679902
4. van de Veerdonk FL, Plantinga TS, Hoischen A, Smeekens SP, Joosten LA, Gilissen C, et al. STAT1 mutations in autosomal dominant chronic mucocutaneous candidiasis. *N Engl J Med.* (2011) 365:54–61. doi: 10.1056/NEJMoa1100102
5. Kobbe R, Kolster M, Fuchs S, Schulze-Sturm U, Jenderny J, Kochhan L, et al. Common variable immunodeficiency, impaired neurological development and reduced numbers of T regulatory cells in a 10-year-old boy with a STAT1 gain-of-function mutation. *Gene.* (2016) 586:234–8. doi: 10.1016/j.gene.2016.04.006
6. Kalina T, Flores-Montero J, van der Velden VH, Martin-Ayuso M, Bottcher S, Ritgen M, et al. EuroFlow standardization of flow cytometer instrument settings and immunophenotyping protocols. *Leukemia.* (2012) 26:1986–2010. doi: 10.1038/leu.2012.122
7. Heeringa JJ, Karim AF, van Laar JAM, Verdijk RM, Paridaens D, van Hagen PM, et al. Expansion of blood IgG4(+) B, TH2, and regulatory T cells in patients with IgG4-related disease. *J Allergy Clin Immunol.* (2018) 141:1831–1843.e1810. doi: 10.1016/j.jaci.2017.07.024
8. van Zelm MC, Smet J, Adams B, Mascart F, Schandene L, Janssen F, et al. CD81 gene defect in humans disrupts CD19 complex formation and leads to antibody deficiency. *J Clin Invest.* (2010) 120:1265–74. doi: 10.1172/JCI39748
9. Chapgier A, Kong XF, Boisson-Dupuis S, Jouanguy E, Averbuch D, Feinberg J, et al. A partial form of recessive STAT1 deficiency in humans. *J Clin Invest.* (2009) 119:1502–14. doi: 10.1172/JCI37083
10. Berkowska MA, Schickel JN, Grosserichter-Wagener C, de Ridder D, Ng YS, van Dongen JJ, et al. Circulating human CD27-IgA+ memory B cells recognize bacteria with polyreactive Igs. *J Immunol.* (2015) 195:1417–26. doi: 10.4049/jimmunol.1402708
11. Tiller T, Meffre E, Yurasov S, Tsuiji M, Nussenzweig MC, Wardemann H. Efficient generation of monoclonal antibodies from single human B cells by single cell RT-PCR and expression vector cloning. *J Immunol Methods.* (2008) 329:112–24. doi: 10.1016/j.jim.2007.09.017

12. de Jong BG, IJspeert H, Marques L, van der Burg M, van Dongen JJ, Loos BG, et al. Human IgG2- and IgG4-expressing memory B cells display enhanced molecular and phenotypic signs of maturity and accumulate with age. *Immunol Cell Biol.* (2017) 95:744–52. doi: 10.1038/icb.2017.43
13. Berglund LJ, Avery DT, Ma CS, Moens L, Deenick EK, Bustamante J, et al. IL-21 signalling via STAT3 primes human naive B cells to respond to IL-2 to enhance their differentiation into plasmablasts. *Blood.* (2013) 122:3940–50. doi: 10.1182/blood-2013-06-506865
14. Zheng J, van de Veerdonk FL, Crossland KL, Smeekens SP, Chan CM, Al Shehri T, et al. Gain-of-function STAT1 mutations impair STAT3 activity in patients with chronic mucocutaneous candidiasis (CMC). *Eur J Immunol.* (2015) 45:2834–46. doi: 10.1002/eji.201445344
15. van de Veerdonk FL, Kullberg BJ, Netea MG. Adjunctive immunotherapy with recombinant cytokines for the treatment of disseminated candidiasis. *Clin Microbiol Infect.* (2012) 18:112–9. doi: 10.1111/j.1469-0691.2011.03676.x
16. Gazendam RP, van de Geer A, van Hamme JL, Tool AT, van Rees DJ, Aarts CE, et al. Impaired killing of Candida albicans by granulocytes mobilized for transfusion purposes: a role for granule components. *Haematologica.* (2016) 101:587–96. doi: 10.3324/haematol.2015.136630
17. van de Veerdonk FL, Koenen HJ, van der Velden WJ, van der Meer JW, Netea MG. Immunotherapy with G-CSF in patients with chronic mucocutaneous candidiasis. *Immunol Lett.* (2015) 167:54–6. doi: 10.1016/j.imlet.2015.05.008
18. Forbes LR, Vogel TP, Cooper MA, Castro-Wagner J, Schussler E, Weinacht KG, et al. Jakinibs for the treatment of immune dysregulation in patients with gain-of-function signal transducer and activator of transcription 1 (STAT1) or STAT3 mutations. *J Allergy Clin Immunol.* (2018) 142:1665–9. doi: 10.1016/j.jaci.2018.07.020
19. Higgins E, Al Shehri T, McAleer MA, Conlon N, Feighery C, Lilic D, et al. Use of ruxolitinib to successfully treat chronic mucocutaneous candidiasis caused by gain-of-function signal transducer and activator of transcription 1 (STAT1) mutation. *J Allergy Clin Immunol.* (2015) 135:551–3. doi: 10.1016/j.jaci.2014.12.1867
20. Meesilpavikkai K, Dik WA, Schrijver B, Nagtzaam NMA, Posthumus-van Sluijs SJ, van Hagen PM, et al. Baricitinib treatment in a patient with a gain-of-function mutation in signal transducer and activator of transcription 1 (STAT1). *J Allergy Clin Immunol.* (2018) 142:328–330.e322. doi: 10.1016/j.jaci.2018.02.045
21. Zimmerman O, Rosler B, Zerbe CS, Rosen LB, Hsu AP, Uzel G, et al. Risks of ruxolitinib in STAT1 gain-of-function-associated severe fungal disease. *Open Forum Infect Dis.* (2017) 4:ofx202. doi: 10.1093/ofid/ofx202
22. Breuer O, Daum H, Cohen-Cymberknoh M, Unger S, Shoseyov D, Stepensky P, et al. Autosomal dominant gain of function STAT1 mutation and severe bronchiectasis. *Respir Med.* (2017) 126:39–45. doi: 10.1016/j.rmed.2017.03.018
23. Huh HJ, Jhun BW, Choi SR, Kim YJ, Yun SA, Nham E, et al. Bronchiectasis and recurrent respiratory infections with a *de novo* STAT1 gain-of-function variant: first case in Korea. *Yonsei Med J.* (2018) 59:1004–7. doi: 10.3349/ymj.2018.59.8.1004

12

Adiponectin Receptors and Pro-inflammatory Cytokines are Modulated in Common Variable Immunodeficiency Patients: Correlation with Ig Replacement Therapy

Rita Polito[1,2†], *Ersilia Nigro*[2,3†], *Antonio Pecoraro*[3], *Maria Ludovica Monaco*[2], *Franco Perna*[4], *Alessandro Sanduzzi*[4], *Arturo Genovese*[3], *Giuseppe Spadaro*[3] and *Aurora Daniele*[1,2*]

[1] *Dipartimento di Scienze e Tecnologie Ambientali Biologiche Farmaceutiche, Università degli Studi della Campania "Luigi Vanvitelli," Caserta, Italy,* [2] *CEINGE-Biotecnologie Avanzate Scarl, Naples, Italy,* [3] *Dipartimento di Scienze Mediche Traslazionali, Allergologia e Immunologia Clinica, Università degli Studi di Napoli Federico II, Naples, Italy,* [4] *Dipartimento di Medicina Clinica e Chirurgia, Università degli Studi di Napoli "Federico II," Naples, Italy*

Correspondence:
Aurora Daniele
aurora.daniele@unicampania.it

† These authors have contributed equally to this work

Adiponectin exerts beneficial pleiotropic effects through three receptors, AdipoR1, AdipoR2, and T-cadherin; it also exerts immunomodulatory effects. We previously demonstrated that adiponectin levels are altered in common variable immunodeficiency disease (CVID). The purpose of the present study was to investigate further the specific involvement of adiponectin in CVID by characterizing (i) the expression profile of adiponectin receptors on peripheral blood mononuclear cells; (ii) the levels of another relevant adipokine, namely leptin; (iii) the levels of five other cytokines (IL-2, IL-6, IL-10, TNFα, and IFNγ) in 24 patients on maintenance therapy, in 18 treatment-naïve patients (before and 24 h after the first Ig infusion) and in 28 healthy controls. We found that (i) adiponectin was down-expressed in patients on maintenance therapy and in treatment-naïve patients, and that it increased in treatment-naïve patients 24 h after the first Ig infusion; (ii) leptin expression did not differ between maintenance patients and controls either before or after the first Ig infusion; (iii) AdipoR1 expression was significantly higher on B lymphocytes, monocytes and NK cells of CVID patients than in controls; (iv) the expression of AdipoR1 and AdipoR2 on B lymphocytes, monocytes and NK cells was higher after the first Ig infusion than in treatment-naïve patients; (v) T-cadherin expression did not differ between treatment- naïve CVID patients and controls, and was not affected by Ig infusion; and (vi) IL-6, IL-8, IL-10, and TNFα levels were differently expressed in CVID patients on therapy maintenance and were not affected by the first Ig replacement therapy. This is the first study to demonstrate that the expression of AdipoRs in peripheral blood mononuclear cells from CVID patients differs from that of controls, and changes after the first Ig infusion. The specificity of adiponectin involvement in CVID is supported by the absence of changes in leptin levels and in the levels of the cytokines investigated.

Taken together, these results suggest that the adiponectin system plays an important and specific role in CVID. A better understanding of adiponectin as a link in the cross-talk between the immune system and adipose tissue may provide additional benefits for the management of CVID patients.

Keywords: adiponectin, common variable immunodeficiency, adiponectin receptors, leptin, cytokines

INTRODUCTION

Common variable immunodeficiency (CVID) comprises a group of heterogeneous disorders characterized by impaired antibody production (1, 2). It is the most common clinically symptomatic primary antibody disorder (prevalence: approximately 1:50.000 to 1:25.000) (3). CVID patients show also deregulation in the secretion of IL-2, IL- 4, IL-10, and IFN-γ by T cells (4). Adipose tissue is a source of adipokines involved in the pathogenesis and progression of metabolic and immune disorders and consequently plays a pivotal role in the control of metabolism and immunity (5). Adiponectin, that is produced by mature adipocytes, exerts beneficial effects on such cellular processes as energy metabolism, insulin sensitivity and inflammation (6). In particular, adiponectin levels are decreased in the metabolic diseases obesity (5, 6) and type 2-diabetes (5–7) but are elevated in classic chronic inflammatory/autoimmune diseases, such as asthma and chronic obstructive pulmonary disease (COPD) (8–10), multiple sclerosis and systemic lupus erythematosus (11, 12).

Adiponectin is a 244 amino acid monomer with a molecular weight of approximately 26 kDa. It is present in the circulation and accounts for up to 0.05% of total serum protein (13). It circulates as three oligomeric isoforms that differ in molecular weight: low molecular weight (LMW) trimers, medium molecular weight (MMW) hexamers and high molecular weight (HMW) multimers (13). The latter have been correlated with the most significant biological activities of adiponectin (13).

Adiponectin acts mainly through two receptors: AdipoR1 and AdipoR2 (14); a third non-signaling receptor has also been identified, T-cadherin (15, 16). AdipoRs are expressed in most tissues and cell lines including cells of the immune system, i.e., monocytes, B cells and NK cells, whereas they are barely expressed on T cells (17). AdipoR1 and AdipoR2 differ in both localization and binding affinity for adiponectin. Indeed, AdipoR1 is mainly expressed in skeletal muscle and binds globular adiponectin while AdipoR2 is mainly expressed in liver and engages the full-length adiponectin (14). Adiponectin negatively regulates lymphocyte functions (17). T-cadherin (also known as CDH13, cadherin 13, and H-cadherin) is abundantly expressed in injured vascular endothelial and smooth muscle cells in atherosclerotic regions (15). It is a receptor for the hexameric and high-molecular-weight species of adiponectin but not for the trimeric or globular species. Whether T-cadherin mediates signaling pathways is still controversial, but it is plausible that it serves as a reservoir of adiponectin (16).

Interest in the role of T-cadherin in human malignancies has recently increased consequent to the finding that it is down-regulated in several types of cancer (15) and that it regulates the progression of malignancies by modulating tumor cell proliferation and migration (16). Adiponectin has recently been found to be a modulator of the immune system that acts by inducing the secretion of the anti-inflammatory cytokines Interleukin (IL)-10 and Interleukin 1 Receptor Antagonist (IL-1RA), and by down-regulating the pro-inflammatory cytokines TNF-α and IL-6 (9, 18).

We recently demonstrated that adiponectin and in particular its HMW oligomers play an immunomodulatory role in CVID (19). In fact, we found that adiponectin levels are decreased, and correlated to IgA levels and associated with CVID phenotypes. In addition, adiponectin and HMW levels quickly and dramatically increased after the first Ig infusion in treatment-naïve CVID patients (19). In the attempt to shed further light on the role of adiponectin in CVID, we analyzed the expression profile of AdipoR1, AdipoR2 and T-cadherin on peripheral blood mononuclear cells (PBMC) from 18 treatment-naïve CVID patients, before and 24 h after the first Ig infusion. In addition, since cytokines are involved in the immunomodulation of CVID, we measured the serum expression of adiponectin, leptin, IL-2, IL-6, IL-10, TNF-α, and IFN-γ in 24 CVID maintenance patients, in 18 treatment-naïve CVID patients (before and after the first Ig infusion) and in 28 healthy controls.

MATERIALS AND METHODS

Recruitment of Subjects

Twenty-four CVID patients on maintenance treatment with Ig (12 men, 12 women) and 18 (10 men and 8 women) treatment-naïve patients, diagnosed according to the European Society for Immunodeficiencies (2), were recruited by the Division of Allergy and Clinical Immunology of the Department of Translational Medical Sciences, University of Naples "Federico II." As controls, we recruited 28 age-, body weight-, and body mass index-matched healthy volunteers from the staff of CEINGE-Biotecnologie Avanzate, Naples. Furthermore, T cell count and B cell subsets and the response to pneumococcal polysaccharide antigens were also measured data on serum Ig levels T cell count and B cell subsets at diagnosis, and clinical history were retrospectively retrieved from the medical files of CVID patients (19).

CVID maintenance patients received continuous Ig replacement therapy (0.4 g/kg/month) at intervals of 3 weeks to maintain Ig levels above 600 mg/dl (768 ± 87 mg/dl). There were no familial cases of CVID in the control group. Treatment-naïve patients received intravenous Ig immunomodulating therapy at a dose of 0.4 g/kg. The research protocol was approved by the Ethics Committee of the School of Medicine, University of Naples "Federico II" and was conducted in accordance with the principles of the Helsinki II Declaration. Written informed consent was obtained from all participants.

Anthropometric and Biochemical Investigations

The height and weight of the patients were measured using standard techniques and the body mass index was calculated as body weight (kg)/height^2 (m^2). Blood samples (5 ml) were taken after 12 h of fasting from maintenance patients, and from treatment-naïve CVID patients before the first Ig replacement therapy (0.4 g/kg) and 24 h after. Serum samples were immediately centrifuged and aliquots were stored at −20°C. The levels of IgG, IgA, IgM, total cholesterol, HDL, and LDL cholesterol, triglycerides, glucose, total proteins, iron, fibrinogen, C reactive protein (CRP) and erythrocyte sedimentation rate (ESR) were determined in all patients with standard enzymatic methods (Hitachi Modular, Roche, Mannheim, Germany).

Measurement of Adiponectin and Leptin

Serum concentrations of adiponectin and leptin were evaluated in 18 naïve CVID patients before and 24 h after the first Ig infusion, in the 24 CVID patients on maintenance therapy and in the 28 healthy controls. The concentration of total adiponectin was measured by enzyme-linked immunosorbent assay (ELISA) as previously reported (20). Leptin levels were measured using an ELISA commercial kit (Elabscience, Houston, Texas, USA).

Assessment of Adiponectin Receptor Expression on Peripheral Blood Mononuclear Cells by Flow Cytometry

Leukocyte adiponectin receptor expression (AdipoR1, AdipoR2, and T cadherin) was evaluated in 18 treatment-naïve CVID patients before and after the first administration of Ig. PBMC were stained with the specific antibodies for 30 min at 4°C. Subsequently, samples were labeled with the relevant secondary conjugated antibodies for 30 min at 4°C. Isotype controls and secondary only conditions served as negative controls. Rabbit anti-human AdipoR1 (357–375) and AdipoR2 (374–386) antibodies (Phoenix Pharmaceuticals, Karlsruhe, Germany) were used at 5 μg/ml and detected using 8 μg/ml goat-anti rabbit Alexa 488 secondary antibody (Life Technologies, Milan, Italy). Gating to measure the expression of AdipoR1 and AdipoR2 on PBMC and B cells was based on the isotype control. Isotype control frequencies were subtracted from the AdipoR1 and AdipoR2 frequencies in each subject. The following antibodies were used to stain human PBMC: CD4-FITC (1:50) (OKT-4), CD3-PerCp-Cy5.5 (1:50) (OKT3), CD19-PECy7 (1:50) (HIB19), CD8-Pacific Blue (1:50) (OKT8), CD56-PE (1:50) (MEM188) (all from E-bioscience, Hatfield, UK), CD4-Pacific orange (1:10) (clone S3.5) (Life Technologies, Milan, Italy) and CD45RO-APC (1:20) (UCHL1) (BD Bioscience, Oxford, UK), α4β1-PE (1:100) (P5D2), αLβ2-FITC (1:100) (212701), DP-2-FITC (1:10) (301108) (R&D Systems, Abingdon, UK.), CXCR3-PE (1:50) (2Ar1) (VWR International PBI S.r.l., Milano, Italy). B cell subsets were labeled using CD19-PerCp-Vio700 (1:30) (LT19), IgM-PE (1:30) (PJ2-22H3), IgD-APC (1:60) (IgD26), CD38-FTIC (1:150) (IB6), and CD27-APC-Vio-770 (1:10) (M-T271) (all from Miltenyi Biotec, Bergisch Gladbach, Germany).

Measurement of Cytokine Levels

The levels of 8 cytokine species (IL-2, IL-4, IL-6, IL-8, IL-10. INFγ, TNFα, GM-CSF) were measured in the serum of the 18 treatment-naïve CVID patients before and 24 h after the first Ig infusion, in the 24 maintenance therapy CVID patients and in 28 healthy controls using a commercially available kit (Bio-Plex Pro™ Human Cytokine 8-plex Assay, Hercules, CA, USA). The assay was performed according to the manufacturer's instructions and the concentrations of cytokines were calculated by comparing reads with a 5-parameter logistic standard curve using a Bioplex-200 instrument (Bio-Rad, Hercules, CA, USA).

Statistical Analysis

Statistical significance was established at $p < 0.05$. Bonferroni and Student's t-tests were used to compare the means of biochemical parameters. Analysis of variance (ANOVA) and the Bonferroni t-test were used to compare mean cytokine levels.

RESULTS

Anthropometric and Biochemical Features of CVID Patients

The anthropometric and biochemical characteristics of the 24 CVID patients on maintenance therapy, and the 28 healthy controls are reported in **Table 1**. The levels of total cholesterol, total proteins and iron were lower in patients than in controls ($p < 0.03$). The results of the ELISA test confirmed the lower total adiponectin levels in CVID patients vs. control subjects ($p = 0.03$), and moreover show that total adiponectin levels increased in treatment-naïve patients 24 h after the first Ig replacement treatment ($p = 0.007$). **Table 2** shows the characteristics of the 18 treatment-naïve CVID patients before and 24 h after the first Ig replacement.

Leptin Concentrations in CVID Patients

To verify the specificity of adiponectin modulation in CVID, we investigated the involvement of leptin, which is one of the most pivotal cytokines produced by adipose tissue. First, to explore whether the levels of leptin are modulated by Ig replacement therapy, we measured their levels in treatment-naïve CVID patients before and 24 h after the first Ig replacement therapy. Interestingly, unlike adiponectin, leptin levels were not affected by Ig infusion (**Table 2**). Accordingly, leptin concentrations did not differ between CVID patients on maintenance therapy and controls (**Table 1**).

Figure 1 shows adiponectin and leptin levels and the adiponectin/leptin ratio in treatment-naïve CVID patients before and 24 h after the first Ig replacement therapy vs. healthy

TABLE 1 | Anthropometric and biochemical features of CIVD patients on maintenance therapy, and in treatment-naïve patients and controls.

	Controls	Maintenance therapy patients	*p-value*	Naive patients n. 18	*p-value*
Sex M/F	14/14	12/12		10/8	
Age (years)	42.67 (15)	45.29 (14.86)	0.53	41.44 (16.18)	0.42
Body Mass Index (kg/m^2)	24.36 (2.74)	25.19 (4.45)	0.45	24.51 (4.47)	0.65
Total Cholesterol (mg/dl)	199.88 (43.17)	161.41 (41.21)	**0.002**	158.37 (28.33)	0.87
Triglycerides (mg/dl)	95.56 (45.25)	95.16 (35.80)	0.97	94.66 (56.52)	0.97
Glycemia (mg/dl)	87.29 (13.86)	80.29 (15.31)	0.09	82.06 (10.79)	0.69
IgG (mg/dl)	–	224.79 (97.56)	–	2.36 (1.85)	**5.47^{-12}**
IgA (mg/dl)	–	12.41 (13.99)	–	0.11 (0.13)	**0.0006**
IgM (mg/dl)	–	23.75 (47.88)	–	0.31 (0.38)	0.07
Total proteins (mg/dl)	7.3 (0.62)	6.48 (0.59)	**0.001**	6.01 (0.54)	
Iron (μg/dl)	95.59 (34)	68.79 (34.12)	**0.01**	55.75 (26.04)	0.20
Fibrinogen (mg/dl)	–	331.54 (99.66)	–	301.81 (66.44)	0.30
C reactive protein (mg/dl)	–	0.678 (0.78)	–	2.21 (2.87)	**0.02**
ESR (mm)	–	10.16 (9.75)	–	8.4 (4.83)	0.59
Adiponectin (μg/ml)	20.17 (8.74)	15.96 (3.63)	**0.03**	6.53 (6.19)	**2.55^{-07}**
Leptin (ng/ml)	9.49 (3.59)	8.38 (3.75)	0.28	8.32 (3.29)	0.95

Data are expressed as mean (sd).
Statistically relevant values are reported in bold.

TABLE 2 | Anthropometric and biochemical features of treatment-naïve CVID patients before and 24 h after the first Ig infusion.

	Naïve patients n.18	Naïve patients—24 h post Ig infusion	*p-value*
Sex M/F	10/8	–	–
Age (years)	41.44 (16.18)	–	–
Body Mass Index (kg/m^2)	24.51 (4.47)	–	–
Total Cholesterol (mg/dl)	158.37 (28.33)	–	–
Triglycerides (mg/dl)	94.66 (56.52)	–	–
Glycemia (mg/dl)	82.06 (10.79)	–	–
IgG (mg/dl)	2.36 (1.85)	7.99 (2.83)	**0.54^{-8}**
IgA (mg/dl)	0.11 (0.13)	0.12 (0.15)	0.78
IgM (mg/dl)	0.31 (0.38)	0.33 (0.35)	0.87
Total proteins (g/dl)	6.01 (0.54)	–	–
Iron (μg/dl)	55.75 (26.04)	–	–
Fibrinogen (mg/dl)	301.81 (66.44)	–	–
C reactive protein (mg/dl)	2.21 (2.87)	–	–
ESR (mm)	8.4 (4.83)	–	–
Adiponectin (μg/ml)	6.53 (6.19)	13.93 (9.22)	**0.007**
Leptin (ng/ml)	8.32 (3.29)	9.01 (4.88)	0.62

Data are expressed as mean (sd).
Statistically relevant values are reported in bold.

controls. The adiponectin-leptin ratio was consistently lower in treatment-naïve patients than in controls. On the contrary, the adiponectin-leptin ratio increased 24 h after the first Ig replacement infusion (**Figure 1**). Given that Ig infusion did not affect leptin levels, we conclude that this difference in ratio values is attributable to variations in adiponectin expression.

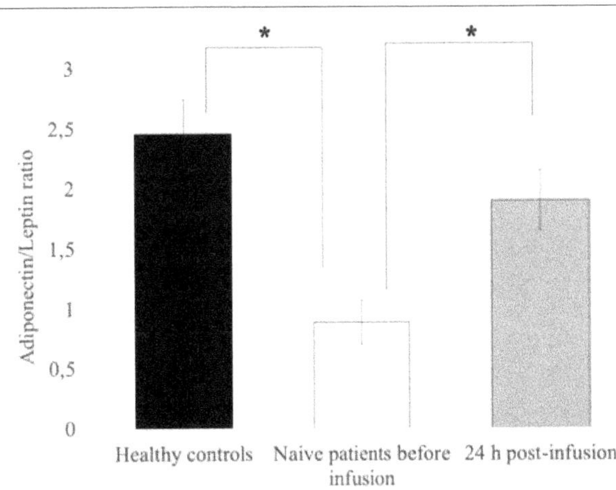

FIGURE 1 | Leptin levels are comparable in controls and patients, and are unchanged after the first Ig infusion. The adiponectin-leptin ratio in patients on maintenance therapy and in 16 treatment-naïve CVID patients before and 24 h after the first Ig infusion. Data represent the mean (±standard deviation of three independent experiments, each performed in triplicate. $^*p \leq 0.05$.

AdipoR1, AdipoR2, and T-Cadherin Expression on PBMC

As shown in **Figure 2**, flow cytometry demonstrated that the expression (in terms of the percentage of positive cells) of AdipoR1 and AdipoR2 on the surface of CD19+ B cells, CD19+CD27+ activated B cells, CD3-CD56+ NK cells, and CD14+ monocytes (**Figures 2A,B**) was higher in treatment-naïve CVID patients than in healthy controls. Notably, AdipoR1 expression on CD19+ B cells, CD3− CD56+NK cells and CD14+ monocytes in CVID patients was significantly higher

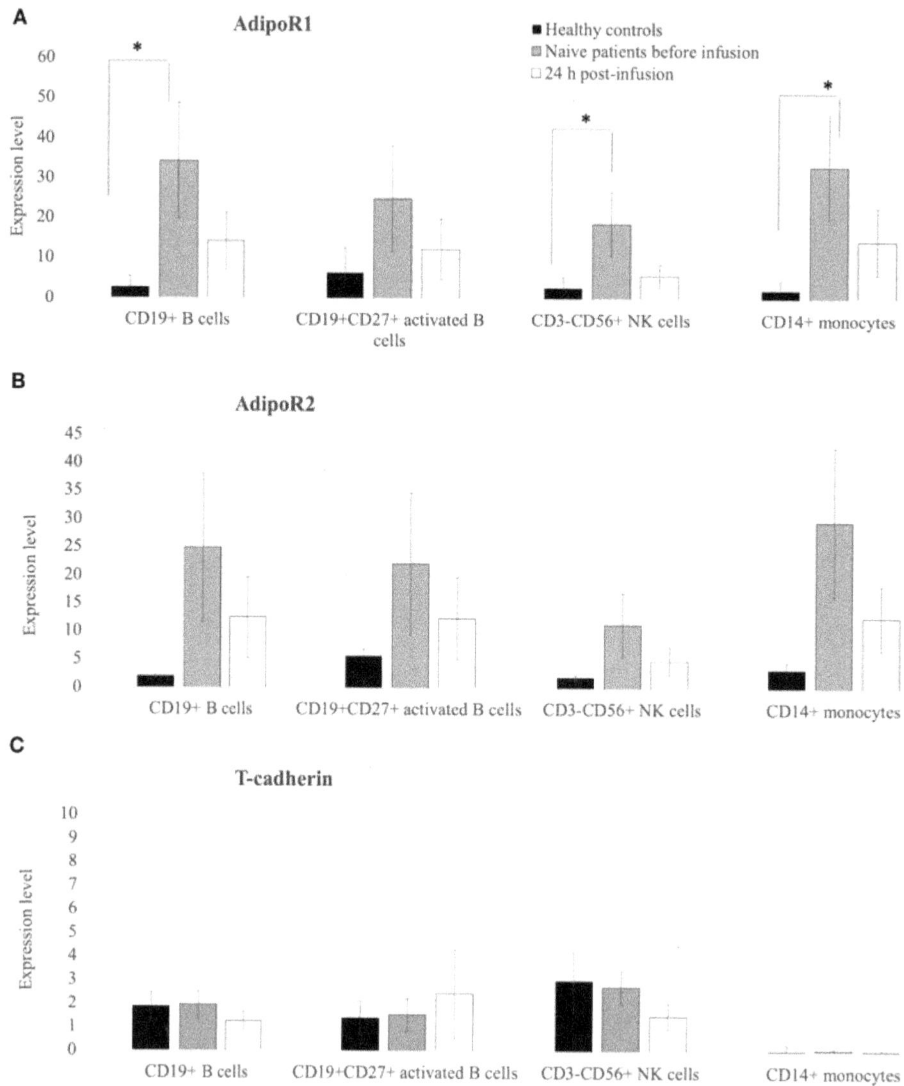

FIGURE 2 | AdipoR1 and AdipoR2 expression was higher in lymphocyte subpopulations of treatment-naïve CVID patients than in those of healthy controls. Their expression decreases 24 h post the first Ig replacement therapy. **(A–C)** Percentage of AdipoR1- AdipoR2- and T-cadherin-positive cells on the lymphocyte subpopulations (CD19+ B cells, CD19+CD27+ B-activated cells, CD3–CD56+ NK lymphocytes and CD14+ monocytes) from healthy controls and treatment-naïve CVID patients before and 24 h after the first Ig infusion. Data obtained from two independent experiments performed by flow-cytometry in triplicate. $^{*}p \leq 0.05$.

than in healthy controls whereas AdipR1 expression on CD27+ B cells did not differ significantly from controls (**Figure 2A**). AdipoR2 expression on CD19+ B cells, CD– CD56+NK, CD14+ monocytes and CD27+ B cells was higher in CVID treatment-naïve patients than in controls although the difference was not significant (**Figure 2B**).

Interestingly, 24 h after the first Ig replacement therapy, the levels of both AdipoR1 and 2 decreased on the surface of CD19+B cells, CD19+CD27+activated B cells, CD3–CD56+ NK cells, and CD14+ monocytes. The expression of T-cadherin on activated B cells, NK or monocytes did not differ between patients and controls after the first Ig replacement therapy (**Figure 2C**). We also collected blood samples from 5 patients and analyzed AdipoRs expression in PBMC at 7, 14, and 21 days post-infusion and found that the data did not differ among the various time points examined (**Supplementary Figure 1**). The expression of AdipoR1, 2, and T-cadherin on T-lymphocytes was barely detectable (data not shown).

The Cytokine Profile in Maintenance Therapy CVID Patients

As shown in **Figure 3**, the levels of IL-6, IL-8, and TNF-α were significantly higher in the two treatment groups than in controls, and IL-10 levels were significantly lower in patients than in controls, while the expression of IL-2, IL-4, and INF-γ did not differ significantly between the two groups of patients (maintenance and naïve) and controls. The levels of IL-6, IL-8, and TNF-α in treatment naïve patients were comparable

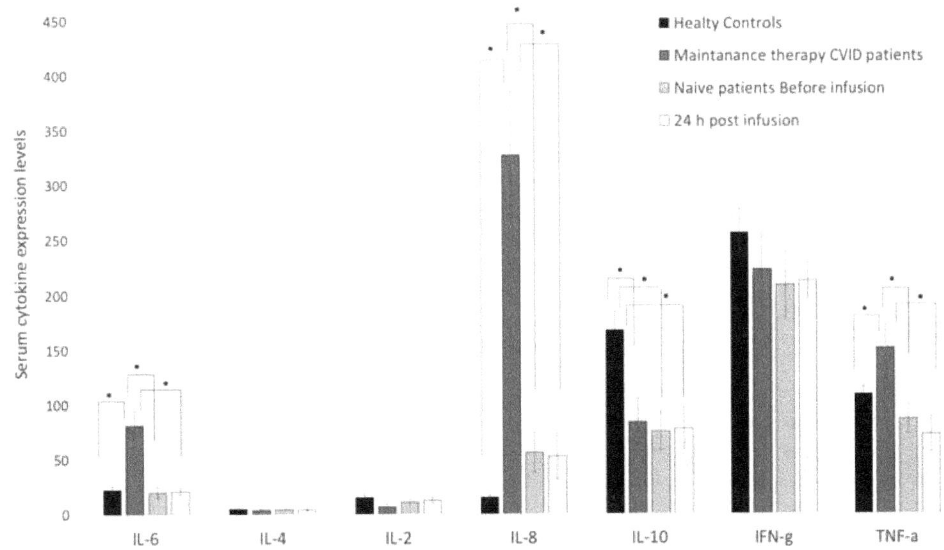

FIGURE 3 | Serum levels of IL-6, IL-8 and TNF-α were higher in CVID patients than in healthy controls. Their levels are barely modified by the replacement therapy. ELISA assay was performed to quantify serum levels of cytokines in CVID patients and healthy controls. IL-6, IL-4, IL-2, IL-8, IL-10, INFγ, and TNF-α were quantified in sera from healthy controls, maintenance CVID patients, and treatment-naïve patients before and 24 h after the first Ig replacement therapy. Data obtained from two independent experiments performed in triplicate $^{*}p \leq 0.05$.

to those of healthy controls. The first infusion of Ig barely modified cytokine levels after 24 h or 7, 14, and 21 days later (**Supplementary Figure 2**). IL-10 serum levels were significantly lower in naïve patients than in controls (**Figure 3**).

DISCUSSION

We recently reported that the expression of total adiponectin and its HMW oligomers is decreased in patients with CVID, that it is associated with CVID activity and that it is correlated to the first Ig infusion (19). Here we demonstrate that the expression of AdipoR1 and AdipoR2 in PBMCs from CVID patients differs from that of controls, and changes after the first Ig infusion. The specificity of adiponectin involvement in CVID is supported by the absence of changes in leptin expression and in the levels of various cytokines tested. Taken together these results suggest that the adiponectin system plays a role in CVID.

The expression of AdipoR1 and AdipoR2 has been studied on B lymphocytes, monocytes, and NK cells but not on T lymphocytes (21). AdipoR1 and AdipoR2 expression was found to be decreased on the surface of B lymphocytes of patients with autoimmune disorders, namely, rheumatoid arthritis and type 1 diabetes (22). Chimen et al. reported an inverse association between adiponectin serum levels and AdipoR expression on immune cells (23). Accordingly, in an earlier study we found that low levels of adiponectin in CVID are accompanied by up-regulation of AdipoR1 and AdipoR2 and, *vice versa*, that high serum levels of adiponectin in autoimmune disorders result in the down-regulation of AdipoR1 and AdipoR2 (5). In addition, our findings suggest that the immune regulation functions of adiponectin in CVID are specifically related to AdipoR1 and 2 but not to T-cadherin signaling.

While T-cadherin expression has been associated with endothelial injuries and cancer progression (24, 25), to our knowledge, there are no data about the expression of T-cadherin on immune cells. The absence of changes in T-cadherin expression on the PBMC of our patients suggests that, in CVID, this receptor is not involved in the immune functions of adiponectin.

Another interesting result of our study concerns the changes in AdipoR1 and AdipoR2 expression, which, similar to the changes in adiponectin levels, were partially restored to "normal" levels after the first Ig treatment. This novel finding strengthens the concept that the adiponectin system plays a pre-eminent role in CVID. To assess the specificity of adiponectin involvement in CVID we looked at leptin. The latter cytokine is produced by adipose tissue, and is reported to play a key role in immunity (26, 27). We found that leptin expression did not differ between maintenance patients and controls, nor before and after the first Ig treatment in treatment naïve CVID patients. In the only study conducted thus far on leptin in CVID, leptin expression was not associated to the disease (28).

Various studies have been devoted to the production of cytokines in CVID, albeit with conflicting results (4, 29, 30). In the present study we found (i) that IL-6, IL-8 and TNF-α levels were higher, (ii) that L-10 levels were lower, and (iii) that IL-2, IL-4, and INF-γ were not differently expressed in patients vs. controls. Moreover, we found that in treatment-naïve patients, the levels of most cytokines were comparable to those of healthy controls with the exception of IL-10, the levels of which were significantly lower in treatment-naïve patients than in controls (31, 32). The different behavior between cytokine levels in maintenance vs. absence of modifications in treatment-naïve patients is probably related to the patient's condition (i.e., infections, cancer, etc.). Indeed, changes in the cytokine expression are evident only after several Ig administrations, as observed in patients on maintenance therapy. IL-6 and IL-8 are mainly produced and secreted by macrophages thereby enhancing the proliferation and the differentiation of B cells into memory or plasma cells (33, 34), while IL-2 and IL-4 are produced in most part by T lymphocytes (35). The up-regulation of IL-6 and IL-8 in CVID maintenance therapy may indicate a primary involvement of macrophages instead of T lymphocytes. We believe that the continuous infusion of Ig might activate Th2 and macrophages, thereby resulting in the release of IL-6 and IL-8. Elevation of IL- 6 and IL-8 was reported in CVID patients by Varzaneh et al. (4) and by Ibanez et al. (36). In addition, persistent activation of macrophages, which are the major sources of IL6 and IL8, was seen in CVID patients on maintenance therapy (37).

IL-10 serum levels are closely related to those of IL-2 and IL-4, which are low in naïve patients due to the alteration of the immune system typical of CVID patients (38). In fact, impaired secretion of IL-10 by the T-cells of CVID patients has been widely reported (32, 39, 40).

In conclusion, this is the first study to demonstrate that adiponectin receptors are differentially expressed on PBMC from CVID patients and that their expression is partially restored after the first Ig infusion. The peculiarity and relevance of the role played by adiponectin in CVID is confirmed by the finding that leptin and the other cytokines tested herein did not change after the first Ig infusion in treatment-naïve CVID patients. Further studies are needed to better understand the molecular mechanisms underlying the effects exerted by adiponectin in the pathogenesis of CVID.

AUTHOR CONTRIBUTIONS

RP, EN, and MM performed the experiments. RP, AD, and EN wrote the manuscript. AP, AG, and GS recruited the patients and samples. FP and AS performed flow-cytometry experiments. GS and AD conceived the study and revised and approved the final version of the manuscript.

ACKNOWLEDGMENTS

We thank Jean Ann Gilder (Scientific Communication srl., Naples, Italy) for revising and editing the text.

REFERENCES

1. Tam JS, Routes JM. Common variable immunodeficiency. *Am J Rhinol Allergy.* (2013) 4:260–5. doi: 10.2500/ajra.2013.27.3899
2. Yazdani R, Habibi S, Sharifi L, Azizi G, Abolhassani H, Olbrich P, et al. Common variable immunodeficiency: epidemiology, pathogenesis, clinical manifestations, diagnosis, classification and management. *J Investig Allergol Clin Immunol.* (2019) doi: 10.18176/jiaci.0388. [Epub ahead of print].
3. Emmaneel A, Bogaert DJ, Van Gassen S, Tavernier SJ, Dullaers M, Haerynck F, et al. A computational pipeline for the diagnosis of CVID patients. *Front Immunol.* (2019) 10:2009. doi: 10.3389/fimmu.2019.02009
4. Varzaneh FN, Keller B, Unger S, Aghamohammadi A, Warnatz K, Rezaei N. Cytokines in common variable immunodeficiency as signs of immune dysregulation and potential therapeutic targets - a review of the current knowledge. *J Clin Immunol.* (2014) 5:524–43. doi: 10.1007/s10875-014-0053-0
5. Francisco V, Ruiz-Fernández C, Pino J, Mera A, González-Gay MA, Gómez R, et al. Adipokines: linking metabolic syndrome, the immune system, and arthritic diseases. *Biochem Pharmacol.* (2019) 165:196–206. doi: 10.1016/j.bcp.2019.03.030
6. Achari AE, Jain SK. Adiponectin, a therapeutic target for obesity, diabetes, and endothelial dysfunction. *Int J Mol Sci.* (2017) 18:6. doi: 10.3390/ijms18061321
7. Yosaee S, Khodadost M, Esteghamati A, Speakman JR, Djafarian K, Bitarafan V, et al. Adiponectin: an indicator for metabolic syndrome. *Iran J Public Health.* (2019) 6:1106–15.
8. Saeed E, Amin X, Jacob G. The multifaceted and controversial immunometabolic actions of adiponectin. *Cell Press.* (2014) 25:9. doi: 10.1016/j.tem.2014.06.001
9. Nigro E, Scudiero O, Sarnataro D, Mazzarella G, Sofia M, Bianco A, et al. Adiponectin affects lung epithelial A549 cell viability counteracting TNFα and IL-1ß toxicity through AdipoR1. *Int J Biochem Cell Biol.* (2013) 6:1145–53. doi: 10.1016/j.biocel.2013.03.003
10. Bianco A, Nigro E, Monaco ML, Matera MG, Scudiero O, Mazzarella G, et al. The burden of obesity in asthma and COPD: role of adiponectin. *Pulm Pharmacol Ther.* (2017) 43:20–5. doi: 10.1016/j.pupt.2017.01.004
11. Signoriello E, Lus G, Polito R, Casertano S, Scudiero O, Coletta M, et al. Adiponectin profile at baseline is correlated to progression and severity of multiple sclerosis. *Eur J Neurol.* (2019) 2:348–55. doi: 10.1111/ene.13822
12. Zhang TP, Zhao YL, Li XM, Wu CH, Pan HF, Ye DQ. Altered mRNA expression levels of vaspin and adiponectin in peripheral blood mononuclear cells of systemic lupus erythematosus patients. *Clin Exp Rheumatol.* (2019) 3:458–64.
13. Waki H, Yamauchi T, Kamon J, Ito Y, Uchida S, Kita S, et al. Impaired multimerization of human adiponectin mutants associated with diabetes. Molecular structure and multimer formation of adiponectin. *J Biol Chem.* (2003) 41:40352–63. doi: 10.1074/jbc.M300365200
14. Yamauchi T, Iwabu M, Okada-Iwabu M, Kadowaki T. Adiponectin receptors: a review of their structure, function and how they work. *Best Pract Res Clin Endocrinol Metab.* (2014) 28:15–23. doi: 10.1016/j.beem.2013.09.003
15. Takeuchi T, Adachi Y, Ohtsuki Y, Furihata M. Adiponectin receptors, with special focus on the role of the third receptor, T-cadherin, in vascular disease. *Med Mol Morphol.* (2007) 3:115–20. doi: 10.1007/s00795-007-0364-9
16. Hug C, Wang J, Ahmad NS, Bogan JS, Tsao TS, Lodish HF. T-cadherin is a receptor for hexameric and high-molecular-weight forms of Acrp30/adiponectin. *Proc Natl Acad Sci USA.* (2004) 101:10308–13. doi: 10.1073/pnas.0403382101
17. Luo Y, Liu M. Adiponectin: a versatile player of innate immunity. *J Mol Cell Biol.* (2016) 2: 120–8. doi: 10.1093/jmcb/mjw012
18. He Y, Lul L, Wei X, Jin D, Qien T, Yu A, et al. The multimerization and secretion of adiponectin are regulated by TNF-alpha. *Endocrine.* (2016) 3:456–68. doi: 10.1007/s12020-015-0741-4
19. Pecoraro A, Nigro E, Polito R, Monaco ML, Scudiero O, Mormile I, et al. Total and high molecular weight adiponectin expression is decreased in patients with common variable immunodeficiency: correlation with Ig

replacement therapy. *Front Immunol.* (2017) 8:895. doi: 10.3389/fimmu.2017.00895

20. Lacedonia D, Nigro E, Matera MG, Scudiero O, Monaco ML, Polito R, et al. Evaluation of adiponectin profile in Italian patients affected by obstructive sleep apnea syndrome. *Pulm Pharmacol Ther.* (2016) 40:104–8. doi: 10.1016/j.pupt.2016.07.008
21. Pang TT, Narendran P. The distribution of adiponectin receptors on human peripheral blood mononuclear cells. immunology of diabetes. *Ann NY Acad Sci.* (2008) 1150:143–5. doi: 10.1196/annals.1447.021
22. Mandal P, Pratt BT, Barnes M, McMullen MR, Nagy LE. Molecular mechanism for adiponectin-dependent M2 macrophage polarization: link between the metabolic and innate immune activity of full-length adiponectin. *J Biol Chem.* (2011) 15:13460–9. doi: 10.1074/jbc.M110.204644
23. Chimen M, McGettrick HM, Apta B, Kuravi SJ, Yates CM, Kennedy A, et al. Homeostatic regulation of T cell trafficking by a B cell-derived peptide is impaired in autoimmune and chronic inflammatory disease. *Nat Med.* (2015) 5:467–75. doi: 10.1038/nm.3842
24. Ren JZ, Huo JR. Correlation between T-cadherin gene expression and aberrant methylation of T-cadherin promoter in human colon carcinoma cells. *Med Oncol.* (2012) 29:915–18. doi: 10.1007/s12032-011-9836-9
25. Ye M, Huang T, Li J, Zhou C, Yang P, Ni C, et al. Role of CDH13 promoter methylation in the carcinogenesis, progression and prognosis of colorectal cancer: a systematic meta-analysis under PRISMA guidelines. *Medicine.* (2017) 96:e5956. doi: 10.1097/MD.0000000000005956
26. Procaccini C, Jirillo E, Matarese G. Leptin as an immunomodulator. *Mol Aspects Med.* (2012) 1:35–45. doi: 10.1016/j.mam.2011.10.012
27. Fantuzzi G, Faggioni R. Leptin in the regulation of immunity, inflammation, and hematopoiesis. *J Leukoc Biol.* (2000) 68:437–46. doi: 10.1189/jlb.68.4.437
28. Goldberg AC, Eliaschewitz FG, Montor WR, Baracho GV, Errante PR, Callero MA, et al. Exogenous leptin restores *in vitro* T cell proliferation and cytokine synthesis in patients with common variable immunodeficiency syndrome. *Clin Immunol.* (2005) 2:147–53. doi: 10.1016/j.clim.2004.09.002
29. Hel Z, Huijbregts RPH, Xu J, Nechvatalova J, Vlkova M, Litzman J. Altered serum cytokine signature in common variable immunodeficiency. *J Clin Immunol.* (2014) 8:971–8. doi: 10.1007/s10875-014-0099-z
30. Zhang JM, An J. Cytokines, Inflammation and Pain. *Int Anesthesiol Clin.* (2007) 2:27–37. doi: 10.1097/AIA.0b013e318034194e
31. Barsotti NS, Almeida RR, Costa PR, Barros MT, Kalil J, Kokron CM. IL-10-producing regulatory B cells are decreased in patients with common variable immunodeficiency. *PLoS ONE.* (2016) 3:e0151761. doi: 10.1371/journal.pone.0151761
32. Holm AM, Aukrust P, Aandahl EM, Müller F, Taskén K, Frøland SS. Impaired secretion of IL-10 by T cells from patients with common variable immunodeficiency–involvement of protein kinase A type I. *J Immunol.* (2003) 11:5772–7. doi: 10.4049/jimmunol.170.11.5772
33. Jego G, Bataille R, Pellat-Deceunynck C. Interleukin-6 is a growth factor for nonmalignant human plasmablasts. *Blood.* (2001) 6:1817–22. doi: 10.1182/blood.V97.6.1817
34. Pandolfi F, Paganelli R, Oliva A, Quinti I, Polidori V, Fanales-Belasio E, et al. Increased IL-6 gene expression and production in patients with common variable immunodeficiency. *Clin Exp Immunol.* (1993) 2:239–44. doi: 10.1111/j.1365-2249.1993.tb03386.x
35. Taraldsrud E, Fevang B, Jørgensen SF, Moltu K, Hilden V, Taskén K, et al. Defective IL-4 signaling in T cells defines severe common variable immunodeficiency. *J Autoimmun.* (2017) 81:110–19. doi: 10.1016/j.jaut.2017.04.004
36. Ibáñez C, Suñé P, Fierro A, Rodríguez S, López M, Álvarez A, et al. Effects of Intravenous Immunoglobulins on serum cytokine levels in patients with primary hypogammaglobulinemia. *BioDrugs.* (2005) 19:59–65. doi: 10.2165/00063030-200519010-00007
37. Paquin-Proulx D, Sandberg JK. Persistent immune activation in CVID and the role of IVIg in its suppression. *Front Immunol.* (2014) 5:637. doi: 10.3389/fimmu.2014.00637
38. Mitchell RE, Hassan M, Burton BR, Britton G, Hill EV, Verhagen J, et al. IL-4 enhances IL-10 production in Th1 cells: implications for Th1 and Th2 regulation. *Sci Rep.* (2017) 12:11315. doi: 10.1038/s41598-017-11803-y
39. Zhou Z, Huang R, Danon M, Mayer L, Cunningham-Rundles C. IL-10 production in common variable immunodeficiency. *Clin Immunol Immunopathol.* (1998) 86:298–304. doi: 10.1006/clin.1997.4483
40. Azizi G, Bagheri Y, Yazdani R, Zaki-Dizaji M, Jamee M, Jadidi-Niaragh F, et al. The profile of IL-4, IL-5, IL-10 and GATA3 in patients with LRBA deficiency and CVID with no known monogenic disease: association with disease severity. *Allergol Immunopathol.* (2019) 47:172–8. doi: 10.1016/j.aller.2018.06.003

13

Non-parametric Heat Map Representation of Flow Cytometry Data: Identifying Cellular Changes Associated with Genetic Immunodeficiency Disorders

*Julia I. Ellyard[1,2], Robert Tunningley[1,2], Ayla May Lorenzo[1,2], Simon H. Jiang[1,2,3], Amelia Cook[1,2], Rochna Chand[1,2,4], Dipti Talaulikar[5], Ann-Maree Hatch[2], Anastasia Wilson[2], Carola G. Vinuesa[1,2], Matthew C. Cook[1,2,4] and David A. Fulcher[1,2]**

[1] Department of Immunology and Infectious Diseases, Australian National University, Canberra, ACT, Australia, [2] Centre for Personalised Immunology, John Curtin School of Medical Research, Australian National University, Canberra, ACT, Australia, [3] Department of Nephrology, The Canberra Hospital, Canberra, ACT, Australia, [4] Department of Immunology, The Canberra Hospital, Canberra, ACT, Australia, [5] Department of Hematology, The Canberra Hospital, Canberra, ACT, Australia

***Correspondence:**
David A. Fulcher
david.fulcher@anu.edu.au

Genetic primary immunodeficiency diseases are increasingly recognized, with pathogenic mutations changing the composition of circulating leukocyte subsets measured by flow cytometry (FCM). Discerning changes in multiple subpopulations is challenging, and subtle trends might be missed if traditional reference ranges derived from a control population are applied. We developed an algorithm where centiles were allocated using non-parametric comparison to controls, generating multiparameter heat maps to simultaneously represent all leukocyte subpopulations for inspection of trends within a cohort or segregation with a putative genetic mutation. To illustrate this method, we analyzed patients with Primary Antibody Deficiency (PAD) and kindreds harboring mutations in *TNFRSF13B* (encoding TACI), *CTLA4*, and *CARD11*. In PAD, loss of switched memory B cells (B-SM) was readily demonstrated, but as a continuous, not dichotomous, variable. Expansion of CXCR5+/CD45RA- CD4+ T cells (X5-Th cells) was a prominent feature in PAD, particularly in TACI mutants, and patients with expansion in CD21-lo B cells or transitional B cells were readily apparent. We observed differences between unaffected and affected TACI mutants (increased B cells and CD8+ T-effector memory cells, loss of B-SM cells and non-classical monocytes), cellular signatures that distinguished *CTLA4* haploinsufficiency itself (expansion of plasmablasts, activated CD4+ T cells, regulatory T cells, and X5-Th cells) from its clinical expression (B-cell depletion), and those that were associated with *CARD11* gain-of-function mutation (decreased CD8+ T effector memory cells, B cells, CD21-lo B cells, B-SM cells, and NK cells). Co-efficients of variation exceeded 30% for 36/54 FCM parameters, but by comparing inter-assay variation with disease-related variation, we ranked each parameter in terms of laboratory precision vs. disease variability, identifying X5-Th cells (and derivatives), naïve, activated, and central memory CD8+ T cells, transitional B cells, memory and SM-B cells, plasmablasts, activated CD4 cells, and total T cells as the 10 most useful cellular parameters. Applying these to cluster analysis of our PAD cohort, we could detect subgroups with the potential to reflect underlying genotypes. Heat mapping of normalized FCM data reveals cellular trends missed by standard reference ranges, identifies changes associating with a phenotype or genotype, and could inform hypotheses regarding pathogenesis of genetic immunodeficiency.

Keywords: flow cytometry, immunodeficiency, common variable immunodeficiency, TACI, CTLA4, TNFSF13B, CARD11

INTRODUCTION

Widespread availability of DNA sequencing has uncovered an expanding array of genetic explanations for primary immunodeficiency disorders (PIDs) (1). Causative mutations can change cellular function and affect the balance between protective immunity and immune tolerance, resulting in clinical phenotypes of recurrent infection with or without autoimmunity. Changes in cellular physiology frequently result in quantitative differences in the composition of circulating leukocyte populations, which can be determined using multiparameter flow cytometry (FCM); indeed the power of this technique to measure an increasing array of specific subpopulations has challenged the ability to depict and analyse potentially important and pathogenically relevant cellular changes that might accompany or even identify a disease phenotype or genotype.

Traditionally, quantitative variations in cell subpopulations have been deemed to be abnormal if they vary significantly from a background control population, with the target range calculated based on two standard deviations either side of the mean, or by using 95% confidence intervals if non-parametric in distribution. Whilst stringent, this approach has the potential to miss less extreme but physiologically relevant cellular changes when found consistently in a cohort of patients, defined either by clinical phenotype or genotype; such subtle cellular changes could be more readily identified if all relevant parameters could be visually presented simultaneously, allowing identification of trends that might be considered for subsequent statistical analysis, and analysis in larger cohorts.

We conceived an analysis technique in which FCM data from 51 cellular parameters in an individual patient were compared non-parametrically to corresponding data from controls, generating centiles which could be depicted in heat maps. Heat maps could then be aligned within a kindred or clinical phenotype, allowing identification of consistent cellular trends. Here we demonstrate this technique by analyzing a cohort of patients with PID, including kindreds with known PID-associated mutations. The same technique should be applicable to guiding the search for new potentially pathogenic mutations uncovered in WGS screens.

METHODS

Patient and Control Subjects

The cohort consisted of 77 control subjects and 199 patients with various immunological diagnoses, including autoimmunity (112), primary immunodeficiency conditions (57), oncology (21), neurological disease (5), sarcoidosis (3), and autoinflammatory conditions (1). Control subjects were aged between 20 and 72 years (median 40.5, mean ± SD: 40.8 ± 12.9) and were 64% female. We studied a subset of 22 patients from the primary immunodeficiency group who had primary antibody deficiency (PAD), 19 of whom met IUIS criteria for Common Variable Immunodeficiency (CVID) (2); the remaining 3 had specific antibody deficiency, 1 of whom was on infliximab (**Supplementary Table 1**). All PAD patients were on immunoglobulin replacement therapy and no other members of the PAD cohort were on immunosuppressives. PAD patients were aged between 10 and 72 years (median 36, mean ± SD: 38.3 ± 16.8) and were 55% female. See **Supplementary Table 1** for details of patients reported in **Figures 3–6**.

Written informed consent was obtained as part of the Australian Point Mutation in Systemic Lupus Erythematosus study (APOSLE), the Centre for Personalized Immunology (CPI) program, the Healthy Blood Donors register and the Hematology Research Tissue Bank (The Canberra Hospital, Canberra, Australia). This study was carried out in accordance with the recommendations of the *National Statement on Ethical Conduct in Human Research (2007)*, National Health and Medical Research Council with written informed consent from all subjects. All subjects gave written informed consent in accordance with the Declaration of Helsinki. The protocol was approved by the Sydney Local Health District HREC at Concord Repatriation General Hospital, ACT Health HREC, ACT Hematology Research Tissue Bank Committee and Australian National University HREC.

Cell Surface Staining Approach and Gating

We processed cells collected from the 276 subjects detailed above, many of whom had already undergone Whole Exome or Whole Genome sequencing under HREC-approved protocols, for flow cytometry. Blood was collected into ACD 9 ml collection tubes and processed within 24 h of collection. Peripheral blood mononuclear cells (PBMCs) were purified by layering blood over Ficoll-Paque, resuspended in RPMI, 10% DMSO and FCS, then stored in liquid nitrogen prior to analysis.

Immunophenotyping of PBMCs was performed using 1×10^6 cells for each staining panel. Cells were thawed at 37°C and washed with FACS buffer (PBS/2% bovine serum/0.05% sodium azide). Fc receptors were blocked using Human TruStain FcX (Cat #422302; Biolegend) and dead cells discrimination performed with LD Fixable Dead Cell stain (Cat #L34962; Invitrogen) according to the manufacturer's instructions. PBMCs were stained with four antibody cocktails (**Supplementary Table 2**) enabling identification of 54 cell parameters (**Figure 1**). Samples were fixed with eBioscience

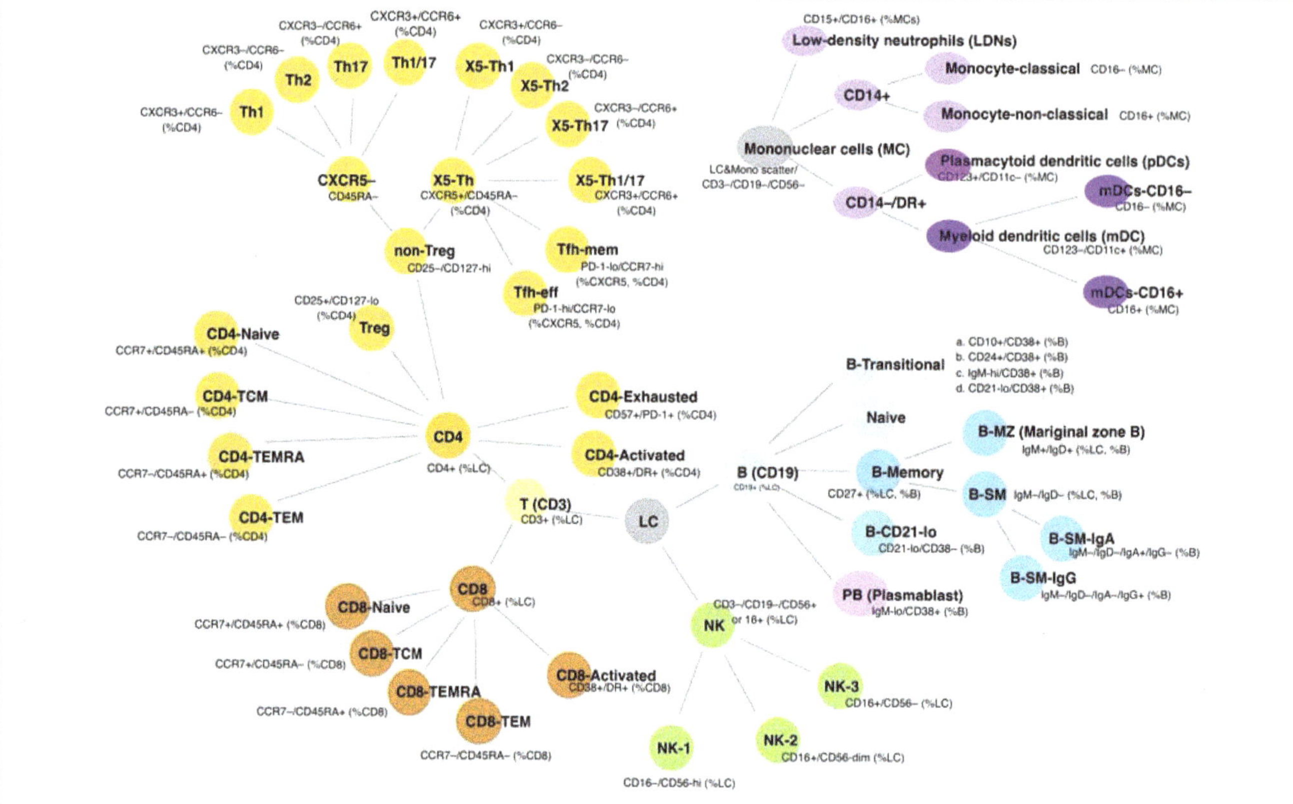

FIGURE 1 | Cellular subpopulations as measured by FCM. Schematic shows the 54 separate cell populations determined using the four antibody panels (see section Methods). Lines show the relationship to parent populations.

FoxP3 Fixation/Permeabilization reagent (Cat #00-5523-00; Invitrogen) according to the manufacturer's protocol. Flow cytometric acquisition was performed using a BD Fortessa FACS analyser at the Microscopy and Cytometry Resource Facility, John Curtin School of Medical Research and data analysis performed in Flowjo (v10; TreeStar). Repeated analysis of stored PBMCs from a single control was included with every FCM run, which allowed experimental variation in each parameter to be measured.

Cell Populations and Methodological Aspects of FCM Analysis

The FCM analysis is shown in **Supplementary Figure 1**; initial gating was on viable singlet cells. Lymphocytes were gated by scatter; for non-lymphocyte populations, a broad leukocyte light scatter gate was used after excluding CD3, CD19, and CD56 expressing cells. Subpopulations were quantitated as a proportion of various parent populations, to generate up to 54 separate parameters per subject. Given varying approaches to defining transitional B cells, four commonly used gating strategies were initially applied: CD38+/CD10+, CD38+/CD24+, CD38+/IgM-hi, and CD38+/CD21-lo (**Figure 1** and **Supplementary Figure 1**), although the latter strategy was abandoned because of its inclusion of circulating plasmablasts. Since the three remaining subsets were highly correlated (**Supplementary Figure 2**), we chose to use the CD38+/CD24+ proportion of B cells to represent the transitional cell population, leaving 51 total FCM parameters. NK cells, defined as CD3-/CD19- lymphocytes that expressed either CD16 or CD56, could be divided into three subpopulations (CD16-/CD56-hi, CD16+/CD56-dim, and CD16+/CD56-), and these were arbitrarily designated NK-1, -2, and -3, respectively (**Figure 1** and **Supplementary Figure 1**). In the process of analysis, we found inconsistencies in CD4 T-helper (Th) chemokine receptor staining, such that values were censored when they were unable to clearly delineate four Th cell populations. We also observed that low density neutrophils appeared to accumulate with increasing time between collection and cryopreservation (data not shown).

In attempting to analyse memory T cell populations, we noted that some subjects over-expressed CD45RA, making precise gating impossible; these samples were censored for memory T cell parameters. This notable phenomenon reflects the action of a synonymous C > G variant at nucleotide position 77 in exon 4 (rs17612648) of the Protein tyrosine phosphatase receptor type C gene (*PTPRC*) that encodes the CD45 pan leukocyte receptor, that has previously been shown to interfere with CD45 splicing in T cells (3, 4). The variant allele, occurring in approximately 8% of individuals, acts in a dominant manner to maintain CD45RA expression on T cells following *in vitro* cell activation (5, 6). Although memory cell formation and function is not affected (5), T cells of individuals carrying this allele do not downregulate CD45RA. Since many subjects in our cohort had had genetic sequencing, we were able to identify seven individuals carrying the *PTPRC*^{C77G} allele who had also undergone immunophenotyping. Consistent with previous reports, we observed that all CD4+ and CD8+ T cells in these individuals expressed high levels of CD45RA (**Supplementary Figure 3**). The effect was more pronounced on CD8+ cells than CD4+ T cells, however a true CD45RA− population was not evident in either subset of T cell. Interestingly, we did not identify any CD45RA over-expressors in our healthy controls.

Description of Normalization Algorithm/Software

Spreadsheet data for all FCM cellular populations from the study population were compared with the comparable data generated from controls. Bespoke software was written to analyse each subject parameter and to generate centiles by comparison with controls. To do this, the software sorted control values in ascending order and each one was allocated a centile value. The lowest value was allocated a centile of 1/(n+1), and the highest was 1−[1/(n+1)], where n is the number of values in the control cohort; this approach allowed extreme 'unprecedented' values, namely those which were never found in the control population, to be emphasized (**Figure 2**). The test parameter value was then compared with the sorted control values and attributed the corresponding centile (0–1), with further adjustment based on interpolation between the two neighboring control values. Centiles from each subject were then color coded in two ways: (i) continuously, where color intensity varied with deviation from the median (0.5 = black), values above the median depicted in intensity of red, and values below the median, in intensity of green; and (ii) discontinuously, where color strata represented variation from normal, differentiating the extreme 5, 10, or 25% in each direction; the central 50% of control values were represented as green (**Figure 2**).

Statistics

All comparisons were performed in GraphPad Prism 8.0 for Mac, using Mann-Whitney non-parameteric comparison of non-paired values; *p*-values below 0.05 were considered significant.

Cluster Analysis

To look for clusters of cellular changes within CVID patients, centile data from selected cellular parameters were generated. These data were loaded onto Morpheus (https://software.broadinstitute.org/morpheus/) and hierarchical clustering applied using 1-Pearson correlation.

RESULTS

Non-parametric Heatmapping to Depict Cellular Changes in Patients With Primary Antibody Deficiency

Flow cytometry has an important role in understanding cellular changes in primary antibody deficiency disorders, particularly Common Variable Immunodeficiency (CVID). Sub-classifications have been based on differences in B-cell maturation patterns, the critical parameters including the proportions of total B cells, switched memory B cells (B-SM), CD21-lo B cells (sometimes referred to as "anergic" B cells) and transitional B cells (7, 8). We applied our analysis technique to our cohort of 22 patients with Primary Antibody Deficiency (PAD), 19 of whom met criteria for CVID (**Supplementary Table 1**), using heat mapping with continuous color shading (**Figure 2A**) to visually represent variations in the measured 51 cellular parameters, sorting patients on the

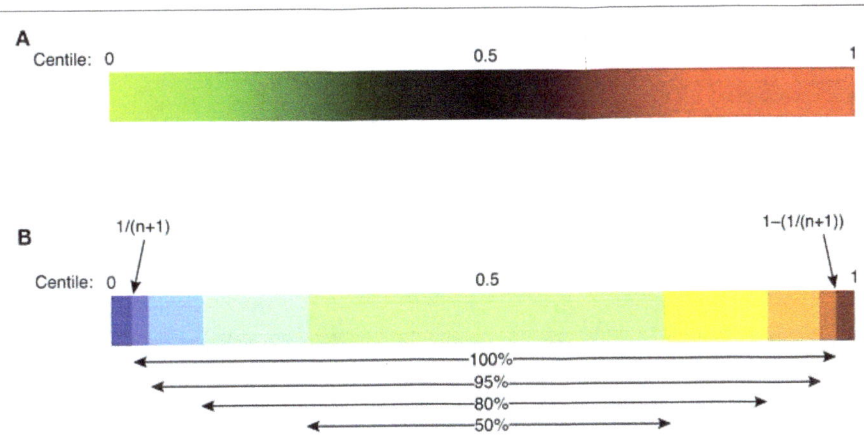

FIGURE 2 | Heat mapping strategy for continuous green-black-red shading **(A)**, or discontinuous shading **(B)**. For continuous shading, colors vary continuously in shades of green (below control median), or red (above control median) with an intensity proportional to the difference from the median (0.5 centile). For discontinuous shading, colors vary stepwise as shown, based on the difference from the median, with the middle 50% of the control population in pale green, then progressively from light to dark blue (below control median), or yellow/orange/red/brown (above control median). Centiles for the control population are defined to vary from 1/(n+1) to 1−[1/(n+1)], depicted as "100%" in **(B)**, where n is the size of the control population; such an approach allows identification of "extreme" or unprecedented values, namely those lying outside the bounds of the control population. Other percentages represent the proportion of the control population included in each indicated color stratum.

basis of an ascending value for B-SM cells. This technique readily identified the known reduction in B-SM cells in CVID (**Figure 3**), but also demonstrated that this parameter was a continuous (rather than dichotomous) variable amongst PAD patients. Thus, whilst 16/22 (74%) subjects fulfilled objective criteria for "deficiency" of B-SM cells—values less or equal to the published cut-off of 0.4% of lymphocytes, also referred to as Freiberg I (9, 10)—the trend to SM-B cell reduction was evident in all but two patients (**Figure 3**, subjects "u" and "v").

The reported expansion in CD21-lo cells could also readily be discerned from the PAD heat-map (**Figure 3**), particularly prominent in three patients (boxed, **Figure 3**), but was found in patients with "normal" as well as statistically deficient B-SM cells. Although our cohort was too small to make firm conclusions about clinical associations, we noted that 2 of the 3 patients with CD21-lo B cell expansions also had clinical lymphoproliferation and autoimmunity (**Figure 3**, subjects "e" and "t," **Supplementary Table 1**), both reported associations (7, 11–13). A subset of patients with expansion of transitional B cells could also readily be appreciated (**Figure 3**) (8).

We could also demonstrate expansion of circulating CXCR5+/CD45RA− CD4+ T helper cells (here termed X5-Th) as a feature of PAD (**Figure 3**) (14, 15). Both the X5-Th cells and as well as the PD-1+/CD45RA-/CCR7-lo subpopulation (here termed Tfh-effector cells), a population that has been shown to correlate more closely with germinal center activity (16, 17), were significantly increased ($p = 0.0021$ and $p = 0.0016$, respectively). In contrast to previous reports (15), we found no correlation between the degree of SM-B cell depletion and the proportion of X5-Th cells (data not shown).

Thus, simultaneous representation of FCM parameters in a heat map, statistically normalized to a control population, can readily identify the known cellular patterns and trends in PAD patients, but also has the potential to facilitate discovery of new cellular changes not previously identified.

Normalized Heat Mapping in Genetic Immunodeficiencies

Cellular changes might be noted in a proportion of patients with PAD, as demonstrated above, but no single change is characteristic. This is likely due to the fact that multiple gene mutations can result in the heterogeneous PAD clinical phenotype, with recent reports suggesting that up 30–40% of patients may have a monogenic disorder (18–21). Stratifying PIDs based on genetic mutation should result in more uniform cellular findings and reduce heterogeneity. Furthermore, since many of the identified causes are autosomal dominant with incomplete penetrance, cellular phenotyping might have the potential to distinguish the clinical phenotype of the mutation from healthy relatives with the same mutation. On the other hand, such changes might be missed if abnormalities are defined

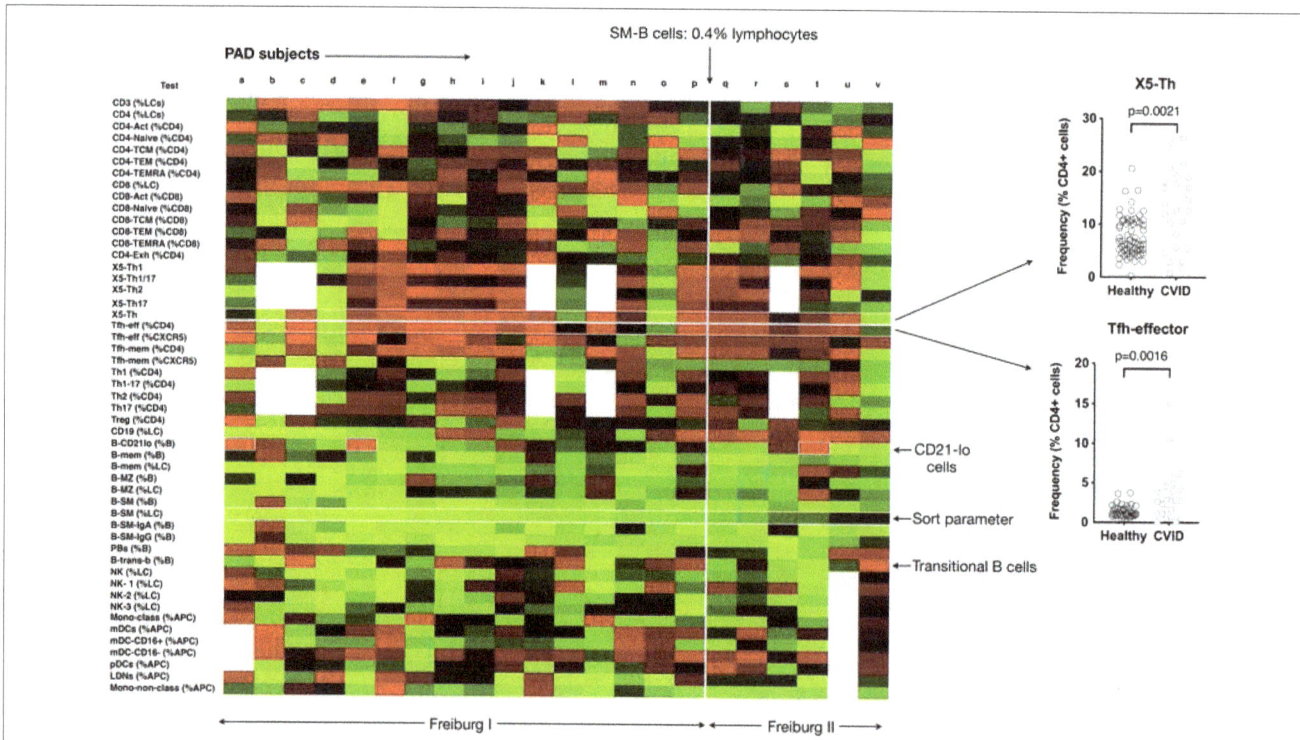

FIGURE 3 | Heat mapping with continuous color shading (as depicted in **Figure 2A**) in PAD patients. Heat maps from individual patients (labeled a to v) are ordered from left to right based on increasing proportions of switched memory B cells (B-SM), with the cut-off of 0.4% of total lymphocytes shown. The expansion of CD21-lo B cells can be readily appreciated (labeled), as can the expansion in CXCR5+/CD45RA–CD4 T cells (X5-Th), and Tfh-effector cells and (as a percentage of CD4 T cells). Inset shows the comparisons between control values ($n = 77$) and PAD patients for X5-Th and Tfh-effector cells. Details of PAD patients presented in **Supplementary Table 2**.

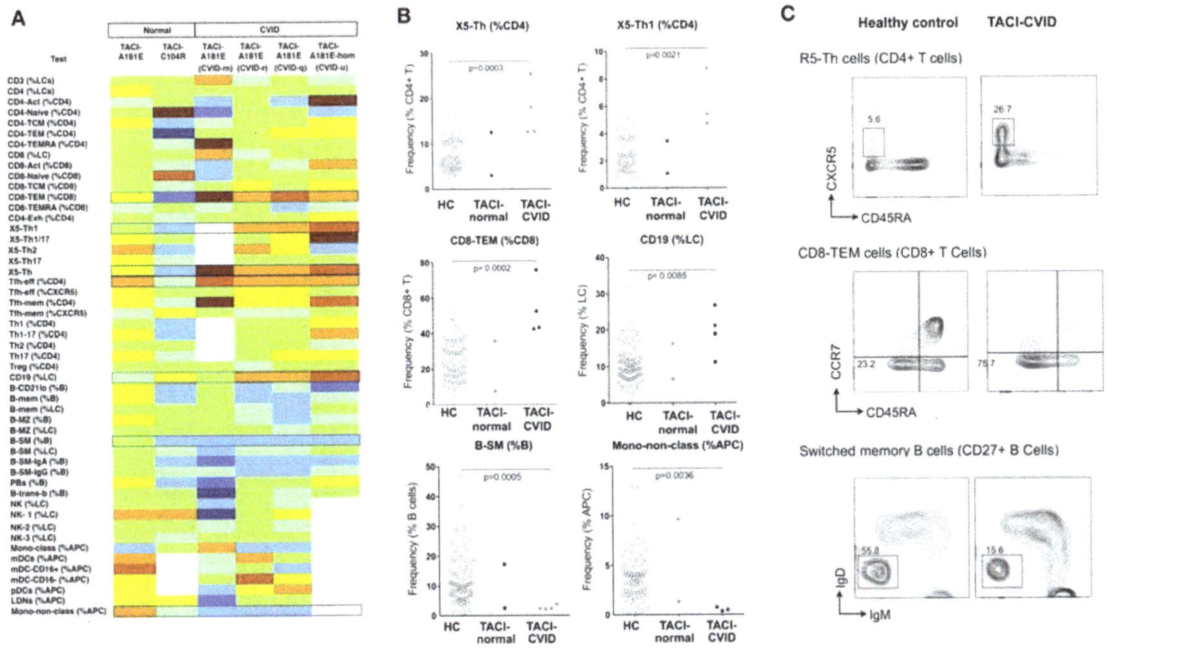

FIGURE 4 | Analysis of cellular parameters in CVID patients carrying TACI variants in comparison to TACI mutant control subjects without CVID. **(A)** Heat mapping with discontinuous shading for four unrelated CVID patients carrying the TACI A181E allele, one homozygous, along with two healthy individuals with A181E, or C104R alleles. Boxes highlight parameters for which cellular changes differ in those with CVID compared with TACI controls. **(B)** Scatter plots showing raw values for populations identified in **(A)**, along with representative FCM contour plots of these critical parameters **(C)**. Raw and centile data is presented in **Supplementary Table 3**.

by and restricted to 95% confidence interval cut-offs. Using heat maps to depict variations from normal in patients with known mutations in *TNFRSF13B*, *CTLA4*, and *CARD11*, we asked whether we could identify trends within defined cellular populations that might be relevant to the genetic pathogenesis of their immunodeficiency.

TACI

Heterozygous and homozygous mutations in *TNFRSF13B* encoding the lymphocyte receptor TACI (transmembrane activator and calcium-modulating cyclophilin ligand interactor) are associated with CVID (22–24). Mutations affecting *TNFRSF13B* are found in 8% of CVID patients, however they are also found in 2% of the normal population (24), indicating that *TNFRSF13B* is a genetic risk factor for CVID, with disease expression presumably dependent on genetic modifiers or environmental triggers. Although *TNFRSF13B* is a highly polymorphic gene, two damaging variants resulting in protein mutations C104R and A181E (25) are most strongly associated with antibody failure (24, 26). We identified four patients with the A181E mutation in our CVID cohort, three heterozygous and one homozygous; we compared the cellular profiles of these four patients with two unaffected members of our cohort who had TACI mutations (one C104R, one A181E) but without antibody deficiency. Depicting the cellular changes as heatmaps, we looked for variations common to TACI mutants that were not present in unaffected individuals, and then statistically analyzed relevant parameters.

TACI mutant patients in our cohort showed consistently higher proportions of X5-Th cells, particularly their Th1 counterparts (X5-Th1), and Tfh-effector cells (**Figure 4** and **Supplementary Table 3**), with the X5-Th cell expansion appearing even more prominently in TACI mutants than in the PAD cohort overall (**Figure 3**); we noted however that the difference found in the PAD cohort remained statistically significant after removal of the TACI mutants (data not shown). TACI mutants also showed expansion of CD8+ effector memory T cells, and total B cells, with reductions in B-SM cells and non-classical monocytes (**Figure 4**). Even though most of these changes did not lie outside the 95% confidence intervals (**Supplementary Table 3**), when analyzed as a group, the differences were significant (**Figure 4B**). Interestingly, we saw a similar increase in X5-Th cell cells in the patient homozygous for TACI mutation as in the heterozygotes, whereas it has been previously reported that only heterozygous TACI patients showed this expansion (27).

CTLA4 Patients

Heterozygosity for loss-of-function mutations in *CTLA4* gives rise to an autosomal dominant autoimmune lymphoproliferative syndrome (Type V MIM# 616100) with incomplete penetrance (28, 29). Clinical features are similar to CVID with an added propensity to autoimmunity. Reported cellular abnormalities have included expansion of CD21-lo B cells, reduction in naive T cells, over-expression of PD-1 by T-cells, and sometimes expansion of regulatory T (Treg) cells (28, 29). We studied

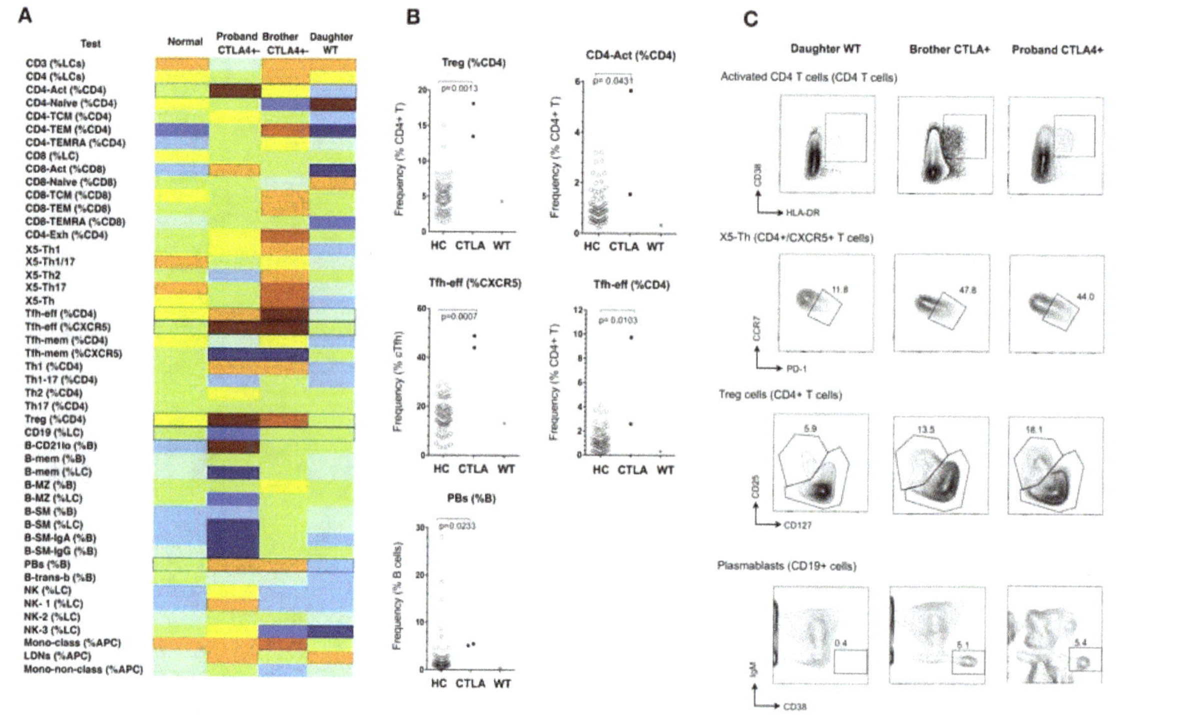

FIGURE 5 | Analysis of cellular parameters in a CTLA4 haploinsufficient kindred. **(A)** Heat mapping with discontinuous shading showing changes in cell populations for the CTLA4 haploinsufficient proband with CVID, in comparison with the clinically normal brother with the CTLA4 mutation, the unaffected proband's adult daughter without CTLA4 mutation and the internal control. Boxes highlight parameters for which cellular changes differ between the two CTLA4 mutants, the unaffected subjects, and between the CTLA4 mutants with or without clinical expression. **(B)** Scatter plots showing raw values for populations identified in **(A)**, along with representative FCM contour plots of these critical parameters **(C)**. Raw and centile data is presented in **Supplementary Table 3**.

a kindred with CTLA4 haploinsufficiency (heterozygous c.152_ins+GA), and generated normalized heat-maps of the heterozygous proband (profound hypogammaglobulinaemia, enteropathy and interstitial lung disease), the heterozygous brother (minimal clinical manifestations), and the unaffected adult daughter who did not carry the variant CTLA4 allele (**Figure 5**). From the resulting heatmap we observed that CTLA4 haploinsufficiency itself resulted in expansion of Treg cells, activated CD4+ cells, Tfh-effector cells (CCR7-lo/PD-1-hi, as a percentage of either CD4+ T cells, or CXCR5+ CD4+ T cells), and circulating plasmablasts, irrespective of the clinical phenotype (**Figure 5** and **Supplementary Table 3**). In contrast, only the hypogammaglobulinaemic proband showed reduction of B cells (<1%).

CARD11

CARD11 is a scaffold protein distal to antigen-receptor engagement in lymphocytes; dominant negative mutations give rise to a diverse clinical phenotype which includes atopic disease, autoimmunity and a combined immunodeficiency involving both B and T cell immunodeficiency (30). Mutations result in defects of T cell activation, NFκB activation and production of cytokines, such as IFN-γ, and IL-2 (20, 31), however changes in cellular phenotype are less established. In a recent multicenter study, we and others reported B-cell defects, including low total and memory B-cells, along with increased naïve and decreased memory T cells, however changes in peripheral lymphocytes differed considerably depending on the specific *CARD11* mutation (30). Using the same technique described above, we studied two unrelated kindreds with two different dominant negative CARD11 mutations (R47H (c.140G>A), and R974C (c.2920C>T), previously reported (30). In the two affected patients, there was reduction in CD8+ effector memory T cells, total NK cells and B cells (the latter two parameters giving rise to a relative increase in total T cell proportion), along with a reduction in the CD21-lo proportion of B cells (**Figure 6** and **Supplementary Table 3**).

Critical Cell Population Changes Determined by Ranking FCM Parameters by Laboratory and Disease Variation

We have demonstrated that cellular trends within a clinical phenotype or genotype can be readily depicted using our approach, but the inherent variability of FCM could challenge the reliability of the technique for general application. Such variability might relate to interlaboratory differences in monoclonal antibodies, their conjugate, the flow cytometer and its set-up, fluorescence compensation settings, and variations in subjective gating strategies between operators, but also to stochastic factors within the laboratory and inherent to the

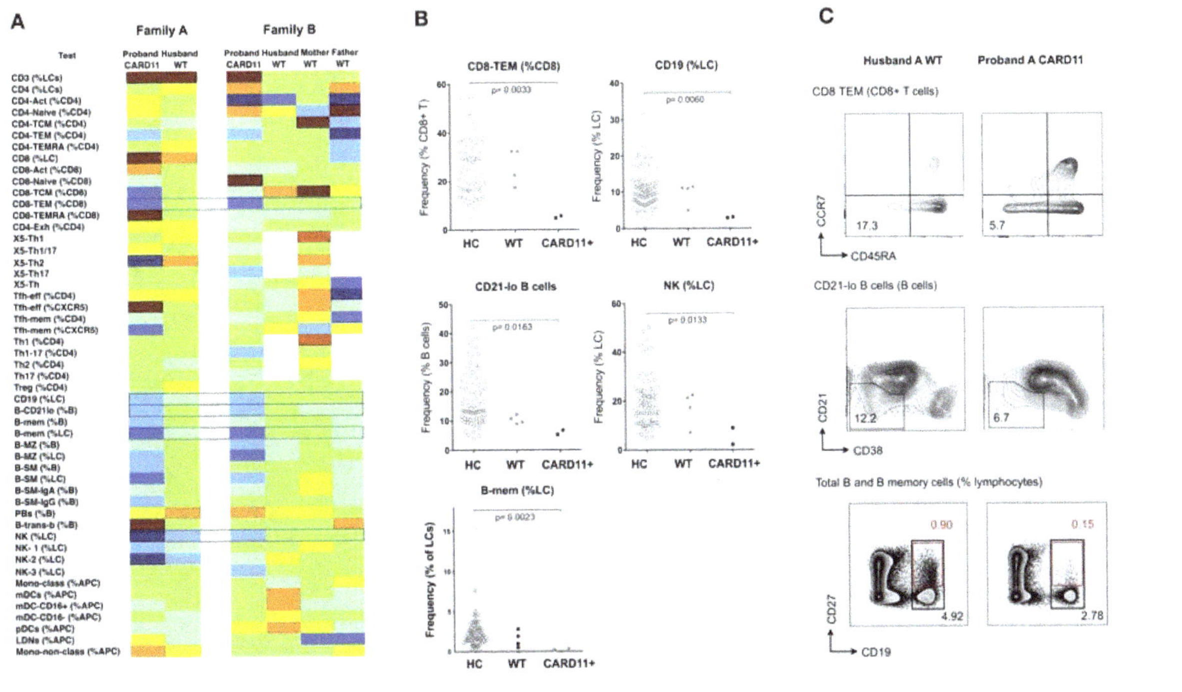

FIGURE 6 | Analysis of cellular parameters in a CARD11 mutant kindred. **(A)** Heat mapping with discontinuous shading showing changes in cell populations for two unrelated patients with dominant negative CARD11 mutations, along with their relative(s) without mutation. Boxes highlight cellular changes common to the two CARD11 mutants, but differing from the family members. **(B)** Scatter plots showing raw values for populations identified in **(A)**, along with representative FCM contour plots of these critical parameters **(C)**; in the B-cell contour plot, black boxes and numbers refer to total CD19+ cells, and red boxes and numbers refer to CD19+/CD27+ memory B cells. Raw and centile data is presented in **Supplementary Table 3**.

methodology itself. To measure inter-assay variation in our laboratory, we analyzed the same frozen cells from a single subject (collected on three separate occasions) in each of 28 runs, and measured the co-efficients of variation (CV) for the 54 original analysis parameters. Despite using the same monoclonal antibodies, conjugate, dilution, flow cytometer, operators (RT, AL) and gating review (DF), more than half of the parameters measured showed significant imprecision, with CV values above 30% for 36/54 parameters (**Supplementary Figure 4**). In the case of CVID, such laboratory variations could have significant implications for assessment, diagnosis and classification; considering only those parameters used for classification of CVID, we still found intra-laboratory CV values around 30% (**Supplementary Figure 4**), meaning that individual patients could vary in whether or not they fulfilled diagnostic criteria for CVID, or else be classified into different sub-groups at different timepoints, depending on random variations in the methodology alone.

Despite challenges posed by intra-laboratory variability, we asked whether parameters could be chosen that show more acceptable laboratory variation yet vary even more widely within patient populations. If so, realistically measurable cell parameters could be prioritized to 'profile' more reliably a specific immune disease phenotype (e.g., CVID, lupus, Sjogren's), or to assist in the diagnosis of immune disease, based on the hypothesis that there exist unique combinations of cellular changes characteristic to a disease or a disease subset.

To identify such critical cell parameters, we plotted co-efficients of variation for the control sample (reflecting intra-laboratory variation) against variation for each test parameter in the entire disease cohort of 199 patients with miscellaneous conditions, including PID, autoimmunity, autoinflammatory disease, and cancer (see section Methods). By calculating the quotient of disease-based variation against inter-assay variation, we identified the top parameters that might be most useful for this purpose (**Figure 7** and inset). Interestingly, X5-Th cells and their derivatives (Tfh-effector and Tfh-memory cells, X5-Th1, X5-Th1/17 cells, and X5-Th17 cells, all as %CD4 T cells), emerged as reproducible cell parameters that were at the same time most variable in disease; as these values all varied in parallel to the parent population (X5-Th cells), the latter parameter was deemed the most independent for cluster analysis (see below). Other critical parameters were naïve, activated and central memory CD8+ T cells, transitional B cells, memory B cells, SM-B cells, plasmablasts, activated CD4 cells, and total T cells (inset, **Figure 7**). On the other hand, the remaining traditional lymphocyte subsets frequently measured in the diagnosis of immune disease, namely CD4, CD8, CD19, and total NK cells, whilst reproducible methodologically, showed much less variation in disease, and hence might be less useful in practice than other cellular populations now quantifiable in the laboratory. Finally, when we restricted analysis of parameter variation to the PID patients alone, IgA-expressing switched memory B cells (B-SM-IgA (%B)) emerged as an important

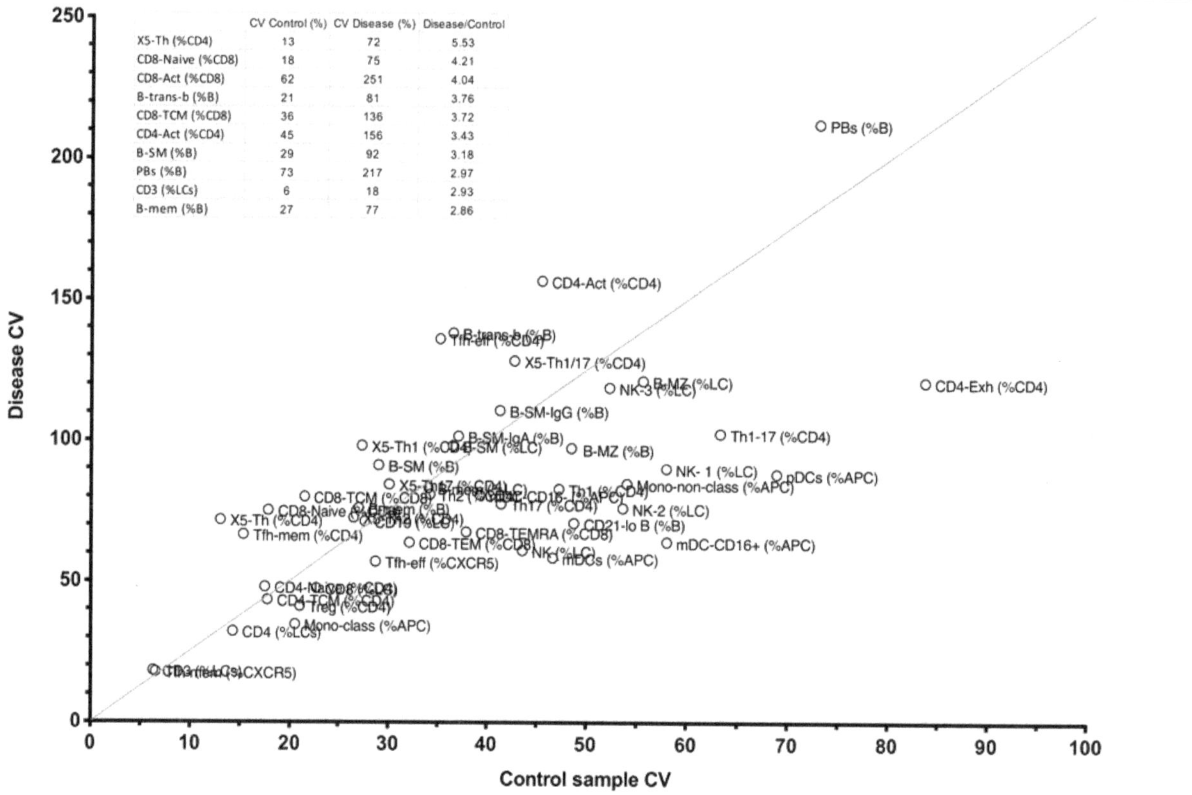

FIGURE 7 | Comparison between CV percentages of 51 cellular parameters derived from the internal FCM control, and the same variation in the entire CPI cohort with widely varying immune conditions (see section Methods). The line shows the cut-off for the top 10 parameters with the highest ratio of disease-driven variation divided by internal variation, and these 10 parameters, and corresponding raw values appear in the table inset.

variable in this cohort, in addition to the those identified above (data not shown).

Finally, we asked the question as to whether restricting analysis to these critical 10 parameters might have the potential to stratify better PAD patients, perhaps giving clues to their genetic pathogenesis. By generating centiles for the 10 most discriminating parameters in our PAD cohort, and submitting them for cluster analysis, we were indeed able to identify a number of subgroups (**Figure 8**). The largest subgroup (I) was characterized by expansion of X5-Th cells with loss of B-SM cells; this subgroup included all TACI heterozygotes. Interestingly, the TACI homozygote clustered with the CTLA heterozygote, a group which were characterized by the above two characteristics along with T-cell (both CD4 and CD8) activation (**Figure 8**, subgroup II). A third subgroup lacked X5-Th cell expansion, but showed expansion of transitional B cells and naïve CD8 cells (**Figure 8**, subgroup III). Finally, the two patients with NFKB2 mutation were distinct from the remaining PAD patients, lacking X5-Th cell expansion, but with expansion of plasmablasts and decreased transitional B cells (subgroup IV). The addition of B-SM-IgA (%B) to the other 10 parameters did not change these subgroups, presumably because all but two of the PAD cohort were depleted of IgA-expressing switched memory B cells (data not shown); nevertheless, including this parameter may be important when analyzing PID cohorts not uniformly selected on the basis of antibody failure.

DISCUSSION

Flow cytometry facilitates rapid quantitation of multiple circulating white blood cell subpopulations, yet depicting variations in these parameters in disease, and associating such changes with corresponding genetic mutations, can be difficult. Here we report a non-parametric method for mapping variations in cellular subpopulations to facilitate detection of relevant cellular trends; raw patient values were converted into centiles based on comparison to controls, the centiles were mapped to color changes, and then the colors were assembled into a heat map. By aligning heat maps within a disease cohort (PAD, **Figure 3**), a genetic cohort (TACI, **Figure 4**) or within one or more genetic kindreds (CTLA4, **Figure 5**; CARD11, **Figure 6**), we have demonstrated how cellular changes can be readily identified, and specific candidate parameters chosen for definitive statistical analysis. For example, reported cellular changes associated with CVID were readily appreciated (**Figure 3**), and cellular fingerprints were successfully identified in the genetic cohorts or kindreds (**Figures 4–6**).

Our method of non-parametric heat mapping thus has the potential to detect more subtle, but nevertheless relevant and consistent, cellular changes than would be detected by applying traditional "normal ranges" based on the control mean plus or minus two standard deviations (parametric distributions), or

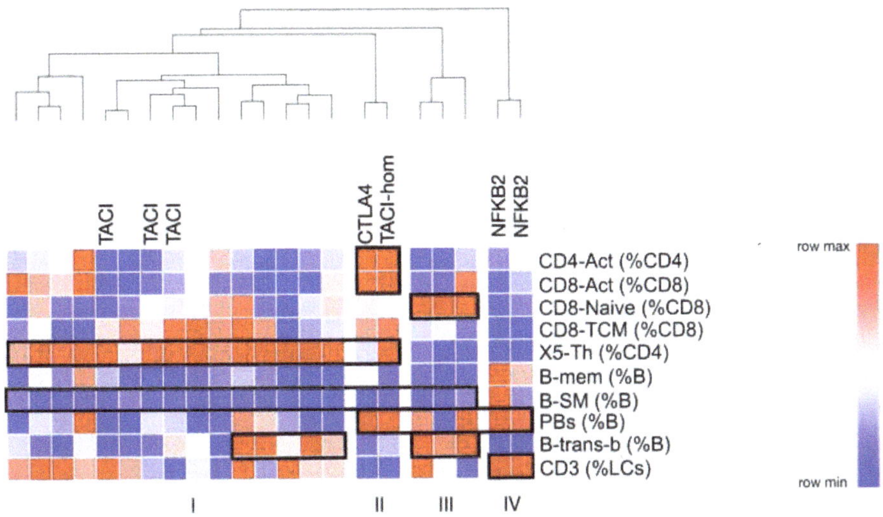

FIGURE 8 | Cluster analysis of PAD patients based on centiles of the top 10 cellular parameters determined as outlined in the legend to **Figure 7** (see text). Hereditary branches show relatedness in terms of cellular similarities, the major ones highlighted in boxes. Known genotypes are shown.

95% confidence intervals (non-parametric distributions). Whilst reference ranges are important for an individual patient, when studying cohorts of patients or kindreds, variations in cellular parameters, either increased or decreased, might show consistent, and pathogenically relevant trends even though individual values might lie within the target range. For example, most of the changes we found in our genetic subgroups were statistically significant despite individually having centiles between 0.025 and 0.975 (**Supplementary Table 3**), which would otherwise represent the non-parametric normal range. Furthermore, when searching out real alterations in cell composition that are dependent on the possible effects of subtle gene changes, one cannot assume that the biological effect on a given cell population will be so extreme that they can be categorized into "expanded" vs. "deficient," based on a defined 95% confidence interval alone.

Defining cellular changes in immune disease could therefore generate hypotheses regarding the pathogenesis of genetic immunodeficiencies. We noted, for example, the expansion of X5-Th cells in CVID patients, particularly in those with *TNFSF13B* mutations. It is perhaps counter-intuitive that patients with antibody deficiency should have increased X5-Th cells (commonly referred to as circulating T-follicular helper cells, cTfh), a phenotype that has been frequently associated with autoimmunity (32). However, studies in TACI deficient mice have shown that expansion of Tfh cells is extrinsically regulated by increased expression of ICOSL on B cells, and that antibody deficiency results from the important role that TACI plays in promoting plasma cell survival (33). Also, whether expansion of X5-Th cells reflects heightened Tfh cell activity or numbers in secondary lymphoid tissues of CVID patients remains unknown. Furthermore, Tfh cells are B cell dependent, and have been shown to be deficient in patients who lack B cells as a result of BTK deficiency (34); this phenomenon was observed in our NFKB2 patients, who also exhibited profound B cell deficiency (subjects "b" and "d," **Figure 3**). Given the association of cTfh cells with autoimmunity, it is tempting to speculate that this change might also play a pathogenic role in the increase propensity to autoimmunity in CVID patients with TACI-deficiency (35). However, it cannot be assumed that an increase in cTfh cell numbers would necessarily correlate with an increase in cTfh cell function; analysis of cTfh cells from a range of different genetic PIDs has revealed that mutations can impact both the quality and quantity of cTfh cells (36), and thus it is relevant to ask whether the increased frequency of cTfh cells in TACI-mutant CVID patients also correlates with changes in function.

We also observed increased Tfh-effector cells and plasmablasts in CTLA4 haploinsufficient subjects (**Figure 5**), which has not previously been reported. Whilst our numbers are small and require further validation in additional kindreds, overactivity of Tfh-effector cells would be consistent with the spontaneous development of germinal centers in CTLA4-deficient mice (37) and might suggest that in addition to the defect in negative regulation due to reduced expression of CTLA4, Tfh effector cells might drive increased germinal centre output and possibly contribute to the increased propensity toward autoimmunity in these patients. The similarity in cellular phenotype in the patient and her unaffected brother does raise questions as to the pathogenesis of the clinical expression in CTLA4 haploinsufficiency, and whether these patients are 'primed' for susceptibility to environmental factors that might be responsible for driving the antibody deficiency and, in this patient, B-cell loss.

Non-parametric heat mapping might also facilitate the search for genetic explanations of immune disease, based on the assumption that a mutation or polymorphism under study is pathogenically relevant and alters cellular subpopulations in the blood. To do this, heat maps from members of a kindred can be assembled, and cell parameters that associate with specific genetic changes identified for further analysis. Should such cellular fingerprints prove to be characteristic of a particular genotype, diagnosis of immunodeficiency diseases could be facilitated by aligning the cellular heatmap of a new patient with an immunodeficiency (or other immune) condition with the heatmaps of other patients with established clinical or genetic diagnoses, similarities in critical parameters prompting a provisional diagnosis prior to confirmatory testing. For example, in the CTLA4 kindred (**Figure 5**), the lack of characteristic cellular changes in the daughter suggested her WT genotype well-before the CTLA4 sequencing results were known. Similarly, the clustering of the two NFKB2-deficient patients together on the basis of 10 critical FCM parameters (**Figure 8**) implies that this approach could also be used to prompt a genetic diagnosis based on cellular phenotype alone.

Analysis of FCM data in this way may however be limited by the wide inter-assay variation that seems intrinsic to FCM as a technique; despite careful control of methodological conditions, we noted high CV values for most cellular parameters measured (**Supplementary Figure 4**). It should be evident that such variation challenges the wide-spread application of defined cut-offs, for example in CVID, since the same patient may change their classification or ability to fulfill diagnostic criteria based on random laboratory variables alone. We have addressed this laboratory variation in two ways. Firstly, we have depicted variation using normalized heat mapping such that trends can be detected even if they do not lie outside reference ranges. Using PAD as an example, we were able to demonstrate known trends without the need to define "normal" vs. "abnormal" (**Figure 3**). Secondly, we selected critical parameters that were both reproducible in the laboratory and also most variable in disease, based on the observation that disease-related cellular variation always exceeded intra-laboratory variations (**Figure 7**), and that cellular parameters could be ranked in terms of their utility for such profiling. We demonstrated this approach in PAD, where clusters of changes could be identified based on a selection of 10 of the most discriminating cellular parameters, and in some cases could be characteristic of a particularly genotype (NFKB2, **Figure 8**, subgroup IV). A similar approach could be used to look for critical commonalities within a heterogeneous immunological disease (e.g., lupus, Sjögren's), carefully selecting or weighting sorting parameters based on both their laboratory reproducibility and simultaneously their greater variation in immunological disease.

There were a few limitations to our study. Numbers within each study population or kindred were relatively small, and it would be important to apply our methodology to larger genetic cohorts. We stress however that the aim of our study was never to develop a new classification system for CVID, nor to provide definitive data on the cellular phenotypes of the genetic PIDs studies, as our relatively small numbers would never have had the power to replicate the findings of more substantial, multicenter cohorts such as those reported in the Freiburg or Euroclass studies (8, 9), particularly in regard to clinical correlations. Nevertheless, our technique of normalizing patient data to control samples may readily be applied to such larger cohorts, and that careful selection of differentiating parameters (**Figure 8**) might facilitate discovery of clustering algorithms that more closely correlate with the expanding array of genetic changes associated with immunologic disease.

Given the methodological variability in the FCM technique itself, it was also difficult to exclude that variations in specific cellular parameters in our cohorts might have arisen through such random variation alone. Nevertheless, the statistical comparisons we did employ were often highly significant, with p-values < 0.01. Since many of our cellular parameters were interdependent, adjustment for multiple comparisons was not feasible, however the False Discovery Rate when comparing 50 parameters would predict that <1 parameter should have p-value ≤ 0.01 by chance alone; given the number of cellular differences we were able to identify, often with p-values below 0.01, we believe that the changes we noted were not only real, but also afforded credence to the techniques used to identify them. Our technique might be less practical however in pediatric settings, given the need for reliable age-dependent control reference values. Some parameters, such as low-density neutrophils, were too methodologically variable to be useful, and few of the myeloid markers emerged as useful candidate parameters, perhaps expected given the focus here on "lymphocyte-centric" immunodeficiency diseases; such parameters might play a role in other (perhaps autoimmune) conditions where innate mechanisms are more prominent pathogenically. Despite these limitations, we were able to fulfill the main aim of our study namely to demonstrate an approach to visually depict trends within small cohorts, trends which can then be used to generate hypotheses for confirmation in larger groups.

Here we illustrate the use of non-parametric normalized heat mapping of FCM parameters to represent changes in cellular parameters in a phenotype or genotype. By relinquishing reliance on reference intervals, this technique can discern trends within a disease or kindred, possibly improve diagnosis or classification, and refine understanding of the pathogenic relevance of gene mutations in established and emerging PID.

AUTHOR CONTRIBUTIONS

DF and JE designed the study, analyzed data, and wrote the manuscript. RT, AL, AC, and RC performed experiments. SJ, DT, DF, and MC recruited patients and blood samples. A-MH and AW recruited patients and healthy controls and maintained clinical data. MC and CV provided intellectual input to the study design and manuscript.

FUNDING

This study was supported by a National Health and Medical Research Council (NHMRC) of Australia Centre of Research Excellence (APP1079648).

ACKNOWLEDGMENTS

We are very grateful to Jonathan Fulcher for coding DF_Phenotyper used in analysis of the FCM data. Dr. Teresa Neeman provided advice regarding the statistical analysis. We also would like to acknowledge Yaoyuan Zhang, Maurice Stanley, Xiangpeng Meng, Katharine Bassett, Pablo Fernandez De Canete Nieto, Grant Brown, and Cynthia Turnbull for purifying and freezing PBMCs; to Dr. Harpreet Vorhra and Michael Devoy of the JCSMR MCF Facility.

SUPPLEMENTARY MATERIAL

Supplementary Figure 1 | Immunophenotyping gating strategies. Flow cytometry plots showing the gating strategy employed to differentiate and quantify each of the 54 cell parameters. Plots are pre-gated on live cells or lymphocytes (as indicated) after removal of doublets. Four antibody FACS panels were used covering T cells **(A,B)**, B cells **(C)**, and myeloid/NK cells **(D)**. Cell populations are named on final gate. Markers used to define each gate are indicated. Arrows between plots indicate sub-gating.

Supplementary Figure 2 | Correlation between values derived from 3 different transitional gating strategies (see section Methods). Scatter plots show the correlation between the frequency of transitional B cell populations in all analyzed patients and controls, as defined by either CD38+/CD24+ B cells ("Trans-b") as the independent variable, in comparison to CD38+/CD10+ B cells ("Trans-a") or CD38+/IgM-hi B cells ("Trans-c").

Supplementary Figure 3 | T cell memory subpopulation gating demonstrating CD45RA over-expression in an individual bearing the variant PTPRC G77 allele (bottom) compared to an individual with the wild type allele (top). Gating on CD4 (left) or CD8 T cells (right).

Supplementary Figure 4 | Coefficients of Variation (CV) for all 54 FCM parameters. Values above 30% were considered to show significant imprecision and are shaded.

Supplementary Table 1 | Details of the PID patients in the four cohorts analyzed in the cited figures.

Supplementary Table 2 | Reagents used for staining cells for flow cytometry, for the four separate panels.

Supplementary Table 3 | Raw percentages and derived centiles for each of the FCM parameters from subjects whose corresponding heatmaps are presented in **Figures 4–6** (Cent. = centiles).

REFERENCES

1. Picard C, Bobby Gaspar H, Al-Herz W, Bousfiha A, Casanova JL, Chatila T, et al. International union of immunological societies: 2017 primary immunodeficiency diseases committee report on inborn errors of immunity. *J Clin Immunol.* (2018) 38:96–128. doi: 10.1007/s10875-017-0464-9
2. Geha RS, Notarangelo LD, Casanova JL, Chapel H, Conley ME, Fischer A, et al. Primary immunodeficiency diseases: an update from the international union of immunological societies primary immunodeficiency diseases classification committee. *J Allergy Clin Immunol.* (2007) 120:776–94. doi: 10.1016/j.jaci.2007.08.053
3. Thude H, Hundrieser J, Wonigeit K, Schwinzer R. A point mutation in the human CD45 gene associated with defective splicing of exon A. *Eur J Immunol.* (1995) 25:2101–6. doi: 10.1002/eji.1830250745
4. Motta-Mena LB, Smith SA, Mallory MJ, Jackson J, Wang J, Lynch KW. A disease-associated polymorphism alters splicing of the human CD45 phosphatase gene by disrupting combinatorial repression by heterogeneous nuclear ribonucleoproteins (hnRNPs). *J Biol Chem.* (2011) 286:20043–53. doi: 10.1074/jbc.M111.218727
5. Schwinzer R, Wonigeit K. Genetically determined lack of CD45R- T cells in healthy individuals. Evidence for a regulatory polymorphism of CD45R antigen expression. *J Exp Med.* (1990) 171:1803. doi: 10.1084/jem.171.5.1803
6. Schwinzer R, Schraven B, Kyas U, Meuer SC, Wonigeit K. Phenotypical and biochemical characterization of a variant CD45R expression pattern in human leukocytes. *Eur J Immunol.* (1992) 22:1095–8. doi: 10.1002/eji.18302 20433
7. Piqueras B, Lavenu-Bombled C, Galicier L, Bergeron-Van Der Cruyssen F, Mouthon L, Chevret S, et al. Common variable immunodeficiency patient classification based on impaired B cell memory differentiation correlates with clinical aspects. *J Clin Immunol.* (2003) 23:385–400. doi: 10.1023/A:1025373601374
8. Wehr C, Kivioja T, Schmitt C, Ferry B, Witte T, Eren E, et al. The EUROclass trial: defining subgroups in common variable immunodeficiency. *Blood.* (2008) 111:77–85. doi: 10.1182/blood-2007-06-091744
9. Warnatz K, Denz A, Dräger R, Braun M, Groth C, Wolff-Vorbeck G, et al. Severe deficiency of switched memory B cells (CD27+IgM-IgD-) in subgroups of patients with common variable immunodeficiency: a new approach to classify a heterogeneous disease. *Blood.* (2002) 99:1544–51. doi: 10.1182/blood.V99.5.1544
10. Berglund LJ, Wong SWJ, Fulcher DA. B-cell maturation defects in common variable immunodeficiency and association with clinical features. *Pathology.* (2008) 40:288–94. doi: 10.1080/00313020801911470
11. Ko J, Radigan L, Cunningham-Rundles C. Immune competence and switched memory B cells in common variable immunodeficiency. *Clin Immunol.* (2005) 116:37–41. doi: 10.1016/j.clim.2005.03.019
12. Vodjgani M, Aghamohammadi A, Samadi M, Moin M, Hadjati J, Mirahmadian M, et al. Analysis of class-switched memory B cells in patients with common variable immunodeficiency and its clinical implications. *J Investig Allergol Clin Immunol.* (2007) 17:321–8.
13. Sánchez-Ramón S, Radigan L, Yu JE, Bard S, Cunningham-Rundles C. Memory B cells in common variable immunodeficiency: clinical associations and sex differences. *Clin Immunol.* (2008) 128:314–21. doi: 10.1016/j.clim.2008.02.013
14. Coraglia A, Galassi N, Fernández Romero DS, Juri MC, Felippo M, Malbrán A, et al. Common variable immunodeficiency and circulating TFH. *J Immunol Res.* (2016) 2016:4951587. doi: 10.1155/2016/4951587
15. Cunill V, Clemente A, Lanio N, Barceló C, Andreu V, Pons J, et al. Follicular T cells from smB- common variable immunodeficiency patients

are skewed toward a Th1 phenotype. *Front Immunol.* (2017) 8:174. doi: 10.3389/fimmu.2017.00174
16. He J, Tsai LM, Leong YA, Hu X, Ma CS, Chevalier N, et al. Circulating precursor CCR7 lo PD-1 hi CXCR5 + CD4 + T cells indicate tfh cell activity and promote antibody responses upon antigen reexposure. *Immunity.* (2013) 39:770–81. doi: 10.1016/j.immuni.2013.09.007
17. Heit A, Schmitz F, Gerdts S, Flach B, Moore MS, Perkins JA, et al. Vaccination establishes clonal relatives of germinal center T cells in the blood of humans. *J Exp Med.* (2017) 214:2139–52. doi: 10.1084/jem.20161794
18. de Valles-Ibáñez G, Esteve-Solé A, Piquer M, Azucena González-Navarro E, Hernandez-Rodriguez J, Laayouni H, et al. Evaluating the genetics of common variable immunodeficiency: monogenetic model and beyond. *Front Immunol.* (2018) 9:636. doi: 10.3389/fimmu.2018.00636
19. Maffucci P, Filion CA, Boisson B, Itan Y, Shang L, Casanova JL, et al. Genetic diagnosis using whole exomesequencing in common variable immunodeficiency. *Front Immunol.* (2016) 7:220. doi: 10.3389/fimmu.2016.00220
20. Dadi H, Jones TA, Merico D, Sharfe N, Ovadia A, Schejter Y, et al. Combined immunodeficiency and atopy caused by a dominant negative mutation in caspase activation and recruitment domain family member 11 (CARD11). *J Allergy Clin Immunol.* (2018) 141:1818–30.e2. doi: 10.1016/j.jaci.2017.06.047
21. Stray-Pedersen A, Sorte HS, Samarakoon P, Gambin T, Chinn IK, Coban Akdemir ZH, et al. Corrigendum: primary immunodeficiency diseases: genomic approaches delineate heterogeneous Mendelian disorders. *J Allergy Clin Immunol.* (2017) 139:232–45. doi: 10.1016/j.jaci.2016.05.042
22. Salzer U, Chapel HM, Webster ADB, Pan-Hammarström Q, Schmitt-Graeff A, Schlesier M, et al. Mutations in TNFRSF13B encoding TACI are associated with common variable immunodeficiency in humans. *Nat Genet.* (2005) 37:820–8. doi: 10.1038/ng1600
23. Castigli E, Wilson SA, Garibyan L, Rachid R, Bonilla F, Schneider L, et al. TACI is mutant in common variable immunodeficiency and IgA deficiency. *Nat Genet.* (2005) 37:829–34. doi: 10.1038/ng1601
24. Salzer U, Bacchelli C, Buckridge S, Pan-Hammarström Q, Jennings S, Lougaris V, et al. Relevance of biallelic versus monoallelic TNFRSF13B mutations in distinguishing disease-causing from risk-increasing TNFRSF13B variants in antibody deficiency syndromes. *Blood.* (2009) 113:1967–76. doi: 10.1182/blood-2008-02-141937
25. Fried AJ, Rauter I, Dillon SR, Jabara HH, Geha RS. Functional analysis of transmembrane activator and calcium-modulating cyclophilin ligand interactor (TACI) mutations associated with common variable immunodeficiency. *J Allergy Clin Immunol.* (2011) 128:226–8.e1 doi: 10.1016/j.jaci.2011.01.048
26. Hammarström L, Bacchelli C, Pan-Hammarström Q, Behrens TW, Grimbacher B, Björkander J, et al. Reexamining the role of TACI coding variants in common variable immunodeficiency and selective IgA deficiency. *Nat Genet.* (2007) 39:429–30. doi: 10.1038/ng0407-429
27. Romberg N, Chamberlain N, Saadoun D, Gentile M, Kinnunen T, Ng YS, et al. CVID-associated TACI mutations affect autoreactive B cell selection and activation. *J Clin Invest.* (2013) 123:4283–93. doi: 10.1172/JCI69854
28. Schubert D, Bode C, Kenefeck R, Hou TZ, Wing JB, Kennedy A, et al. Autosomal dominant immune dysregulation syndrome in humans with CTLA4 mutations. *Nat Med.* (2014) 20:1410–6. doi: 10.1038/nm.3746
29. Kuehn HS, Ouyang W, Lo B, Deenick EK, Niemela JE, Avery DT, et al. Immune dysregulation in human subjects with heterozygous germline mutations in CTLA4. *Science.* (2014) 345:1623–7. doi: 10.1126/science.1255904
30. Dorjbal B, Stinson JR, Ma CA, Weinreich MA, Miraghazadeh B, Hartberger JM, et al. Hypomorphic caspase activation and recruitment domain 11 (CARD11) mutations associated with diverse immunologic phenotypes with or without atopic disease. *J Allergy Clin Immunol.* (2018) 143:1482–95. doi: 10.1016/j.jaci.2018.08.013
31. Ma CA, Stinson JR, Zhang Y, Abbott JK, Weinreich MA, Hauk PJ, et al. Germline hypomorphic CARD11 mutations in severe atopic disease. *Nat Genet.* (2017) 49:1192–201. doi: 10.1038/ng.3898
32. Vinuesa CG, Sanz I, Cook MC. Dysregulation of germinal centres in autoimmune disease. *Nat Rev Immunol.* (2009) 9:845–57. doi: 10.1038/nri2637
33. Ou X, Xu S, Lam K-P. Deficiency in TNFRSF13B (TACI) expands T-follicular helper and germinal center B cells via increased ICOS-ligand expression but impairs plasma cell survival. *Proc Natl Acad Sci USA.* (2012) 109:15401–6. doi: 10.1073/pnas.1200386109
34. Martini H, Enright V, Perro M, Workman S, Birmelin J, Giorda E, et al. Importance of B cell co-stimulation in CD4+ T cell differentiation: X-linked agammaglobulinaemia, a human model. *Clin Exp Immunol.* (2011) 164:381–7. doi: 10.1111/j.1365-2249.2011.04377.x
35. Zhang Y, Li J, Zhang YM, Zhang XM, Tao J. Effect of TACI signaling on humoral immunity and autoimmune diseases. *J Immunol Res.* (2015) 2015:247426. doi: 10.1155/2015/247426
36. Ma CS, Wong N, Rao G, Avery DT, Torpy J, Hambridge T, et al. Monogenic mutations differentially affect the quantity and quality of T follicular helper cells in patients with human primary immunodeficiencies. *J Allergy Clin Immunol.* (2015) 136:993–1006.e1. doi: 10.1016/j.jaci.2015.05.036
37. Wang CJ, Heuts F, Ovcinnikovs V, Wardzinski L, Bowers C, Schmidt EM, et al. CTLA-4 controls follicular helper T-cell differentiation by regulating the strength of CD28 engagement. *Proc Natl Acad Sci USA.* (2015) 112:524–9. doi: 10.1073/pnas.1414576112

14

Complete Multilineage CD4 Expression Defect Associated with Warts Due to an Inherited Homozygous CD4 Gene Mutation

Rosa Anita Fernandes[1†], Martin Perez-Andres[2,3,4†], Elena Blanco[2,3,4], Maria Jara-Acevedo[3,4,5], Ignacio Criado[2,3,4], Julia Almeida[2,3,4], Vitor Botafogo[2,3,4], Ines Coutinho[6], Artur Paiva[7,8,9], Jacques J. M. van Dongen[10], Alberto Orfao[2,3,4‡] and Emilia Faria[1‡] on behalf of the EuroFlow Consortium*

[1] Allergy and Clinical Immunology Department, Centro Hospitalar e Universitário de Coimbra, Coimbra, Portugal, [2] Department of Medicine, Cancer Research Centre (IBMCC, USAL-CSIC), Cytometry Service (NUCLEUS), University of Salamanca (USAL), Salamanca, Spain, [3] Institute of Biomedical Research of Salamanca (IBSAL), Salamanca, Spain, [4] Biomedical Research Networking Centre on Cancer-CIBER-CIBERONC (CB16/12/00400), Institute of Health Carlos III, Madrid, Spain, [5] Sequencing DNA Service, NUCLEUS, University of Salamanca, Salamanca, Spain, [6] Dermatology Department, Centro Hospitalar e Universitário de Coimbra, Coimbra, Portugal, [7] Flow Cytometry Unit—Clinical Pathology Department, Centro Hospitalar e Universitário de Coimbra, Coimbra, Portugal, [8] Ciências Biomédicas Laboratoriais, ESTESC-Coimbra Health School, Instituto Politécnico de Coimbra, Coimbra, Portugal, [9] Faculty of Medicine, Coimbra Institute for Clinical and Biomedical Research (iCBR), University of Coimbra, Coimbra, Portugal, [10] Department of Immunohematology and Blood Transfusion, Leiden University Medical Center, Leiden, Netherlands

***Correspondence:**
Alberto Orfao
orfao@usal.es

† These authors have contributed equally to this work and share first authorship

‡ These authors have contributed equally to this work and share last authorship

Idiopathic T-CD4 lymphocytopenia (ICL) is a rare and heterogeneous syndrome characterized by opportunistic infections due to reduced CD4 T-lymphocytes (<300 cells/μl or <20% T-cells) in the absence of HIV infection and other primary causes of lymphopenia. Molecular testing of ICL has revealed defects in genes not specific to CD4 T-cells, with pleiotropic effects on other cell types. Here we report for the first time an absolute CD4 lymphocytopenia (<0.01 $CD4^+$ T-cells/μl) due to an autosomal recessive CD4 gene mutation that completely abrogates CD4 protein expression on the surface membrane of T-cells, monocytes, and dendritic cells. A 45-year-old female born to consanguineous parents consulted because of exuberant, relapsing, and treatment-refractory warts on her hands and feet since the age of 10 years, in the absence of other recurrent infections or symptoms. Serological studies were negative for severe infections, including HIV 1/2, HTLV-1, and syphilis, but positive for CMV and EBV. Blood analysis showed the absence of $CD4^+$ T-cells (<0.01%) with repeatedly increased counts of B-cells, naïve $CD8^+$ T-lymphocytes, and particularly, CD4/CD8 double-negative (DN) $TCR\alpha\beta^+$ $TCR\gamma\delta^-$ T-cells (30% of T-cells; 400 cells/μl). Flow cytometric staining of CD4 using monoclonal antibodies directed against five different epitopes, located in two different domains of the protein, confirmed no cell surface membrane or intracytoplasmic expression of CD4 on T-cells, monocytes, and dendritic cells but normal soluble CD4 plasma levels. DN T-cells showed a phenotypic and functional profile similar to normal $CD4^+$ T-cells as regards expression of maturation markers, T-helper and T-regulatory chemokine receptors, TCRvβ repertoire, and *in vitro* cytokine production against polyclonal and antigen-specific stimuli. Sequencing of the

CD4 gene revealed a homozygous (splicing) mutation affecting the last bp on intron 7–8, leading to deletion of the juxtamembrane and intracellular domains of the protein and complete abrogation of CD4 expression on the cell membrane. These findings support previous studies in CD4 KO mice suggesting that surrogate DN helper and regulatory T-cells capable of supporting antigen-specific immune responses are produced in the absence of CD4 signaling and point out the need for better understanding the role of CD4 on thymic selection and the immune response.

Keywords: CD4, warts, double-negative T-cells (DNTs), CD4 lymphopenia, idiopathic CD4 lymphocytopenia

BACKGROUND

CD4 is a monomeric type I transmembrane glycoprotein consisting of four immunoglobulin-like extracellular domains connected by a short stalk to a transmembrane domain and a short cytoplasmic tail (1–4). Although rare polymorphisms have been described in humans that suppress reactivity with the anti-CD4 OKT4 antibody clone (5, 6), comparison of CD4 sequences from different animal species indicates that the basic structure of this molecule was highly preserved during evolution for more than 400 million years (7). The CD4 molecule is mostly known because it has long been used to define helper T-cells and, more recently, regulatory T-cells (Tregs). These represent two functionally unique T-cell populations responsible for driving humoral and cytotoxic responses through production of different cytokine profiles (8, 9) and suppressing the immune response (10), respectively. In addition, lower CD4 expression is also detected on antigen-presenting cells such as monocytes and dendritic cells (DCs) (11) and on megakaryocytic precursors (12).

Multiple studies have demonstrated that CD4 serves as a co-receptor during T-cell receptor (TCR) recognition of major histocompatibility complex MHC/HLA class II–associated peptides (1–3). Binding of the membrane-distal D1 domain of CD4 to non-polymorphic residues of MHC/HLA class II molecules provides a more potent stimulus for the T-cell than simply ligating the TCR alone (1–3). Thus, ligation of CD4 to MHC/HLA class II has been shown to induce positive selection of helper T-cells during thymic differentiation (4) and supports activation of helper T-cells and Tregs in blood and other lymphoid and non-lymphoid tissues (1–3). However, CD4–MHC/HLA class II affinity is low, leading to weak binding between the two proteins (2, 3). As a consequence, other molecules are required for productive interactions with downstream effects. In fact, it has been confirmed in murine models that differentiation of helper T-cells can occur in the absence of CD4 expression, suggesting that signaling via this co-receptor might be dispensable (13, 14). Thus, in CD4 knock-out (KO) mice, an expanded subpopulation of CD4/CD8 double-negative (DN) TCR$\alpha\beta^+$ T-cells with T-helper ability is generated at abnormally high numbers, which functionally replace conventional CD4$^+$ T-cells (13, 14).

A limited number of cases ($n \approx 100$) of persistent CD4$^+$ T-cell lymphopenia in the absence of human immunodeficiency virus 1 (HIV 1) infection have been reported so far. Of note, none of these patients have been associated with a specific defect of CD4 expression. Most of the cases display clinical manifestations that are characteristic of combined immunodeficiencies (15, 16). Although in the majority of the cases, the genetic etiology of Idiopathic T-CD4 lymphocytopenia (ICL) has not been investigated, preliminary molecular genetic studies in 20 patients suggest that, at least in some patients, there are mutations in several genes other than CD4 (i.e., RAG1, DOCK8, MAGT1), with pleotropic effects not restricted to CD4$^+$ T-cells (17–19). Altogether, these findings suggest that the clinical and immunological alterations reported in ICL are most likely associated with a helper T-cell defect potentially combined with defects on other cell lineages, rather than with a lack of expression of the CD4 molecule.

Here we report for the first time in human a selective CD4 molecule deficiency associated with a homozygous autosomal recessive mutation in the CD4 gene that completely abrogates expression of the CD4 protein. The immunological and clinical features of this case support previous studies on CD4 KO mice suggesting that, although the immune response is affected in these cases, surrogate CD4-negative CD8-negative helper T-cells and Tregs can be produced in the absence of CD4 signaling, which are capable of replacing most of the functional roles of CD4$^+$ T-cells.

CASE PRESENTATION

A 45-year-old Caucasian female born to first-cousin parents, with two healthy children and without any relevant family history record of prior diseases, was seen at the service of Dermatology (University of Coimbra, Coimbra, Portugal) in March 2014 because of persistent extensive, skin-colored, exuberant, and disfiguring warts in both feet and hands since the age of 10 years (**Figure 1**). Warts were refractory to treatment with keratolytic agents, cryosurgery, and excision, with minor improvement after treatment with acitretin in association with topical 50% urea cream. Apart from this, the patient did not describe recurrent infection-related episodes or diseases, except for past medical history of measles and mumps during her infancy and varicella infection during her first pregnancy, which all resolved without complications. Of note, such past history of infections is not rare among the patient age-matched Portuguese population since vaccination for these diseases was introduced in the Portuguese national vaccination program years after she was born (1969): in 1974 for measles, in 1987 for mumps, and in 2004 for varicella

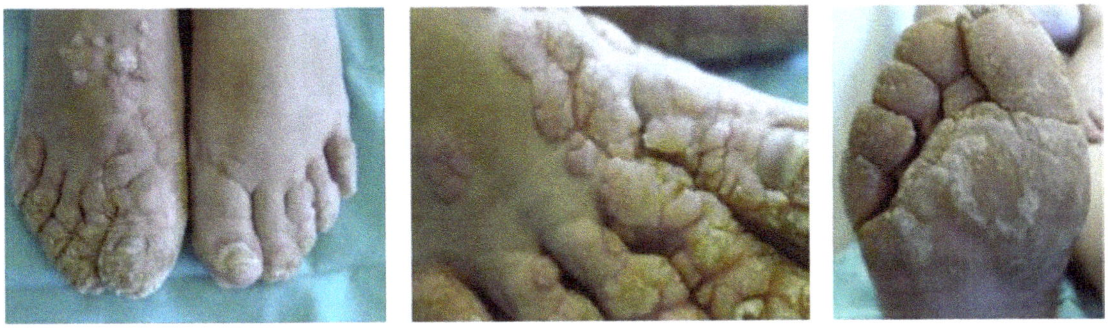

FIGURE 1 | Photographs of warts present in the patient's feet.

(20–22). In fact, outbreaks of measles and mumps have been reported in Portugal until the late 80s to mid-90s, with peaks of >10,000 cases per year (20, 21).

In addition, she referred allergic rhino-conjunctivitis treated with cetirizine and fluticasone, and chronic polyarthralgias in the absence of impaired functionality. Serological studies were negative for (severe) infections, including HIV 1/2, HTLV-1, and syphilis. In turn, she showed IgG antibodies for ubiquitous pathogens including CMV >250 arbitrary units (AU/ml) (positive threshold >6AU/ml) and *Epstein-Barr* virus VCA = 192 U/ml (positive threshold >20 U/ml) and EBNA = 24 U/ml (positive threshold >20 U/ml) in the absence of serum IgM antibodies for these pathogens (0.06 AU/ml; positive threshold >6AU/ml). Slightly increased serum IgG levels (IgG: 1,430 mg/dl), associated with normal IgA (278 mg/dl), IgM (67 mg/dl), C3 (1.4 g/L), C4 (0.33 g/L), and C1 inhibitor (0.318 g/L) serum levels, were detected. In addition, anti-neutrophil and anti-double-strand DNA autoantibodies were negative, while antinuclear autoantibodies were weakly positive. Screening for immunological alterations by flow cytometry (**Supplementary Material**) (23–25) using the EuroFlow Primary Immunodeficiency Orientation Tube (PIDOT) (26, 27) showed an absolute defect of CD4-expressing T-cells (<0.01 cells/μl), with normal total T-cell, $CD8^+$ $TCR\gamma\delta^-$ T-cell, and NK-cell (absolute) numbers, associated with consistently increased B-cell counts vs. age-matched normal reference values. Importantly, ($TCR\alpha\beta^+$ $TCR\gamma\delta^-$) DN T-cells were significantly expanded (**Table 1**). Signs/symptoms associated with primary immunodeficiency other than persistent warts in the feet and hands were not observed either at presentation or during the subsequently 5-year follow-up period. Of note, peripheral blood (PB) monocytes and DCs showed no cell surface expression of CD4.

LABORATORY INVESTIGATIONS AND DIAGNOSTIC TESTS

Expression of CD4 on T-Cells, Monocytes, and DCs

Since rare CD4 polymorphisms that abrogate reactivity of some monoclonal antibodies (MoAbs) with the CD4 molecule have been described (5, 6), CD4 expression was evaluated using eight different MoAb clones. These eight CD4 MoAb clones were directed against five different epitopes located in two distinct domains of the CD4 protein (**Supplementary Material**; **Figure 2A**), as confirmed in competitive staining inhibition experiments (data not shown), in line with previous data in the literature (32–34). Detectable levels of either surface membrane (sm) or intracytoplasmic (cy) CD4 expression were observed in none of the cell lineages that usually express this protein in blood of healthy controls, such as T-cells, monocytes, and DCs (**Figure 2B**). A lack of CD4 expression was confirmed for both classical T-cells and invariant MAIT and iNKT cells (data not shown). In contrast, the expression of other molecules previously associated with CD4 lymphopenia, such as CD3 and HLA-DR (35), was normal and comparable to that observed in healthy donors (data not shown). Besides no cellular CD4 protein being detected, normal soluble CD4 levels in plasma were observed in the patient using an ELISA assay with a pair of antibodies directed against the extracellular domains of CD4 (amino acids 26–390; **Table 2**).

CD4 Gene DNA and cDNA Sequencing

CD4 gene sequencing of patient DNA revealed an isolated homozygous mutation (**Figure 3**; **Supplementary Table 1**) in the last bp of the 7-8 intron (NC_000012.12: g6818420 G>A), corresponding to the juxtamembrane domain of the CD4 protein. This alteration was considered by the Variant Effect Predictor Tool (VEP) (36) as a splice acceptor variant with a high impact on CD4 protein transcription. No wild type CD4 DNA sequence was detected based on the analysis of the sequence of the amplicon products obtained after PCR amplification of DNA from the patient. Instead, two truncated forms of CD4 RNA/cDNA were detected. Both truncated forms of CD4 RNA presented with a frameshift deletion starting at the juxtamembrane region at the first bp of exon 8 and a premature stop codon associated with a truncated protein with normal extracellular domains in the absence of the anchoring domain to the membrane (**Figure 3**). The first frameshift deletion (NM_000616: c.1157_1278del) consisted of a complete deletion of exon 8 (122 pb), resulting in a 399-amino-acid protein. In turn, the second frameshift deletion produced a 430-amino-acid protein because of (only) a 29 bp deletion (NM_000616: c.1157_1185del) (**Figure 3**) that ended just before a 5 bp

TABLE 1 | Distribution of distinct populations of innate immune cells T- and B-lymphocytes in the CD4^{null} patient here reported compared to age-matched reference values.

Leucocyte subsets	Patient	Age reference values
T-cells	1,700 ± 733	(743–2,379)
CD4$^+$ CD8$^-$ TCRγδ$^-$ T-cells	**0 ± 0**	(501–1,654)
Naïve	**0 ± 0**	(83–1,057)
Central memory/transitional memory	**0 ± 0**	(235–784)
Effector memory	**0 ± 0**	(25–208)
Terminally differentiated	**0 ± 0**	(0–663)
CD4$^-$ CD8$^+$ TCRγδ$^-$ T-cells	902 ± 367	(133–1,432)
Naïve	**556 ± 226**	(29–386)
Central memory/transitional memory	217 ± 98	(59–453)
Effector memory CD27$^-$	105 ± 26	(6–323)
Effector CD27^{dim}	**4 ± 6**	(7–457)
Terminally differentiated	33 ± 14	(0–500)
TCRγδ$^+$ T-cells	**238 ± 96**	(7–231)
CD4$^-$ CD8$^-$ TCRγδ$^-$ T-cells	**560 ± 287**	(4–24)
Treg-like (CD8$^-$/TCRγδ$^-$/CD25^{++}/CD127$^-$)	66	(22–141)*
TFH-like (CD8$^-$/TCRγδ$^-$/CXCR5$^+$)	134	(45–240)*
Th1-like (CD8$^-$/TCRγδ$^-$/CXCR3$^+$/CCR4$^-$/CCR6$^-$/CXCR5$^-$)	139	(57–704)*
Th2-like (CD8$^-$/TCRγδ$^-$/CXCR3$^-$/CCR4$^+$/CCR6$^-$/CXCR5$^-$)	55	(24–123)*
Th17-like (CD8$^-$/TCRγδ$^-$/CXCR3$^-$/CCR4$^+$/CCR6$^+$/CXCR5$^-$)	43	(14–93)*
Th1/Th17-like (CD8$^-$/TCRγδ$^-$/CXCR3$^+$/CCR4$^-$/CCR6$^+$/CXCR5$^-$)	**146**	(20–124)*
NK-cells	603 ± 134	(150–672)
Classical monocytes	610 ± 258	(343–1,104)
CD62L$^+$ cMo	249	(2–731)*
CD62L$^-$ cMo	220	(19–473)
Non-classical monocytes (CD16^{++})	169 ± 102	(26–141)
iMo (CD14$^+$/CD16^{++})	21	(0–89)
Late ncMo (CD14$^-$/CD16^{++})	120	(0–160)
SLAN$^-$ Late ncMo	96	(0–155)
SLAN$^+$ Late ncMo	24	(0–52)
Plasmacytoid DCs	6 ± 3	(4–29)
Neutrophils	3,872 ± 787	(1,800–6,782)
Eosinophils	213 ± 64	(0–648)
Basophils	62 ± 15	(10–64)
B-cells	**517 ± 241**	(48–413)
Immature B-cells	7.5 ± 2.1	(0.8–23)
Naïve B-cells	**394 ± 155**	(26–244)
CD21$^+$	**388 ± 151**	(24–372)
CD21$^-$	5.5 ± 3.5	(0.3–31)
Memory B-cells	**209 ± 77**	(25–173)
CD27$^+$	**194 ± 71**	(19–160)
CD27$^-$	15 ± 5.7	(1.4–17)
CD21$^+$	**201 ± 76**	(16–144)
CD21$^-$	8.0 ± 1.4	(2.8–33)
IgM^{++}D$^+$	82 ± 38	(12–114)
IgG1$^+$	**42 ± 11**	(2.8–30)
IgG2$^+$	**17 ± 3.5**	(0.6–14)
IgG3$^+$	**9.0 ± 4.2**	(0.7–6)
IgG4$^+$	0.8	(<0.01–4.1)
IgA1$^+$	**44 ± 18**	(2.5–27)
IgA2$^+$	13 ± 1.4	(0.4–14)
Only IgD$^+$	0.7 ± 1.0	(<0.01–0.9)
Plasmablasts	6.6 ± 6.2	(0.6–9.7)
IgM$^+$	0.07	(0.04–1)
IgG1$^+$	0.3	(<0.01–1.7)
IgG2$^+$	<0.01	(<0.01–0.7)
IgG3$^+$	0.08	(<0.01–0.2)
IgG4$^+$	<0.01	(<0.01–0.1)
IgA1$^+$	**6.2**	(0.2–3.8)
IgA2$^+$	0.4	(0.04–2.9)
Only IgD$^+$	<0.01	(<0.01–0.1)

(Continued)

TABLE 1 | Continued

*Results expressed as (mean ± standard deviation) absolute cell counts per μl of peripheral blood, obtained from repeated analysis performed during the last 5 years following diagnosis. Normal reference values expressed as minimum and maximum of age-matched healthy donors (40–59 years) based on previously published data (20, 21, 26, 28) are also shown between brackets (). Populations that showed abnormal absolute numbers compared to age-reference values are depicted in bold. *Reference values obtained from CD4$^+$ CD8$^-$ TCRγδ$^-$ T-cells of age-matched healthy donors. DNT, double-negative T-cell; Tregs, regulatory T-cells; TFH, follicular helper T-cells; DCs, dendritic cells; cMo, classical monocytes; iMo, intermediate monocytes; ncMo, non-classical monocytes.*

combination (TGCAG), homologous to the sequence observed at the end of the 7–8 intron (**Figure 3**).

In order to investigate the origin of the mutation, DNA from four first-degree patient relatives (all asymptomatic) was also analyzed. Thus, the mutation identified in the patient (NC_000012.12: g6818420 G>A) was also found in heterozygosis in DNA from each of her two children and each of her parents. In contrast, her brother's DNA only showed wild type CD4 gene sequences. Further cDNA sequencing from her children and her parents revealed two CD4 mRNA sequences, one carrying the large deletion observed in the patient (NM_000616: c.1156_1278del) and another with the unmutated (wild type) CD4 allele sequence (**Figure 3**). These results are fully consistent with a germinal mutation in the patient inherited from her parents and transmitted to her children. In contrast, in the patient's brother, both alleles were found to be wild type. Analysis of CD4 protein levels by flow cytometry confirmed that, although normal CD4$^+$ T-cell counts were observed in the patient's children and parents (**Table 3**), the amount of expression of the CD4 protein on CD4$^+$ T-cells, monocytes, and pDCs was reduced to around half when compared to healthy controls ($n = 3$) and the patient's brother, stained in parallel (**Supplementary Table 2**).

Immunophenotypic and Functional Characterization of Expanded CD4/CD8 DN T-Cells

As described above, a lack of CD4 expression on patient T-cells was associated with abnormally expanded DN TCRγδ$^-$ TCRαβ$^+$

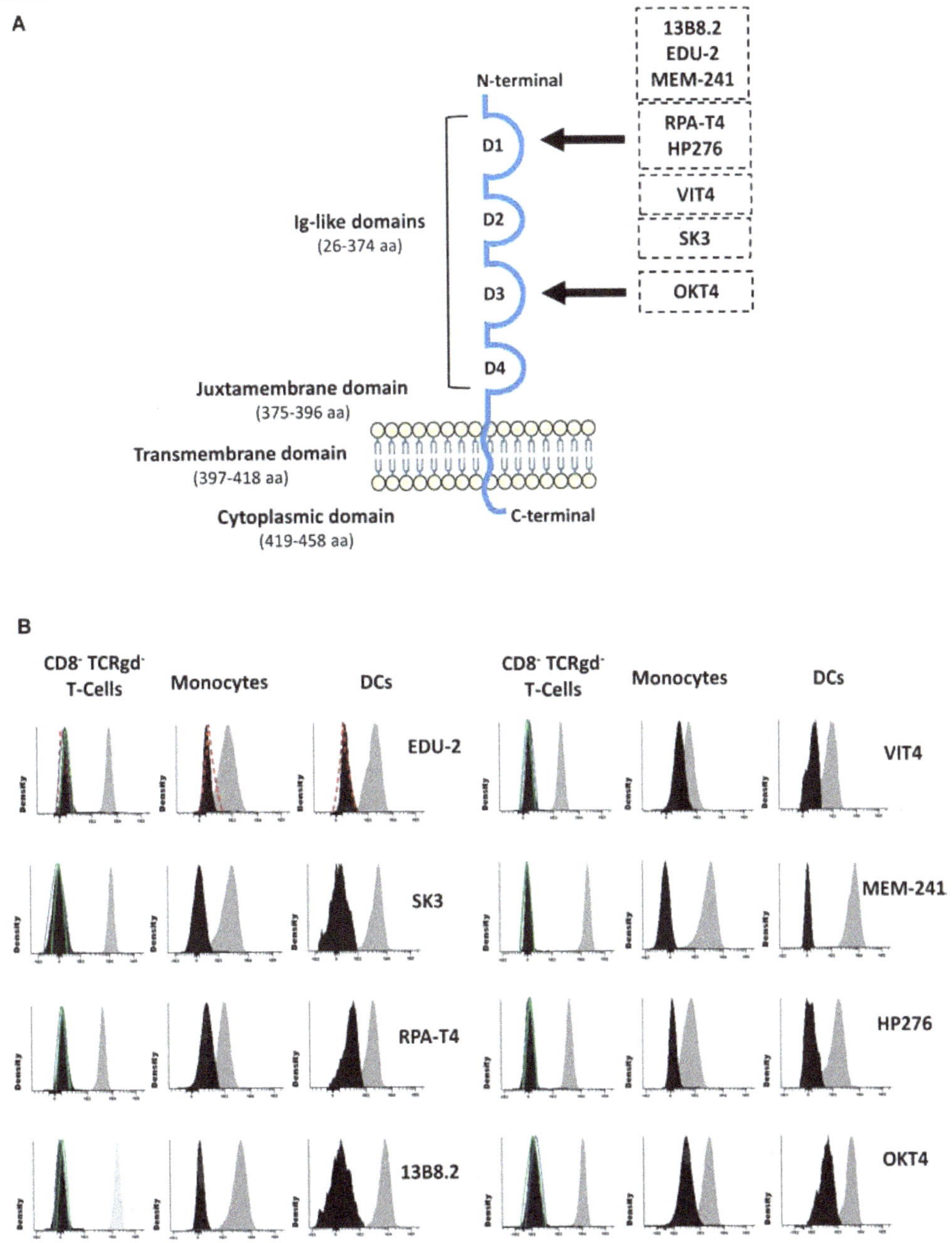

FIGURE 2 | Schematic representation of the CD4 protein molecule **(A)** and CD4 surface membrane expression in the patient's (vs. healthy donor) blood CD8$^-$ TCR$\gamma\delta^-$ T-cells, monocytes, and dendritic cells **(B)**. Panel **(A)** shows a schematic representation of the CD4 protein molecule including the localization of epitopes identified by the distinct antibody clones used in this study (29–31). Amino acid positions that conform each domain are indicated between brackets. Black arrows depict the domain that contains those epitopes that the antibody clones are directed to. Panel **(B)** shows CD4 surface membrane expression levels for CD8$^-$ TCR$\gamma\delta^-$ T-cells, monocytes, and dendritic cells for the different anti-CD4 antibody clones tested in the patient (black histogram) compared to a representative healthy donor (gray histogram) and an isotype control (red dash line), and the staining for a negative population (CD8$^+$ T-cells) in the patient (green line) and the healthy control (blue line). DCs, dendritic cells.

T-cell counts in PB (>30% of all T-cells; **Table 1**), compared to age-matched normal reference values (26, 27). Based on CD27, CD45RA, and CCR7 expression, these DN T-cells showed a similar distribution per maturation stage to that of CD4$^+$ T-cells from age-matched healthy controls, both in relative and absolute numbers: (i) naïve: 27% and 240 cells/μ (6–66% and 83–676 cells/μl), (ii) central memory: 66% and 587 cells/μl (18–71% and 235–589 cells/μl), and (iii) effector memory: 7% and 62 cells/μl (2–66% and 14–221 cells/μl) (26, 27). In addition, expanded DN T-cells showed a polyclonal TCRVβ repertoire with a distribution per TCR family evaluated, fully consistent with reference TCRVβ repertoire values observed in HLA class II-restricted CD4$^+$

TABLE 2 | Soluble CD4 plasma levels detected in the patient and her children compared to two healthy donors.

	CD4 concentration (ng/ml)
Patient	7.61
Daughter	13.36
Son	10.64
Healthy donor 1	11.7
Healthy donor 2	9.20

T-cells from healthy donors (37) (**Supplementary Figure 1**). More extended phenotypic analysis of central/effector memory DN T-cells from the patient showed Treg and Th surrogate marker expression profiles for Tregs, TFH, Th1, Th2, Th17, and Th1/Th17 CD4$^+$ helper T-cell to be present at frequencies similar to those observed for normal CD4$^+$ T-cells (**Table 1**) from age-matched healthy donors (Botafogo et al., submitted).

Short-term *in vitro* stimulation, for 4 and 6 h, showed that the expanded DN T-cells were capable of producing cytokines from the main Th patterns (e.g., IFNγ, IL-4/IL-5, and IL-17A/IL-17F) at frequencies similar to CD4$^+$ helper T-cells from age-matched healthy controls, when either polyclonal (i.e., PMA) or antigen-specific (i.e., CMV) stimuli that required antigen presentation were used (**Table 4**). In contrast, the percentage of DN T-cells expressing markers of cytotoxic T-cells (cyGranzyme B or cyPerforin) was decreased below <1% (normal age-matched range of <1–21% of DN T-cells).

Immunophenotypic and Functional Evaluation of Cytotoxic, Humoral, and Innate Immune Cells and Immune Responses

Normal total CD8+ T-cell, TCR$\gamma\delta^+$ T-cell, and NK-cell counts were found in the patient blood, although the latter two were increased in some of the monitoring time points tested during the 5-year follow-up period. In contrast, consistently increased naïve CD8+ T-cell counts (**Table 1**) vs. age-matched reference values (26, 27), associated with normal central and effector memory CD8+ T-cell numbers, were found in the patient's blood at different time points. Expression of cytolytic enzymes (cyGranzyme B and cyPerforin) was detected in CD8$^+$ T-cells (13 and 9% of CD8$^+$ T-cells) and NK-cells (>99%) at normal values (15–65% and 10–53% of CD8$^+$ T-cells, respectively; >99% of NK-cells). In addition, CD8$^+$ TCR$\alpha\beta^+$ T-cells also showed a normal polyclonal TCRVβ repertoire (vs. normal age-matched reference values, shown in **Supplementary Figure 1**) (37) and a normal cytokine production profile in response to PMA and CMV (**Table 4**) (29).

Detailed dissection of the PB B-cell compartment from the patient showed persistently increased total B-cell counts due to increased naïve (CD21$^+$) B-cells, IgG_{1-3} and IgA_1 memory B-cells, and IgA_1 plasmablasts, with normal immature/transitional B-cell numbers (**Table 1**) (28, 38), in line with the observed higher serum IgG levels.

Analysis of circulating PB monocytes based on expression of CD14 (LPS receptor) and CD16 (low-affinity Fc IgG receptor) showed normal absolute counts for all subsets (**Table 1**) (39), including: (1) CD14$^+$ CD16$^-$ classical monocytes (cMo), (2) CD14$^+$ CD16$^+$ intermediate monocytes (iMo), and (3) CD14$^-$ CD16$^+$ non-classical monocytes (ncMo). Further dissection of cMo and ncMo based on the expression of the CD62L and SLAN selectins, respectively, did not show significant differences vs. normal age-matched reference values (39). In addition, CD4-negative monocytes and DCs were capable of producing cytokines at frequencies similar to their CD4$^+$ counterparts from age-matched healthy control blood, after stimulation with LPS and γ-IFN (**Supplementary Table 3**) (40).

Clinical Records and Immunophenotypic and Functional Features of Immune Cells of Patient Relatives

All patient relatives were completely asymptomatic, and they have no past history of recurrent infections or cancer. The father of the patient has had type diabetes since he was 45 years old. They do not have other records of autoimmunity. No significant consistent alterations were found as regards the distribution of immune cell subsets (n > 50) in the blood of the relatives of the patient, once compared to age-matched reference values, except for a slight increase in IgG_1, IgG_4, and IgD-only memory B-cells in the patient's daughter (**Table 3** and **Supplementary Tables 4, 5**). In addition, a normal TCRvβ repertoire distribution (data not shown) together with normal *in vitro* cytokine production profiles in response to both PMA and CMV (**Table 4**) were observed among the patient's parents, children, and brother.

DISCUSSION

Here we describe for the first time in the literature a patient carrying an inherited homozygous autosomal recessive mutation in the CD4 gene leading to complete absence of CD4 expression on the surface membrane of blood T-cells, monocytes, and DCs. This was associated with a relatively mild clinical phenotype consisting of extensive (treatment-refractory) warts in both feet and hands. Lack of CD4 expression was confirmed by flow cytometry on both the surface and cytoplasm of T-cells (<0.01 CD4$^+$ cells/μl) and other CD4$^+$ myeloid immune innate cells (<0.01 CD4$^+$ monocytes and DCs/μl). Despite this, normal soluble CD4 protein levels were found in plasma by ELISA. Rare CD4 polymorphisms that abrogate reactivity of some MoAbs with the CD4 molecule have been described (5, 6). However, in our patient, we demonstrated a lack of reactivity for eight different MoAb clones directed against five distinct epitopes located in two different domains of the CD4 protein, which confirms that the lack of CD4 expression was not due to any previously described single-nucleotide polymorphism in the CD4 gene (5, 6).

In contrast, CD4 gene sequencing of patient DNA revealed that the lack of CD4 expression at the cell surface membrane was associated with a homozygous mutation of the CD4 gene in

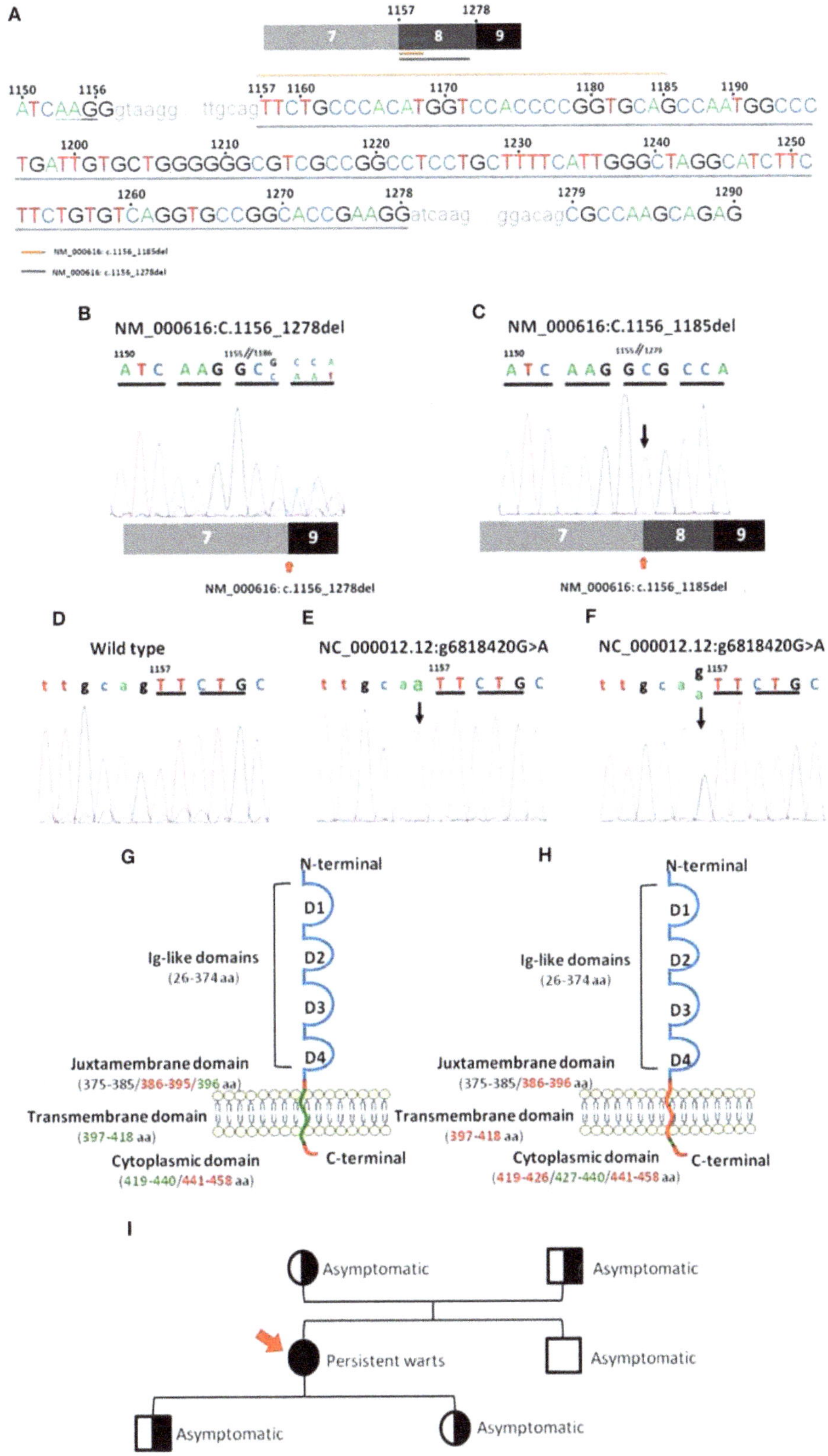

FIGURE 3 | Nucleotide sequences of CD4 PCR products for the regions of interest and their localization in the CD4 gene. Panel **(A)** shows a representative sequence of CD4 focused on the region of interest. Gray underlining shows the nucleotide sequence affected by the major deletion (NM_000616: r.1157_1278del), and orange top line shows the nucleotide sequence affected by the minor deletion (NM_000616: r.1157_1185del). Panels **(B,C)** show mRNA electropherograms obtained from *(Continued)*

FIGURE 3 | analysis of the minor (NM_000616: r.1157_1185del) and major (NM_000616: r.1157_1278del) deletions detected in the patient's CD4 cDNA, respectively, and the patient's relatives **(C)**. Panels **(D–F)** show genomic DNA electropherograms from: **(D)**, wild type CD4 gene; **(E)**, patient's homozygous mutated CD4 gene; and **(F)**, heterozygous mutated CD4 gene from the patient's parents and children. Panels **(G,H)** display a schematic representation of the localization in wild type CD4 protein of the mutated (green) nucleotide bases and the deleted (red) amino acid sequences, including the minor **(G)** and major **(H)** deletions, observed in the truncated CD4 cDNA molecules detected in the CD4^{null} patient here reported. Panel **(I)** shows the family pedigree (men are represented as squares and women as circles), including the key clinical manifestations and, between brackets, the results of CD4 DNA analysis in a coded/graphic format: half-shaded circles and squares, heterozygous DNA; fully shaded circles and squares, homozygous mutated DNA; and unshaded circles and squares, wild type DNA.

TABLE 3 | PB distribution of distinct populations of innate immune cells T- and B-lymphocytes in the patient relatives as analyzed with the EuroFlow Primary Immunodeficiency Orientation Tube (PIDOT) vs. age-matched reference values.

	Daughter$^{mut/wt}$ (normal range)	Son$^{mut/wt}$ (normal range)	Mother$^{mut/wt}$ (normal range)	Father$^{mut/wt}$ (normal range)	Brother$^{wt/wt}$ (normal range)
T-cells	1,470 (564–2,935)	1,159 (564–2,935)	1,561 (636–3,030)	1,910 (636–3,030)	1,056 (564–2,935)
CD4$^+$	663 (207–1,900)	726 (207–1,900)	900 (345–1,474)	1,293 (345–1,474)	556 (207–1,900)
Naïve	288 (74–1,173)	129 (74–1,173)	145 (27–939)	251 (27–939)	**73** (74–1,173)
Central memory/transitional memory	307 (117–886)	421 (117–886)	634 (173–764)	630 (173–764)	370 (117–886)
Effector memory	53 (14–500)	174 (14–500)	118 (30–539)	410 (30–539)	90 (14–500)
Terminally differentiated	15 (0–87)	1.5 (0–87)	3.9 (0–219)	2.8 (0–219)	24 (0–87)
CD8$^+$	611 (160–1,103)	370 (160–1,103)	567 (202–1,571)	487 (202–1,571)	335 (160–1,103)
Naïve	356 (33–737)	192 (33–737)	19 (2–223)	14 (2–223)	**30** (33–737)
Central memory/transitional memory	186 (54–424)	108 (54–424)	235 (42–321)	245 (42–321)	137 (54–424)
Effector memory	20 (2–515)	18 (2–515)	242 (11–925)	118 (11–925)	10 (2–515)
Effector CD27^{dim}	1.1 (0–144)	1 (0–144)	27 (4–576)	11 (4–576)	5 (0–144)
Terminally differentiated	48 (1–273)	50 (1–273)	44 (0–905)	99 (0–905)	153 (1–273)
CD4$^-$ CD8$^-$ TCR$\gamma\delta^-$	36 (5–79)	30 (5–79)	15 (2–27)	**73** (2–27)	8.7 (5–79)
TCR$\gamma\delta^+$	160 (11–470)	33 (11–470)	80 (4–1,060)	57 (4–1,060)	156 (11–470)
NK-cells	233 (161–672)	242 (161–672)	195 (124–1,737)	733 (124–1,737)	**122** (161–672)
Neutrophils	5,468 (1,875–6,483)	**7,222** (1,875–6,483)	3,408 (1,904–5,516)	3,955 (1,904–5,516)	3,019 (1,875–6,483)
Eosinophils	133 (17–2,353)	82 (17–2,353)	468 (40–508)	**635** (40–508)	49 (17–2,353)
Basophils	36 (6–124)	43 (6–124)	42 (0–97)	**162** (0–97)	22 (6–124)
Monocytes	413 (198–1,048)	486 (198–1,048)	438 (201–840)	**1,480** (201–840)	363 (198–1,048)
Non-classical monocytes (CD16^{++})	91 (7–147)	109 (7–147)	188 (10–249)	**409** (10–249)	99 (7–147)
Plasmacytoid DCs	16 (2.7–27)	6.6 (2.7–27)	8.8 (4–19)	7.9 (4–19)	5.2 (2.7–27)

Results expressed as absolute cell counts per μ of peripheral blood. Normal reference values are expressed as minimum and maximum values previously reported for age-matched healthy donors (20, 21). Altered cell numbers are depicted in bold. mut, mutated allele; wt, wild type allele, PB, peripheral blood.

the first bp of the 7–8 intron. This mutation affected downstream coding sequences corresponding to regions located between the juxtamembrane and transmembrane domains of the *CD4* gene. As a result of the mutation, two frameshift deletions from NM_000616: c.1157 onward were found in the mRNA/cDNA sequences of both alleles of CD4. In line with these findings, VEP analysis (36) predicted that the genomic alteration detected (NC_000012.12: g6818420 G>A) would cause the observed cDNA deletions due to modifications in the corresponding splicing site. Identification of a 5 bp sequence at the end of the minor deletion (NM_000616: c.1157_1185del), homologous to the end sequence of wild type intron 7, suggests that in this patient, a new alternative splicing variant might have occurred 29 pb downstream of the mutation. This might reflect a "repair" attempt to produce a functional CD4 protein capable of anchoring CD4 to the cell surface membrane. However, further studies are necessary to confirm this hypothesis and explain the presence of the minor deletion variant identified here at the mRNA level.

Further analysis of the patient's parents and children confirmed that the presence of the mutation identified in the patient was an inherited germline mutation (NC_000012.12: g6818420 G>A), as it was also found in heterozygosis in the two parents and in her two children. Thus, in all four family members two cDNAs were detected: a wild type and a truncated (NM_000616: c.1157_1278del) CD4 cDNA. Most interestingly, the presence of the mutation in heterozygosis resulted in decreased levels of CD4 protein expression in all CD4$^+$ cell types to around half of normal CD4 levels per cell. This further confirms the direct association between the (NC_000012.12: g6818420 G>A) CD4 gene mutation and CD4 expression levels on immune cells in the blood for a codominant gene expression profile. In contrast, this or other CD4 gene mutations were not found in the brother of the patient, who only showed wild type

TABLE 4 | *In vitro* cytokine production by PB T-cells of the patient and her relatives after polyclonal (PMA + ionomycin) and after antigen-specific stimulation (whole CMV lysate).

Cytokine	Subset	Healthy adults (n = 5)	Patient	Daughter	Son	Mother	Father	Brother
POLYCLONAL STIMULATION (PMA + IONOMYCIN)								
IFNγ	CD8+ T-cells	26–67%	39%	26%	32%	81%	76%	76%
	CD4+ T-cells	19–32%	44%*	22%	45%	38%	27%	34%
IL-4/IL-5	CD8+ T-cells	0.1–0.3%	0.5%	0.1%	0.3%	0.4%	0.1%	0.6%
	CD4+ T-cells	1.6–2.9%	4%*	1.1%	2.6%	1.7%	1%	2.1%
IL-17A/IL-17F	CD8+ T-cells	0.2–1.3%	5%	0.7%	3.2%	6.3%	9%	5.7%
	CD4+ T-cells	1.4–2.5%	5%*	3%	14%	5.8%	6%	7.2%
ANTIGEN-SPECIFIC STIMULATION (CMV)								
IFNγ	CD8+ T-cells	0.3–0.7%	0.8%	0%	0.2%	1%	2.9%	0.3%
	CD4+ T-cells	0.5–5%	0.4%*	0.4%	4.8%	1.6%	1.6%	1%
IL-4/IL-5	CD8+ T-cells	0–0%	0%	0%	0%	0%	0%	0.6%
	CD4+ T-cells	0–0.2%	0.1%*	0%	0%	0%	0.2%	0%
IL-17A/IL-17F	CD8+ T-cells	0–0%	0%	0%	0%	0%	0%	0.05%
	CD4+ T-cells	0–0%	0.4%*	0%	0%	0%	0%	0.08%

*Results expressed as percentage of cells positive for each cytokine in CD8$^+$, CD4$^+$ T-cells and double-negative T-cells (DNTs). *Results from double CD4$^-$ CD8$^-$ TCRγδ$^-$ T-cells.*

cDNA and normal levels of cellular CD4 expression in blood T-cells, monocytes, and DCs.

Despite no cases of CD4^{null} mutation having been previously reported in humans, the immunological consequences of a lack of CD4 expression have been extensively analyzed in CD4 KO mice (13, 14, 41). Although it is well-established that CD4 plays an important role in differentiation, maturation, and the functionality of MHC/HLA class II–restricted T-lymphocytes, previous studies in CD4 KO mice indicate that this molecule is not absolutely required for (i) positive selection of T-cells (41, 42) and (ii) the effector function of MHC/HLA class II-restricted helper T-cells (13, 14, 41, 43). Thus, CD4 KO mice are apparently healthy, fertile, and indistinguishable from wild type littermates on gross physical inspection (13). In fact, except for a lack of CD4$^+$ T-cells, defects in the *CD4* gene did not show a major impact on leukocyte production and differentiation, with normal CD8$^+$ T-cell, B-cell, and myeloid cell counts in CD4 KO mice (13, 14, 41). Here, we confirmed that, also in our patient, apart from a lack of CD4$^+$ T-cells and CD4$^+$ innate cells, the CD4 mutation was associated with overall normal lymphocyte and myeloid cell counts, including normal monocyte and DC counts and functionality.

Failure to control infections has been observed in mice (and humans) that lack CD4$^+$ T-cells, after sustained CD4$^+$ T-cell depletion, or due to MHC/HLA class II defects (35, 44). In contrast, CD4 KO mice are able to control infections at levels similar to wild type animals for virtually all pathogens investigated, including viral (13, 45–47), bacterial (43, 48, 49), and parasite (14) infections. The ability of CD4 KO mice to mount normal immune responses has been consistently associated with a subset of MHC/HLA class II–restricted T-cells that emerge from the thymus as DN TCRγδ$^-$ TCRαβ$^+$ T-cells that fully replace the functional role of conventional CD4$^+$ T-helper cells (13, 14, 41, 43). These DN T-cells are expanded in PB of CD4 KO mice (10–20% of the T-cell pool in blood) (13) and other immune tissues, including the spleen (14), lymph nodes (13, 41), and mucosa (50). Interestingly, expanded DN T-cells in CD4 KO mice have been shown to efficiently help to mount potent cytotoxic and humoral immune responses, including those involving immunoglobulin class-switch recombination (13, 41). Similar to CD4 KO mice, our patient also showed an expansion of DN T-cells. Like their CD4 KO mouse counterpart, DN T-cells from the CD4^{null} patient here reported were capable of producing Th1, Th2, and Th17 cytokines at similar levels to those of normal conventional CD4$^+$ T-cells, in response to both unspecific and specific stimuli requiring antigen presentation. In addition, they showed identical expression profiles for Th surrogate markers, including markers of Tregs, TFH, Th1, Th2, Th17, and Th1/Th17, compared to age-matched normal CD4$^+$ blood T-cells (26, 27) (Botafogo et al., submitted). Despite this, the patient persistently showed abnormally increased naïve CD8 T-cell numbers in the blood with an inverted helper/cytotoxic T-cell ratio (0.6 for total T-cells, 0.3 for naïve T-cells). Previous studies in mice have shown that positive selection of CD4$^+$ T-helper thymocytes is around fivefold less efficient in the absence of CD4, due to inefficient positive selection (42). These results suggest that the lack of CD4 might provide a competitive advantage to the CD8 lineage in the thymus, consistent with the increased naïve CD8 T-cell numbers found in our patient. However, the clonal diversity of DN helper T-cells was not affected, and, like in CD4 KO mice (14), a polyclonal TCRVβ repertoire was found among DN T-cells, similar to that of conventional CD4$^+$ helper T-cells. Such a polyclonal DN T-cell repertoire as found in our CD4-deficient patient (and in CD4 KO mice) is different from the typically restricted TCRVβ repertoire observed in DN T-cells from healthy mice and humans (51) and from autoimmune lymphoproliferative syndrome (ALPS) patients (52), which usually contain expanded clones of MHC/HLA class I-related T-cells. Of note, the lack of CD4 expression by DN T-cells did not appear to significantly affect differentiation of cytotoxic T-cells, since normal antigen-experienced memory and effector $CD8^+$ T-cell and NK-cell counts associated with normal expression profiles of cytolytic enzymes were observed in PB except for borderline low $TCR\alpha\beta^+$ $CD8^+$ $CD27^{lo}$ effector T-cells. Likewise, we did not observe any significant global effect of the CD4 defect on the humoral immune response, as normal (or even slightly increased) IgM, IgG_{1-3}, and IgA_{1-2} memory B-cell and plasmablast subset counts (associated with normal or slightly increased serum antibody levels) were observed in our patient. These findings suggest that DN T-cells from our patient are also capable of supporting T-cell–dependent B-cell activation and immunoglobulin isotype switching, as previously reported for CD4 KO mice (41). Altogether, these results support the notion that CD4 is dispensable for commitment of thymocyte precursors to the helper T-cell lineage as long as the affinity threshold for positive selection is sustained (53). At the same time, they strongly argue against an essential role for CD4 in delivering a unique instructional signal for T-helper cell lineage commitment. Although no cell surface membrane or intracytoplasmic expression of CD4 protein was detected in our patient, we found expression of truncated CD4 mRNA and normal soluble CD4 plasma levels evaluated with MoAb against extracellular domains of the protein. Further studies would be necessary to characterize the amino acid sequence of this soluble CD4 protein. Altogether, these findings support the notion that ($TCR\gamma\delta^-$ $TCR\alpha\beta^+$) DN T-cells committed to the CD4 T-cell lineage/compartment are produced even in the absence of CD4 expression. These cells may overall contribute to maintaining normal immune surveillance based on otherwise normal primary and secondary immune responses associated with fast clearance of infection, against both intracellular and extracellular pathogens, as previously observed in KO mice (13, 14, 43, 45, 49). However, a few studies have previously reported a decreased ability of these DN T-cells to induce long-term cytotoxic memory cells and prevent viral persistence in specific situations (44, 54, 55), which might contribute to explaining the recurrent skin lesions observed in our patient. Further studies are necessary to elucidate the precise mechanisms involved in the overall higher naïve and memory B-cell counts and the presence of potentially dysfunctional helper and regulatory antigen-associated/specific DN T-cells.

While the function of CD4 on T-cells has been characterized in detail, the functional role of CD4 on human monocytes is much less understood (56). At present, it is well-established that monocytes do not express lck (an src-family kinase) that interacts with the intracellular domain of CD4 in T-cells. Thus, it has been suggested that CD4 activation via interaction with MCH-II might contribute to cytokine production and differentiation of human blood cMo into ncMo and macrophages (56, 57). In our patient, the lack of CD4 expression did not show a significant impact either on the PB counts of DCs, cMo, and ncMo or on the profile and amount of inflammatory cytokines produced by these cells after *in vitro* stimulation vs. age-matched controls (26, 39). However, further functional studies are still required to determine the impact of this mutation on the distinct subsets of monocytes' functionality, including their susceptibility to be infected by HIV.

In fact, the most striking sign of immunodeficiency found in our patient is the presence of extensive verrucous lesions since she was 10 years-old, which were resistant to treatment with topical keratolytic agents, cryosurgery, and excision. Despite no CD4 gene defect having been previously reported in humans, several case reports have previously described the association of persistent idiopathic $CD4^+$ T-cell lymphopenia, in the absence of infection with HIV 1 or HTLV-1/2, and/or of a well-defined (primary or secondary) immunodeficiency disease, with recalcitrant warts and generalized verrucosis (58–64). Thus, more than half of idiopathic $CD4^+$ T-cell lymphopenia cases present with mucocutaneous lesions (15, 16). Disseminated warts have also been frequently found in several autosomal recessive genetic defects that present with CD4 lymphopenia (e.g., RAG1, RHOH, MST1, CORO1A, DOCK8) (17–19). However, none of these genetic defects are specific for the CD4 T-cell lineage, and Idiopathic CD4 lymphopenia patients typically display additional clinical and immunological features in common with other combined immunodeficiencies (65–68). In fact, detailed analysis of idiopathic CD4 lymphopenia cases reported in the literature shows that many of them are not selective CD4 T-cell deficiencies, since they commonly show additional immunologic defects including decreased $CD8^+$ T-cell, B-cell, and NK-cell counts in PB and/or low immunoglobulin levels (15, 16). In these patients, the presence of such immune alterations other than CD4 lymphopenia is associated with a higher risk of severe opportunistic infections and a greater mortality (15, 16). In contrast, patients with selective depletion of $CD4^+$ T-cells but normal $CD8^+$ T-cell and B-cell counts, as well as normal serum antibody levels, have been reported to display clinical manifestations restricted to cutaneous or genital infections (69, 70), in the absence of a broader susceptibility to more severe infections. Further studies are therefore required to understand the apparently close association between the lack of expression of CD4 and persistent and recurrent warts, which points out a still-unraveled (critical) role of the CD4 protein.

In summary, here we report for the first time ever a patient carrying a CD4 gene mutation that translates into complete abrogation of CD4 expression in multiple lymphoid and myeloid cell lineages, associated with recurrent, treatment-refractory warts in both hands and feet, in the absence of other clinically relevant manifestations of disease. In contrast to individuals depleted in $CD4^+$ T-cells due to an external agent (e.g., HIV infection) or an associated combined immunodeficiency involving other immune cell compartments, defective CD4 expression was associated in our patient with milder immunological and clinical manifestations, except for refractory and recurrent skin lesions. This unique case provides insight about the role of CD4 in human T-cell differentiation, T-cell selection in the thymus, and effector T-helper and Treg functions that supports previous observations in CD4 KO mice. Altogether, our findings suggest that although CD4 contributes to MHC/HLA class II binding and signal transduction, it is not essential to generate MHC/HLA-II–restricted helper T-cells and T-helper–dependent cytotoxic and humoral immune responses.

AUTHOR CONTRIBUTIONS

RF, MP-A, AO, and EF contributed to the conception and design of the study. RF, ICo, and EF collected and analyzed the clinical and serological information of the patient and relatives. MP-A, EB, ICr, JA, VB, and AP performed the flow cytometry data acquisition and data analysis. MJ-A and EB performed the molecular biology data acquisition and data analysis. RF, MP-A, JA, AP, JD, AO, and EF critically reviewed the data. RF, MP-A, EB, MJ-A, AO, and EF wrote the manuscript. All authors contributed to manuscript revision and read and approved the submitted version.

FUNDING

EB was supported by a grant from the Junta de Castilla y León (Fondo Social Europeo, ORDEN EDU/346/2013, Valladolid, Spain). This work was supported by: the CB16/12/00400 grant (CIBERONC, Instituto de Salud Carlos III, Ministerio de Economía y Competitividad, Madrid, Spain and FONDOS FEDER), the FIS PI12/00905-FEDER grant (Fondo de Investigación Sanitaria of Instituto de Salud Carlos III, Madrid, Spain), and a grant from Fundación Mutua Madrileña (Madrid, Spain).

REFERENCES

1. Janeway CA Jr. The T cell receptor as a multicomponent signaling machine: CD4/CD8 coreceptors and T cell activation. *Annu Rev Immunol.* (1992) 10:645–54. doi: 10.1146/annurev.iy.10.040192.003241
2. Zamoyska R. CD4 and CD8: Modulators of T-cell receptor recognition of antigen and of immune responses? *Curr Opin Immunol.* (1998) 10:82–7. doi: 10.1016/s0952-7915(98)80036-8
3. Li Y, Yin Y, Mariuzza RA. Structural and biophysical insights into the role of CD4 and CD8 in T cell activation. *Front Immunol.* (2013) 4:206. doi: 10.3389/fimmu.2013.00206
4. Singer A, Bosselut R. CD4/CD8 coreceptors in thymocyte development, selection, and lineage commitment: analysis of the CD4/CD8 lineage decision. *Adv Immunol.* (2004) 83:91–131. doi: 10.1016/s0065-2776(04)83003-7
5. Fuller TC, Trevithick JE, Fuller AA, Colvin RB, Cosimi AB, Kung PC. Antigenic polymorphism of the T4 differentiation antigen expressed on human T helper/inducer lymphocytes. *Hum Immunol.* (1984) 9:89–102. doi: 10.1016/0198-8859(84)90031-4
6. Lederman S, DeMartino JA, Daugherty BL, Foeldvari I, Yellin MJ, Cleary AM, et al. A single amino acid substitution in a common African allele of the CD4 molecule ablates binding of the monoclonal antibody, OKT4. *Mol Immunol.* (1991) 28:1171–81. doi: 10.1016/0161-5890(91)90003-3
7. Laing KJ, Zou JJ, Purcell MK, Phillips R, Secombes CJ, Hansen JD. Evolution of the CD4 family: teleost fish possess two divergent forms of CD4 in addition to lymphocyte activationgene-3. *J Immunol.* (2006) 177:3939–51. doi: 10.4049/jimmunol.177.6.3939
8. Mahnke YD, Brodie TM, Sallusto F, Roederer M, Lugli E. The who's who of T-cell differentiation: human memory T-cell subsets. *Eur J Immunol.* (2013) 43:2797–809. doi: 10.1002/eji.201343751
9. Sallusto F. Heterogeneity of Human CD4+ T cells against microbes. *Annu Rev Immunol.* (2016) 34:317–34. doi: 10.1146/annurev-immunol-032414-112056
10. Caramalho Í, Nunes-Cabaço H, Foxall RB, Sousa AE. Regulatory T-cell development in the human thymus. *Front Immunol.* (2015) 6:395. doi: 10.3389/fimmu.2015.00395
11. Almeida J, Bueno C, Algueró MC, Sanchez ML, de Santiago M, Escribano L, et al. Comparative analysis of the morphological, cytochemical, immunophenotypical, and functional characteristics of normal human peripheral blood lineage(-)/CD16(+)/HLA-DR(+)/CD14(-/lo) cells, CD14(+) monocytes, and CD16(-) dendritic cells. *Clin Immunol.* (2001) 100:325–38. doi: 10.1006/clim.2001.5072
12. Basch RS, Kouri YH, Karpatkin S. Expression of CD4 by human megakaryocytes. *Proc Natl Acad Sci USA.* (1990) 87:8085–9. doi: 10.1073/pnas.87.20.8085
13. Rahemtulla A, Fung-Leung WP, Schilham MW, Kündig TM, Sambhara SR, Narendran A, et al. Normal development and function of CD8+ cells but markedly decreased helper cell activity in mice lacking CD4. *Nature.* (1991) 353:180–4. doi: 10.1038/353180a0
14. Locksley RM, Reiner SL, Hatam F, Littman DR, Killeen N. Helper T cells without CD4: control of leishmaniasis in CD4-deficient mice. *Science.* (1993) 261:1448–51. doi: 10.1126/science.8367726
15. Zonios DI, Falloon J, Bennett JE, Shaw PA, Chaitt D, Baseler MW, et al. Idiopathic CD4+ lymphocytopenia: natural history and prognostic factors. *Blood.* (2008) 112:287–94. doi: 10.1182/blood-2007-12-127878
16. Régent A, Autran B, Carcelain G, Cheynier R, Terrier B, Charmeteau-De Muylder B, et al. Idiopathic CD4 lymphocytopenia: clinical and immunologic characteristics and follow-up of 40 patients. *Medicine.* (2014) 93:61–72. doi: 10.1097/MD.0000000000000017
17. Li FY, Chaigne-Delalande B, Kanellopoulou C, Davis JC, Matthews HF, Douek DC, et al. Second messenger role for Mg2+ revealed by human T-cell immunodeficiency. *Nature.* (2011) 475:471–6. doi: 10.1038/nature 10246
18. Kuijpers TW, Ijspeert H, van leeuwen EM, Jansen MH, Hazenberg MD, Weijer KC, et al. Idiopathic CD4+ T lymphopenia without autoimmunity or granulomatous disease in the slipstream of rag mutations. *Blood.* (2011) 117:5892–6. doi: 10.1182/blood-2011-01-329052
19. de Jong SJ, Imahorn E, Itin P, Uitto J, Orth G, Jouanguy E, et al. Epidermodysplasia verruciformis: inborn errors of immunity to human beta-papillomaviruses. *Front Microbiol.* (2018) 9:1222. doi: 10.3389/fmicb.2018.01222
20. Republic of Portugal - Directorate-General of Health (DGS). *Programa Nacional para a Eliminação do Sarampo [National Programme for Measles Elimination].* Lisbon: DGS (Portuguese). Available online at: https://www.dgs.pt/documentose-publicacoes/programa-nacional-de-eliminacao-do-sarampojpg.aspx
21. Goncalves G, De Araujo A, Monteiro Cardoso ML. Outbreak of mumps associated with poor vaccine efficacy - Oporto Portugal 1996. *Euro Surveill.* (1998) 3:119–21. doi: 10.2807/esm.03.12.00101-en
22. Maia C, Fonseca J, Carvalho I, Santos H, Moreira D. Clinical and epidemiological study of complicated infection by varicella-zoster virus in the pediatric age. *Acta Med Port.* (2015) 28:741–8. doi: 10.20344/amp.6264
23. Flores-Montero J, Sanoja-Flores L, Paiva B, Puig N, García-Sánchez O, Böttcher S, et al. Next Generation Flow for highly sensitive and standardized detection of minimal residual disease in multiple myeloma. *Leukemia.* (2017) 31:2094–103. doi: 10.1038/leu.2017.29
24. Kalina T, Flores-Montero J, van der Velden VH, Martin-Ayuso M, Böttcher S, Ritgen M, et al. EuroFlow standardization of flow cytometer instrument settings and immunophenotyping protocols. *Leukemia.* (2012) 26:1986–2010. doi: 10.1038/leu.2012.122
25. van Dongen JJ, Lhermitte L, Böttcher S, Almeida J, van der Velden VH, Flores-Montero J, et al. EuroFlow antibody panels for standardized n-dimensional flow cytometric immunophenotyping of normal, reactive and malignant leukocytes. *Leukemia.* (2012) 26:1908–75. doi: 10.1038/leu. 2012.120

26. Van der Burg M, Kalina T, Perez-Andres M, VLkova M, Lopez-Granados E, Blanco E et al. The EuroFlow PID orientation tube for flow cytometric diagnostic screening of primary immunodeficiencies of the lymphoid system. *Front Immunol.* (2019) 10:246. doi: 10.3389/fimmu.2019.00246
27. van Dongen JJM, van der Burg M, Kalina T, Perez-Andres M, Mejstrikova E, Vlkova M, et al. EuroFlow based flowcytometric diagnostic screening and classification of primary immunodeficiencies of the lymphoid system. *Front Immunol.* (2019) 10:1271. doi: 10.3389/fimmu.2019.01271
28. Blanco E, Perez-Andres M, Sanoja-Flores L, Wentink M, Pelak O, Martín-Ayuso M, et al. Selection and validation of antibody clones against IgG and IgA subclasses in switched memory B-cells and plasma cells. *J Immunol Methods.* (2017). doi: 10.1016/j.jim.2017.09.008. [Epub ahead of print].
29. Pérez-Andres M, Almeida J, Martin-Ayuso M, Moro MJ, Martin-Nuñez G, Galende J, et al. Characterization of bone marrow T cells in monoclonal gammopathy of undetermined significance, multiple myeloma, and plasma cell leukemia demonstrates increased infiltration by cytotoxic/Th1 T cells demonstrating a squed TCR-Vbeta repertoire. *Cancer.* (2006) 106:1296–305. doi: 10.1002/cncr.21746
30. Nomura LE, Walker JM, Maecker HT. Optimization of whole blood antigen-specific cytokine assays for CD4$^+$ T cells. *Cytometry.* (2000) 40:60–8. doi: 10.1002/(SICI)1097-0320(20000501)40:1<60::AID-CYTO8>3.0.CO;2-J
31. Rodríguez-Caballero A, García-Montero AC, Bueno C, Almeida J, Varro R, Chen R, et al. A new simple whole blood flow cytometry-based method for simultaneous identification of activated cells and quantitative evaluation of cytokines released during activation. *Lab Invest.* (2004) 84:1387–98. doi: 10.1038/labinvest.3700162
32. Sattentau QJ, Dalgleish AG, Weiss RA, Beverley PC. Epitopes of the CD4 antigen and HIV infection. *Science.* (1986) 234:1120–3. doi: 10.1126/science.2430333
33. Sattentau QJ, Arthos J, Deen K, Hanna N, Healey D, Beverley PC, et al. Structural analysis of the human immunodeficiency virus-binding domain of CD4. Epitope mapping with site-directed mutants and anti-idiotypes. *J Exp Med.* (1989) 170:1319–34. doi: 10.1084/jem.170.4.1319
34. Helling B, König M, Dälken B, Engling A, Krömer W, Heim K, et al. A specific CD4 epitope bound by tregalizumab mediates activation of regulatory T cells by a unique signaling pathway. *Immunol Cell Biol.* (2015) 93:396–405. doi: 10.1038/icb.2014.102
35. Hanna S, Etzioni A. MHC class I and II deficiencies. *J Allergy Clin Immunol.* (2014) 134:269–75. doi: 10.1016/j.jaci.2014.06.001
36. McLaren W, Gil L, Hunt SE, Riat HS, Ritchie GR, Thormann A, et al. The ensemble variant effect predictor. *Genome Biol.* (2016) 17:122. doi: 10.1186/s13059-016-0974-4
37. van den Beemd R, Boor PP, van Lochem EG, Hop WC, Langerak AW, Wolvers-Tettero IL, et al. Flow cytometric analysis of the Vbeta repertoire in healthy controls. *Cytometry.* (2000) 40:336–45. doi: 10.1002/1097-0320(20000801)40:4<336::AID-CYTO9>3.0.CO;2-0
38. Blanco E, Pérez-Andrés M, Arriba-Méndez S, Contreras-Sanfeliciano T, Criado I, Pelak O, et al. Age-associated distribution of normal B-cell and plasma cell subsets in peripheral blood. J *Allergy Clin Immunol.* (2018) 141:2208–19.e16. doi: 10.1016/j.jaci.2018.02.017
39. Damasceno D, Teodosio C, van den Bossche WBL, Perez-Andres M, Arriba-Méndez S, Muñoz-Bellvis L, et al. Distribution of subsets of blood monocytic cells throughout life. *J Allergy Clin Immunol.* (2019) 144:320–3.e6. doi: 10.1016/j.jaci.2019.02.030
40. Martín-Ayuso M, Almeida J, Pérez-Andrés M, Cuello R, Galende J, González-Fraile MI, et al. Peripheral blood dendritic cell subsets from patients with monoclonal gammopathies show an abnormal distribution and are functionally impaired. *Oncologist.* (2008) 13:82–92. doi: 10.1634/theoncologist.2007-0127
41. Rahemtulla A, Kündig TM, Narendran A, Bachmann MF, Julius M, Paige CJ, et al. Class II major histocompatibility complex-restricted T cell function in CD4-deficient mice. *Eur J Immunol.* (1994) 24:2213–8. doi: 10.1002/eji.1830240942
42. Strong J, Wang Q, Killeen N. Impaired survival of T helper cells in the absence of CD4. *Proc Natl Acad Sci USA.* (2001) 98:2566–71. doi: 10.1073/pnas.051329698
43. Derrick SC, Evering TH, Sambandamurthy VK, Jalapathy KV, Hsu T, Chen B, et al. Characterization of the protective T-cell response generated in CD4-deficient mice by a live attenuated *Mycobacterium tuberculosis* vaccine. *Immunology.* (2007) 120:192–206. doi: 10.1111/j.1365-2567.2006.02491.x
44. Trautmann T, Kozik JH, Carambia A, Richter K, Lischke T, Schwinge D, et al. CD4+ T-cell help is required for effective CD8+ T cell-mediated resolution of acute viral hepatitis in mice. *PLoS ONE.* (2014) 9:e86348. doi: 10.1371/journal.pone.0086348
45. von Herrath MG, Yokoyama M, Dockter J, Oldstone MB, Whitton JL. CD4-deficient mice have reduced levels of memory cytotoxic T lymphocytes after immunization and show diminished resistance to subsequent virus challenge. *J Virol.* (1996) 70:1072–9.
46. Moretto M, Casciotti L, Durell B, Khan IA. Lack of CD4(+) T cells does not affect induction of CD8(+) T-cell immunity against Encephalitozoon cuniculi infection. *Infect Immun.* (2000) 68:6223–32. doi: 10.1128/IAI.68.11.6223-6232.2000
47. Fang M, Remakus S, Roscoe F, Ma X, Sigal LJ. CD4+ T cell help is dispensable for protective CD8+ T cell memory against mousepox virus following vaccinia virus immunization. *J Virol.* (2015) 89:776–83. doi: 10.1128/jvi.02176-14
48. Pearce EL, Shedlock DJ, Shen H. Functional characterization of MHC class II-restricted CD8+CD4- and CD8-CD4- T cell responses to infection in CD4-/- mice. *J Immunol.* (2004) 173:2494–9. doi: 10.4049/jimmunol.173.4.2494
49. Wang J, Santosuosso M, Ngai P, Zganiacz A, Xing Z. Activation of CD8 T Cells by mycobacterial vaccination protects against pulmonary tuberculosis in the absence of CD4 T Cells. *J Immunol.* (2004) 173:4590–7. doi: 10.4049/jimmunol.173.7.4590
50. Hörnquist CE, Ekman L, Grdic KD, Schön K, Lycke NY. Paradoxical IgA immunity in CD4-Deficient mice. *J Immunol.* (1995) 155:2877-87.
51. Niehues T, Gulwani-Akolkar B, Akolkar PN, Tax W, Silver J. Unique phenotype and distinct TCR V beta repertoire in human peripheral blood alpha beta TCR+, CD4-, and CD8-double negative T cells. *J Immunol.* (1994) 152:1072–81.
52. Bristeau-Leprince A, Mateo V, Lim A, Magerus-Chatinet A, Solary E, Fischer A, et al. Human TCR alpha/beta+ CD4-CD8- double-negative T cells in patients with autoimmune lymphoproliferative syndrome express restricted Vbeta TCR diversity and are clonally related to CD8+ T cells. *J Immunol.* (2008) 181:440–8. doi: 10.4049/jimmunol.181.1.440
53. Kao H, Allen PM. An antagonist peptide mediates positive selection and CD4 lineage commitment of MHC class II–restricted T cells in the absence of CD4. *J Exp Med.* (2005) 201:149–58. doi: 10.1084/jem.20041574
54. Battegay M, Moskophidis D, Rahemtulla A, Hengartner H, Mak TW, Zinkernagel RM. Enhanced establishment of a virus carrier state in adult CD4+ T-cell-deficient mice. *J Virol.* (1994) 68:4700–4.
55. Shedlock DJ, Shen H. Requirement for CD4 T cell help in generating functional CD8 T cell memory. *Science.* (2003) 300:337–9. doi: 10.1126/science.1082305
56. Glatzová D, Cebecauer M. Dual Role of CD4 in peripheral T lymphocytes. *Front Immunol.* (2019) 10:618. doi: 10.3389/fimmu.2019.00618
57. Zhen A, Krutzik SR, Levin BR, Kasparian S, Zack JA, Kitchen SG. CD4 ligation on human blood monocytes triggers macrophage differentiation and enhances HIV infection. *J Virol.* (2014) 88:9934–46. doi: 10.1128/JVI.00616-14
58. Manchado LP, Ruiz de Morales JM, Ruiz Gonzalez I, Rodriguez Prieto MA. Cutaneous infections by papillomavirus, herpes zoster, and *Candida albicans* as the only manifestation of idiopathic CD4+ T lymphocytopenia. *Int J Dermatol.* (1999) 38:119–21. doi: 10.1046/j.1365-4362.1999.00364.x
59. Van Wagoner JA, Khan DA. Selective CD4+ T cell lymphocytopenia and recalcitrant warts in an 8-year-old child. *Ann Allergy Astham Immunol.* (2001) 87:373–78. doi: 10.1016/S1081-1206(10)62917-1
60. Stetson CL, Rapini RP, Tyring SK, Kimbrough RC. CD4+ T lymphocytopenia with disseminated HPV. *J Cutan Pathol.* (2002) 29:502–05. doi: 10.1034/j.1600-0560.2002.290809.x
61. Fischer LA, Norgaard A, Permin H, Ryder LP, Marquart H, Svejgaard A, et al. Multiple flat warts associated with idiopathic CD4-positive T lymphocytopenia. *J Am Acad Dermatol.* (2008) 58:S37–8. doi: 10.1016/j.jaad.2006.04.026

62. Ladoyanni E, North J, Tan CY. Idiopathic CD4+ T-cell lymphocytopaenia associated with recalcitrant viral warts and squamous malignancy. *Acta Derm Venereol.* (2008) 87:76–7. doi: 10.2340/00015555-0150
63. Alisjahbana B, Dinata R, Sutedja E, Suryahudaya I, Soedjana H, Hidajat NN, et al. Disfiguring generalized verrucosis in an Indonesian man with idiopathic CD4 lymphopenia. *Arch Dermatol.* (2010) 146:69–73. doi: 10.1001/archdermatol.2009.330
64. Cheung L, Weinstein M. Idiopathic CD4 T-Cell Lymphocytopenia: a case report of a young boy with recalcitrant warts. *J Cutan Med Surg.* (2016) 20:470–3. doi: 10.1177/1203475416638045
65. Crequer A, Picard C, Patin E, D'Amico A, Abhyankar A, Munzer M, et al. Inherited MST1 deficiency underlies susceptibility to EV-HPV infections. *PLoS ONE.* (2012) 7:e44010. doi: 10.1371/journal.pone.0044010
66. Crequer A, Troeger A, Patin E, Ma CS, Picard C, Pedergnana V, et al. Human RHOH deficiency causes T cell defects and susceptibility to EV-HPV infections. *J Clin Invest.* (2012) 122:3239–47. doi: 10.1172/JCI62949
67. Stray-Pedersen A, Jouanguy E, Crequer A, Bertuch AA, Brown BS, Jhangiani SN, et al. Compound heterozygous CORO1A mutations in siblings with a mucocutaneous-immunodeficiency syndrome of epidermodysplasia verruciformis-HPV, molluscum contagiosum and granulomatous tuberculoid leprosy. *J Clin Immunol.* (2014) 34:871–90. doi: 10.1007/s10875-014-0074-8
68. Tahiat A, Badran YR, Chou J, Cangemi B, Lefranc G, Labgaa ZM, et al. Epidermodysplasia verruciformis as a manifestation of ARTEMIS deficiency in a young adult. *J Allergy Clin Immunol.* (2017) 139:372–5.e4. doi: 10.1016/j.jaci.2016.07.024
69. Borgogna C, Landini MM, Lanfredini S, Doorbar J, Bouwes Bavinck JN, et al. Characterization of skin lesions induced by skin-tropic α- and β-papillomaviruses in a patient with epidermodysplasia verruciformis. *Br J Dermatol.* (2014) 171:1550–4. doi: 10.1111/bjd.13156
70. Landini MM, Borgogna C, Peretti A, Colombo E, Zavattaro E, Boldorini R, et al. α- and β-Papillomavirus infection in a young patient with an unclassified primary T-cell immunodeficiency and multiple mucosal and cutaneous lesions. *J Am Acad Dermatol.* (2014) 71:108–15.e1. doi: 10.1016/j.jaad.2014.01.859

15

Phenotypical T Cell Differentiation Analysis: A Diagnostic and Predictive Tool in the Study of Primary Immunodeficiencies

Enrico Attardi[1,2†], *Silvia Di Cesare*[1,3*†], *Donato Amodio*[1,3], *Carmela Giancotta*[1], *Nicola Cotugno*[3,4], *Cristina Cifaldi*[1], *Maria Chiriaco*[1], *Paolo Palma*[4], *Andrea Finocchi*[1,3], *Gigliola Di Matteo*[1,3], *Paolo Rossi*[1,3] and *Caterina Cancrini*[1,3*]

[1] *Unit of Immunology and Infectious Diseases, Academic Department of Pediatrics, Bambino Gesù Children's Hospital, Rome, Italy,* [2] *Department of Experimental and Clinical Medicine, University of Florence, Florence, Italy,* [3] *Department of Systems Medicine, University of Rome Tor Vergata, Rome, Italy,* [4] *Research Unit of Congenital and Perinatal Infection, Academic Department of Pediatrics, Children's Hospital Bambino Gesù, Rome, Italy*

Correspondence:
Silvia Di Cesare
di.cesare@med.uniroma2.it
Caterina Cancrini
cancrini@med.uniroma2.it

† These authors have contributed equally to this work

Multiparametric flow cytometry (MFC) represents a rapid, highly reproducible, and sensitive diagnostic technology for primary immunodeficiencies (PIDs), which are characterized by a wide range of T cell perturbations and a broad clinical and genetic heterogeneity. MFC data from CD4+ and CD8+ T cell subsets were examined in 100 patients referred for Primary Immunodeficiencies to our center. Naïve, central memory, effector memory, and terminal effector memory cell differentiation stages were defined by the combined expression CD45RA/CD27 for CD4 and CD45RA/CCR7 for CD8. Principal component analysis (PCA), a non-hypothesis driven statistical analysis, was applied to analyze MFC data in order to distinguish the diverse PIDs. Among severe lymphopenic patients, those affected by severe combined and combined immunodeficiency (SCID and CID) segregated in a specific area, reflecting a homogenous, and a more severe T cell impairment, compared to other lymphopenic PID, such as thymectomized and partial DiGeorge syndrome patients. PID patients with predominantly antibody defects were distributed in a heterogeneous pattern, but unexpectedly PCA was able to cluster some patients' resembling CID, hence warning for additional and more extensive diagnostic tests and a diverse clinical management. In conclusion, PCA applied to T cell MFC data might help the physician to estimate the severity of specific PID and to diversify the clinical and diagnostic approach of the patients.

Keywords: flow cytometric immunophenotyping, T cell subsets, primary immunodeficiencies, multivariate data analysis, diagnostic markers

INTRODUCTION

Primary Immunodeficiencies Disorders (PIDs) are a heterogeneous group of congenital disorders, caused by defects in development and/or function of the immune system, associated with an increased susceptibility to infections, immune-dysregulation, and a higher risk of malignancy (1, 2). Currently, about 340 genetic disorders responsible for defects in the immune system have been identified (3). The T cell compartment plays a key role in coordinating innate and adaptive immune responses upon antigen stimulation. Its impairment leads to a broad spectrum of immune diseases, which require rapid and defined diagnosis in order to adopt the targeted therapeutic management. Severe combined immunodeficiency (SCID) are caused by a severe defect in T cells differentiation, variably associated with B cell, natural killer (NK) cell, and/or myeloid lineage impairment, with the first symptoms usually manifesting within the first year of life and the only curative therapy is represented by haematopoietic stem cell transplantation and/or gene therapy for defined diseases (4, 5). Conversely, CID manifest later with a more heterogeneous clinical picture, often associated with immune-dysregulation manifestations (6, 7). Although few observational studies on CID are in progress, a commonly accepted clinical and diagnostic management for these patients has not been defined yet, and it often relies on the local center expertise, rather than on evidence based systematic experiences (8, 9). Moreover, humoral defects, classified as a predominantly antibody defects and common variable immunodeficiency (CVID) are characterized by recurrent infections, hypogammaglobulinemia, poor response to vaccines, and can be associated to diverse T cell abnormalities (10). Currently, the most accepted T cell maturation model suggests a progressive differentiation from naïve T cells to the memory phenotype, ending with the generation of T effector cells (11, 12). Multiparametric flow cytometry (MFC) allows an extensive and detailed characterization of lymphocytes subsets (13, 14). In this study, we analyzed by MFC the T cell immunophenotypes in a large group of PID patients, clinically classified according to ESID (European Society for Immunodeficiencies) criteria (15). T cell subsets frequencies were then investigated by principal component analysis (PCA) in order to test if this analysis could estimate the relative disease severity and could possibly support the clinical and diagnostic approach (16, 17).

MATERIALS AND METHODS

Study Population

Study cohort is composed of 100 patients affected by PID and 30 healthy donors followed at Bambino Gesù Childrens' Hospital between 2013 and 2017 and diagnosed for PID by ESID criteria (15). Patients' data were collected retrospectively and the study groups are described in **Table 1** while their clinical and molecular characteristics are reported in **Supplementary Tables 1a–c**.

Moreover, the study cohort includes 10 patients affected, respectively, by: selective IgM deficiency, NEMO (NF-kappa-B essential modulator) deficiency, not determined agammaglobulinemia, undefined T-defect, DOCK8-deficiency (dedicator of cytokinesis 8 gene), XIAP deficiency (X-linked inhibitor of apoptosis), XL-HIGM1 (X-linked Hyper IgM type 1), STING (STimulator of INterferon Genes) associated vasculopathy with onset in infancy (SAVI). Patients did not receive any corticosteroid treatment or immunosuppressive therapy at enrollment. Patients' median age was 10 years (range 3,6 months–36 years) while healthy donors' median age was 6,1 years (range 5 months–30 years). Healthy donors were immunocompetent individuals. The work was conducted in accordance with the ethical standards of the institutional research committee and with the 1964 Helsinki declaration and its later amendments or comparable ethical standards. Informed consent, approved by the Ethical Committee of the Children's Hospital Bambino Gesù and Policlinico Tor Vergata, was obtained from either patients or their parents/legal guardians, if minors.

TABLE 1 | Demographics of the study groups.

PID groups	Number	Age (years) median–interquartile range	Male:Female
SCID	5	0.8 (0.35–1.6)	5:0
CID	15	12.6 (3–8)	8:7
TE	5	4 (2.5–7)	2:3
DGS	12	12 (9–16)	9:3
LOF STAT3 (AD–HIES)	5	15 (6.7–27.7)	3:2
CGD	13	16 (7–23)	13:0
CVID	16	15.5 (6–18.5)	9:7
Selective IgM Deficiency	1	19	1:0
NEMO Deficiency	2	13 (10–16)	2:0
XLA	5	16 (6–23.5)	5:0
Not determined Agammablobulinemia	1	28	0:1
SIgAD	14	5.5 (3–8.5)	9:5
DOCK8 (AR–HIES) Deficiency	1	2	0:1
SAVI	1	1	0:1
XL–HIGM1	2	12.5 (6–19)	2:0
XIAP Deficiency	1	7	1:0
Undefined T–Defect	1	4	1:0
Healthy Donors	30	6.1 (2.2–12.6)	21:9
Total	130		

SCID, Severe Combined Immunodeficiency; CID, Combined Immunodeficiency; TE, Thymic Excision; DGS, DiGeorge Syndrome; LOF STAT3 (AD–HIES), Loss Of Function STAT3 (Autosomal Dominat Hyper–IgE Syndrome); CVID, Common Variable Immunodeficiency; CGD, Chronic Granulomatous Disease; XLA, X–linked Agammaglobulinemia; SigAD, Selective IgA deficiency; NEMO Deficiency, Nuclear factor–kappa B Essential Modulator Deficiency; DOCK8 (AR–HIES), Dedicator Of Cytokinesis 8 (Autosomal Recessive Hyper–IgE Syndrome) Deficiency; XL-HIGM1, X-Linked Hyper IgM type 1; SAVI, STING–Associated Vasculopathy with onset in Infancy; XIAP Deficiency, X–Linked Inhibitor of Apoptosis Protein Deficiency.

Multiparametric Flow Cytometric Analysis

T cell development can be phenotypically assessed by the combined cell surface expression of CD45RA, CD31, CCR7, and

Abbreviations: SCID, severe combined immunodeficiency; CID, combined immunodeficiency; TE, thymic excision; DGS, DiGeorge syndrome; LOF STAT3 (AD-HIES), loss of function STAT3 (autosomal dominant hyper-IgE syndrome); CVID, common variable immunodeficiency; CGD, chronic granulomatous disease; XLA, X-linked agammaglobulinemia; SIgAD, selective IgA deficiency; NEMO deficiency, nuclear factor-kappa B essential modulator deficiency; DOCK8 (AR-HIES) deficiency, dedicator Of cytokinesis 8 (autosomal recessive hyper-IgE syndrome) deficiency; XL-HIGM1, X-linked HyperIgM type1; SAVI, STING-associated vasculopathy with onset in infancy; XIAP, X-linked inhibitor of apoptosis protein; TACI, transmembrane activator and calcium-modulator and cyclophilin-ligand Interactor, CTLA4, cytotoxic T-lymphocyte-associated protein 4.

CD27 molecules. CD4 subsets are identified as naïve (CD4+ T_N: CD45RA+CD27+), central memory (CD4+ T_{CM}: CD45RA-CD27+), effector memory (CD4+ T_{EM}: CD45RA-CD27–) and terminally differentiated (CD4+ T_{EMRA}: CD45RA+CD27-). Moreover, CD4+ naïve T cells coexpressing CD31+ are highly enriched in recent thymic emigrants (RTE), a naïve T CD4+ cell subpopulation that have just egressed the thymus and characterized by higher signal joint T-cell receptor excision circle (sjTREC) content (18, 19). Similarly CD8 subsets are defined by the expression of lymph node homing receptor CCR7 in naïve (CD8+ T_N: CD45RA+CCR7+), central memory (CD8+ T_{CM}: CD45RA-CCR7+), effector memory (CD8+ T_{EM}: CD45RA-CCR7-), and terminally differentiated (CD8+ T_{EMRA}: CD45RA+CCR7-). All flow cytometric analysis were performed on ethylenediamine tetraacetic acid (EDTA) blood samples within 24 h of venipuncture. After red blood cells lysis with ammonium chloride the lymphocytes were stained with the following previously titrated monoclonal Abs: CD3 PerCP (clone BW264/56, Miltenyi Biotec), CD45RA APC-H7 (clone T6D11, Miltenyi Biotec), CCR7 PE (clone 3D12, Ebioscience), CD4 APC (clone OKT4, Becton Dickinson), CD8 PE-Cy7 (clone RPA-T8, Becton Dickinson), CD19 PE-CY7 (clone SJ25C1, Becton Dickinson), CD16 PE (clone 3G8), CD56 (clone NCAM16.2) PE, CD27 FITC (clone M-T271, Becton Dickinson), TCR alpha-beta APC (clone T10B9, Becton Dickinson), TCR gamma-delta FITC (11F3, Miltenyi Biotec). Cells were incubated with the appropriate antibody cocktail for 30 min at 4°C, washed with PBS and suspended in PBS. At least 50,000 events in the lymphocyte live gate were acquired for each sample. Samples were acquired on FACSCANTO II (BD Biosciences, San Diego, CA, USA) and analyzed with FlowJo software (Tree Star Inc, version 8.8.6, Ashland, Ore). Some patients of our cohort presented with severe lymphopenia and to avoid this bias, we have considered the cell subsets frequencies, instead of absolute counts. Details of the gating strategy are shown in **Supplementary Figure 1**.

Statistical Analysis

Unpaired *t*-test was used to compare the patients and controls for variables with normal distribution. For non-parametric variables, the unpaired two-tailed non-parametric Mann-Whitney test was used. All graphical representations and statistical analyses were performed using Prism 6.0 (GraphPad). The relative T subsets frequencies were subjected to PCA analysis, using PAST (PAleontological STatistics, version 3.22, University of Oslo) to visualize and to estimate the correlation among variables.

RESULTS

T subsets frequencies were diversely perturbed in most PIDs in univariate analysis, while those of STAT3, XLA, and SIgAD patients were all comparable to healthy donors. Moreover, no significant differences were evident between all lymphopenic groups (CID, DGS, TE) (**Figure 1**). T cell subsets frequencies were then interrogated by PCA: STAT3, XLA, and SIgAD groups did not show any evident alteration (**Supplementary Figures S4A,B**), with the exception of one SIgAD patient with severe autoimmune cytopenia clustering far from the SIgAD group (A13) and two XLA patients (X2 and X4) with $T_{EM/EMRA}$ CD8+ cell expansion (**Supplementary Figure 4B**).

Most of the CID patients clearly segregated far from healthy donors, similarly to SCID (**Figures 2A,B** and **Supplementary Figures 2, 5A**) and the main discriminating variables were the T_{CM} CD4+ and T_{EM} CD8+ and to a lesser extent T_{EMRA} CD8+ cell subsets, as clearly evident in the CID patients (C9, C13, C14, C15) diagnosed as APDS (activated PI3K delta syndrome) (**Figure 2B**). While 13 patients out of 15 segregated uniformly, two patients (C3 and C7) classified as CID, with recurrent respiratory infections but in absence of immune dysregulation phenomena, segregated differently: C7 lied inside the HD area and C3 was skewed toward naive cells and low memory subsets in PCA (**Figure 2B**). Indeed, patient C3 had normal TREC levels, despite a reduction in CD4+CD31+CD45RA+ T cells and an increase in the CD4+CD31-CD27+CD45RA+ (>20%), suggesting a defective T cell maturation. Some other patients were clearly identifiable, like the DOCK8 (AR-HIES) deficiency patient (K1) showing a trend vs. T_{EMRA} CD8+ expansion and the patient (R1) with an undefined T cell defect clustering toward T_{EM} CD4+ differentiation. Conversely, the immunophenotype of the two XL-HIGM1 patients (L1, L2) and XIAP deficiency patient (P1) segregated more closely to HD, although their clinical picture mimicked a CID (**Figure 2B**). In patient S1, admitted at 14 months of age for a severe dermatitis, chronic diarrhea, and anemia associated with a profound alteration in T cell distribution, PCA showed clearly a peculiar localization near HD area and far from CID group, excluding a combined immunodeficiency. Later targeted next generation sequencing (NGS) analysis revealed a STING (STimulator of INterferon Genes) mutation, justifying her severe course due to a deficiency in the interferon pathway (20).

CVID immunophenotypes did not segregate uniformly (**Figure 3**), but when analyzed by age groups and compared to CID (**Figures 4A,B** and **Supplementary Figure 3**), PCA showed one 4-year-old patient (V1) with a CID-like clinical phenotype, characterized by recurrent infections, bronchiectasis, and facial dysmorfism that clustered far from HD near the CID age matched patients' area (**Supplementary Figure 3**). Furthermore, two 6–16-year-old CVID patients (V4 and V8, **Figure 4A**) presented a severe clinical course and could be distinguished by T_{EMRA} CD8+ expansion in V4, probably related to persistent viral infections, and T_{CM} CD4+ and T_{EM} CD8+ in V8; patient V8 developed overtime a MAS (Macrophage Activated Syndrome), leading eventually to death. On the other hand, in the same 6–16 year age range three CVID patients (V2, V5, V10) with increased T_N CD4+ clustered nearby but showed diverse molecular diagnosis: in V2 was reported a dominant heterozygous mutation c.2557CNT (p.Arg853*) in the *NFKB2* gene, in V5 was detected a mutation in Transmembrane Activator and Calcium-Modulator and Cyclophilin-Ligand Interactor (*TACI*), while V10 is still without a definite diagnosis (**Figure 4A**).

The immunoprofile of two NEMO deficiency relatives patients in age range 6–16 year (N1 and N2) (**Figure 4A**) and bearing a splice site mutation in the 59 UTR of the *NEMO* transcript, was skewed differently: N1 more vs. T_{CM} CD4+ while N2 showed a trend vs. $T_{EM/EMRA}$ CD8+.

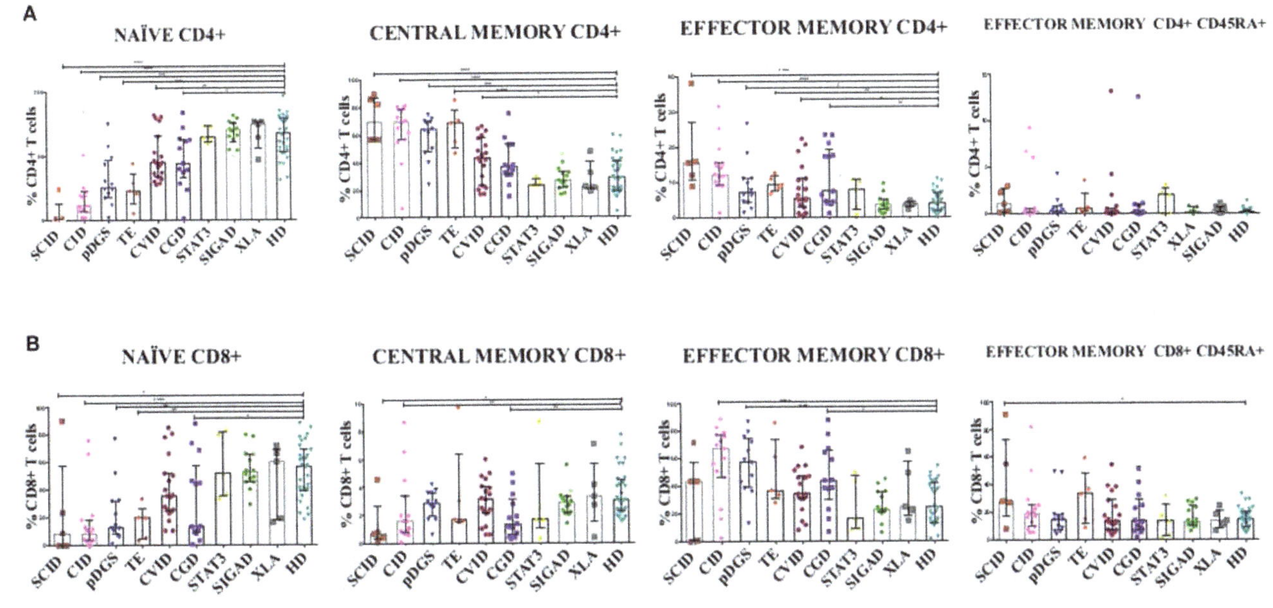

FIGURE 1 | (A) CD4+ and **(B)** CD8+ T cell subsets in patients with primary immunodeficiency diseases. Unpaired two-tailed non-parametric Mann-Whitney test was used to compare the patients and controls. The columns and error bars indicate median and interquantile ranges (25°–75°). *$P \leq 0.05$, **$P \leq 0.01$, ***$P \leq 0.001$, ****$P \leq 0.0001$. SCID and CID patients showed a severe reduction in frequency of T_N CD4+ and CD8+ cells and a corresponding increase in T_{CM} and T_{EM} CD4+ and CD8+, while in CVID patients the same reduction is reported only in CD4+ subsets. DGS and Thymic-excision patients present the same distributions pattern, except for T_{CM} and T_{EM} CD8+. In CGD group there is a reduction in the frequency of T_N CD4+ cells and an increase T_{EM} CD4+ cells, while T_N and T_{CM} CD8+ T cell compartment are significantly reduced accompanied by T_{EM} CD8+ expansion. Symbol with a cross in the SIgAD groups represents the SIgAD patient with the severe clinical presentation. SCID, Severe Combined Immunodeficiency; CID, Combined Immunodeficiency; TE, Thymic Excision; DGS, DiGeorge Syndrome; STAT3, Loss Of Function STAT3 (Autosomal Dominat Hyper-IgE Syndrome); CVID, Common Variable Immunodeficiency; CGD, Chronic Granulomatous Disease; XLA, X-linked Agammaglobulinemia; SIgAD, Selective IgA deficiency; HD, Healthy Donors.

The older than 16 year CVID patient (V16), mother of patient V2 and bearing the same *NFKB2* mutation of her child, outlied far in the upper right quadrant, influenced by the highly increased T_N CD4+ frequencies (**Figure 4B**). In the same age range two CVID patients (V11, V15), segregated according to their relative T_{CM} CD4+ expansion, maintaining normal T_N CD8+ frequencies: V15 carried a Cytotoxic T-Lymphocyte-Associated protein 4 deficiency (CTLA4) while patient V11 is still under investigation (**Figure 4B**). The single selective IgM deficiency patient (M1) was not characterized by a distinctive differentiation pattern, although segregating outside HD area (**Figure 4B**).

DGS and Thymic excision patients were distributed in a broad area between controls and CID group (**Figure 5** and **Supplementary Figure 5B**) mirroring the reported variable T cell defect severity and highlighting those with a CID-like phenotype (D4 and D12). Consistently, patient D1, the only one affected by complete DGS, resembling a SCID phenotype, clustered close to SCID area.

Notably, CGD patients showed a trend vs. effector memory subsets, more evident in older patients and in the younger ones (G5 and G6) with a more severe clinical presentation (**Figure 6**).

DISCUSSION

Several attempts have been used to categorize PIDs based on clinical manifestations, humoral immune defects and T cell phenotypes. Standardized disease definitions are still lacking in the current classification for PIDs, especially in pediatric age (15, 21). Unsupervised clustering methods applied to immunophenotype data might provide additional information regarding the diagnostic and clinical criteria of PIDs, which do not fulfill any classification. We particularly focused our analysis on specific categories of patients, as well as CID and CVID given their high clinical heterogeneity, which increases the complexity of the diagnostic approach and the clinical management. Indeed, according to PCA analysis, most of CID patients clearly segregated from healthy donors and the principal discriminating variables resulted the T_{CM} $CD4^+$ and T_{EM} $CD8^+$ and to a lesser extent T_{EMRA} CD8+ cell subsets, suggesting an imbalance between CD4+ helper and CD8+ cytotoxic function in peripheral sites (22, 23). Their expansion in the majority of CID patients is partially explained by a lymphopenia-induced proliferation process (24, 25), but also revealed a trend to an accelerated T cell exhaustion leading to an inefficient immune response and the risk to develop immunedysregulation phenomena (6). This is particularly evident in APDS patients (C9, C13, C14, C15) (**Figure 2B**), in which their T cell senescence leads to a higher risk of chronic infection, such as EBV replication, and therefore to lymphoproliferative disease/malignancy susceptibility (26). At the same time PCA clearly identified two CID patients (C3, C7) with milder clinical course

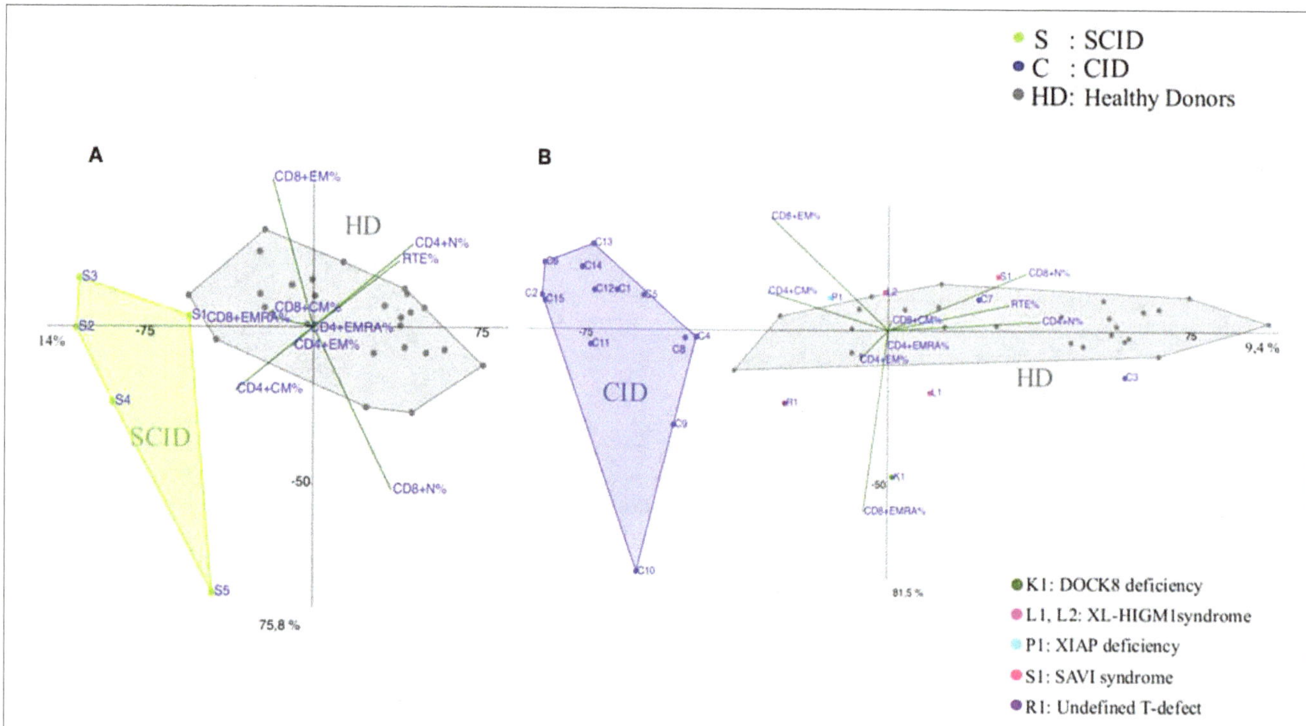

FIGURE 2 | PCA Scatter plots of T cell subpopulations frequencies of **(A)** Severe Combined Immunodeficiency (SCID), **(B)** Combined Immunodeficiency (CID) patients compared to healthy donors (HD). Each sample (subject) is represented by the combination of variables (T subsets) and allocated in a Cartesian space. Samples are plotted, and similarities and differences can be visualized. The overlay of the 2D (2 Dimensional) plot of the scores (subjects) with the 2D plot of the loadings (combination of T subsets) allows the identification of the variables that most contribute to the characterization of a specific subject, since they lie in the same area of the graphs. PCA identifies directions, called principal components, along which the variation in the data is maximal, reported as percentages near the axis. SCID patients are indicated by green dots and the letter S, CID patients by blue dots and the letter C and healthy donors (HD) are represented by gray dots. Individual patients are represented as: C3 and C7 (blue dots) diagnosed as Combined Immunodeficiency patients (CID), K1 (dark green dot) is a DOCK8 Deficiency patient (AR-HIES), L1 and L2 (fuchsia dots) are X-Linked HyperIgM type1 patients (XL-HIGM1), P1 (light blue) is a patient with X-Linked Inhibitor of Apoptosis Protein deficiency (XIAP), S1 (magenta dot) is a SAVI patient (STING-Associated Vasculopathy with onset in Infancy: STING), R1 (purple dot) is a patient with a not determined T cell defect.

segregating far from CID area and close to HD (**Figure 4A**), distinguishing them from those at higher risk to develop severe complications.

A highly heterogeneous pattern of T cell abnormalities has been observed in CVID group (**Figures 3**, **4A,B** and **Supplementary Figure 3**) and PCA clustered some CVID immunophenotypes in proximity to CID area, providing a clue for a deeper monitoring in these patients. Recent ESID Registry-Working Definitions for Clinical Diagnosis shows that some patients, previously diagnosed as CVID, were reclassified as CID and unclassified antibody deficiency (15, 27). Indeed, V8 patient, initially identified as CVID, showed a marked T_{CM} CD4+ and T_{EM} CD8+ expansion (**Figure 4A**), suggesting that a more aggressive treatment should have been considered, before developing fatal complications. In patient V15 segregating far from HD due to T_{CM} CD4+ increase (**Figure 4B**) a *CTLA4* haploinsufficiency responsible for a perturbed T CD4+ cell homeostasis was eventually confirmed by NGS (28).

Interestingly V2 (**Figure 4A**) and V16 patients (**Figure 4B**) currently diagnosed as CVID clustered far from either HD

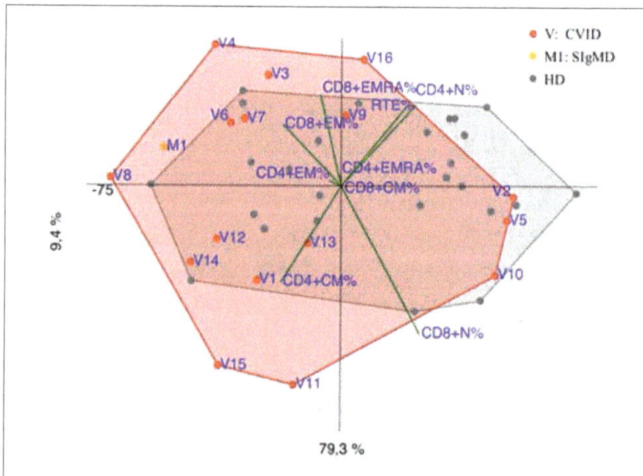

FIGURE 3 | PCA Scatter plot of T cell subpopulations frequencies of CVID patients (shown as red dots and the letter V) and SIgMD patient (orange dot) compared to healthy donors (HD gray dots) show overlapping areas except for V3,V4, V8, V11, V15, V16 and M1.

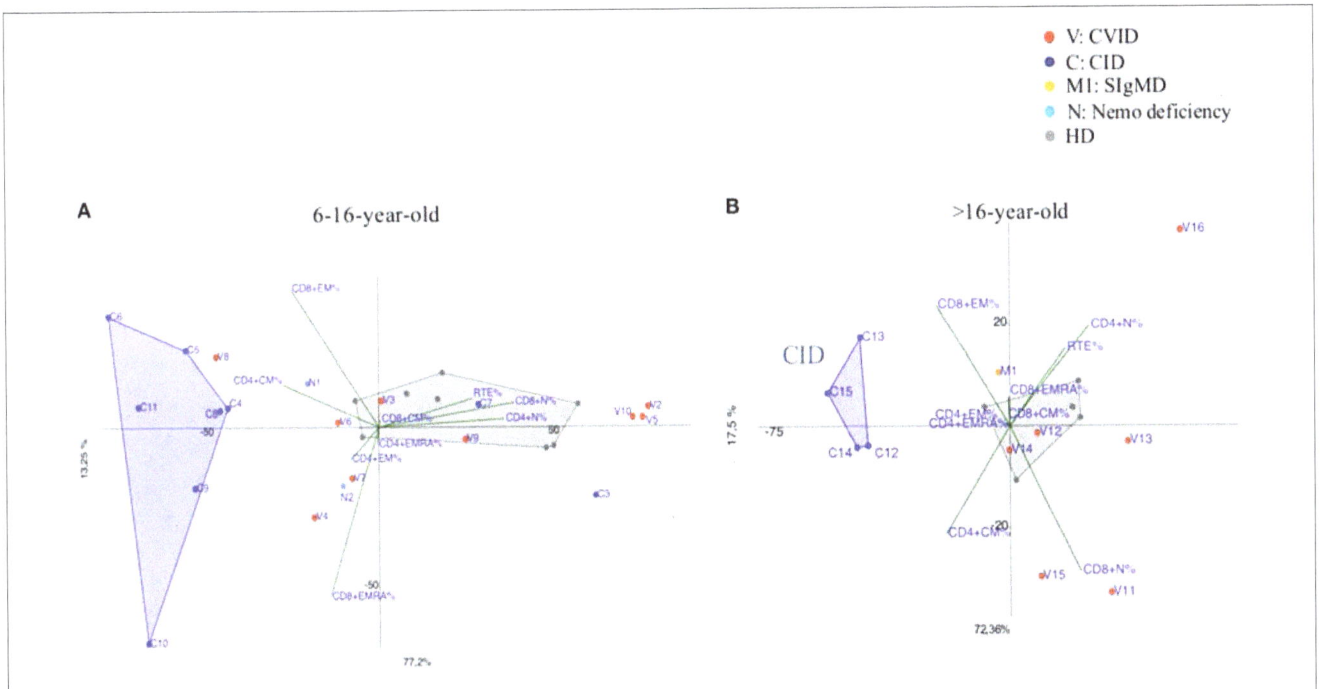

FIGURE 4 | (A) 6–16-year-old CVID patients (shown as red dots and with the letter V) compared to 6–16 year old CID patients (distinguished by blue dots and the letter C) and age matched HDs (shown as gray dots). CVID patients (V2, V5, V10) showed immunoprofile with increased T_N CD4+ although they do not have the same diagnosis. N1 and N2 (light blue dots) patients bearing a splice site mutation NEMO transcript are differently identified: N1 more vs. T_{CM} CD4+ while N2 showed a trend vs. $T_{EM/EMRA}$ CD8+. **(B)** more than 16-year-old CVID patients (shown as red dots and the letter V) compared to more than 16-year CID patients (drawn as blue dots and the letter C) and age matched HD (shown as gray dots). CID patients (C13, C14, C15) diagnosed as APDS (activated PI3K delta syndrome) and C12 cluster together due to the main discriminating variables such as T_{CM} CD4+ and T_{EM} CD8+ and to T_{EMRA} CD8+ cell subsets. M1 (orange dot) is a selective IgM deficiency (SIgMD) patient with an immunoprofile showing a trend vs. late memory differentiation in both CD4+ and CD8+ subsets.

and CVID group reflecting their own peculiar *NFKB2* driven differentiation defect (T_N cell expansion) (29, 30). NEMO deficiency patients (N1, N2) (**Figure 4A**) showed a different trend vs. T_{CM} CD4+ and $T_{EM/EMRA}$ CD8+ respectively, confirming the high variability in the clinical and immunological disease expression (31). IgM deficiency patient (M1) (**Figure 4B**) showed a trend vs. late memory differentiation in both CD4+ and CD8+ subsets that could influence B cell subset, as reported in a larger cohort (32).

As largely described (33), immunoprofiles of patients with partial DGS and Thymic excisions resulted extremely heterogeneuos in PCA (**Figure 5**), as well as in their clinical course. Patients who underwent to total thymic excision during cardiac surgery in neonatal age show a clinical improvement with age in terms of frequency/severity of infections, suggesting a peripheral recovery of the T-cell compartment (34). Interestingly two patients partial DGS (D4 and D12) with a more severe clinical phenotype (refractory autoimmune cytopenia and recurrent bacterial infections) clustered in CID area suggesting the need of a stricter follow up.

Although CGD is primarily a phagocytes disorder, recent evidence showed a defect in adaptive immunity in both T and B cell compartment (35–37), as shown in PCA by an early T cell senescence evident in older CGD patients (**Figure 6**), probably related to chronic inflammation. PCA could be useful to consider and to monitor an immunomodulating treatment whenever necessary in CGD patients to reduce the T cell exhaustion (38).

No evident alterations and specific segregation were detected in XL-HIGM1, XIAP, LOF STAT3 (AD-HIES), and SIgAD patients (**Supplementary Figures 4A,B**), except for one SIgAD patient (A13) with a severe autoimmune cytopenia which segregated outside the HD area (39–42). Although reduction in CD4+ memory T cell subsets was previously reported in XLA patients (43), this data was not confirmed in our limited cohort and a longer follow up is necessary. Only two XLA patients (X2 and X4) segregated accordingly to their $T_{EM/EMRA}$ CD8+ cell expansion, likely associated to recent infections (**Supplementary Figure 4B**).

In order to test the PCA potentiality, we applied it in three patients (K1, R1, and S1) with a severe clinical presentation not easily classifiable (**Figure 2B** and **Table 1**). Patient K1, with a history of endocarditis, vasculitis and sepsis, apparently normal T cell count, showed a high and evident terminal effector CD8+ T cells expansion and later DOCK8 deletion was detected using multiple genetic approaches (44, 45). Patient R1, with a history of interstitial pneumonia and lymphocytes lung infiltration, showed T_{EM} CD4+ expansion, alerting us for a severe but still undefined T cell defect. Finally, child S1

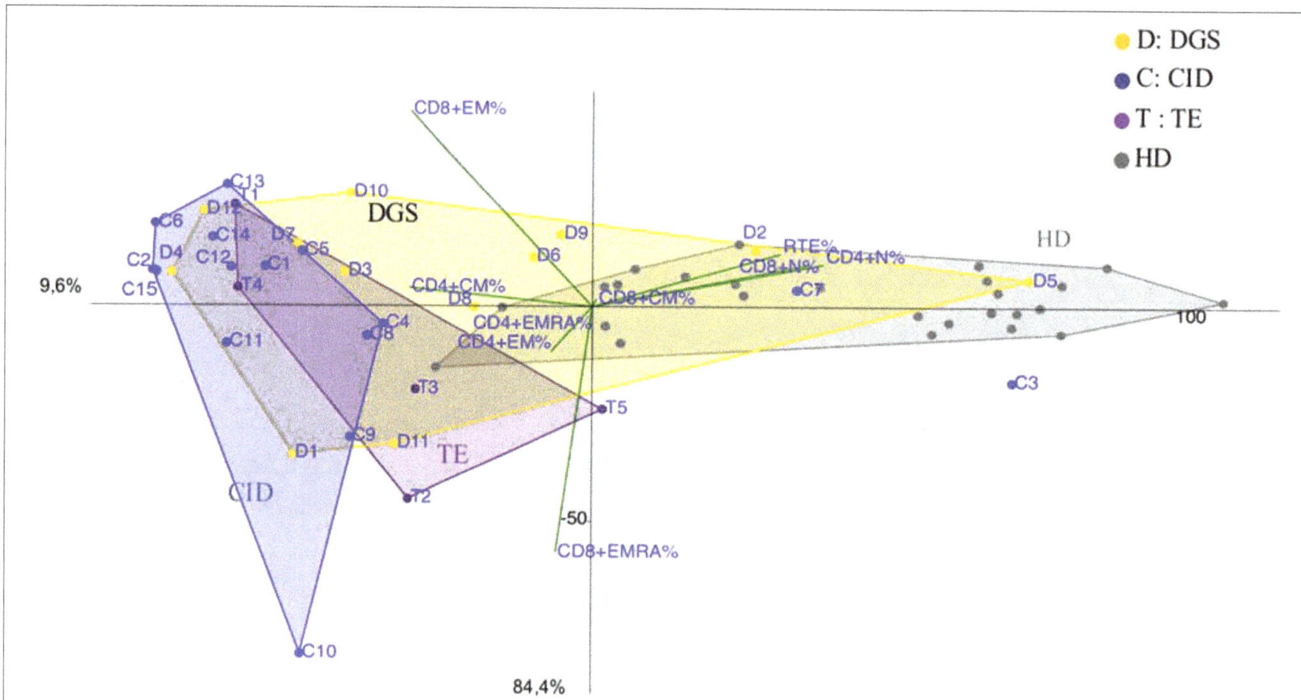

FIGURE 5 | PCA Scatter plots of T cell subpopulations frequencies of DiGeorge Syndrome (DGS, yellow dots and letter D) patients, Thymic Excision patients (TE, distinguished by purple dots and letter T), Combined Immunodeficiency (CID, represented by blue dots and the letter C) patients and healthy donors are shown as gray dots. D1 is the complete DGS patient, D4 and D12 are partial DGS patients with a CID-like clinical presentation.

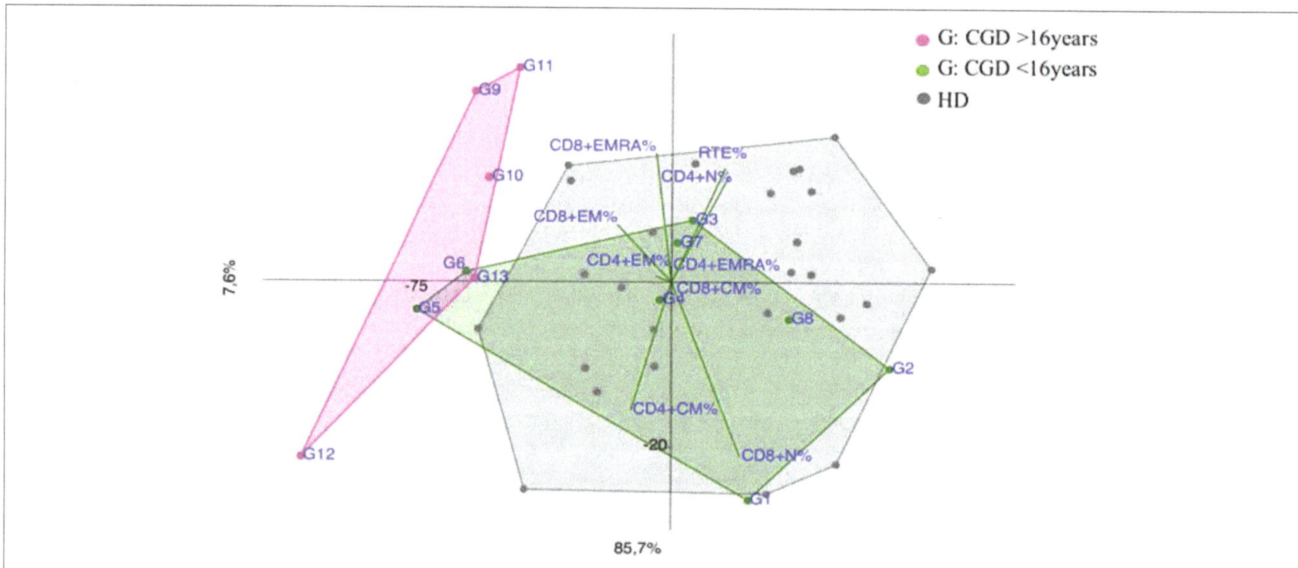

FIGURE 6 | PCA Scatter plots of T cell subpopulations frequencies of Chronic Granulomatous Disease (CGD) patients divided by age: younger CGD patients (G1, G2, G3, G4, G5, G6, G7, G8 represented by green dots) are <16 year old; they cluster inside HD area with the exception of G5 and G6, that are two twin brothers with a severe clinical presentation. The older than 16 year CGD patients (G9, G10, G11, G12, G13 drawn as fuchsia dots), show a CID-like immunoprofile.

with a picture mimicking a CID, in PCA segregated close to healthy donors' area, ruling out a severe immunodeficiency. Mutation in STING gene was detected by NGS targeted panel for autoinflammatory inborn error allowing the start of a specific treatment (46).

CONCLUSIONS

The multivariate data processing techniques could be used as a diagnostic and prognostic tool to identify peculiar immune profiles, to screen atypical PID with higher risk for severe disease progression and monitor the response to personalized therapeutic approaches.

AUTHOR CONTRIBUTIONS

SD performed the experiments, analyzed, and interpreted the results and wrote the manuscript. EA analyzed and interpreted the results and wrote the manuscript. GD and CCi performed the molecular analysis. EA, NC, DA, CG, CCi, PP, and AF provided or referred clinical samples and patient's clinical data. EA, SD, and CCa designed the work, participated to the study design and data interpretation. NC, DA, MC, GD, CCi, and PR revised critically the manuscript.

FUNDING

The study was supported by grants of the Italian Ministero della Salute (NET-2011-02350069) to CCa and Ricerca Corrente from Childrens' Hospital Bambino Gesù, Rome, Italy (201702P003966) to CCa. We are grateful to Yu Nee Lee for providing advice regarding the multivariate analysis and Prof. Notarangelo Luigi for helpful suggestions.

SUPPLEMENTARY MATERIAL

Supplementary Figure 1 | Naïve and memory T-cell subsets gating strategy. PBMC from lysed whole blood were gated on live lymphocytes and identified as CD45+. Then after sequential gating on CD3+CD4+ subset, the naïve (T_N) cells were distinguished as CD45RA+CD27+, central memory cells (T_{CM}) as CD45RA-CD27+, effector memory cells (T_{EM}) as CD45RA-CD27-, and terminally differentiated cells (T_{EMRA}) as CD45RA+CD27-. Among CD3+CD4+ T cells, recent thymic emigrants (RTE) were identified as CD31++CD45RA+. Similarly after gating on CD3+CD8+ subset, the naïve (T_N) cells were gated as CD45RA+CCR7+, central memory cells (T_{CM}) as CD45RA-CCR7+, effector memory cells (T_{EM}) as CD45RA-CCR7-, and terminally differentiated cells (T_{EMRA}) as CD45RA+CCR7-.

Supplementary Figure 2 | PCA Scatter plot of T cell subpopulations frequencies in SCID patients and HD < 6-year-old. Healthy donors <6-year-old are represented by gray dots and SCID patients by green dots and the letter S. PCA identifies directions along which the variation in the data is maximal, in this analysis represented by T_{CM} CD4+ cells inversely correlated to T_N CD4+ as variables that most contribute to the characterization of different subjects.

Supplementary Figure 3 | Less than 6-year-old Common Variable Immunodeficiency (CVID) aged patient (V1) indicated by red dot and the letter V compared to aged matched Combined Immunodeficiency (CID) patients, represented by blue dots and the letter C and age matched healthy donors (HD) shown as gray dots.

Supplementary Figure 4 | PCA Scatter plot of T cell subpopulations frequencies in **(A)** Loss of Function STAT3 (LOF STAT3) (Autosomal Dominant Hyper-IgE Syndrome) (AD-HIES) patients represented by green dots and the letter E and healthy donors by gray dots, showing the complete overlapping of the areas. **(B)** X-linked Agammaglobulinemia (XLA) patients by light blue dots and the letter X, Selective IgA deficiency (SIgAD) patients by yellow dots and the letter A, one not defined Agammaglobulinemia patient (n.d) by brown dot and letter Y, healthy donors are represented by gray dots. The X2 and X4 patients' immunoprofiles segregated outside HD area, accordingly to their $T_{EM/EMRA}$ CD8+ cell expansion. Not defined Agammaglobulinemia (Y1) patient clustered in the HD area, not revealing any peculiar pattern.

Supplementary Figure 5 | PCA Scatter plots of T cell subpopulations frequencies of **(A)** Severe Combined Immunodeficiency (SCID) compared to Combined Immunodeficiency (CID) patients. SCID patients are indicated by green dots and the letter S and CID patients by blue dots and the letter C. **(B)** DiGeorge Syndrome (DGS) patients (represented by yellow dots and letter D), Thymic excision patients (TE) (by purple dots and letter T) compared to CID patients (by blue dots and the letter C).

Supplementary Tables 1a–c | Clinical and molecular diagnosis of the patients.

REFERENCES

1. Notarangelo LD. Primary immunodeficiencies. *J Allergy Clin Immunol.* (2010) 125:S182–94. doi: 10.1016/j.jaci.2009.07.053
2. Lehman HK. Autoimmunity and immune dysregulation in primary immune deficiency disorders. *Curr Allergy Asthma Rep.* (2015) 15:53. doi: 10.1007/s11882-015-0553-x
3. Bousfiha A, Jeddane L, Picard C, Ailal F, Bobby Gaspar H, Al-Herz W, et al. The 2017 IUIS phenotypic classification for primary immunodeficiencies. *J Clin Immunol.* (2018) 38:129–43. doi: 10.1007/s10875-017-0465-8
4. Fischer A. Severe Combined Immunodeficiencies (SCID). *Clin Exp Immunol.* (2000) 122:143–9. doi: 10.1046/j.1365-2249.2000.01359.x
5. Cifaldi C, Alessandro F, Caterina A, Email C. *Hematopoietic Stem Cell Gene Therapy for the Cure of Blood Diseases: Primary Immunodeficiencies.* Rendiconti Lincei. Scienze Fisiche e Naturali. Available online at: doi: 10.1007/s12210-018-0742-3 (accessed October 30, 2018).
6. Delmonte OM, Castagnoli R, Calzoni E, Notarangelo LD. Inborn errors of immunity with immune dysregulation: from bench to bedside. *Front Pediatr.* (2019) 7:353. doi: 10.3389/fped.2019.00353
7. Picard C, Al-Herz W, Bousfiha A, Casanova JL, Chatila T, Conley ME, et al. Primary immunodeficiency diseases: an update on the classification from the international union of immunological societies expert committee for primary immunodeficiency 2015. *J Clin Immunol.* (2015) 35:696–726. doi: 10.3389/fimmu.2014.00162
8. Speckmann C, Doerken S, Aiuti A, Albert MH, Al-Herz W, Allende LM, et al. A prospective study on the natural history of patients with profound combined immunodeficiency: an interim analysis. *J Allergy Clin Immunol.* (2017) 139:1302–10.e4. doi: 10.1016/j.jaci.2016.07.040
9. pCID study (DRKS00000497). Available online at: https://www.uniklinik-freiburg.de/cci/studien/p-cid.htm
10. Bateman EA, Ayers L, Sadler R, Lucas M, Roberts C, Woods A, et al. T cell phenotypes in patients with common variable immunodeficiency disorders: associations with clinical phenotypes in comparison with other groups with recurrent infections. *Clin Exp Immunol.* (2012) 170:202–11. doi: 10.1111/j.1365-2249.2012.04643.x
11. Fritsch RD, Shen X, Sims GP, Hathcock KS, Hodes RJ, Lipsky PE. Stepwise differentiation of CD4 memory T cells defined by expression of CCR7 and CD27. *J Immunol.* (2005) 175:6489–97. doi: 10.4049/jimmunol.175.10.6489
12. Maecker HT, McCoy JP, Nussenblatt R. Standardizing immunophenotyping for the human immunology project. *Nat Rev Immunol.* (2012) 12:191–200. doi: 10.1038/nri3229
13. Garcia-Prat M, Álvarez-Sierra D, Aguiló-Cucurull A, Salgado-Perandrés S, Briongos-Sebastian S, Franco-Jarava C, et al. Extended immunophenotyping

reference values in a healthy pediatric population. *Cytometry B Clin Cytom.* (2019) 96:223–33. doi: 10.1002/cyto.b.21728
14. van der Burg M, Kalina T, Perez-Andres M, Vlkova M, Lopez-Granados E, Blanco E, et al. The EuroFlow PID orientation tube for flow cytometric diagnostic screening of primary immunodeficiencies of the lymphoid system. *Front Immunol.* (2019) 10:246. doi: 10.3389/fimmu.2019.00246
15. Seidel MG, Kindle G, Gathmann B, Quinti I, Buckland M, van Montfrans J, et al. The European Society for Immunodeficiencies (ESID) registry working definitions for the clinical diagnosis of inborn errors of immunity. *J Allergy Clin Immunol Pract.* (2019) 7:1763–70. doi: 10.1016/j.jaip.2019.02.004
16. Genser B, Cooper PJ, Yazdanbakhsh M, Barreto ML, Rodrigues LC. A guide to modern statistical analysis of immunological data. *BMC Immunol.* (2007) 8:27. doi: 10.1186/1471-2172-8-27
17. Lugli E, Roederer M, Cossarizza A. Data analysis in flow cytometry: the future just started. *Cytometry A.* (2010) 77:705–13. doi: 10.1002/cyto.a.20901
18. Hazenberg MD, Verschuren MC, Hamann D, Miedema F, van Dongen JJ. T cell receptor excision circles as markers for recent thymic emigrants: basic aspects, technical approach, and guidelines for interpretation. *J Mol Med.* (2001) 79:631–40. doi: 10.1007/s001090100271
19. Junge S, Kloeckener-Gruissem B, Zufferey R, Keisker A, Salgo B, Fauchere JC, et al. Correlation between recent thymic emigrants and CD31+ (PECAM-1) CD4+ T cells in normal individuals during aging and in lymphopenic children. *Eur J Immunol.* (2007) 37:3270–80. doi: 10.1002/eji.200636976
20. Crow YJ, Casanova JL. STING-associated vasculopathy with onset in infancy–a new interferonopathy. *N Engl J Med.* (2014) 371:568–71. doi: 10.1056/NEJMe1407246
21. Farmer JR, Ong MS, Barmettler S, Yonker LM, Fuleihan R, Sullivan KE, et al. Common variable immunodeficiency non-infectious disease endotypes redefined using unbiased network clustering in large electronic datasets. *Front Immunol.* (2018) 8:1740. doi: 10.3389/fimmu.2017.01740
22. Sallusto F, Geginat J, Lanzavecchia A. Central memory and effector memory T cell subsets: function, generation, and maintenance. *Annu Rev Immunol.* (2004) 22:745–63. doi: 10.1146/annurev.immunol.22.012703.104702
23. Lanzavecchia A, Sallusto F. Understanding the generation and function of memory T cell subsets. *Curr Opin Immunol.* (2005) 17:326–32. doi: 10.1016/j.coi.2005.04.010
24. Delphine S, Larsen M, Fastenackels S, Roux A, Gorochov G, Katlama C, et al. Lymphopenia-driven homeostatic regulation of naive T cells in elderly and thymectomized young adults. *J Immunol.* (2012) 189:5541–8. doi: 10.4049/jimmunol.1201235
25. Saidakova EV, Shmagel KV, Korolevskaya LB, Shmage NG, Chereshnev VA. Lymphopenia-induced proliferation of CD4 T-cells is associated with CD4 T-lymphocyte exhaustion in treated HIV-infected patients. *Indian J Med Res.* (2018) 147:376–83. doi: 10.4103/ijmr.IJMR_1801_15
26. Wentink MWJ, Mueller YM, Dalm VASH, Driessen GJ, van Hagen PM, van Montfrans JM, et al. Exhaustion of the CD8+ T cell compartment in patients with mutations in phosphoinositide 3-kinase delta. *Front Immunol.* (2018) 9:446. doi: 10.3389/fimmu.2018.00446
27. De Valles-Ibáñez G, Esteve-Solé A, Piquer M, González-Navarro EA, Hernandez-Rodriguez J, Laayouni H, et al. Evaluating the genetics of common variable immunodeficiency: monogenetic model and beyond. *Front Immunol.* (2018) 9:636. doi: 10.3389/fimmu.2018.00636
28. Schwab C, Gabrysch A, Olbrich P, Patiño V, Warnatz K, Wolff D, et al. Phenotype, penetrance, and treatment of 133 cytotoxic T-lymphocyte antigen 4-insufficient subjects. *J Allergy Clin Immunol.* (2018) 142:1932–46. doi: 10.1016/j.jaci.2018.02.055
29. Maccari E, Scarselli A, Di Cesare S, Floris M, AngiusA, Deodati A, et al. Severe *Toxoplasma gondii* infection in a member of a NFKB2-deficient family with T and B cell dysfunction. *Clin Immunol.* (2017) 183:273–7. doi: 10.1016/j.clim.2017.09.011
30. Klemann C, Camacho-Ordonez N, Yang L, Eskandarian Z, Rojas-Restrepo JL, Frede N, et al. Clinical and immunological phenotype of patients with primary immunodeficiency due to damaging mutations in NFKB2. *Front Immunol.* (2019) 10:297. doi: 10.3389/fimmu.2019.00297
31. Fusco F, Pescatore A, Conte MI, Mirabelli P, Paciolla M, Esposito E, et al. EDA-ID and IP, two faces of the same coin: how the same IKBKG/NEMO mutation affecting the NF-κB pathway can cause immunodeficiency and/or inflammation. *Int Rev Immunol.* (2015) 34:445–59. doi: 10.3109/08830185.2015.1055331
32. Louis AG, Agrawal S, Gupta S. Analysis of subsets of B cells, Breg, CD4Treg and CD8Treg cells in adult patients with primary selective IgM deficiency. *Am J Clin Exp Immunol.* (2016) 5:21–32.
33. Javier C, Rosenblatt HM, O'Brian Smith E, Shearer WT, Noroski LM. Long-term assessment of T-cell populations in DiGeorge syndrome. *J Allergy Clin Immunol.* (2003) 111:573–9. doi: 10.1067/mai.2003.165
34. van Gent R, Schadenberg AWL, Otto SA, Nievelstein RAJ, Sieswerda GT, Haas F, et al. Long-term restoration of the human T-cell compartment after thymectomy during infancy: a role for thymic regeneration? *Blood.* (2011) 118:627–34. doi: 10.1182/blood-2011-03-341396
35. Chiriaco M, Casciano F, Di Matteo G, Gentner B, Claps A, Di Cesare S, et al. Impaired X-CGD T cell compartment is gp91phox-NADPH oxidase independent. *Clin Immunol.* (2018) 193:52–9. doi: 10.1016/j.clim.2018.01.010
36. Albuquerque AS, Fernandes SM, Tendeiro R, Cheynier R, Lucas M, Silva SL, et al. Major CD4 T-Cell Depletion and Immune Senescence in a Patient with Chronic Granulomatous Disease. *Front Immunol.* (2017) 8:543. doi: 10.3389/fimmu.2017.00543
37. Cotugno N, Finocchi A, Cagigi A, Di Matteo G, Chiriaco M, Di Cesare S, et al. Defective B-cell proliferation and maintenance of long-term memory in patients with chronic granulomatous disease. *J Allergy Clin Immunol.* (2015) 135:753–61.e2. doi: 10.1016/j.jaci.2014.07.012
38. Weisser M, Demel UM, Stein S, Chen-Wichmann L, Touzot F, Santilli G, et al. Hyperinflammation in patients with chronic granulomatous disease leads to impairment of hematopoietic stem cell functions. *J Allergy Clin Immunol.* (2016) 138:219–28.e9. doi: 10.1016/j.jaci.2015.11.028
39. Egwuagu CE. STAT3 in CD4+ T helper cell differentiation and inflammatory diseases. *Cytokine.* (2009) 47:149–56. doi: 10.1016/j.cyto.2009.07.003
40. Ma CS, Chew GYJ, Simpson N, Priyadarshi A, Wong M, Grimbacher B, et al. Deficiency of Th17 cells in hyper IgE syndrome due to mutations in STAT3. *J Exp Med.* (2008) 205:1551–5. doi: 10.1084/jem.20080218
41. Lougaris V, Lanzi G, Baronio M, Gazzurelli L, Vairo D, Lorenzini T, et al. Progressive severe B cell and NK cell deficiency with T cell senescence in adult CD40L deficiency. *Clin Immunol.* (2018) 190:11–14. doi: 10.1016/j.clim.2018.02.008
42. Rebecca A. Marsh, MD, Bleesing JJ, Filipovich AH. Using flow cytometry to screen patients for X-linked lymphoproliferative disease due to SAP deficiency and XIAP deficiency. *J Immunol Methods.* (2010) 362:1–9. doi: 10.1016/j.jim.2010.08.010
43. Martini H, Enright V, Perro M, Workman S, Birmelin J, Giorda E, et al. Importance of B cell co-stimulation in CD4(+) T cell differentiation: X-linked agammaglobulinaemia, a human model. *Clin Exp Immunol.* (2011) 164:381–7. doi: 10.1111/j.1365-2249.2011.04377.x
44. Randall KL, Chan SSY, Ma CS, Fung I, Mei Y, Yabas M, et al. DOCK8 deficiency impairs CD8 T cell survival and function in humans and mice. *J Exp Med.* (2011) 208:2305–20. doi: 10.1084/jem.201 10345
45. Janssen E, Tsitsikov E, Al-Herz W, Lefranc G, Megarbane A, Dasouki M, et al. Flow cytometry biomarkers distinguish DOCK8 deficiency from severe atopic dermatitis. *Clin Immunol.* (2013) 150:220–4. doi: 10.1016/j.clim.2013.12.006
46. Volpi S, Insalaco A, Caorsi R, Santori E, Messia V, Sacco O, et al. Efficacy and adverse events during janus kinase inhibitor treatment of SAVI syndrome. *J Clin Immunol.* (2019) 39:476–85. doi: 10.1007/s10875-019-00645-0

16

Monozygotic Twins Concordant for Common Variable Immunodeficiency: Strikingly Similar Clinical and Immune Profile Associated with a Polygenic Burden

Susana L. Silva[1,2,3], Mariana Fonseca[1,2], Marcelo L. M. Pereira[4], Sara P. Silva[1,2,3], Rita R. Barbosa[1], Ana Serra-Caetano[1,2], Elena Blanco[5,6], Pedro Rosmaninho[1,2], Martin Pérez-Andrés[5,6], Ana Berta Sousa[1,2,3], Alexandre A. S. F. Raposo[1,2], Margarida Gama-Carvalho[4], Rui M. M. Victorino[1,2,3], Lennart Hammarstrom[7] and Ana E. Sousa[1,2]*

[1] Faculdade de Medicina, Instituto de Medicina Molecular João Lobo Antunes, Universidade de Lisboa, Lisbon, Portugal, [2] Centro de Imunodeficiências Primárias, Centro Académico de Medicina de Lisboa, Centro Hospitalar Universitário Lisboa Norte and Faculdade de Medicina da Universidade de Lisboa and Instituto de Medicina Molecular, Lisbon, Portugal, [3] Centro Hospitalar Universitário Lisboa Norte, Hospital de Santa Maria, Lisbon, Portugal, [4] Faculty of Sciences, BioISI-Biosystems & Integrative Sciences Institute, University of Lisboa, Lisbon, Portugal, [5] Department of Medicine, Cancer Research Centre (IBMCC, USAL-CSIC), Cytometry Service (NUCLEUS), Institute of Biomedical Research of Salamanca (IBSAL), University of Salamanca (USAL), Salamanca, Spain, [6] Biomedical Research Networking Centre on Cancer-CIBER-CIBERONC, Number CB16/12/00400, Institute of Health Carlos III, Madrid, Spain, [7] Department of Laboratory Medicine, Karolinska Institutet, Stockholm, Sweden

****Correspondence:***
Susana L. Silva
susanasilva@medicina.ulisboa.pt

Monozygotic twins provide a unique opportunity to better understand complex genetic diseases and the relative contribution of heritable factors in shaping the immune system throughout life. Common Variable Immunodeficiency Disorders (CVID) are primary antibody defects displaying wide phenotypic and genetic heterogeneity, with monogenic transmission accounting for only a minority of the cases. Here, we report a pair of monozygotic twins concordant for CVID without a family history of primary immunodeficiency. They featured a remarkably similar profile of clinical manifestations and immunological alterations at diagnosis (established at age 37) and along the subsequent 15 years of follow-up. Interestingly, whole-exome sequencing failed to identify a monogenic cause for CVID, but unraveled a combination of heterozygous variants, with a predicted deleterious impact. These variants were found in genes involved in relevant immunological pathways, such as *JUN*, *PTPRC*, *TLR1*, *ICAM1,* and *JAK3*. The potential for combinatorial effects translating into the observed disease phenotype is inferred from their roles in immune pathways, namely in T and B cell activation. The combination of these genetic variants is also likely to impose a significant constraint on environmental influences, resulting in a similar immunological phenotype in both twins, despite exposure to different living conditions. Overall, these cases stress the importance of integrating NGS data with clinical and immunological phenotypes at the single-cell level, as provided by multi-dimensional flow-cytometry, in order to understand the complex genetic landscape underlying the vast majority of patients with CVID, as well as those with other immunodeficiencies.

Keywords: CVID, flow-cytometry, polygenic disease, genetics, WES, monozygotic twins

BACKGROUND

Monozygotic twins provide a unique opportunity to evaluate the relative contribution of genome and environment to the development and evolution of the immune system throughout life (1–3). A recent study on a large twin cohort suggests that life experience is the main determinant, challenging the importance of genetic background (2). Monozygotic twins (MZ) also provide a valuable tool to investigate complex diseases of the immune system like Common Variable Immunodeficiency (CVID).

CVID is defined overall by a marked decrease in serum IgG and IgA, normal or decreased serum IgM, poor antibody responses to vaccines and absence of other identifiable causes for hypogammaglobulinemia (4). However, almost all components of the immune system may feature alterations, with high heterogeneity between patients (5, 6). Given the marked clinical heterogeneity, multiparametric flow-cytometry is instrumental to detail the individual immune profile (7–10), allowing personalized approaches to treatment and monitoring of co-morbidities (7, 10).

A genetic basis for CVID was already recognized in 1968 (11), though the identification of the underlying molecular defects has been hampered in the majority of patients, which usually do not have a family history. In recent years, next generation sequencing (NGS) strategies, including genome-wide association and whole-exome/genome sequencing studies (WES/WGS) (9, 12–19), have facilitated the identification of an increasing list of genes, with heterozygous or biallelic variants associated with monogenic CVID (9, 12–20). Nevertheless, monogenic transmission is currently assumed in only 15–25% of the patients with CVID, in association with pathogenic variants in genes related mostly to B-cell activation, T-cell signaling and cytokine expression (14, 15, 17, 20). Conversely, CVID is likely to be polygenic in the majority of patients, resulting from multiple epistatic interactions with cumulative effects (12, 21). Consistently, CVID may develop clinically at any age, suggesting progressive and cumulative deterioration of B-cell functions, in a putative multifactorial pathogenic process (8, 22).

The contribution of non-heritable influences, such as infectious exposure, to the establishment of the clinical and immunological phenotypes in CVID is also recognized (23). The possible role of viral infections as triggers to disease onset, and the impact of microbiome are illustrative ongoing debates (23, 24). Twin studies thus provide a powerful model to dissect the relative contributions of heritable and non-heritable variables to the establishment of clinical and immunological profiles, but have so far been poorly explored, given the rarity of these cases (2, 3).

We provide here the first report of MZ twins concordant for CVID. Extensive phenotypic profile of circulating B and T-cell subsets was obtained by flow-cytometry at diagnosis and during 15-years follow-up. The twins featured a remarkably similar immunologic and clinical profile, despite the absence of a recognizable monogenic cause, being 50 years-old, and having lived apart for many years. Importantly, WES allowed us to identify a combination of variants with putative impact in the immune system that is not shared by their progenitors or progeny, supporting a polygenic basis for the CVID phenotype and their concordant immune evolution.

CASE PRESENTATION

CVID diagnosis was performed at 37 years of age in a pair of Caucasian MZ twins, living in Lisbon, Portugal, born from non-consanguineous parents and with no family history of primary immunodeficiency. They presented a remarkably similar clinical and immunological profile throughout 15 years of follow-up, despite distinct living conditions (jobs, housing, and nuclear families) since age 25.

At diagnosis, both twins featured severe hypogammaglobulinemia, with very low serum IgG (<0.3 and 1.65 g/L, cases 1 and 2, respectively), undetectable IgA (<0.25 g/L) and IgM (<0.19 g/L), and no increase in titres of specific IgG upon polysaccharide pneumococcal and conjugated *Haemophilus influenzae* vaccinations. They had a low frequency of circulating total and memory B cells, particularly of switched-memory B cells, with no expansions of transitional B cells or of cells expressing low levels of CD21 (**Figure 1A**), thus featuring an identical EuroClass classification $B^{+}smB^{-}Tr^{norm}21^{norm}$ (25). They also exhibited comparable naïve/memory subset distribution and expression of activation markers in CD4 and CD8 T cells (**Figure 1B**), with a defect in CD45 alternative splicing leading to the persistence of CD45RA in memory/effector T cells. Functional studies in T cells revealed an equal production of IL-2, IL-4, IFNγ, and IL-17 (**Figure 1B**) and impairment of proliferative responses to recall antigens, despite the relative high levels of proliferative responses to mitogens (**Figure 1C**).

Along the follow-up there was concordant evolution of their immunological profile, shown by the PCAs obtained at age 50 with the EuroFlow protocols (**Figure 2A**). The detailed phenotypic evaluation of circulating B cells revealed severe B-cell depletion (total B cells <1%) in both, with residual preservation of $IgG3^{+}CD27^{-}$ memory B cells detected by high-sensitivity methods (7, 26, 27) (**Figure 2B**). This profile, which reflects extreme deterioration of IgG-switching capacity in memory B cells, is compatible with the most severe (CVID-6) subgroup, as recently reported in the literature (7).

The type and severity of clinical manifestations before diagnosis and during follow-up have also been very similar. Both twins featured upper and lower respiratory infections since their twenties, with progressively increased frequency leading to several hospital admissions for pneumonia; bilateral bronchiectasis; and nasal polypectomy at age 32 in both. Upon diagnosis, intravenous IgG replacement was initiated, leading to serum IgG levels above 800–900 mg/dL and a marked decline in the frequency of infectious episodes. Both maintained persistent sinusitis, with recurrent exacerbations mostly in conjunction with *H. influenza* infection, and intermittent non-infectious diarrhea compatible with minor chronic lymphocytic infiltration, observed in duodenal and colon mucosa.

This remarkably similar profile in MZ twins strongly suggested that the genetic background is the main contributor

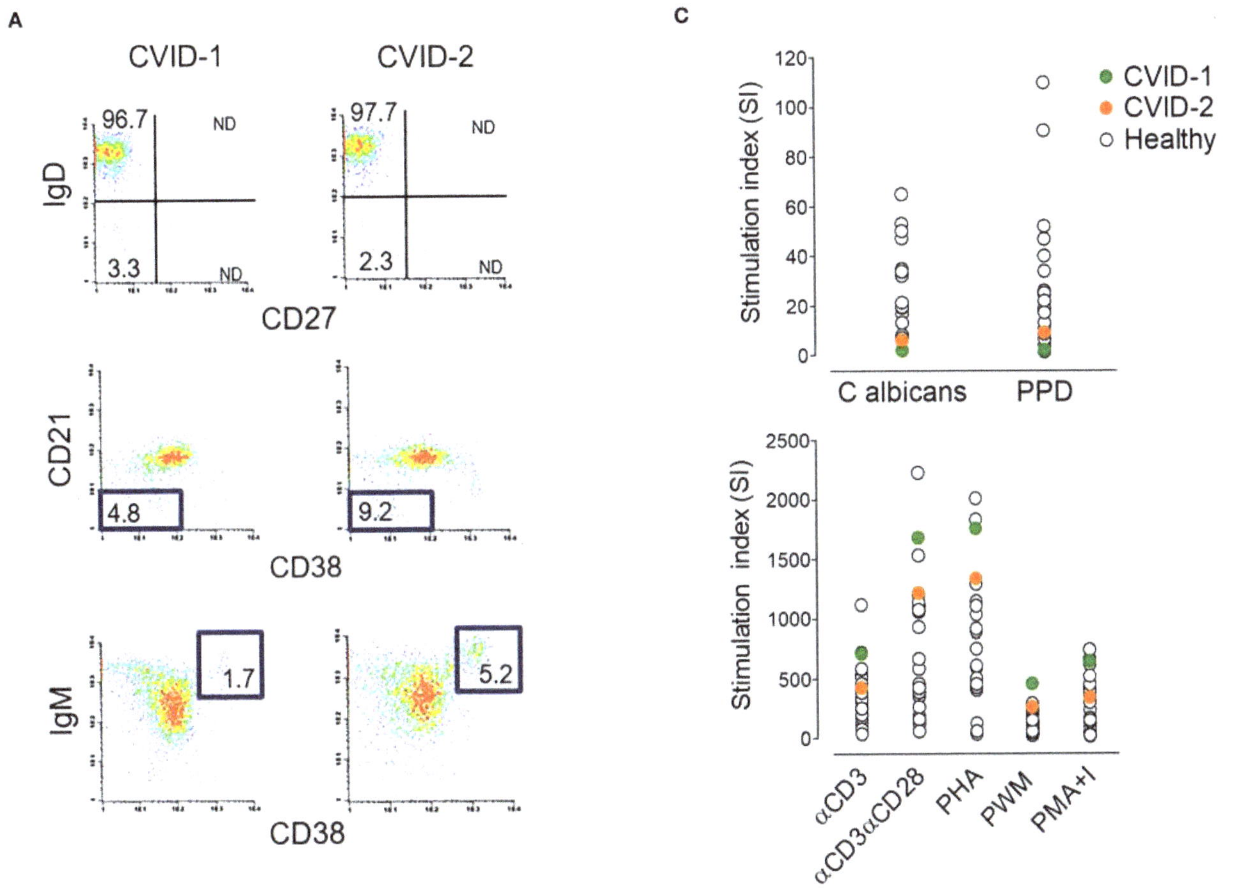

B

		Naïve	RO+27+	RO+27-	HLA-DR+	IL-2+	IL-4+	IFN-γ+	IL-17+
% within CD4 T-cells	CVID-1	64.4	33.7	1.9	8.6	35.3	1.2	5.7	0.4
	CVID-2	61.3	36.8	1.8	9.3	43.9	1.9	6.9	0.5
% within CD8 T-cells	CVID-1	56.1	15.9	10.6	32.1	14.4	0.5	24.6	<0.1
	CVID-2	59.5	17.4	9.1	35.4	21.7	1.1	24.7	<0.1

FIGURE 1 | Immune phenotype at CVID diagnosis at age 37 in the MZ twins. **(A)** Representative plots of the flow-cytometry analysis of switched-memory B cells (top), $CD21^{low}CD38^{low}$ B cells (middle) and transitional B cells (bottom). Numbers represent the percentage of the given population within $CD19^{+}$ cells (3.0%/4.2% in case-1/case-2, respectively). **(B)** Frequency of naïve and memory subpopulations, expression of activation marker $HLA\text{-}DR^{+}$, and frequency of cells producing IL-2, IL-4, IFN-γ, and IL-17 within CD4 and CD8 T cells (1,777/1,380 lymphocytes/μL; CD4 T cells 42.2%/43.6%; CD8 T cells 44.1%/39.8%; in cases 1/2, respectively) **(C)** Lymphoproliferative responses upon culture with antigens (top) and mitogens (bottom) in comparison with healthy adult individuals.

to their clinical and immunological evolution. We therefore sequenced their whole exome (WES) using DNA extracted from blood samples. We focused the analysis on genes involved in immunological pathways, identifying SNVs with a non-synonymous coding effect predicted to be either probably damaging or deleterious (28, 29), or frame shift variants (see Methods). We also looked for variants affecting mRNA splice sites, but we found no variants in genes reported as monogenic causes of CVID. In fact, WES analysis was unable to reveal a monogenic cause for CVID. However, we identified in both a combination of 7 heterozygous SNVs, occurring in *JAK3, JUN, LYST, MBL2, ICAM1, and TLR1* (**Table 1** and **Figure 3A**). None of these 6 genes has previously been shown to be associated with *monogenic* CVID (15, 32). A compound heterozygous change, combining one variant from each parent, was found in *ICAM1*.

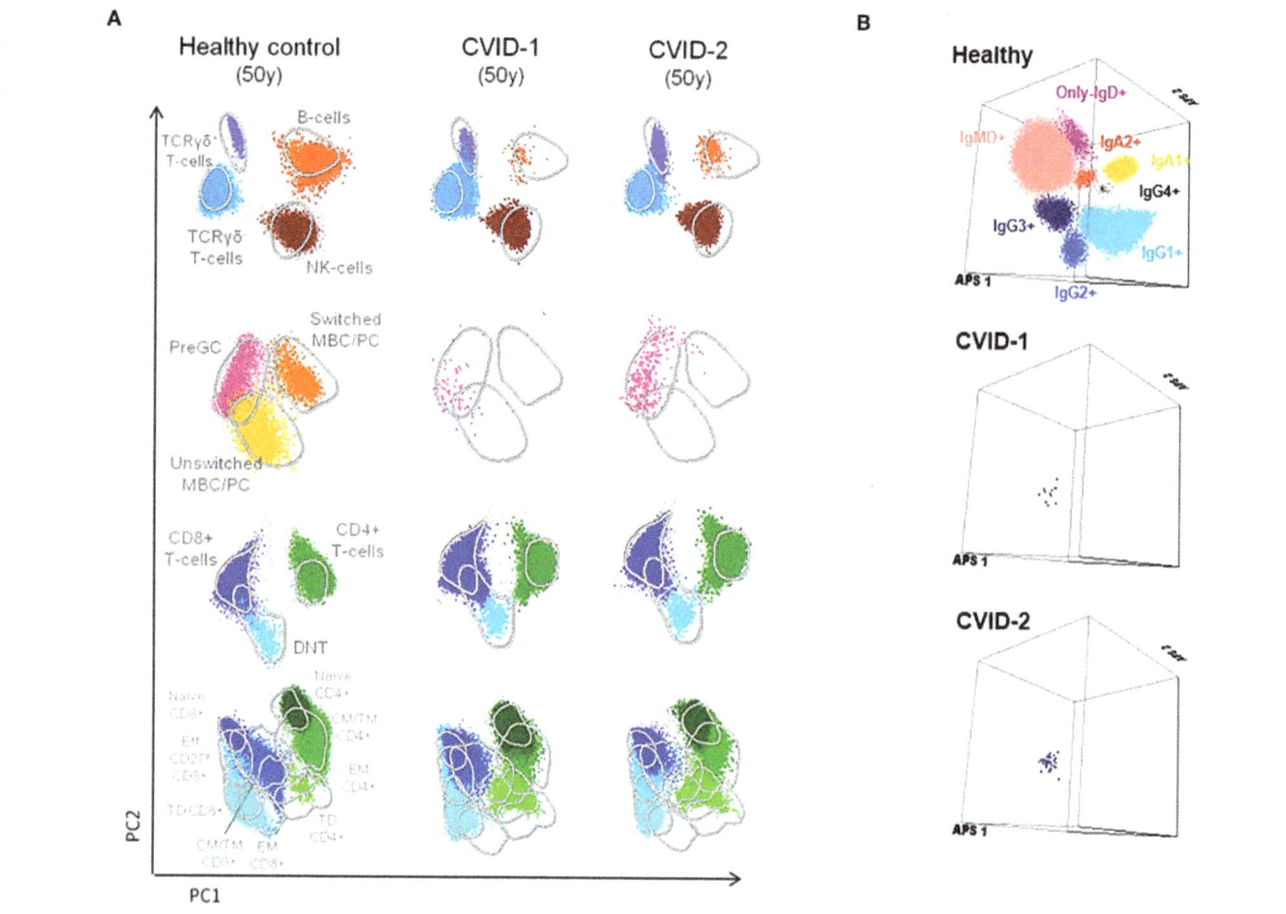

FIGURE 2 | Supervised flow-cytometric analysis of blood lymphocytes in MZ twins concordant for CVID at age 50. **(A)** Principal component analysis (PCA) multidimensional view of the distribution of major lymphocyte subsets analyzed with the EuroFlow PID orientation tube in 1 × 10^6 peripheral blood leukocytes. **(B)** Distribution of memory B cells according to the surface membrane expression of the IgH-isotypes (IgM, IgD, IgG1, IgG2, IgG3, IgG4, IgA1, and IgA2) in 5 × 10^6 peripheral blood leukocytes analyzed from an age-matched healthy donor and the two twins with CVID (7, 8, 26).

In face of the defect in CD45 alternative splicing observed in T cells, we additionally looked at variants in *PTPRC (CD45)*. We found the twins were heterozygous carriers of C77G (**Table 1** and **Figure 3A**), a heterozygous variant that was previously reported in heterozigosity in CVID patients (33, 34).

In order to elucidate the segregation of the identified variants and their possible associations with clinical manifestations and/or immunological profile, their parents and children were also evaluated. Neither the progenitors nor the progeny had any severe/recurrent infections or immune-mediated diseases, and all had normal levels of serum IgG, IgA, and IgM, except for one son with a past-history of autoimmune thrombocytopenia (III:3, **Figure 3A**). Parents and children were genotyped for the 8 genetic variants (**Figure 3A**) and the variants considered were found to be split between parents, and none of the descendants inherited the combination of variants observed in the twins. Due to the frequent onset of CVID-associated clinical manifestations in adulthood, prospective follow-up of the offspring, particularly of the son with a past-history of autoimmune thrombocytopenia, will be important to complete our current interpretation of NGS data.

METHODS

Patients and Relatives

Longitudinal data obtained from a pair of MZ twins followed at Centro de Imunodeficiências Primárias, of Lisbon Academic Medical Center. The patients met the European Society for Immunodeficiencies (ESID) diagnostic criteria for CVID at the time of enrolment (35). Patients and relatives gave written informed consent. The study was approved by the ethical boards of the Faculty of Medicine of University of Lisbon and Centro Hospitalar Universitário Lisboa Norte.

Immunological Studies

Phenotypic analysis was performed by flow-cytometry during follow-up using previously described protocols (8, 36, 37) and different cytometers (FACSCalibur, FACSCanto and

TABLE 1 | Selected SNVs with impact in the immune system identified by WES.

Gene	Change coordinates	Ensembl transcript ID	Protein variant (HGVS)	dbSNP ID	ExAC (MAF EUR)	PolyPhen	SIFT	Immunological role of the gene-encoded protein
JAK3	chr19:17952472 T/C	ENST00000428406 ENST00000458235 ENST00000527670 ENST00000534444	T321A	NA	NA	PD	T	Member of Janus kinase family of tyrosine kinases; Cytokine receptor-mediated intracellular signal transduction
ICAM1	chr19:10394792 G/A	ENST00000264832	G241R	rs1799969	0,1102	PD	D	Cell surface glycoprotein with major role in cell-cell adhesion, in endothelia and immune cells
	chr19:10395468 G/A	ENST00000423829 ENST00000264832	R397Q	rs5497	0,0006	PD	D	
JUN	chr1:59248405 C/G	ENST00000371222	G113A	rs1462279538	NA	PD	D	Transcription Factor AP-1 interacts with specific target DNA sequences to regulate gene expression in the immune system
LYST	chr1:235972992 G/T	ENST00000536965 ENST00000389794 ENST00000389793	P376T	rs770362521	3×10^{-5}	PD	T	Regulates intracellular protein trafficking in endosomes; Mutations associated with Chediak-Higashi syndrome with impaired cytotoxic lymphocyte function (30)
TLR1	chr4: 38799956; NM_003263.4:c.497del	ENST00000308979 ENST00000502213	K166fs	rs761749628	0,0003454	NA	D	Member of the Toll-like receptor family, with a role in pathogen recognition and activation of innate immunity. Identified as a critical mediator of intestinal immunity
MBL2	chr10:54531242 G/A	ENST00000373968	R52C	rs5030737	0,076	PD	D	Belongs to collectin family. Important element in the innate immune system Variants associated with susceptibility to autoimmunity and infections (31)
PTPRC	chr1:198665917 C/G	ENST00000352140 ENST00000367376 ENST00000418674 ENST00000442510 ENST00000529828	C77G	rs17612648	0,016	S	N/A	Important for efficient T and B-cell antigen receptor signal transduction CD45RA persistence in memory T cells in alternative splicing defect

HGVS, human genome variation society; NA, not available; MAF, minor allele frequency; EUR, European; PD, probably damaging; S, synonimous; T, tolerated; D, deleterious.

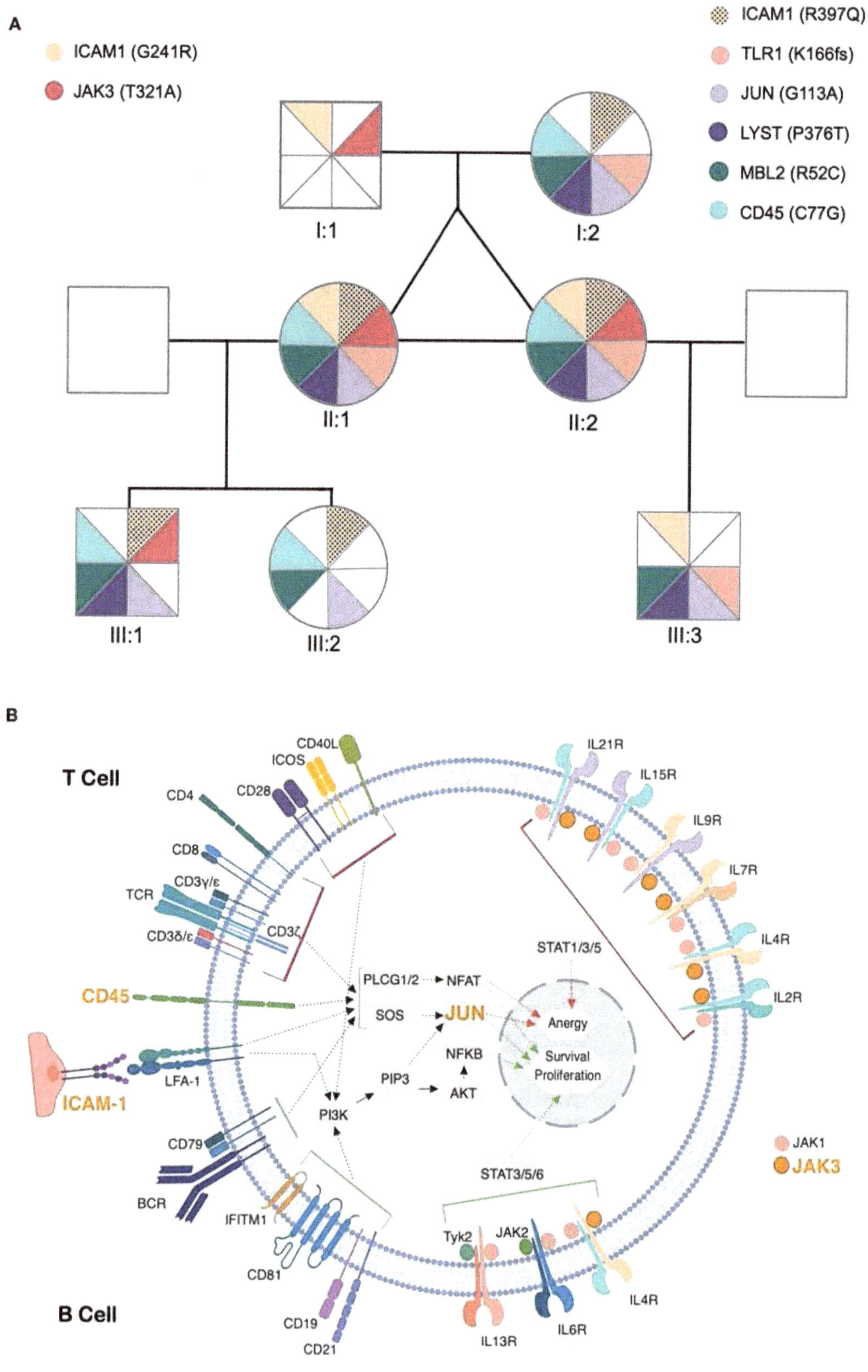

FIGURE 3 | Identified genetic variants and predicted functional impact on B and T-cell activation pathways. **(A)** Family tree of the patients. The sectors and color patterns represent the 8 genetic variants identified in the 7 listed genes, and their presence/absence in both the progenitors and the children of the two siblings. Each *(Continued)*

FIGURE 3 | sector corresponds to one specific variant. Paternally inherited variants are represented on the left, and maternal variants on the right, with a color code per gene, next to the gene ID and identified variant (in parenthesis). The black dotted pattern highlights the maternal variant in the case of *ICAM*, for which the patients have two altered alleles. **(B)** Role of affected genes in T and B-cell activation processes. The figure represents a generic lymphoid cell with the major membrane receptors, signaling molecules and transcription factors (identified by their names) and intracellular signaling pathways (identified by arrows) involved in the activation process. Red and green arrows represent the final stages of the lymphocyte activation pathways leading to the expression of genes that promote anergy (red) or survival/proliferative responses (green) within the cell nucleus. The top half of cell highlights proteins and processes specific for T cell activation and the bottom half those specific for B-cell activation. The names of proteins encoded by genes that present potentially pathogenic variants are presented in orange. The figure compiles all the information that was retrievable from pathways databases and literature search regarding the connections between genes presented in **(A)** and the B and T cell activation pathways. Of these 7 genes, *LYST* did not present any connection to these processes, whereas two others (*MBL2* and *TLR1*) have reported functions in lymphocyte activation but their connection to signaling pathways remains unclear and are thus not represented in the figure.

LSR-Fortessa X-20 flow-cytometers, Becton/Dickinson Biosciences (BD), San José, CA). Briefly, stainings with monoclonal antibodies were performed in whole blood after red blood cells lysis using BD FACS Lysing Solution (BD Biosciences), and a minimum of 100,000 lymphocytes were acquired per sample with data analyzed using CellQuest Software (BD Biosciences) and FlowJo Software (Tree Star Inc., Ashland, OR). More recently, 10^7 nucleated cells were stained with the EuroFlow 12-color Ig-isotype B-cell tube and bulk-lyse standard operating procedure (SOP; www.EuroFlow.org), $\geq 5 \times 10^6$ leukocytes were acquired in LSR-Fortessa X-20, with instrument set-up and calibration performed according to the EuroFlow SOP (38), and data analyzed with Infinicyt software (Cytognos S.L., Salamanca, Spain).

Cytokine production was assessed at the single-cell level in peripheral blood mononuclear cells (PBMC) freshly isolated by Ficoll-Hypaque density gradient (Amersham Pharmacia Biotech, Uppsala, Sweden), as described (39). Briefly, after a 4-h culture with phorbol myristate acetate (PMA; 50 ng/mL, Sigma-Aldrich) plus ionomycin (500 ng/mL; Calbiochem, Merck Biosciences, Nottingham, U.K.), in the presence of brefeldin A (10 μg/mL; Sigma-Aldrich), PBMC were surface stained, fixed, permeabilized, and stained intracellularly with monoclonal antibodies against IL-2, IL-4, IFN-γ, and IL-17, as described (36). Flow-cytometric analysis was subsequently performed as described above.

Lymphocyte proliferation was evaluated as follows: 10^5 freshly isolated PBMCs were cultured in a 96-well plate in the absence or presence of mitogens PHA (20 μg/mL), anti-CD3 (1 μg/mL), anti-CD3 anti-CD28 (1 μg/mL), PWM (1 μg/mL) and PMA (50 ng/mL)+ ionomycin (500 ng/mL) and antigens *Candida albicans* (40 μg/mL) and PPD (5 μg/mL), for 3 and 6 days, respectively, at 37°C, 5% CO_2. Proliferation was assessed by 3H-Thy (Amersham Pharmacia Biotech) incorporation in the last 8 h of culture. Results were expressed as stimulation indexes (SI) which represents the ratio of the mean counts per minute (cpm) in the presence of a given mitogen or antigen over the mean cpm in the absence of the stimulus.

Whole Exome Sequencing

Genomic DNA was extracted from peripheral blood, subjected to library construction using the Agilent Sure Select Human All Exon 50 Mb kit (Agilent Technologies) and sequenced on a Hiseq2000 Illumina sequencer (BGI-Shenzhen, China) (40). Low-coverage and low-quality Single-Nucleotide Variants (SNVs) were removed as described (41). High-quality reads were aligned to the reference human genome (GRCh37/hg 19) and annotated with SnpEff Tool. Non-synonymous SNVs predicted to be probably damaging or deleterious [either by PolyPhen 2.2.2 (28) or SIFT 5.1.1 (29)], or frameshift variants, regardless of the minor allele frequency were filtered and prioritized. Criteria to further narrow down the candidate gene list were applied as previously described (42). Extensive search was performed in the literature, interactome and pathways databases regarding the roles of identified genes in the immune system, particularly concerning their involvement in B and T-cell activation pathways, illustrated in **Figure 3B**.

DISCUSSION

Here we report the first study of a pair of MZ twins concordant for CVID. They featured remarkable similarity in clinical and immunological phenotypes at diagnosis and during 15-year follow-up, and the analysis of WES data did not identify pathogenic variants in genes previously reported in association with monogenic CVID. In contrast, we identified 7 non-synonymous coding variants with predicted damaging/deleterious impact on the 6 proteins coded by the involved genes. These genes integrate relevant immune pathways and are therefore likely to have a clinical impact, supporting a polygenic burden for CVID, as well as to constrain the evolution of immunological profiles, leading to the high degree of similarity observed between the twins, despite having led separate lives for over 25 years. The clinical and immunological outcome in the twins likely results from the accumulation of distinct functional impairments, due to variants in genes related to critical immunological pathways (12, 21), as none of the identified heterozygotic variants can independently explain their clinical/immunological picture. Consistent with this polygenic model, there is a potential combinatorial impact of the observed SNVs in B and T-cell activation, as illustrated in **Figure 3B**. The absence of clinical and immunological manifestations in close family members also argues in favor of a pathogenic burden derived from the unique combination of variants shared by the twins.

There are previous reports of CVID patients who are heterozygous carriers of C77G in *CD45* (33, 34). CD45 is known to be important for efficient T and B-cell antigen receptor signal transduction and for control of signaling thresholds through TCR (31, 43). C77G is the most common cause of *CD45* abnormal splicing in European populations (44), which leads to the persistence of CD45RA in memory T cells (45, 46). The twins are heterozygous for C77G and exhibit a strong mitogenic response to anti-CD3, but markedly diminished proliferative responses to the tested recall antigens. Our data add to previous reports (33, 34) favoring a role for this SNV in a polygenic scenario for CVID, although the frequency of (heterozygous) carriers of C77G in *CD45* was not increased in a large CVID cohort (33) and different clinical phenotypes have been associated with C77G in *CD45*.

Obviously, we cannot exclude a role for other variants, such as non-coding variants, in the genes that we mentioned, nor in other genes, that may impact in the clinical and immunological phenotype of the twins. Nevertheless, it is worth noting that 4 out of the 7 selected genes with variants act on both T and B-cell receptor signaling-pathways, namely *JUN*, *CD45* (*PTPRC*), and *ICAM1* (**Figure 3B**); and *MBL2* and *TLR1*, influence these processes through as yet unidentified mechanisms (see below) (30, 31, 46–53). Furthermore, the presence of a potentially damaging variant in the *JAK3* kinase may influence the cytokine receptor-mediated intracellular signal transduction, with crucial implications in the differentiation, function and survival of B and T cells (**Figure 3B**) (54). Other immune pathways that may be influenced by this group of variants are: Fcγ R-mediated phagocytosis (*CD45),* TNF signaling-pathway (*ICAM1*, *JUN*), Toll-like receptor signaling-pathway (*TLR1*, *JUN*) and innate immune responses (*ICAM1*, *TLR1*, *MBL2*) (55). *TLR1* encodes for a member of the Toll-like receptor family, and plays a fundamental role in pathogen recognition and activation of innate immunity (30, 56). *TLR1* was identified as a critical innate receptor for protective intestinal Th17 immunity (57) but, to our knowledge, has not been previously associated with increased susceptibility to infections, or hypogammaglobulinemia.

Two potentially damaging variants were identified in *ICAM1*, which encodes a cell surface glycoprotein involved in cell-cell adhesion, expressed on endothelial cells and cells of the immune system, and has a prominent role in several types of immune responses (51, 52). Variants in *ICAM1* have been associated with inflammatory bowel disease (58). The p.G241R variant, which the twins inherited from their father, has been associated with adult onset celiac disease in a French cohort (59).

Flow-cytometry is crucial to the functional validation of genetic variants, allowing adequate interpretation of NGS data and stratification of patients (25, 26, 60). Notably, we documented a synchronous progressive B-cell depletion throughout follow-up. Taking advantage of the EuroFlow strategy for highly-sensitive Ig-subclass analysis of blood B cells and plasma cells, six subgroups of patients were recently identified in CVID, with different IgG-switching patterns and clinical profiles, even in patients with <1% B cells (7). The immunological phenotype of both twins at 50, was compatible with the CVID-6 subgroup, the most severe, defined by markedly decreased $CD27^+$ unswitched and switched-memory B cells, with very low $CD27^-IgG3^+$ memory B cells. CVID-6 patients also show significantly reduced pre-germinal B cells, reflecting defective B-cell production in the bone marrow (61, 62). These recently developed standardized flow-cytometry assays to analyse memory B-cell immunoglobulin isotypes and IgH-subclasses will be very important in longitudinal studies to investigate the progression of B-cell defects, that has been hypothesized, but not yet supported by solid immunological data (7, 8).

The remarkable similarity between the immune profiles of the MZ twins, at age 50, even though they have lived in different households since they were 25, with distinct jobs and nuclear families, is even more striking in light of studies that have emphasized the dominant contribution of non-heritable influences to the shape and function of the immune system (1, 2). Although they live in the same geographical region, the impact of co-habitation has been considered very relevant in the shaping of the immune system, as illustrated by the immunological data from non-related housemates (63, 64). This debate on relative contributions of "nature" vs. "nurture" was addressed in a study that included 105 pairs of healthy MZ twins, which shows that variation in immune cell frequencies and serum proteins between twins increases with age, likely due in large part to exposure to pathogens, namely CMV (2). Notably, there has been no evidence of CMV infection in the MZ twins, both with negative PCR for CMV in blood on different occasions, and no evidence of CMV infection in gut biopsies.

Epigenetic modifications necessarily contribute to the discordance in clinical and immunological phenotype between MZ twins (1, 3). In line with this, a pair of MZ twins discordant for CVID was previously reported (3), with a significant increase in DNA methylation of B cells in the affected sister (3, 65). Consistent with this finding, a recent study showed that impaired demethylation in B-cell key genes is associated with the reduction of memory B cells in CVID patients (66). In our context, it will be interesting to explore the epigenetic landscape of the MZ concordant twins in order to confirm its contribution to the disease and add a new layer of insight to our clinical, immunological, and genomic data.

CONCLUDING REMARKS

The clinical, immunologic and genetic profile of a pair of monozygotic twins concordant for CVID provides further support to the hypothesis that a combination of allelic variants can additively predispose to non-familial CVID. Moreover, these data suggest that genetic variants may impose a significant constraint on the impact of the environment, as attested by the remarkably similar immunological phenotype observed in both twins, despite prolonged exposure to different living conditions. The integration of NGS data with clinical and immunological phenotypes at the single-cell level, as provided by multi-dimensional flow-cytometry, is crucial to further expose the complex genetic landscape underlying the vast majority of patients with CVID, and patients with other immunodeficiencies.

AUTHOR CONTRIBUTIONS

SLS, MF, ABS, RV, and AES designed the study. SLS, MF, SPS, and RV collected the clinical data. MF, RB, AS-C, EB, and MP-A performed the immunological studies. MF, MP, PR, AR, MG-C, and LH analyzed WES data and investigated the selected variants. SLS, MF, ABS, AR, MG-C, LH, and AES discussed the results. SLS and AES supervised the study. SLS wrote the paper.

FUNDING

This work received funding from PAC - PRECISE - LISBOA-01-0145-FEDER-016394, co-funded by FEDER through POR Lisboa 2020 - Programa Operacional Regional de Lisboa PORTUGAL 2020 and Fundação para a Ciência e a Tecnologia; and UID/BIM/50005/2019, project funded by Fundação para a Ciência e a Tecnologia (FCT)/Ministério da Ciência, Tecnologia e Ensino Superior (MCTES) through Fundos do Orçamento de Estado. Work in MG-C lab is supported by UID/MULTI/04046/2019 Research Unit grant from FCT, Portugal (to BioISI) and FCT research grant PTDC/BIA-CEL/29257/2017.

REFERENCES

1. Brodin P, Davis MM. Human immune system variation. *Nat Rev Immunol.* (2017) 17:21–9. doi: 10.1038/nri.2016.125
2. Brodin P, Jojic V, Gao T, Bhattacharya S, Angel CJ, Furman D, et al. Variation in the human immune system is largely driven by non-heritable influences. *Cell.* (2015) 160:37–47. doi: 10.1016/j.cell.2014.12.020
3. Rodríguez-Cortez VC, Del Pino-Molina L, Rodríguez-Ubreva J, Ciudad L, Gómez-Cabrero D, Company C, et al. Monozygotic twins discordant for common variable immunodeficiency reveal impaired DNA demethylation during naive-to-memory B-cell transition. *Nat Commun.* (2015) 6:7335. doi: 10.1038/ncomms8335
4. Ameratunga R, Brewerton M, Slade C, Jordan A, Gillis D, Steele R, et al. Comparison of diagnostic criteria for common variable immunodeficiency disorder. *Front Immunol.* (2014) 5:415. doi: 10.3389/fimmu.2014.00415
5. Bonilla FA, Barlan I, Chapel H, Costa-Carvalho BT, Cunningham-Rundles C, de la Morena MT, et al. International Consensus Document (ICON): common variable immunodeficiency disorders. *J Allergy Clin Immunol Pract.* (2016) 4:38–59. doi: 10.1016/j.jaip.2015.07.025
6. Jolles S. The variable in common variable immunodeficiency: a disease of complex phenotypes. *J Allergy Clin Immunol Pract.* (2013) 1:545–56; quiz 557. doi: 10.1016/j.jaip.2013.09.015
7. Blanco E, Pérez-Andrés M, Arriba-Méndez S, Serrano C, Criado I, Del Pino-Molina L, et al. Defects in memory B-cell and plasma cell subsets expressing different immunoglobulin-subclasses in CVID and Ig-subclass deficiencies. *J Allergy Clin Immunol.* (2019) 144:809–24. doi: 10.1016/j.jaci.2019.02.017
8. Blanco E, Pérez-Andrés M, Arriba-Méndez S, Contreras-Sanfeliciano T, Criado I, Pelak O, et al. Age-associated distribution of normal B-cell and plasma cell subsets in peripheral blood. *J Allergy Clin Immunol.* (2018) 141:2208–19.e16. doi: 10.1016/j.jaci.2018.02.017
9. Abolhassani H, Aghamohammadi A, Fang M, Rezaei N, Jiang C, Liu X, et al. Clinical implications of systematic phenotyping and exome sequencing in patients with primary antibody deficiency. *Genet Med.* (2019) 21:243–51. doi: 10.1038/s41436-018-0012-x
10. von Spee-Mayer C, Koemm V, Wehr C, Goldacker S, Kindle G, Bulashevska A, et al. Evaluating laboratory criteria for combined immunodeficiency in adult patients diagnosed with common variable immunodeficiency. *Clin Immunol.* (2019) 203:59–62. doi: 10.1016/j.clim.2019.04.001
11. Kamin RM, Fudenberg HH, Douglas SD.Kamin RM, Fudenberg HH, Douglas SD. A genetic defect in "acquired" agammaglobulinemia. *Proc Natl Acad Sci USA.* (1968) 60:881–5. doi: 10.1073/pnas.60.3.881
12. Wu L, Schaid DJ, Sicotte H, Wieben ED, Li H, Petersen GM. Case-only exome sequencing and complex disease susceptibility gene discovery: study design considerations. *J Med Genet.* (2015) 52:10–6. doi: 10.1136/jmedgenet-2014-102697
13. Orange JS, Glessner JT, Resnick E, Sullivan KE, Lucas M, Ferry B, et al. Genome-wide association identifies diverse causes of common variable immunodeficiency. *J Allergy Clin Immunol.* (2011) 127:1360–7.e6. doi: 10.1016/j.jaci.2011.02.039
14. Maffucci P, Filion CA, Boisson B, Itan Y, Shang L, Casanova JL, et al. Genetic diagnosis using whole exome sequencing in common variable immunodeficiency. *Front Immunol.* (2016) 7:220. doi: 10.3389/fimmu.2016.00220
15. de Valles-Ibáñez G, Esteve-Solé A, Piquer M, González-Navarro EA, Hernandez-Rodriguez J, Laayouni H, et al. Evaluating the genetics of common variable immunodeficiency: monogenetic model and beyond. *Front Immunol.* (2018) 9:636. doi: 10.3389/fimmu.2018.00636
16. van Schouwenburg PA, Davenport EE, Kienzler AK, Marwah I, Wright B, Lucas M, et al. Application of whole genome and RNA sequencing to investigate the genomic landscape of common variable immunodeficiency disorders. *Clin Immunol.* (2015) 160:301–14. doi: 10.1016/j.clim.2015.05.020
17. Yazdani R, Abolhassani H, Kiaee F, Habibi S, Azizi G, Tavakol M, et al. Comparison of common monogenic defects in a large predominantly antibody deficiency cohort. *J Allergy Clin Immunol Pract.* (2019) 7:864–78.e9. doi: 10.1016/j.jaip.2018.09.004
18. Kojima D, Wang X, Muramatsu H, Okuno Y, Nishio N, Hama A, et al. Application of extensively targeted next-generation sequencing for the diagnosis of primary immunodeficiencies. *J Allergy Clin Immunol.* (2016) 138:303–5.e3. doi: 10.1016/j.jaci.2016.01.012
19. Stray-Pedersen A, Sorte HS, Samarakoon P, Gambin T, Chinn IK, Coban Akdemir ZH, et al. Primary immunodeficiency diseases: genomic approaches delineate heterogeneous Mendelian disorders. *J Allergy Clin Immunol.* (2017) 139:232–45. doi: 10.1016/j.jaci.2016.05.042
20. Kienzler AK, Hargreaves CE, Patel SY. The role of genomics in common variable immunodeficiency disorders. *Clin Exp Immunol.* (2017) 188:326–32. doi: 10.1111/cei.12947
21. Lvovs D, Favorova OO, Favorov AV. A polygenic approach to the study of polygenic diseases. *Acta Nat.* (2012) 4:59–71. doi: 10.32607/20758251-2012-4-3-59-71
22. van de Ven AA, Compeer EB, van Montfrans JM, Boes M. B-cell defects in common variable immunodeficiency: BCR signaling, protein clustering and hardwired gene mutations. *Crit Rev Immunol.* (2011) 31:85–98. doi: 10.1615/CritRevImmunol.v31.i2.10
23. Jørgensen SF, Fevang B, Aukrust P. Autoimmunity and inflammation in CVID: a possible crosstalk between immune activation, gut microbiota, and epigenetic modifications. *J Clin Immunol.* (2019) 39:30–6. doi: 10.1007/s10875-018-0574-z
24. Berbers RM, Nierkens S, van Laar JM, Bogaert D, Leavis HL. Microbial dysbiosis in common variable immune deficiencies: evidence, causes, and consequences. *Trends Immunol.* (2017) 38:206–16. doi: 10.1016/j.it.2016.11.008

25. Wehr C, Kivioja T, Schmitt C, Ferry B, Witte T, Eren E, et al. The EUROclass trial: defining subgroups in common variable immunodeficiency. *Blood.* (2008) 111:77–85. doi: 10.1182/blood-2007-06-091744
26. van der Burg M, Kalina T, Perez-Andres M, Vlkova M, Lopez-Granados E, Blanco E, et al. The EuroFlow PID orientation tube for flow cytometric diagnostic screening of primary immunodeficiencies of the lymphoid system. *Front Immunol.* (2019) 10:246. doi: 10.3389/fimmu.2019.00246
27. van der Velden VH, Flores-Montero J, Perez-Andres M, Martin-Ayuso M, Crespo O, Blanco E, et al. Optimization and testing of dried antibody tube: the EuroFlow LST and PIDOT tubes as examples. *J Immunol Methods.* (2017) 2017:e11. doi: 10.1016/j.jim.2017.03.011
28. Sunyaev S, Ramensky V, Koch I, Lathe W, Kondrashov AS, Bork P. Prediction of deleterious human alleles. *Hum Mol Genet.* (2001) 10:591–7. doi: 10.1093/hmg/10.6.591
29. Kumar P, Henikoff S, Ng PC. Predicting the effects of coding non-synonymous variants on protein function using the SIFT algorithm. *Nat Protoc.* (2009) 4:1073–81. doi: 10.1038/nprot.2009.86
30. Lancioni CL, Li Q, Thomas JJ, Ding X, Thiel B, Drage MG, et al. *Mycobacterium tuberculosis* lipoproteins directly regulate human memory $CD4^+$ T cell activation via Toll-like receptors 1 and 2. *Infect Immun.* (2011) 79:663–73. doi: 10.1128/IAI.00806-10
31. Do HT, Baars W, Borns K, Windhagen A, Schwinzer R. The 77C->G mutation in the human CD45 (PTPRC) gene leads to increased intensity of TCR signaling in T cell lines from healthy individuals and patients with multiple sclerosis. *J Immunol.* (2006) 176:931–8. doi: 10.4049/jimmunol.176.2.931
32. Picard C, Bobby Gaspar H, Al-Herz W, Bousfiha A, Casanova JL, Chatila T, et al. International union of immunological societies: 2017 primary immunodeficiency diseases committee report on inborn errors of immunity. *J Clin Immunol.* (2018) 38:96–128. doi: 10.1007/s10875-017-0464-9
33. Vorechovsky I, Kralovicova J, Tchilian E, Masterman T, Zhang Z, Ferry B, et al. Does 77C->G in PTPRC modify autoimmune disorders linked to the major histocompatibility locus? *Nat Genet.* (2001) 29:22–3. doi: 10.1038/ng723
34. Tchilian EZ, Gil J, Navarro ML, Fernandez-Cruz E, Chapel H, Misbah S, et al. Unusual case presentations associated with the CD45 C77G polymorphism. *Clin Exp Immunol.* (2006) 146:448–54. doi: 10.1111/j.1365-2249.2006.03230.x
35. Conley ME, Dobbs AK, Farmer DM, Kilic S, Paris K, Grigoriadou S, et al. Primary B cell immunodeficiencies: comparisons and contrasts. *Annu Rev Immunol.* (2009) 27:199–227. doi: 10.1146/annurev.immunol.021908.132649
36. Barbosa RR, Silva SP, Silva SL, Melo AC, Pedro E, Barbosa MP, et al. Primary B-cell deficiencies reveal a link between human IL-17-producing CD4 T-cell homeostasis and B-cell differentiation. *PLoS ONE.* (2011) 6:e22848. doi: 10.1371/journal.pone.0022848
37. Flores-Montero J, Sanoja-Flores L, Paiva B, Puig N, García-Sánchez O, Böttcher S, et al. Next Generation Flow for highly sensitive and standardized detection of minimal residual disease in multiple myeloma. *Leukemia.* (2017) 31:2094–103. doi: 10.1038/leu.2017.29
38. Kalina T, Flores-Montero J, van der Velden VH, Martin-Ayuso M, Böttcher S, Ritgen M, et al. EuroFlow standardization of flow cytometer instrument settings and immunophenotyping protocols. *Leukemia.* (2012) 26:1986–2010. doi: 10.1038/leu.2012.122
39. Sousa AE, Chaves AF, Loureiro A, Victorino RM. Comparison of the frequency of interleukin (IL)-2-, interferon-gamma-, and IL-4-producing T cells in 2 diseases, human immunodeficiency virus types 1 and 2, with distinct clinical outcomes. *J Infect Dis.* (2001) 184:552–9. doi: 10.1086/322804
40. Abolhassani H, Wang N, Aghamohammadi A, Rezaei N, Lee YN, Frugoni F, et al. A hypomorphic recombination-activating gene 1 (RAG1) mutation resulting in a phenotype resembling common variable immunodeficiency. *J Allergy Clin Immunol.* (2014) 134:1375–80. doi: 10.1016/j.jaci.2014.04.042
41. Romano R, Zaravinos A, Liadaki K, Caridha R, Lundin J, Carlsson G, et al. NEIL1 is a candidate gene associated with common variable immunodeficiency in a patient with a chromosome 15q24 deletion. *Clin Immunol.* (2017) 176:71–6. doi: 10.1016/j.clim.2017.01.006
42. Fang M, Abolhassani H, Lim CK, Zhang J, Hammarström L. Next generation sequencing data analysis in primary immunodeficiency disorders—future directions. *J Clin Immunol.* (2016) 36 (Suppl. 1):68–75. doi: 10.1007/s10875-016-0260-y
43. Tchilian EZ, Beverley PC. Altered CD45 expression and disease. *Trends Immunol.* (2006) 27:146–53. doi: 10.1016/j.it.2006.01.001
44. Gil J, Ruiz-Tíscar JL, Rodríguez-Sainz C, Hernández A, Santamaría B, García-Sánchez F, et al. [Prevalence of C77G polymorphism in exon 4 of the CD45 gene in the Spanish population]. *Med Clin.* (2005) 125:10–1. doi: 10.1157/13076408
45. Zikherman J, Weiss A. Alternative splicing of CD45: the tip of the iceberg. *Immunity.* (2008) 29:839–41. doi: 10.1016/j.immuni.2008.12.005
46. Wu Z, Yates AL, Hoyne GF, Goodnow CC. Consequences of increased CD45RA and RC isoforms for TCR signaling and peripheral T cell deficiency resulting from heterogeneous nuclear ribonucleoprotein L-like mutation. *J Immunol.* (2010) 185:231–8. doi: 10.4049/jimmunol.0903625
47. Foletta VC, Segal DH, Cohen DR. Transcriptional regulation in the immune system: all roads lead to AP-1. *J Leukoc Biol.* (1998) 63:139–52. doi: 10.1002/jlb.63.2.139
48. Eisen DP, Minchinton RM. Impact of mannose-binding lectin on susceptibility to infectious diseases. *Clin Infect Dis.* (2003) 37:1496–505. doi: 10.1086/379324
49. Sanui T, Inayoshi A, Noda M, Iwata E, Stein JV, Sasazuki T., et al.SDOCK2 regulates Rac activation and cytoskeletal reorganization through interaction with ELMO1. *Blood.* (2003) 102:2948–50. doi: 10.1182/blood-2003-01-0173
50. Nishihara H, Maeda M, Tsuda M, Makino Y, Sawa H, Nagashima K, et al. DOCK2 mediates T cell receptor-induced activation of Rac2 and IL-2 transcription. *Biochem Biophys Res Commun.* (2002) 296:716–20. doi: 10.1016/S0006-291X(02)00931-2
51. Verma NK, Kelleher D. Not just an adhesion molecule: LFA-1 contact tunes the T lymphocyte program. *J Immunol.* (2017) 199:1213–21. doi: 10.4049/jimmunol.1700495
52. Wingren AG, Parra E, Varga M, Kalland T, Sjogren HO, Hedlund G, et al. T cell activation pathways: B7, LFA-3, and ICAM-1 shape unique T cell profiles. *Crit Rev Immunol.* (2017) 37:463–81. doi: 10.1615/CritRevImmunol.v37.i2-6.130
53. Gil-Krzewska A, Wood SM, Murakami Y, Nguyen V, Chiang SCC, Cullinane AR, et al. Chediak-Higashi syndrome: lysosomal trafficking regulator domains regulate exocytosis of lytic granules but not cytokine secretion by natural killer cells. *J Allergy Clin Immunol.* (2016) 137:1165–77. doi: 10.1016/j.jaci.2015.08.039
54. Ban SA, Salzer E, Eibl MM, Linder A, Geier CB, Santos-Valente E, et al. Combined immunodeficiency evolving into predominant $CD4^+$ lymphopenia caused by somatic chimerism in JAK3. *J Clin Immunol.* (2014) 34:941–53. doi: 10.1007/s10875-014-0088-2
55. Kanehisa M, Furumichi M, Tanabe M, Sato Y, Morishima K. KEGG: new perspectives on genomes, pathways, diseases and drugs. *Nucleic Acids Res.* (2017) 45:D353–61. doi: 10.1093/nar/gkw1092
56. Whitmore LC, Hook JS, Philiph AR, Hilkin BM, Bing X, Ahn C, et al. A common genetic variant in TLR1 enhances human neutrophil priming and impacts length of intensive care stay in pediatric sepsis. *J Immunol.* (2016) 196:1376–86. doi: 10.4049/jimmunol.1500856
57. DePaolo RW, Kamdar K, Khakpour S, Sugiura Y, Wang W, Jabri B. A specific role for TLR1 in protective T(H)17 immunity during mucosal infection. *J Exp Med.* (2012) 209:1437–44. doi: 10.1084/jem.20112339
58. Braun C, Zahn R, Martin K, Albert E, Folwaczny C. Polymorphisms of the ICAM-1 gene are associated with inflammatory bowel disease, regardless of the p-ANCA status. *Clin Immunol.* (2001) 101:357–60. doi: 10.1006/clim.2001.5118
59. Abel M, Cellier C, Kumar N, Cerf-Bensussan N, Schmitz J, Caillat-Zucman S. Adulthood-onset celiac disease is associated with intercellular adhesion molecule-1 (ICAM-1) gene polymorphism. *Hum Immunol.* (2006) 67:612–7. doi: 10.1016/j.humimm.2006.04.011
60. Warnatz K, Denz A, Dräger R, Braun M, Groth C, Wolff-Vorbeck G, et al. Severe deficiency of switched memory B cells ($CD27^+IgM^-IgD^-$) in subgroups of patients with common variable immunodeficiency: a new approach to classify a heterogeneous disease. *Blood.* (2002) 99:1544–51. doi: 10.1182/blood.V99.5.1544
61. Driessen GJ, van Zelm MC, van Hagen PM, Hartwig NG, Trip M, Warris A, et al. B-cell replication history and somatic hypermutation status identify distinct pathophysiologic backgrounds in common variable immunodeficiency. *Blood.* (2011) 118:6814–23. doi: 10.1182/blood-2011-06-361881
62. Ochtrop ML, Goldacker S, May AM, Rizzi M, Draeger R, Hauschke D, et al. T and B lymphocyte abnormalities in bone marrow biopsies

of common variable immunodeficiency. *Blood.* (2011) 118:309–18. doi: 10.1182/blood-2010-11-321695

63. Carr EJ, Dooley J, Garcia-Perez JE, Lagou V, Lee JC, Wouters C, et al. The cellular composition of the human immune system is shaped by age and cohabitation. *Nat Immunol.* (2016) 17:461–8. doi: 10.1038/ni.3371
64. Liston A, Carr EJ, Linterman MA. Shaping variation in the human immune system. *Trends Immunol.* (2016) 37:637–46. doi: 10.1016/j.it.2016.08.002
65. Li J, Wei Z, Li YR, Maggadottir SM, Chang X, Desai A, et al. Understanding the genetic and epigenetic basis of common variable immunodeficiency disorder through omics approaches. *Biochim Biophys Acta.* (2016) 1860 (11 Pt B):2656–63. doi: 10.1016/j.bbagen.2016.06.014
66. Del Pino-Molina L, Rodríguez-Ubreva J, Torres Canizales J, Coronel-Díaz M, Kulis M, Martín-Subero JI, et al. Impaired CpG demethylation in common variable immunodeficiency associates with B cell phenotype and proliferation rate. *Front Immunol.* (2019) 10:878. doi: 10.3389/fimmu.2019.00878

17

Flow Cytometric-Based Analysis of Defects in Lymphocyte Differentiation and Function Due to Inborn Errors of Immunity

Cindy S. Ma [1,2,3*] *and Stuart G. Tangye* [1,2,3*]

[1] *Immunology Division, Garvan Institute of Medical Research, Sydney, NSW, Australia,* [2] *Faculty of Medicine, St. Vincent's Clinical School, UNSW Sydney, Sydney, NSW, Australia,* [3] *Clincial Immunogenomics Research Consortium Australia, Darlinghurst, NSW, Australia*

Correspondence:
Cindy S. Ma
c.ma@garvan.org.au
Stuart G. Tangye
s.tangye@garvan.org.au

The advent of flow cytometry has revolutionized the way we approach our research and answer specific scientific questions. The flow cytometer has also become a mainstream diagnostic tool in most hospital and pathology laboratories around the world. In particular the application of flow cytometry has been instrumental to the diagnosis of primary immunodeficiencies (PIDs) that result from monogenic mutations in key genes of the hematopoietic, and occasionally non-hematopoietic, systems. The far-reaching applicability of flow cytometry is in part due to the remarkable sensitivity, down to the single-cell level, of flow-based assays and the extremely user-friendly platforms that enable comprehensive analysis, data interpretation, and importantly, robust and rapid methods for diagnosing PIDs. A prime example is the absence of peripheral blood B cells in patients with agammaglobulinemia due to mutations in *BTK* or related genes in the BCR signaling pathway. Similarly, the development of intracellular staining protocols to detect expression of SAP, XIAP, or DOCK8 expedites the rapid diagnosis of the X-linked lymphoproliferative diseases or an autosomal recessive form of hyper-IgE syndrome (HIES), respectively. It has also become evident that distinct cohorts of PID patients exhibit unique "lymphocyte phenotypic signatures" that are often diagnostic even prior to identifying the genetic lesion. Flow cytometry-based sorting provides a technique for separating specific subsets of immune cells such that they can be studied in isolation. Thus, flow-based assays can be utilized to measure immune cell function in patients with PIDs, such as degranulation by cytotoxic cells, cytokine expression by many immune cells (i.e., CD4$^+$ and CD8$^+$ T cells, macrophages etc.), B-cell differentiation, and phagocyte respiratory burst *in vitro*. These assays can also be performed using unfractionated PBMCs, provided the caveat that the composition of lymphocytes between healthy donors and the PID patients under investigation is recognized. These functional deficits can assist not only in the clinical diagnosis of PIDs, but also reveal mechanisms of disease pathogenesis. As we move into the next generation of multiparameter flow cytometers, here we review some of our experiences in the use of flow cytometry in the study, diagnosis, and unraveling the pathophysiology of PIDs.

Keywords: flow cytometry, B cells, T cells, immunodeficencies, phenotpye

INTRODUCTION

The Role of Technological Developments in Understanding Immunology and Immunodeficiency

The application of new technologies to basic research and clinical investigations has greatly improved biochemical and molecular analyses of cellular physiology and identified defects in these processes that underpin human disease. Thus, technological advances have enabled not only fundamental discoveries of basic immunology, but also a greater understanding of disease pathogenesis, rapid diagnoses of these conditions as well as providing opportunities for the development and/or implementation of improved therapies. Great examples of this can be found in the fields of clinical immunology and immunodeficiency.

Using electrophoretic analysis of serum from a young boy with severe and recurrent bacterial infections led to the discovery by Col Ogden Bruton of the first case of agammaglobulinemia (1). Importantly, treating this patient with monthly subcutaneous infusions of concentrated human immune serum globulin prevented further infections (1). These observations established that agammaglobulinemia caused this patient's recurrent infections, and that the gammaglobulin fraction of serum contained antibodies capable of prophylactically preventing infection. Critically, this finding in a single patient—which pre-dated the discovery of B cells by more than a decade (2)—led to the identification 40 years later that mutations in *BTK*, encoding Bruton's tyrosine kinase, cause X-linked agammaglobulinemia (XLA) (3).

Extending this work by Bruton, the advent of serological reagents capable of reacting with specific lymphocyte subsets—such as polyclonal antisera raised against surface Ig molecules—enabled the identification of B cells in the peripheral blood of healthy individuals, and the absence of Ig-expressing cells in XLA (4–7). Importantly, XLA patients were found to have near-normal frequencies of precursor B cells in their bone marrow (BM), the site of B-cell development (8), establishing that the very early—but not later—stages of B-cell development were intact in XLA patients. Similarly, advances in techniques to fractionate human peripheral blood leukocyte subsets by density gradient centrifugation allowed the isolation of populations enriched for B cells, T cells and monocytes. This elegant approach also revealed a stark paucity of B cells in XLA (9). These analytical approaches demonstrating an absence of peripheral blood Ig-expressing B cells in XLA patients provided a clear explanation for their agammaglobulinemia.

These serological studies using anti-Ig not only defined B cells as the cellular deficiency in XLA, but also gave greater clarity to other immune deficient conditions. For instance, investigation of X-linked or autosomal recessive (AR) severe combined immunodeficiency (SCID) revealed that, despite persistent lymphopenia and hypogammaglobulinemia, the majority (>90%) of lymphocytes in these individuals were actually B cells (7, 10). This established that these conditions were likely due to a deficiency of T cells, thus defining $T^{-}B^{+}$ SCID. Likewise, studies of males who were hypo- or agammaglobulinemic but had normal frequencies of B cells, along with T cells, delineated an X-linked PID distinct from XLA that probably represented X-linked hyper-IgM syndrome (6, 7).

Monoclonal Abs Enabled Further Delineation, and Prognosis, of Immunodeficiencies

The ability to generate immortalized cells lines (hybridomas) producing monoclonal Abs (mAbs) with defined and distinct specificities (11) led to quantum leaps in basic and clinical immunology. Thus, it quickly became possible to identify immune cell populations and subsets not only according to the differential expression of surface Ig, but also by the presence, or absence of other cell surface molecules. By using mAbs against surface markers that are coordinately expressed during B-cell development, it was found that the very few B cells present in the circulation of XLA patients resembled immature B cells in BM and were distinct from mature B cells in the peripheral blood of healthy donors (12). This finding was critical in identifying the stage at which B cell development is blocked by inactivating mutations in *BTK* (3).

This approach of studying immune cell subsets by immunofluorescent microscopy was also critical in understanding pathophysiology of HIV infection and subsequent progression to AIDS. Here, a reduction in the number of peripheral blood $CD4^{+}$ T cells, and a corresponding inversion of the CD4:CD8 T cell ratio, became a defining clinical characteristic of individuals infected with HIV (13–16). Furthermore, the steady decline in numbers of $CD4^{+}$ T cells in HIV infection became predictive of progression to full blown AIDS, revealing the need to longitudinally track $CD4^{+}$ T cells as a biomarker of disease progression following HIV infection (16, 17).

Flow Cytometry Revolutionized Immunology and the Study of Immunodeficiencies

While methodologies such as density gradient centrifugation and immunofluorescent microscopy advanced our understanding of basic immunology and disease, they were laborious and often lacked the level of sensitivity and quantitation required to make definitive interpretations of the data. By simultaneously enabling the rapid analysis of large numbers of immune cells, flow cytometry has had a profound impact on immunology (18), including its application to the study of primary and acquired immunodeficiencies.

It became possible to quickly assess the status of $CD4^{+}$ T cells in HIV infection (17), accurately define the stages and phenotypes of B cell development in human BM and how mutations in genes such as *BTK*, *BLNK*, *IGHM*, *IGLL1*, *CD79A*, *CD79B*, *PIK3R1*, and *TCF3* differentially affect this process (3, 19, 20), and delineate distinct types of SCID due to different gene mutations according to the presence and absence of specific lymphocyte populations, such as $B^{+}T^{-}NK^{-}$ SCID (*IL2RG*, *JAK3*), $B^{-}T^{-}NK^{+}$ SCID (*RAG1*, *RAG2*), $B^{+}T^{-}NK^{+}$ SCID (*IL7RA*), or $B^{-}T^{-}NK^{-}$ SCID (*ADA*) (20, 21).

The discoveries of surface molecules that are induced on activated lymphocytes, or distinguish discrete subsets of T and B cells, also led to major advances in the discovery, diagnosis, management, and classification of PIDs (20). Thus, males with X-linked hyper IgM syndrome could be identified by the inability of their CD4$^+$ T cells to upregulate expression of functional CD40L following anti-CD3/CD28 or PMA/ionomycin-mediated activation (22, 23). Common variable immunodeficiency (CVID) due to *ICOS* mutations was discovered by the identification of a small number of patients whose T cells lacked ICOS expression following *in vitro* stimulation (24). The finding that CD27 is expressed on human memory, but not naïve, B cells (25, 26) enabled an entirely new stratification system of CVID that could reliably classify patients with various pathologies (27, 28).

We have also exploited this finding, together with the availability of patients with PIDs, to identify non-redundant molecular and cellular requirements for the generation and/or maintenance of memory B cells in humans. Thus, mutations that disrupt (i) CD4$^+$ T cell/B cell interactions and thus delivery of CD4$^+$ T cell-mediated B cell help (e.g., loss of function [LOF] *CD40L, ICOS, CD40, NEMO, SH2D1A, RLTPR [CARMIL2], CD27/CD70*), (ii) cytokine signaling particularly through IL-21 and STAT3 (i.e., *IL21, IL21R, IL2RG, ZNF341, IL10R* LOF; *STAT3* dominant negative [DN]; *STAT1* gain of function [GOF]), or (iii) other intracellular signaling pathways (*STK4, DOCK8, SP110* LOF; *PIK3CD* GOF) all reduce memory B cells (defined as CD19$^+$CD20$^+$CD10$^-$CD27$^+$ cells) in affected individuals (29–41) (**Figure 1**). Similar studies performed by other investigators have established that signaling via CARD11/BCL10/MALT1 (45), CD19/CD81 (46), and NIK/NFKB2 (47, 48) are also key regulators of the generation and/or maintenance of human memory B cells. Importantly, this approach also established that, for instance, IL12Rβ1/2, IL-23R, TYK2, and STAT1 signaling (32, 42), nor SPPL2A (43) or GINS1 (44), are required for generating and/or maintaining the memory B cell pool in humans (**Figure 1**).

Further advances in flow cytometric methodologies enabled detection of intracellular proteins (49), as well as post-translational modifications to proteins involved in cell signaling (50). These developments were also embraced by the clinical immunology field to facilitate rapid diagnosis of PIDs and discover patients with novel immune defects. The ability to quantify expression of SAP, XIAP, BTK, FOXP3, and DOCK8 proteins by intracellular staining and flow cytometric analysis expedited detection and diagnosis of patients with X-linked lymphoproliferative disease (XLP) type 1 (LOF mutations in *SH2D1A*), XLP-2 (LOF mutations in *XIAP/BIRC4*), XLA (BTK), IPEX (*FOXP3*), and an AR form of HIES (*DOCK8*), respectively (51–56) (**Figure 2**). Furthermore, this facilitated the identification of female carriers of some X-linked traits, such as XLP-1, XLP-2, and XLA (51, 55–57, 59) (**Figure 2**), as well as the discovery of somatic reversion in XLP-1 (60), DOCK8-deficiency (54), and leukocyte adhesion deficiency-1 due to mutations in *ITGB2* encoding CD18 (61, 62). Similarly, the detection of intracellular phosphorylated STAT proteins in response to cytokine-mediated stimulation of lymphocyte populations has been developed as a functional screen to identify individuals with LOF mutations in *IL10R, IL12RB1,* or *IFNGR1* (63–65), or GOF mutations in *STAT1* (66). Importantly, this technique has been applied to discover patients with novel inborn errors of immunity, including LOF mutations in *IL21R* (67), *IL6ST* (68), and *IL6R* (69). Clinical flow cytometry has also played a valuable role in studying PIDs affecting innate immunity. Assessing respiratory burst in phagocytes using oxidation of fluorescent probes such as dihydrorhodamine 123 (DHR) following leukocyte activation *in vitro* is the gold standard for diagnosing individuals with either X-linked or AR forms of chronic granulomatous disease (70), as well as females carriers of the X-linked form of this condition (59). Lastly, the use of cell permeable fluorescent dyes such as carboxyfluorescein succinimidyl ester (CFSE), Cell trace violet and Cell trace yellow, to label intracellular molecules and then track the dilution and concomitant reduction in fluorescence intensity of these dyes with each cell division (71, 72) has enabled detailed analysis of the role of cell division in lymphocyte differentiation and how these events can be uncoupled or compromised in various PIDs (29–31, 33, 35–37, 40, 58, 60, 73–76).

However, there are important caveats to consider when using flow cytometry to determine potential molecular causes of PIDs. While the vast majority of gene variants found to cause PIDs abolish protein expression, and thus a lack of the encoded protein can be used as a surrogate to confirm the pathogenicity of a mutation, several variants do not affect protein expression and are pathogenic due to them being LOF. An example of this can be found in one of the original descriptions of mutations in *CD40LG*, which reported detectable expression of CD40L on activated CD4$^+$ T cells from one patient with X-linked hyper-IgM syndrome despite the presence of a predicted inactivating mutation (23). Similarly, pathogenic mutations have been identified in *SH2D1A* (77), *DOCK8* (78), *BTK* (55, 56), and *IL10RA* (65) in patients with XLP, AR HIES, XLA and very early onset inflammatory bowel disease, respectively, yet expression of the encoded proteins is unaffected. Despite this, flow cytometry was still valuable in some of these cases to establish the LOF nature of variants that did not affect protein expression. Here, quantifying binding of soluble CD40 to the surface of activated CD4$^+$ T cells established that a specific mutation in *CD40LG* that preserved protein expression, as determined flow cytometrically using an anti-CD40L mAb, was unable to bind CD40L (23). Likewise, LOF of expressed but mutant IL-10RA was confirmed by demonstrating an inability of IL-10 to induce phosphorylation of STAT3 in PBMCs from this patient (65). Thus, like all aspects of research and clinical immunology, awareness of the limitations of specific assays needs to be borne in mind, and multiple approaches adopted to ensure the most accurate and clinically-actionable results are obtained. But the contribution of flow cytometry to clinical medicine remains central and unquestioned.

Delineation of Human Peripheral Blood Lymphocytes by Flow Cytometry

To study the impact of gene mutations on the human immune system of individuals with PIDs, it is important to first be able to identify distinct populations of immune cells in peripheral blood

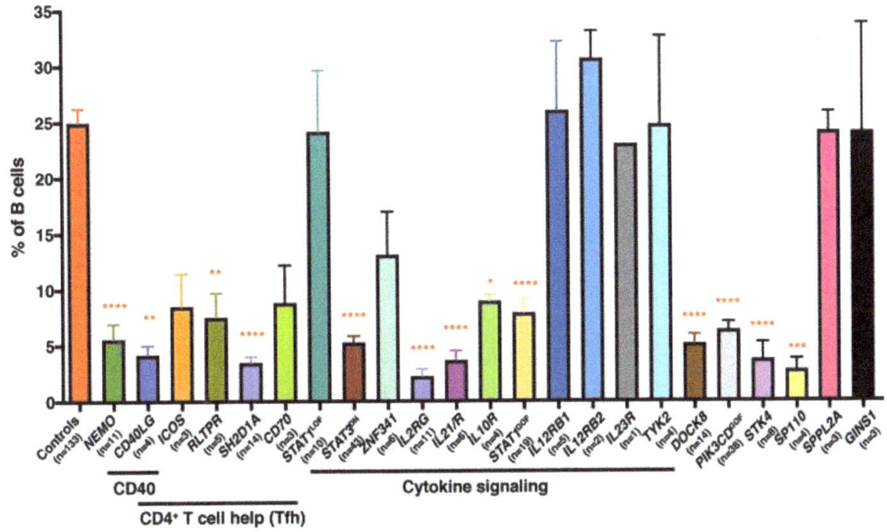

FIGURE 1 | Impact of inborn errors of immunity on the generation of memory B cells. PBMCs from the indicated numbers of healthy donor controls or from individuals with pathogenic mutations in the indicated genes were stained with mAbs against CD19, CD20, CD10, and CD27. The proportions of B cells exhibiting a $CD19^{+}CD10^{-}CD27^{+}$ memory phenotype was determined by flow cytometric gating and analysis. Significant differences were determined by ANOVA ($^{*}p < 0.05$; $^{**}p < 0.01$; $^{***}p < 0.001$; $^{****}p < 0.0001$). The age range of the healthy donors is from birth (cord blood) to ~65 years old. These data are compiled from findings previously reported in the following publications: (29–37, 39–44).

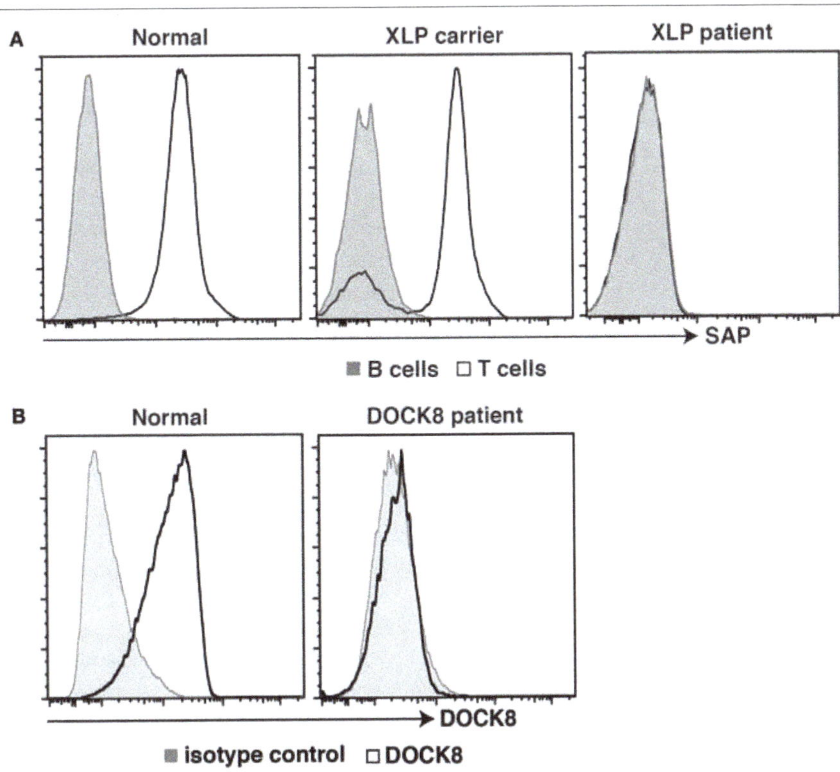

FIGURE 2 | Intracellular staining for SAP and DOCK8 in controls, patients, and female carriers. **(A)** PBMCs from healthy donors, female carriers of the XLP trait, or individuals with pathogenic mutations in *SH2D1A*, or were stained with mAbs against CD3, CD20, and SAP. Expression of SAP in B cells (tinted histogram) and T cells (open histogram) was then determined. **(B)** PBMCs from healthy donors, or from an individual suspected of having DOCK8-deficiency were stained with an isotype control Ab (tinted histogram) or a mAb against DOCK8 (open histogram). Expression of DOCK8 in lymphocytes was then determined. These data are compiled from findings previously reported in the following publications: (37, 57, 58).

TABLE 1 | Immune cell populations identified in human peripheral blood according to specific phenotypes.

Immune cell	Surface markers
$CD4^+$ T CELLS	
Total $CD4^+$ T cells	$CD3^+CD4^+$
Naïve	$CD3^+CD4^+CCR7^+CD45RA^+$
Central memory	$CD3^+CD4^+CCR7^+CD45RA^-$
Effector memory	$CD3^+CD4^+CCR7^-CD45RA^-$
Treg	$CD3^+CD4^+CD25^{hi}CD127^{lo}FoxP3^+$
Tfh	$CD3^+CD4^+CD45RA^-CXCR5^+$
Th1	$CD3^+CD4^+CD45RA^-CXCR5^-CXCR3^+$
Other Th cells including Th2 and Th9 cells	$CD3^+CD4^+CD45RA^-CXCR5^-CXCR3^-CCR6^-$
Th17	$CD3^+CD4^+CD45RA^-CXCR5^-CCR6^+$
$CD8^+$ T CELLS	
Total $CD8^+$ T cells	$CD3^+CD8^+$
Naïve	$CD3^+CD8^+CCR7^+CD45RA^+$
Central memory	$CD3^+CD8^+CCR7^+CD45RA^-$
Effector memory	$CD3^+CD8^+CCR7^-CD45RA^-$
TEMRA	$CD3^+CD8^+CCR7^-CD45RA^+$
B CELLS	
Total $CD20^+$ B cells	$CD20^+$
Transitional	$CD20^+CD10^+CD27^-$
Early transitional	$CD20^+CD10^+CD27^-CD21^{lo}CD44^{-/lo}$
Late transitional	$CD20^+CD10^+CD27^-CD21^+CD44^+$
Naïve	$CD20^+CD10^-CD27^-IgM^+IgD^{hi}$
Memory	$CD20^+CD10^-CD27^+$
IgM memory	$CD20^+CD10^-CD27^+IgM^{hi}IgD^{\pm}$
IgG memory	$CD20^+CD10^-CD27^+IgG^+$
IgA memory	$CD20^+CD10^-CD27^+IgA^+$
Plasmablasts/cells	$CD20^{\pm}CD19^+CD38^{hi}CD27^{hi}$
Atypical/aged memory B cells	$CD19^{hi}CD21^{lo}Tbet^+CD11c^+FCRL5^+$
Innate-like lymphocytes	
NK cells	$CD3^-CD56^+$
NKT cells	$CD3^+V\alpha24^+V\beta11^+$
MAIT cells	$CD3^+V\alpha7.2^+CD161^+$
$\gamma\delta$ T cells	$CD3^+V\alpha\beta^-V\gamma\delta^+$

(PB), as this is the predominant source of cells that is readily obtainable from patients. In line with this, mAbs directed against a myriad of cell surface markers can be used to identify, isolate, and characterize distinct *in vivo*-generated immune cell subsets (**Table 1**). Of the main conventional lymphocyte populations CD3, CD4, CD8, CD20, and CD56 have been used to identify total $CD3^+$ T, $CD4^+$ helper T (Th), $CD8^+$ cytotoxic T, $CD20^+$ B, and $CD3^-CD56^+$ natural killer (NK) cells (**Table 1**). In addition to this, unconventional T cell subsets, which contribute to both innate and adaptive immune responses, have been identified within the T cell compartment as $CD3^+V\alpha24^+V\beta11^+$ NKT, $CD3^+\gamma\delta^+\alpha\beta^-$ $\gamma\delta$ T and $CD3^+V\alpha7.2^+CD161^+$ mucosal associated invariant T (MAIT) cells (79) (**Table 1**).

Importantly, differential expression of specific cell surface markers can be used to determine the maturation status of distinct subsets of $CD4^+$ and $CD8^+$ T and B cells. Specifically CCR7 and CD45RA delineate naive ($CD45RA^+CCR7^+$), central memory (T_{CM}; $CD45RA^-CCR7^+$), and effector memory (T_{EM}; $CD45RA^-CCR7^-$) $CD4^+$ T cells, and naive ($CD45RA^+CCR7^+$), T_{CM} ($CD45RA^-CCR7^+$), T_{EM} ($CD45RA^-CCR7^-$), and revertant memory (T_{EMRA}; $CD45RA^+CCR7^-$) $CD8^+$ T cell populations (80, 81) (**Table 1**). The $CD4^+$ T cell compartment can also be resolved into different "helper" subsets based on expression of CD25, CD127, CD45RA, CXCR5, CXCR3, and CCR6. As such, $CD4^+$ T cell populations corresponding to regulatory T cells (Tregs; $CD25^{hi}CD127^{lo}$), T follicular helper (Tfh; $CD45RA^-CXCR5^+$), Th1 ($CD45RA^-CXCR5^-CXCR3^+CCR6^-$), Th2 ($CD45RA^-CXCR5^-CXCR3^-CCR6^-$), and Th17 ($CD45RA^-CXCR5^-CXCR3^-CCR6^+$) subsets can be identified in PB of healthy individuals (32, 81, 82).

$CD20^+$ human B cells can be divided into transitional ($CD10^+CD27^-$), naïve ($CD10^-CD27^-$), and memory ($CD10^-CD27^+$) subsets by their differential expression of CD10 and CD27 (25, 26, 83, 84). Early/immature and late/mature subsets of transitional B cells can also be identified according to differential expression of CD21 or CD44 (35, 83, 84). Furthermore, memory B cells can remain IgM^{hi} or undergo Ig isotype switching to become IgG- or IgA-expressing cells (25, 26) (**Table 1**). Plasmablasts ($CD19^+CD38^{hi}CD27^{hi}CD20^{lo}$) can also be detected, though these cells persist at very low frequencies in the PB at the basal state (85). A population of $CD19^{hi}CD21^{lo}$ B cells can also be detected within the B cell compartment. These $CD19^{hi}CD21^{lo}$ have been referred to as "atypical" and/or "aged memory" B cells, and have been associated with both health and disease (86–88) (**Table 1**). Thus, on one hand they have been proposed as being plasmablast precursors that are rapidly re-activated and differentiate into plasmablasts during anamnestic immune responses to specific Ag (86). On the other hand they have been considered to be pathogenic in the setting of chronic infection (e.g., HIV, malaria, Hepatitis B) as they are "exhausted" and unable to clear these pathogens, or self-reactive in Ab-mediated autoimmune disease (SLE, RA, Sjogren's syndrome) (27, 87, 88).

Insights Into Disease Pathogenesis in PIDs

Over the past two decades, our flow cytometric-based studies of various PIDs have provided substantial insight and understanding into the non-redundant roles of specific genes, molecules, and signaling pathways in the development, differentiation and effector function of human B cells, $CD4^+$ T cells, $CD8^+$ T cells and innate-like lymphocytes. These findings have not only identified critical requirements for establishing robust primary and long-lived immunity against various pathogens, but have elucidated mechanisms underlying infectious susceptibility in the setting of these PIDs, and defined specialized functions of discrete subsets of immune cells host defense. Some of our key findings from these studies are summarized below:

Autosomal Dominant Hyper IgE Syndrome Due to STAT3 Mutations

AD HIES is characterized by recurrent opportunistic bacterial (*Staphylococcal*) and fungal (*Candida* sps.) infections, recurrent cyst-forming pneumonia and impaired generation of Ag-specific Abs following vaccination or infection, despite dramatically increased levels of serum IgE (89). Affected individuals also present with non-immune connective tissue defects such as broad facial features, high palate, retention of primary teeth, hyperextensibility, scoliosis, osteoporosis, and recurrent fractures (89). AD-HIES was found to result from heterozygous germline DN mutations in *STAT3* (STAT3^{DN}) (90, 91). Examination of PBMCs from these patients has revealed a "lymphocyte phenotype signature" that is distinct from healthy donors.

Specifically, while there were normal frequencies of total CD4^{+} T cells in STAT3^{DN}, we found increases in proportions of naïve and decreases in proportions of T_{CM} cells (**Figures 3A,B, 4A,B**) (32). Further investigations into CD4^{+} T cell subsets revealed a significant decrease in CXCR5^{+} Tfh and CCR6^{+} Th17 cells and to a lesser extent an increase in the CXCR5^{-}CXCR3^{-}CCR6^{-} memory population (32, 92, 94, 95), which contains Th2 cells, in patients with STAT3^{DN} mutations (**Figures 3C, 4C,D**). Frequencies of total CD8^{+} T cells are comparable in healthy donors and STAT3^{DN} patients (**Figure 3D**), however STAT3^{DN} patients have an increase in naïve and a corresponding decrease in T_{CM}, T_{EM}, and T_{EMRA} CD8^{+} T cells (**Figures 3E, 4E,F**) (73). Examination of the B cell compartment of STAT3^{DN} patients also revealed stark differences to healthy donors. Despite normal frequencies of total B cells (**Figure 3F**), they tended to be more immature as revealed by an increase in transitional and naïve B cells and a concurrent decrease in memory B cells (**Figures 1, 3G**) (31, 32, 74). Interestingly, despite the severe reduction in memory B cells, those that do develop in STAT3^{DN} patients have undergone Ig isotype switching, albeit with a trend toward IgG and away from IgA (**Figure 3H**) (31, 74).

In regards to innate-like lymphocytes, the frequencies of NK and $\gamma\delta$ T cells in the PB of STAT3^{DN} patients is normal (**Figures 3I,K**). However, we found a severe reduction in NKT and MAIT cells in the absence of intact STAT3 signaling (**Figures 3J,L**) (93, 95). Taken together this analysis revealed a distinct phenotype for STAT3^{DN} lymphocytes compared to healthy controls. This lymphocyte signature has not only aided in the identification of potential STAT3^{DN} patients, but also provided valuable insights into disease susceptibility and a cellular and molecular explanation for the clinical features of STAT3 deficiency. For instance, CCR6^{+} Th17 cells are implicated in protective immunity against fungal infections (81, 95). Thus, the severe reduction in Th17 cells in STAT3^{DN} patients explains their extreme susceptibility to *Candida albicans* and subsequent chronic mucocutaneous candidiasis. Furthermore, the significant reductions in memory B cells and Tfh cells due to STAT3 deficiency are likely to account for defects in long-lived humoral immunity in STAT3^{DN} patients (95).

While these findings established critical roles for STAT3 signaling in the generation and/or maintenance of various populations of effector lymphocytes, they did not directly identify the upstream STAT3-activating cytokine(s) required for these processes. However, this has now been achieved by the identification and analysis of PID patients with inactivating mutations in specific cytokines or their receptors that signal through STAT3. Thus, IL-21/IL-21R/STAT3 signaling is required for establishing the pool of memory B cells (31, 32, 74, 95) and NKT cells (93, 95), IL-23R/IL-12Rβ1/STAT3 (but not IL-12Rβ2) signaling is necessary for MAIT cells (42, 93), and IL-23R/IL-12Rβ1/STAT3 and IL-21/IL-21R/STAT3 signaling likely co-operate to generate Th17 cells (32, 42, 95).

Mutations in the Novel Transcription Factor ZNF341 Underlie a Form of Autosomal Recessive HIES That Phenotypically and Functionally Resembles STAT3 Deficiency

Recently, 2 studies identified 19 patients with an AR form of HIES who essentially clinically phenocopied individuals with STAT3^{DN} mutations (40, 96). The molecular lesion underlying this form of recessive HIES was found to be bi-allelic mutations in the novel transcription factor *ZNF341*. The link between ZNF341 and STAT3 function was provided by the finding that ZNF341 binds to the *STAT3* promoter and regulates STAT3 expression. Consequently, ZNF341-deficient patients have low levels of *STAT3* mRNA and protein and poor responses following stimulation with STAT3-activating cytokines (40, 96).

When PBMCs from ZNF341-deficient patients were examined, we identified a lymphocyte signature very similar to that of STAT3^{DN} patients. The CD4^{+} T cell compartment was comprised of increased frequencies of naïve and decreased frequencies of T_{CM} cells (**Figures 4A,B**) (32, 40). This could be further broken down to reveal decreases in CCR6^{+} Th17 (**Figures 4C,D**) and CXCR5^{+} Tfh cells and increases in Th2 cells (40, 96). The paucity of Th17 phenotype cells in ZNF341- and STAT3-deficient patients (i.e., CD4^{+}CCR6^{+}CXCR3^{-} memory T cells) was confirmed functionally by demonstrating by flow cytometry reductions in proportions of their memory CD4^{+} T cells that expressed intracellular IL17A, IL17F, and IL22 (**Figures 5A,B**) (32, 40, 92), canonical cytokines produced by Th17 cells (81, 95). Similarly, ZNF341-deficient and STAT3^{DN} patients had increased proportions of memory CD4^{+} T cells expressing the characteristic Th2 cytokines IL-4 and IL-13 (**Figures 5C,D**) (40), consistent with the finding of increased CD4^{+}CD45RA^{-}CXCR5^{-}CCR6^{-}CXCR3^{-} memory cells (**Figure 3C**), as well as the hyper-IgE phenotype and Th2-associated pathologies, in these individuals (40, 95, 96). However, in contrast to STAT3^{DN} patients, the CD8^{+} T cell compartment in ZNF341-deficient patients was relatively comparable to that of normal donors (**Figures 4E,F**) (40, 73). ZNF341-deficient patients have similar decreases in memory B cells as STAT3^{DN} patients (**Figure 1**), and their few memory B cells are predominantly IgG^{+} rather than IgA^{+} (31, 40, 74). When populations of innate-like T cells were examined, ZNF341-deficient patients had comparable frequencies of $\gamma\delta$ T and NKT cells, but fewer MAIT cells than healthy donors (40). In contrast to STAT3, ZNF341 is likely to be important for NK cell development, as these cells are significantly decreased in ZNF341-deficient patients compared to healthy controls (40).

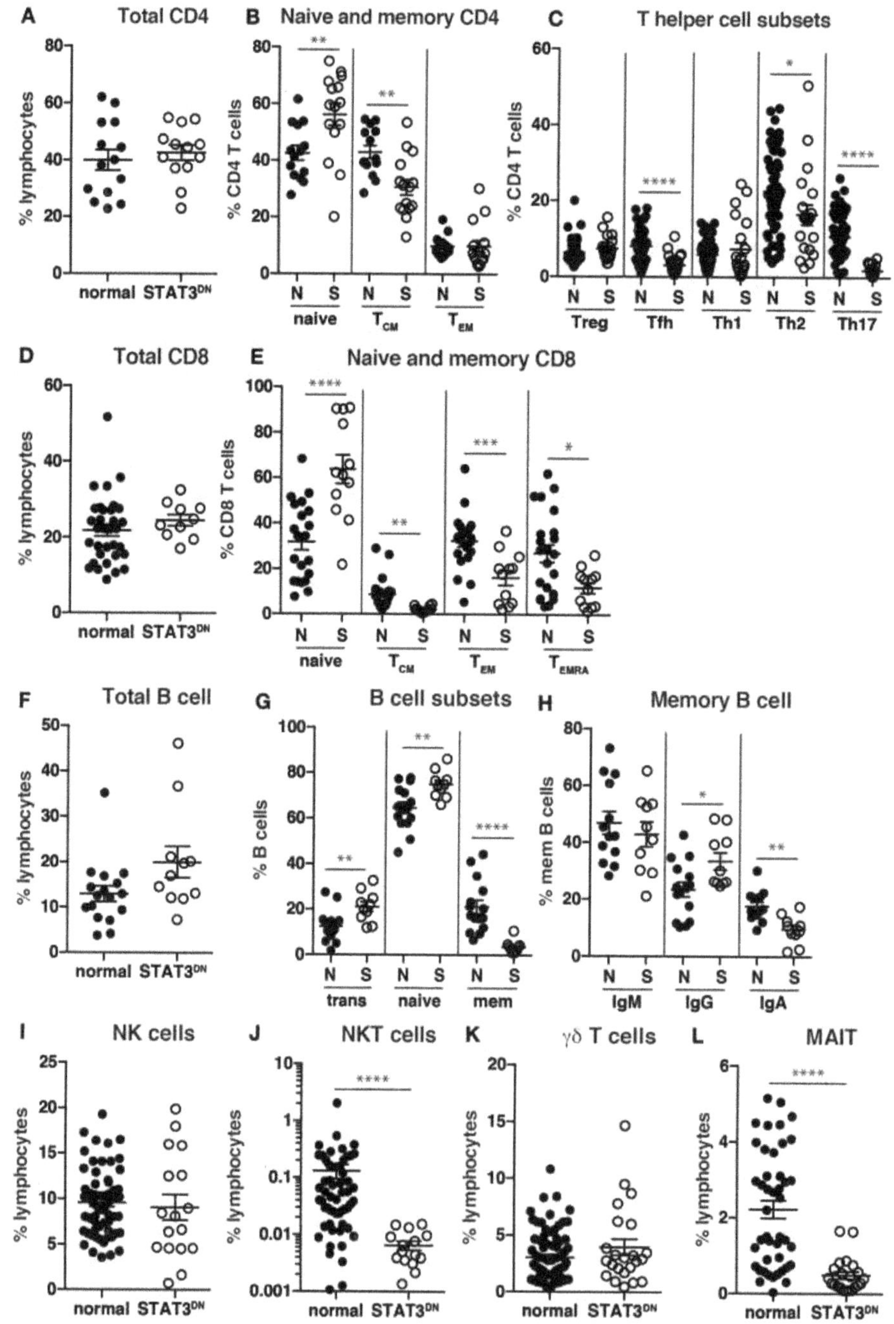

FIGURE 3 | Identification of immune cell populations in $STAT3^{DN}$ patients. **(A)** Total CD4 T cells, **(B)** naïve, central memory (T_{CM}), effector memory (T_{EM}) $CD4^{+}$ T cells, **(C)** regulatory T cells (Treg) T follicular helper (Tfh) cells, Th1, Th2, Th17 $CD4^{+}$ T cells, **(D)** total $CD8^{+}$ T cells, **(E)** naïve, T_{CM}, T_{EM}, and revertant memory (T_{EMRA}) $CD8^{+}$ T cells, **(F)** total B cells, **(G)** transitional, naive and memory B cells, **(H)** IgM, IgG and IgA memory B cells, **(I)** NK cells, **(J)** NKT cells, **(K)** γδ T cells and **(L)** mucosal associated invariant T (MAIT) cells were identified in normal donors (N) and $STAT3^{DN}$ patients (S). Each point represents a different sample and horizontal line represents the average; statistics were performed in Prism using *t*-test ($^{*}p < 0.05$; $^{**}p < 0.01$; $^{***}p < 0.001$; $^{****}p < 0.0001$). These data are compiled from findings previously reported in the following publications: (31, 32, 73–75, 92, 93).

DOCK8-Deficiency

Dedicator of cytokinesis 8 (DOCK8) deficiency is a combined immunodeficiency caused by AR LOF mutations in *DOCK8* (97). This disorder is characterized by recurrent cutaneous viral, bacterial and fungal infections, increased serum IgE levels, and severe atopic disease, including food-induced anaphylaxis (97). Similar to SAP expression in XLP, the use of mAbs to detect DOCK8 expression has been crucial for the diagnosis of

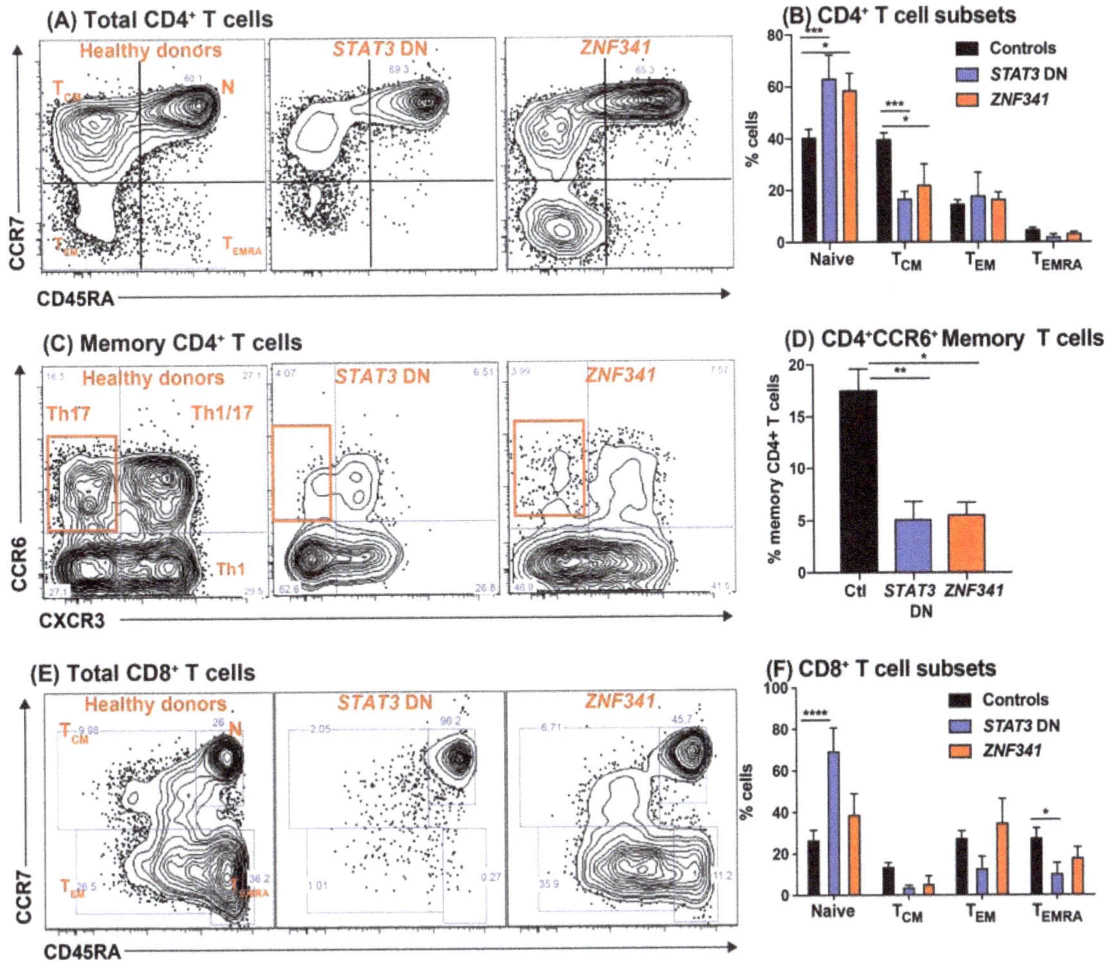

FIGURE 4 | Recessive mutations in *ZNF341* phenocopy clinical and cellular defects due to autosomal dominant *STAT3* mutations to cause AR HIES. PBMCs from healthy donors or from individuals with pathogenic *STAT3* DN or *ZNF341* LOF mutations were stained with mAbs against CD4, CD8, CD45RA, CCR7, CXCR3, CCR6, CXCR5, CD127, and CD25. **(A,B)** Total $CD4^+$ T cells were identified as $CD4^+CD8^-$ cells, and then proportions of naïve, T_{CM}, T_{EM}, and T_{EMRA} cells were determined. **(C,D)** the memory compartment ($CD4^+CD45RA^-$) of $CD4^+$ T cells was analyzed to quantify the proportions of cells with a $CXCR3^-CCR6^+$ Th17-, $CXCR3^+CCR6^-$ Th1-, $CXCR3^+CCR6^+$ Th1/17-, and $CXCR3^-CCR6^-$ Th2-type phenotype. **(E,F)** Total $CD8^+$ T cells were identified as $CD4^-CD8^+$ cells, and then proportions of naïve, T_{CM}, T_{EM}, and T_{EMRA} cells were determined. The contour plots in **(A,C,E)** are representative of 1 healthy donor, and 1 patient each with mutations in *STAT3* or *ZNF341*. The graphs represent the mean ± sem of $CD4^+$ and $CD8^+$ T cell subsets detected in the PB of 17 healthy donors, 8 $STAT3^{DN}$ patients or 4 *ZNF341*-deficient patients. Significant differences were determined by ANOVA ($^*p < 0.05$; $^{**}p < 0.01$; $^{***}p < 0.001$; $^{****}p < 0.0001$). These data are compiled from our findings previously reported in Beziat et al. (40).

DOCK8-deficient patients (37, 53, 97) (**Figure 2**). Intracellular flow cytometry for DOCK8 expression has also detected somatic reversion in these patients (54).

DOCK8-deficient patients also have a unique lymphocyte phenotype, with decreased frequencies of $CD4^+$ T cells, but normal frequencies of $CD8^+$ T cells, resulting in an inverted CD4:CD8 ratio compared to healthy donors (37, 58, 76). When DOCK8-deficient $CD4^+$ and $CD8^+$ T cells were further investigated, we found a decrease in naïve $CD4^+$ and $CD8^+$ T cells and a corresponding increase in $CD4^+$ T_{EM} and $CD8^+$ T_{EM} and T_{EMRA} populations compared to healthy donors (37, 58, 76). Furthermore, memory T cells in DOCK8-deficiency contained reduced frequencies of $CD27^+$, $CD28^+$, and $CD127^+$ and higher frequencies of $CD57^+$, $CD95^+$, and $PD1^+$ cells, indicating these cells had undergone premature exhaustion or senescence compared to their counterparts in healthy donors (37, 58, 76). There were also reductions in frequencies of $CD4^+CCR6^+$ memory T cells in DOCK8-deficient patients, suggesting a role for DOCK8 in Th17 cells (37, 58, 78). This loss of $CCR6^+$ Th17 cells also provides a cellular explanation for increased susceptibility of DOCK8-deficient patients to infections with *Candida* sp. (81, 95). The B cell compartment in DOCK8-deficient patients comprises normal frequencies of total and transitional B cells, however there are increases in naïve and decreases in memory B cells compared to healthy donors (37, 98), thus highlighting a requirement for DOCK8 for B cell differentiation. DOCK8-deficient patients were also found to have decreased αβ T, NKT, and MAIT cells, normal frequencies of

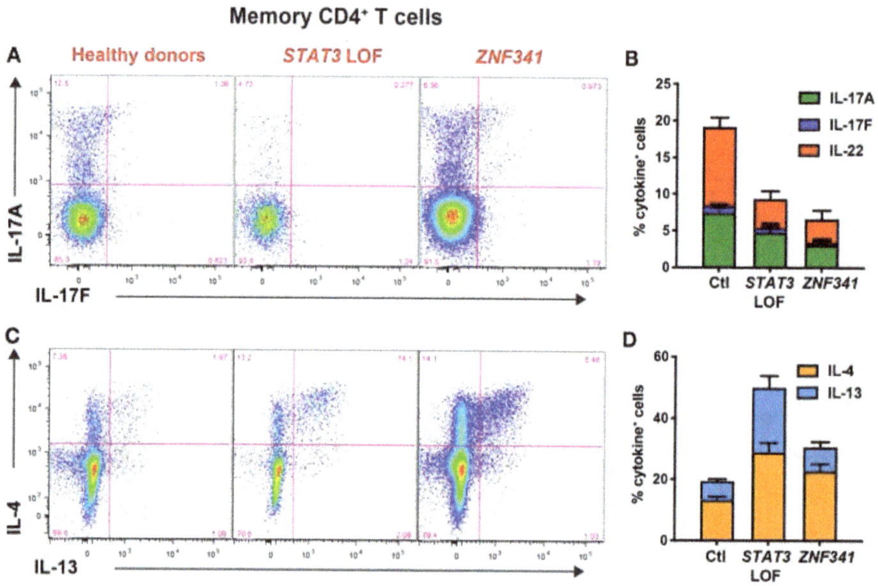

FIGURE 5 | CD4$^+$ T cell defects detectable by immunophenotyping of $STAT3^{DN}$ and *ZNF341*-deficient patients correlate with compromised function determined flow cytometrically *in vitro*. Sort-purified CD4+ memory T cells isolated from healthy donors or individuals with pathogenic *STAT3* DN or *ZNF341* LOF mutations were cultured *in vitro* with anti-CD2/CD3/CD28 mAb conjugated to beads. Following 5 days, the cells were harvested, washed, and then restimulated with PMA/ionomycin for 6 h, with Brefeldin A being added for the final 4 h of culture. Cells were then harvested, fixed, permeabilised, and stained with fluorescently-labeled mAbs specific for **(A,B)** IL-17A and IL-17F, or **(C,D)** IL-4 and IL-13. The proportions of cytokine-expressing cells were then determined by flow cytometric analysis. Contour plots **(A,C)** are representative of 1 healthy donor, and 1 patient with mutations in *STAT3* or *ZNF341*. The graphs **(B,D)** represent the mean ± sem of CD4$^+$ memory T cells expressing the indicated cytokine from 23–28 healthy donors, 6–7 $STAT3^{DN}$ patients or 4–6 *ZNF341*-deficient patients. These data are compiled from our findings previously reported in Beziat et al. (40).

NK cells, but increased γδ T cells (37). Importantly, this cellular phenotype has been able to predict individuals with AR HIES who may have pathogenic mutations in *DOCK8*, and provide explanations for clinical features of this condition (37, 58, 76).

X-Linked Lymphoproliferative Disease

XLP-1 is a rare X-linked PID whereby affected males present with extreme sensitivity to disease resulting from Epstein-Barr virus (EBV) infection. Following exposure to EBV, XLP patients develop severe infectious mononucleosis, leading to often-fatal hemophagocytic lymphohistiocytosis (99). XLP-1 patients also exhibit hypogammaglobulinemia and a heightened risk of developing B-cell lymphoma, both of which occur independently of exposure to EBV (99). XLP-1 results from LOF mutations in *SH2D1A*, encoding signaling lymphocytic activation molecule (SLAM)-associated protein (SAP) (20). SAP is a small intracellular adaptor protein that binds to tyrosine-based motifs in the intracellular domain of SLAM family members and regulates signaling downstream of these receptors (99). The availability of mAbs specific for SAP has been instrumental in expanding our knowledge of this condition. Thus, flow cytometry has (i) accurately defined the cell types that express SAP (predominantly T, NK, and NKT cells, but rarely B cells), (ii) offered a rapid and sensitive diagnostic tool to detect not only XLP patients whom lack SAP expression, but also female carriers of the XLP trait who have bimodal SAP expression in their T and NK cells (**Figure 2**) (57), and (3) revealed lymphocyte defects in XLP-1, thereby providing insight into disease pathogenesis. XLP patients have a paucity for CD27$^+$ memory B cells (**Figure 1**), and the few memory B cells detected express IgM, thereby indicating an inability to undergo class switching to express IgG or IgA (29, 30). Within the CD4$^+$ T cell compartment, XLP patients have a comparable frequency of naïve, T_{CM} and T_{EM} populations to healthy donors (29). Although XLP patients have a normal frequency of Tfh cells (100, 101), the inability of these cells to support B cell differentiation in an *in vitro* helper assay indicates defective B-helper function (30). Together, these observations identify defective CD4$^+$ T cell help as the cellular basis for hypogammaglobulinemia in XLP-1 patients, rather than a B-cell intrinsic defect. This is indeed consistent with the fact that B cells do not express SAP (57, 60) and XLP B cells function normally when provided with the correct T-dependent stimuli *in vitro* (30).

CD8$^+$ T cells from XLP patients are skewed toward T_{EM} and T_{EMRA} cells, usually at the expense of naïve T cells. Interestingly, by utilizing intracellular flow cytometry to detect SAP expression, we were able to show that some XLP patients undergo somatic reversion and a population of SAP$^+$ CD45RA$^-$CCR7$^-$ T_{EM} cells is detectable within their CD8$^+$ T cells (60). These reverted SAP$^+$ CD8$^+$ T cells in XLP patients could respond to EBV and kill-EBV infected B cells, suggesting they were able to provide protective immunity against ongoing EBV infection (60). These functional features were detected by concomitantly tracking proliferation and degranulation of EBV-specific $CD8^+$ T cells (60), further illustrating the utility of flow cytometry in establishing functionality of immune cells in PIDs.

XLP patients also lack NKT cells, revealing an essential role for SAP in the development of this cell type and potentially implicating NKT cells in some of the clinical manifestations of XLP such as impaired anti-viral and anti-tumor immune responses (102). Consistent with this essential role of SAP in NKT cell development, female XLP carriers undergo X chromosome inactivation within NKT cells, but not T or NK cells, resulting in all NKT cells in these carriers expressing only the WT allele (57, 102).

FINAL REMARKS

Flow cytometry has been central to enhancing our understanding of PIDs. It has enabled diagnoses and provided mechanistic insights into disease pathogenesis in many PIDs. For example, the severe reduction in Th17 cells and memory B cells in *STAT3*^{DN}, *ZNF341*-, and *DOCK8*-deficient patients explains susceptibility to recurrent opportunistic bacterial and fungal infections, and impaired long-lived protective humoral immunity, respectively. While our focus has been on lymphocyte populations, flow cytometry has been used to identify other populations such as monocytes ($CD14^+$), dendritic cell (DC) subsets [plasmacytoid DCs (pDCs; $lineage^-HLA\text{-}DR^+CD123^+$), $CD1c^+$ myeloid DCs ($CD1c^+$ mDCs; $lineage^-HLA\text{-}DR^+CD11c^+CD1c^+$), and $CD141^+$ mDC ($CD141^+$ mDC; $lineage^-HLA\text{-}DR^+CD11c^+CD141^+$)], and innate lymphoid cells [(ILCs), ILC1, ILC2, and ILC precursors (ILCPs)]. Beyond deep immunophenotypic analysis by examining expression of specific cell surface molecules, flow cytometry has also been used to diagnose PIDs by assessing expression of specific intracellular proteins (SAP, DOCK8, XIAP, BTK) as well as quantifying cytokine-induced STAT phosphorylation and Ag-receptor induced calcium flux. As we move toward the next generation of flow cytometers, which are capable of simultaneously detecting upward of 28 fluorochromes, the future is looking brighter, fluorescent even, in terms of the applicability of flow cytometry in the study and diagnosis of PIDs.

AUTHOR CONTRIBUTIONS

CM and ST designed, conceptualized, and wrote this review.

FUNDING

Research performed in the Tangye/Ma lab has been supported by the National Health and Medical Council of Australia, the Office of Health and Medical Research of the New South Wales Government, the Jeffrey Modell Foundation, the Job Research Foundation, and the Cancer Council NSW.

ACKNOWLEDGMENTS

We thank our many clinical colleagues and collaborators, as well as the many patients and families, who have made it possible for our laboratories to pursue many of the questions discussed in this review. We are particularly indebted to Jean-Laurent Casanova, Anne Puel, Stephanie Boisson-Dupuis, Emmanuelle Jouanguy, Vivien Beziat, Satoshi Okada, Peter Arkwright, Kaan Boztug, Isabelle Meyts, Qiang Pan-Hammarstrom, Melanie Wong, Paul Gray, Steve Holland, Gulbu Uzel, and Elissa Deenick for ongoing support and input into these projects, and members of our lab who have contributed to these studies over the years!

REFERENCES

1. Bruton OC. Agammaglobulinemia. *Pediatrics.* (1952) 9:722–8.
2. Cooper MD, Peterson RD, Good RA. Delineation of the thymic and bursal lymphoid systems in the chicken. *Nature.* (1965) 205:143–6. doi: 10.1038/205143a0
3. Conley ME, Dobbs AK, Farmer DM, Kilic S, Paris K, Grigoriadou S, et al. Primary B cell immunodeficiencies: comparisons and contrasts. *Annu Rev Immunol.* (2009) 27:199–227. doi: 10.1146/annurev.immunol.021908.132649
4. Cooper MD, Lawton AR, Bockman DE. Agammaglobulinaemia with B lymphocytes. Specific defect of plasma-cell differentiation. *Lancet.* (1971) 2:791–4. doi: 10.1016/S0140-6736(71)92742-5
5. Grey HM, Rabellino E, Pirofsky B. Immunoglobulins on the surface of lymphocytes. IV. Distribution in hypogammaglobulinemia, cellular immune deficiency, and chronic lymphatic leukemia. *J Clin Invest.* (1971) 50:2368–75. doi: 10.1172/JCI106735
6. Siegal FP, Pernis B, Kunkel HG. Lymphocytes in human immunodeficiency states: a study of membrane-associated immunoglobulins. *Eur J Immunol.* (1971) 1:482–6. doi: 10.1002/eji.1830010615
7. Cooper MD, Lawton AR. Circulating B-cells in patients with immunodeficiency. *Am J Pathol.* (1972) 69: 513–28.
8. Pearl ER, Vogler LB, Okos AJ, Crist WM, Lawton AR III, Cooper MD. B lymphocyte precursors in human bone marrow: an analysis of normal individuals and patients with antibody-deficiency states. *J Immunol.* (1978) 120:1169–75.
9. Geha RS, Rosen FS, Merler E. Identification and characterization of subpopulations of lymphocytes in human peripheral blood after fractionation on discontinuous gradients of albumin. The cellular defect in X-linked agammaglobulinemia. *J Clin Invest.* (1973) 52:1726–34. doi: 10.1172/JCI107354
10. Griscelli C, Durandy A, Virelizier JL, Ballet JJ, Daguillard F. Selective defect of precursor T cells associated with apparently normal B lymphocytes in severe combined immunodeficiency disease. *J Pediatr.* (1978) 93:404–11. doi: 10.1016/S0022-3476(78)81146-9
11. Kohler G, Milstein C. Continuous cultures of fused cells secreting antibody of predefined specificity. *Nature.* (1975) 256:495–7. doi: 10.1038/256495a0
12. Conley ME. B cells in patients with X-linked agammaglobulinemia. *J Immunol.* (1985) 134:3070–4.
13. Stahl RE, Friedman-Kien A, Dubin R, Marmor M, Zolla-Pazner S. Immunologic abnormalities in homosexual men. Relationship to Kaposi's sarcoma. *Am J Med.* (1982) 73:171–8. doi: 10.1016/0002-9343(82)90174-7
14. Ammann AJ, Abrams D, Conant M, Chudwin D, Cowan M, Volberding P, Lewis B, Casavant C. Acquired immune dysfunction in homosexual men: immunologic profiles. *Clin Immunol Immunopathol.* (1983) 27:315–25. doi: 10.1016/0090-1229(83)90084-3
15. Modlin RL, Meyer PR, Hofman FM, Mehlmauer M, Levy NB, Lukes RJ, et al. T-lymphocyte subsets in lymph nodes from homosexual men. *JAMA.* (1983) 250:1302–5. doi: 10.1001/jama.250.10.1302

16. Detels R, Visscher BR, Fahey JL, Sever JL, Gravell M, Madden DL, et al. Predictors of clinical AIDS in young homosexual men in a high-risk area. *Int J Epidemiol.* (1987) 16:271–6. doi: 10.1093/ije/16.2.271
17. Fauci AS, Macher AM, Longo DL, Lane HC, Rook AH, Masur H, et al. NIH conference. Acquired immunodeficiency syndrome: epidemiologic, clinical, immunologic, and therapeutic considerations. *Ann Intern Med.* (1984) 100:92–106. doi: 10.7326/0003-4819-100-1-92
18. Herzenberg LA, Herzenberg LA. Genetics, FACS, immunology, and redox: a tale of two lives intertwined. *Annu Rev Immunol.* (2004) 22:1–31. doi: 10.1146/annurev.immunol.22.012703.104727
19. Boisson B, Wang YD, Bosompem A, Ma CS, Lim A, Kochetkov T, et al. A recurrent dominant negative E47 mutation causes agammaglobulinemia and BCR(-) B cells. *J Clin Invest.* (2013) 123:4781–5. doi: 10.1172/JCI71927
20. Picard C, Bobby Gaspar H, Al-Herz W, Bousfiha A, Casanova JL, Chatila T, et al. International union of immunological societies: 2017 primary immunodeficiency diseases committee report on inborn errors of immunity. *J Clin Immunol.* (2018) 38:96–128. doi: 10.1007/s10875-017-0464-9
21. Buckley RH. Molecular defects in human severe combined immunodeficiency and approaches to immune reconstitution. *Annu Rev Immunol.* (2004) 22:625–55. doi: 10.1146/annurev.immunol.22.012703.104614
22. DiSanto JP, Bonnefoy JY, Gauchat JF, Fischer A, de Saint Basile G. CD40 ligand mutations in x-linked immunodeficiency with hyper-IgM. *Nature.* (1993) 361:541–3. doi: 10.1038/361541a0
23. Korthauer U, Graf D, Mages HW, Briere F, Padayachee M, Malcolm S, et al. Defective expression of T-cell CD40 ligand causes X-linked immunodeficiency with hyper-IgM. *Nature.* (1993) 361:539–41. doi: 10.1038/361539a0
24. Grimbacher B, Hutloff A, Schlesier M, Glocker E, Warnatz K, Drager R, et al. Homozygous loss of ICOS is associated with adult-onset common variable immunodeficiency. *Nat Immunol.* (2003) 4:261–8. doi: 10.1038/ni902
25. Klein U, Rajewsky K, Kuppers R. Human immunoglobulin (Ig)M+IgD+ peripheral blood B cells expressing the CD27 cell surface antigen carry somatically mutated variable region genes: CD27 as a general marker for somatically mutated (memory) B cells. *J Exp Med.* (1998) 188:1679–89. doi: 10.1084/jem.188.9.1679
26. Tangye SG, Liu YJ, Aversa G, Phillips JH, de Vries JE. Identification of functional human splenic memory B cells by expression of CD148 and CD27. *J Exp Med.* (1998) 188:1691–703. doi: 10.1084/jem.188.9.1691
27. Warnatz K, Denz A, Drager R, Braun M, Groth C, Wolff-Vorbeck G, et al. Severe deficiency of switched memory B cells (CD27(+)IgM(-)IgD(-)) in subgroups of patients with common variable immunodeficiency: a new approach to classify a heterogeneous disease. *Blood.* (2002) 99:1544–51. doi: 10.1182/blood.V99.5.1544
28. Wehr C, Kivioja T, Schmitt C, Ferry B, Witte T, Eren E, et al. The EUROclass trial: defining subgroups in common variable immunodeficiency. *Blood.* (2008) 111:77–85. doi: 10.1182/blood-2007-06-091744
29. Ma CS, Hare NJ, Nichols KE, Dupre L, Andolfi G, Roncarolo MG, et al. Impaired humoral immunity in X-linked lymphoproliferative disease is associated with defective IL-10 production by CD4+ T cells. *J Clin Invest.* (2005) 115:1049–59. doi: 10.1172/JCI23139
30. Ma CS, Pittaluga S, Avery DT, Hare NJ, Maric I, Klion AD, et al. Selective generation of functional somatically mutated IgM+CD27+, but not Ig isotype-switched, memory B cells in X-linked lymphoproliferative disease. *J Clin Invest.* (2006) 116:322–33. doi: 10.1172/JCI25720
31. Deenick EK, Avery DT, Chan A, Berglund LJ, Ives ML, Moens L, et al. Naive and memory human B cells have distinct requirements for STAT3 activation to differentiate into antibody-secreting plasma cells. *J Exp Med.* (2013) 210:2739–53. doi: 10.1084/jem.20130323
32. Ma CS, Wong N, Rao G, Avery DT, Torpy J, Hambridge T, et al. Monogenic mutations differentially affect the quantity and quality of T follicular helper cells in patients with human primary immunodeficiencies. *J Allergy Clin Immunol.* (2015) 136:993–1006 e1. doi: 10.1016/j.jaci.2015.05.036
33. Wang Y, Ma CS, Ling Y, Bousfiha A, Camcioglu Y, Jacquot S, et al. Dual T cell- and B cell-intrinsic deficiency in humans with biallelic RLTPR mutations. *J Exp Med.* (2016) 213:2413–35. doi: 10.1084/jem.20160576
34. Abolhassani H, Edwards ES, Ikinciogullari A, Jing H, Borte S, Buggert M, et al. Combined immunodeficiency and Epstein-Barr virus-induced B cell malignancy in humans with inherited CD70 deficiency. *J Exp Med.* (2017) 214:91–106. doi: 10.1084/jem.20160849
35. Avery DT, Kane A, Nguyen T, Lau A, Nguyen A, Lenthall H, et al. Germline-activating mutations in PIK3CD compromise B cell development and function. *J Exp Med.* (2018) 215:2073–95. doi: 10.1084/jem.20180010
36. Moran I, Avery DT, Payne K, Lenthall H, Davies EG, Burns S, et al. B cell-intrinsic requirement for STK4 in humoral immunity in mice and human subjects. *J Allergy Clin Immunol.* (2019) 143:2302–5. doi: 10.1016/j.jaci.2019.02.010
37. Pillay BA, Avery DT, Smart JM, Cole T, Choo S, Chan D, et al. Hematopoietic stem cell transplant effectively rescues lymphocyte differentiation and function in DOCK8-deficient patients. *JCI Insight.* (2019) 5:127527. doi: 10.1172/jci.insight.127527
38. Warnatz K, Bossaller L, Salzer U, Skrabl-Baumgartner A, Schwinger W, van der Burg M, et al. Human ICOS deficiency abrogates the germinal center reaction and provides a monogenic model for common variable immunodeficiency. *Blood.* (2006) 107:3045–52. doi: 10.1182/blood-2005-07-2955
39. Recher M, Berglund LJ, Avery DT, Cowan MJ, Gennery AR, Smart J, et al. IL-21 is the primary common gamma chain-binding cytokine required for human B-cell differentiation *in vivo*. *Blood.* (2011) 118:6824–35. doi: 10.1182/blood-2011-06-362533
40. Beziat V, Li J, Lin JX, Ma CS, Li P, Bousfiha A, et al. A recessive form of hyper-IgE syndrome by disruption of ZNF341-dependent STAT3 transcription and activity. *Sci Immunol.* (2018) 3:eaat4956. doi: 10.1126/sciimmunol.aat4956
41. Cliffe ST, Bloch DB, Suryani S, Kamsteeg EJ, Avery DT, Palendira U, et al. Clinical, molecular, and cellular immunologic findings in patients with SP110-associated veno-occlusive disease with immunodeficiency syndrome. *J Allergy Clin Immunol.* (2012) 130:735–42 e6. doi: 10.1016/j.jaci.2012.02.054
42. Martinez-Barricarte R, Markle JG, Ma CS, Deenick EK, Ramirez-Alejo N, Mele F, et al. Human IFN-gamma immunity to mycobacteria is governed by both IL-12 and IL-23. *Sci Immunol.* (2018) 3:eaau6759. doi: 10.1126/sciimmunol.aau6759
43. Kong XF, Martinez-Barricarte R, Kennedy J, Mele F, Lazarov T, Deenick EK, et al. Disruption of an antimycobacterial circuit between dendritic and helper T cells in human SPPL2a deficiency. *Nat Immunol.* (2018) 19:973–85. doi: 10.1038/s41590-018-0178-z
44. Cottineau J, Kottemann MC, Lach FP, Kang YH, Vely F, Deenick EK, et al. Inherited GINS1 deficiency underlies growth retardation along with neutropenia and NK cell deficiency. *J Clin Invest.* (2017) 127:1991–2006. doi: 10.1172/JCI90727
45. Lu HY, Bauman BM, Arjunaraja S, Dorjbal B, Milner JD, Snow AL, et al. The CBM-opathies-a rapidly expanding spectrum of human inborn errors of immunity caused by mutations in the CARD11-BCL10-MALT1 complex. *Front Immunol.* (2018) 9:2078. doi: 10.3389/fimmu.2018.02078
46. Wentink MWJ, van Zelm MC, van Dongen JJM, Warnatz K, van der Burg M. Deficiencies in the CD19 complex. *Clin Immunol.* (2018) 195:82–7. doi: 10.1016/j.clim.2018.07.017
47. Klemann C, Camacho-Ordonez N, Yang L, Eskandarian Z, Rojas-Restrepo JL, Frede N, et al. Clinical and immunological phenotype of patients with primary immunodeficiency due to damaging mutations in NFKB2. *Front Immunol.* (2019) 10:297. doi: 10.3389/fimmu.2019.00297
48. Willmann KL, Klaver S, Dogu F, Santos-Valente E, Garncarz W, Bilic I, et al. Biallelic loss-of-function mutation in NIK causes a primary immunodeficiency with multifaceted aberrant lymphoid immunity. *Nat Commun.* (2014) 5:5360. doi: 10.1038/ncomms6360
49. Pala P, Hussell T, Openshaw PJ. Flow cytometric measurement of intracellular cytokines. *J Immunol Methods.* (2000) 243:107–24. doi: 10.1016/S0022-1759(00)00230-1
50. Krutzik PO, Nolan GP. Intracellular phospho-protein staining techniques for flow cytometry: monitoring single cell signaling events. *Cytometry A.* (2003) 55:61–70. doi: 10.1002/cyto.a.10072
51. Marsh RA, Bleesing JJ, Filipovich AH. Using flow cytometry to screen patients for X-linked lymphoproliferative disease due to SAP deficiency and XIAP deficiency. *J Immunol Methods.* (2010) 362:1–9. doi: 10.1016/j.jim.2010.08.010

52. Torgerson TR, Ochs HD. Immune dysregulation, polyendocrinopathy, enteropathy, X-linked: forkhead box protein 3 mutations and lack of regulatory T cells. *J Allergy Clin Immunol.* (2007) 120:744–50; quiz 51–2. doi: 10.1016/j.jaci.2007.08.044
53. Pai SY, de Boer H, Massaad MJ, Chatila TA, Keles S, Jabara HH, et al. Flow cytometry diagnosis of dedicator of cytokinesis 8 (DOCK8) deficiency. *J Allergy Clin Immunol.* (2014) 134:221–3. doi: 10.1016/j.jaci.2014.02.023
54. Jing H, Zhang Q, Zhang Y, Hill BJ, Dove CG, Gelfand EW, et al. Somatic reversion in dedicator of cytokinesis 8 immunodeficiency modulates disease phenotype. *J Allergy Clin Immunol.* (2014) 133:1667–75. doi: 10.1016/j.jaci.2014.03.025
55. Futatani T, Miyawaki T, Tsukada S, Hashimoto S, Kunikata T, Arai S, et al. Deficient expression of Bruton's tyrosine kinase in monocytes from X-linked agammaglobulinemia as evaluated by a flow cytometric analysis and its clinical application to carrier detection. *Blood.* (1998) 91:595–602.
56. Kanegane H, Futatani T, Wang Y, Nomura K, Shinozaki K, Matsukura H, et al. Clinical and mutational characteristics of X-linked agammaglobulinemia and its carrier identified by flow cytometric assessment combined with genetic analysis. *J Allergy Clin Immunol.* (2001) 108:1012–20. doi: 10.1067/mai.2001.120133
57. Palendira U, Low C, Chan A, Hislop AD, Ho E, Phan TG, et al. Molecular pathogenesis of EBV susceptibility in XLP as revealed by analysis of female carriers with heterozygous expression of SAP. *PLoS Biol.* (2011) 9:e1001187. doi: 10.1371/journal.pbio.1001187
58. Tangye SG, Pillay B, Randall KL, Avery DT, Phan TG, Gray P, et al. Dedicator of cytokinesis 8-deficient CD4(+) T cells are biased to a TH2 effector fate at the expense of TH1 and TH17 cells. *J Allergy Clin Immunol.* (2017) 139:933–49. doi: 10.1016/j.jaci.2016.07.016
59. Marciano BE, Zerbe CS, Falcone EL, Ding L, DeRavin SS, Daub J, et al. X-linked carriers of chronic granulomatous disease: illness, lyonization, and stability. *J Allergy Clin Immunol.* (2018) 141:365–71. doi: 10.1016/j.jaci.2017.04.035
60. Palendira U, Low C, Bell AI, Ma CS, Abbott RJ, Phan TG, et al. Expansion of somatically reverted memory CD8+ T cells in patients with X-linked lymphoproliferative disease caused by selective pressure from Epstein-Barr virus. *J Exp Med.* (2012) 209:913–24. doi: 10.1084/jem.20112391
61. Tone Y, Wada T, Shibata F, Toma T, Hashida Y, Kasahara Y, et al. Somatic revertant mosaicism in a patient with leukocyte adhesion deficiency type 1. *Blood.* (2007) 109:1182–4. doi: 10.1182/blood-2007-08-039057
62. Uzel G, Tng E, Rosenzweig SD, Hsu AP, Shaw JM, Horwitz ME, et al. Reversion mutations in patients with leukocyte adhesion deficiency type-1 (LAD-1). *Blood.* (2008) 111:209–18. doi: 10.1182/blood-2007-04-082552
63. Fleisher TA, Dorman SE, Anderson JA, Vail M, Brown MR, Holland SM. Detection of intracellular phosphorylated STAT-1 by flow cytometry. *Clin Immunol.* (1999) 90:425–30. doi: 10.1006/clim.1998.4654
64. Uzel G, Frucht DM, Fleisher TA, Holland SM. Detection of intracellular phosphorylated STAT-4 by flow cytometry. *Clin Immunol.* (2001) 100:270–6. doi: 10.1006/clim.2001.5078
65. Lee CH, Hsu P, Nanan B, Nanan R, Wong M, Gaskin KJ, et al. Novel *de novo* mutations of the interleukin-10 receptor gene lead to infantile onset inflammatory bowel disease. *J Crohns Colitis.* (2014) 8:1551–6. doi: 10.1016/j.crohns.2014.04.004
66. Uzel G, Sampaio EP, Lawrence MG, Hsu AP, Hackett M, Dorsey MJ, et al. Dominant gain-of-function STAT1 mutations in FOXP3 wild-type immune dysregulation-polyendocrinopathy-enteropathy-X-linked-like syndrome. *J Allergy Clin Immunol.* (2013) 131:1611–23. doi: 10.1016/j.jaci.2012.11.054
67. Kotlarz D, Zietara N, Uzel G, Weidemann T, Braun CJ, Diestelhorst J, et al. Loss-of-function mutations in the IL-21 receptor gene cause a primary immunodeficiency syndrome. *J Exp Med.* (2013) 210:433–43. doi: 10.1084/jem.20111229
68. Schwerd T, Twigg SRF, Aschenbrenner D, Manrique S, Miller KA, Taylor IB, et al. A biallelic mutation in IL6ST encoding the GP130 co-receptor causes immunodeficiency and craniosynostosis. *J Exp Med.* (2017) 214:2547–62. doi: 10.1084/jem.20161810
69. Spencer S, Kostel Bal S, Egner W, Lango Allen H, Raza SI, Ma CA, et al. Loss of the interleukin-6 receptor causes immunodeficiency, atopy, and abnormal inflammatory responses. *J Exp Med.* (2019). doi: 10.1084/jem.20190344. [Epub ahead of print].
70. Vowells SJ, Sekhsaria S, Malech HL, Shalit M, Fleisher TA. Flow cytometric analysis of the granulocyte respiratory burst: a comparison study of fluorescent probes. *J Immunol Methods.* (1995) 178:89–97. doi: 10.1016/0022-1759(94)00247-T
71. Hasbold J, Gett AV, Rush JS, Deenick E, Avery D, Jun J, et al. Quantitative analysis of lymphocyte differentiation and proliferation *in vitro* using carboxyfluorescein diacetate succinimidyl ester. *Immunol Cell Biol.* (1999) 77:516–22. doi: 10.1046/j.1440-1711.1999.00874.x
72. Tempany JC, Zhou JH, Hodgkin PD, Bryant VL. Superior properties of CellTrace Yellow as a division tracking dye for human and murine lymphocytes. *Immunol Cell Biol.* (2018) 96:149–59. doi: 10.1111/imcb.1020
73. Ives ML, Ma CS, Palendira U, Chan A, Bustamante J, Boisson-Dupuis S, et al. Signal transducer and activator of transcription 3 (STAT3) mutations underlying autosomal dominant hyper-IgE syndrome impair human CD8(+) T-cell memory formation and function. *J Allergy Clin Immunol.* (2013) 132:400–11 e9. doi: 10.1016/j.jaci.2013.05.029
74. Avery DT, Deenick EK, Ma CS, Suryani S, Simpson N, Chew GY, et al. B cell-intrinsic signaling through IL-21 receptor and STAT3 is required for establishing long-lived antibody responses in humans. *J Exp Med.* (2010) 207:155–71. doi: 10.1084/jem.20091706
75. Ma CS, Avery DT, Chan A, Batten M, Bustamante J, Boisson-Dupuis S, et al. Functional STAT3 deficiency compromises the generation of human T follicular helper cells. *Blood.* (2012) 119:3997–4008. doi: 10.1182/blood-2011-11-392985
76. Randall KL, Chan SS, Ma CS, Fung I, Mei Y, Yabas M, et al. DOCK8 deficiency impairs CD8 T cell survival and function in humans and mice. *J Exp Med.* (2011) 208:2305–20. doi: 10.1084/jem.20110345
77. Morra M, Simarro-Grande M, Martin M, Chen AS, Lanyi A, Silander O, et al. Characterization of SH2D1A missense mutations identified in X-linked lymphoproliferative disease patients. *J Biol Chem.* (2001) 276:36809–16. doi: 10.1074/jbc.M101305200
78. Keles S, Charbonnier LM, Kabaleeswaran V, Reisli I, Genel F, Gulez N, et al. Dedicator of cytokinesis 8 regulates signal transducer and activator of transcription 3 activation and promotes TH17 cell differentiation. *J Allergy Clin Immunol.* (2016) 138:1384–94 e2. doi: 10.1016/j.jaci.2016.04.023
79. Godfrey DI, Uldrich AP, McCluskey J, Rossjohn J, Moody DB. The burgeoning family of unconventional T cells. *Nat Immunol.* (2015) 16:1114–23. doi: 10.1038/ni.3298
80. Sallusto F, Lenig D, Forster R, Lipp M, Lanzavecchia A. Two subsets of memory T lymphocytes with distinct homing potentials and effector functions. *Nature.* (1999) 401:708–12. doi: 10.1038/44385
81. Sallusto F. Heterogeneity of human CD4(+) T cells against microbes. *Annu Rev Immunol.* (2016) 34:317–34. doi: 10.1146/annurev-immunol-032414-112056
82. Morita R, Schmitt N, Bentebibel SE, Ranganathan R, Bourdery L, Zurawski G, et al. Human blood CXCR5(+)CD4(+) T cells are counterparts of T follicular cells and contain specific subsets that differentially support antibody secretion. *Immunity.* (2011) 34:108–21. doi: 10.1016/j.immuni.2010.12.012
83. Cuss AK, Avery DT, Cannons JL, Yu LJ, Nichols KE, Shaw PJ, et al. Expansion of functionally immature transitional B cells is associated with human-immunodeficient states characterized by impaired humoral immunity. *J Immunol.* (2006) 176:1506–16. doi: 10.4049/jimmunol.176.3.1506
84. Suryani S, Fulcher DA, Santner-Nanan B, Nanan R, Wong M, Shaw PJ, et al. Differential expression of CD21 identifies developmentally and functionally distinct subsets of human transitional B cells. *Blood.* (2010) 115:519–29. doi: 10.1182/blood-2009-07-234799
85. Medina F, Segundo C, Campos-Caro A, Gonzalez-Garcia I, Brieva JA. The heterogeneity shown by human plasma cells from tonsil, blood, and bone marrow reveals graded stages of increasing maturity, but local profiles of adhesion molecule expression. *Blood.* (2002) 99:2154–61. doi: 10.1182/blood.V99.6.2154
86. Lau D, Lan LY, Andrews SF, Henry C, Rojas KT, Neu KE, et al. Low CD21 expression defines a population of recent germinal center graduates primed for plasma cell differentiation. *Sci Immunol.* (2017) 2:eaai8153. doi: 10.1126/sciimmunol.aai8153

87. Karnell JL, Kumar V, Wang J, Wang S, Voynova E, Ettinger R. Role of CD11c(+) T-bet(+) B cells in human health and disease. *Cell Immunol.* (2017) 321:40–5. doi: 10.1016/j.cellimm.2017.05.008
88. Portugal S, Obeng-Adjei N, Moir S, Crompton PD, Pierce SK. Atypical memory B cells in human chronic infectious diseases: an interim report. *Cell Immunol.* (2017) 321:18–25. doi: 10.1016/j.cellimm.2017.07.003
89. Kane A, Deenick EK, Ma CS, Cook MC, Uzel G, Tangye SG. STAT3 is a central regulator of lymphocyte differentiation and function. *Curr Opin Immunol.* (2014) 28C:49–57. doi: 10.1016/j.coi.2014.01.015
90. Holland SM, DeLeo FR, Elloumi HZ, Hsu AP, Uzel G, Brodsky N, et al. STAT3 mutations in the hyper-IgE syndrome. *N Engl J Med.* (2007) 357:1608–19. doi: 10.1056/NEJMoa073687
91. Minegishi Y, Saito M, Tsuchiya S, Tsuge I, Takada H, Hara T, et al. Dominant-negative mutations in the DNA-binding domain of STAT3 cause hyper-IgE syndrome. *Nature.* (2007) 448:1058–62. doi: 10.1038/nature 06096
92. Ma CS, Chew GY, Simpson N, Priyadarshi A, Wong M, Grimbacher B, et al. Deficiency of Th17 cells in hyper IgE syndrome due to mutations in STAT3. *J Exp Med.* (2008) 205:1551–7. doi: 10.1084/jem.20080218
93. Wilson RP, Ives ML, Rao G, Lau A, Payne K, Kobayashi M, et al. STAT3 is a critical cell-intrinsic regulator of human unconventional T cell numbers and function. *J Exp Med.* (2015) 212:855–64. doi: 10.1084/jem.201 41992
94. Ma CS, Deenick EK, Batten M, Tangye SG. The origins, function, and regulation of T follicular helper cells. *J Exp Med.* (2012) 209:1241–53. doi: 10.1084/jem.20120994
95. Tangye SG, Pelham SJ, Deenick EK, Ma CS. Cytokine-mediated regulation of human lymphocyte development and function: insights from primary immunodeficiencies. *J Immunol.* (2017) 199:1949–58. doi: 10.4049/jimmunol.1700842
96. Frey-Jakobs S, Hartberger JM, Fliegauf M, Bossen C, Wehmeyer ML, Neubauer JC, et al. ZNF341 controls STAT3 expression and thereby immunocompetence. *Sci Immunol.* (2018) 3:eaat4941. doi: 10.1126/sciimmunol.aat4941
97. Su HC, Jing H, Angelus P, Freeman AF. Insights into immunity from clinical and basic science studies of DOCK8 immunodeficiency syndrome. *Immunol Rev.* (2019) 287:9–19. doi: 10.1111/imr.12723
98. Jabara HH, McDonald DR, Janssen E, Massaad MJ, Ramesh N, Borzutzky A, et al. DOCK8 functions as an adaptor that links Toll-like receptor–MyD88 signaling to B cell activation. *Nat Immunol.* (2012) 13:612–20. doi: 10.1038/ni.2305
99. Tangye SG. XLP: clinical features and molecular etiology due to mutations in SH2D1A encoding SAP. *J Clin Immunol.* (2014) 34:772–9. doi: 10.1007/s10875-014-0083-7
100. Deenick EK, Chan A, Ma CS, Gatto D, Schwartzberg PL, Brink R, et al. Follicular helper T cell differentiation requires continuous antigen presentation that is independent of unique B cell signaling. *Immunity.* (2010) 33:241–53. doi: 10.1016/j.immuni.2010.07.015
101. He J, Tsai LM, Leong YA, Hu X, Ma CS, Chevalier N, et al. Circulating precursor CCR7(lo)PD-1(hi) CXCR5(+) CD4(+) T cells indicate Tfh cell activity and promote antibody responses upon antigen reexposure. *Immunity.* (2013) 39:770–81. doi: 10.1016/j.immuni.2013.09.007
102. Nichols KE, Hom J, Gong SY, Ganguly A, Ma CS, Cannons JL, et al. Regulation of NKT cell development by SAP, the protein defective in XLP. *Nat Med.* (2005) 11:340–5. doi: 10.1038/nm1189

18

Predominantly Antibody-Deficient Patients with Non-infectious Complications Have Reduced Naive B, Treg, Th17, and Tfh17 Cells

*Emily S. J. Edwards[1,2], Julian J. Bosco[2,3], Pei M. Aui[1,2], Robert G. Stirling[2,3], Paul U. Cameron[2,3], Josh Chatelier[2,3], Fiona Hore-Lacy[2,3], Robyn E. O'Hehir[1,2,3] and Menno C. van Zelm[1,2,3]**

[1] Department of Immunology and Pathology, Central Clinical School, Monash University and The Alfred Hospital, Melbourne, VIC, Australia, [2] The Jeffrey Modell Diagnostic and Research Centre for Primary Immunodeficiencies in Melbourne, Melbourne, VIC, Australia, [3] Allergy, Asthma and Clinical Immunology Service, Department of Respiratory, Allergy and Clinical Immunology (Research), Central Clinical School, The Alfred Hospital, Melbourne, VIC, Australia

Correspondence:
Menno C. van Zelm
menno.vanzelm@monash.edu

Background: Patients with predominantly antibody deficiency (PAD) suffer from severe and recurrent infections that require lifelong immunoglobulin replacement and prophylactic antibiotic treatment. Disease incidence is estimated to be 1:25,000 worldwide, and up to 68% of patients develop non-infectious complications (NIC) including autoimmunity, which are difficult to treat, causing high morbidity, and early mortality. Currently, the etiology of NIC is unknown, and there are no diagnostic and prognostic markers to identify patients at risk.

Objectives: To identify immune cell markers that associate with NIC in PAD patients.

Methods: We developed a standardized 11-color flow cytometry panel that was utilized for in-depth analysis of B and T cells in 62 adult PAD patients and 59 age-matched controls.

Results: Nine males had mutations in Bruton's tyrosine kinase (BTK) and were defined as having X-linked agammaglobulinemia. The remaining 53 patients were not genetically defined and were clinically diagnosed with agammaglobulinemia (n = 1), common variable immunodeficiency (CVID) (n = 32), hypogammaglobulinemia (n = 13), IgG subclass deficiency (n = 1), and specific polysaccharide antibody deficiency (n = 6). Of the 53, 30 (57%) had one or more NICs, 24 patients had reduced B-cell numbers, and 17 had reduced T-cell numbers. Both PAD–NIC and PAD+NIC groups had significantly reduced Ig class-switched memory B cells and naive CD4 and CD8 T-cell numbers. Naive and IgM memory B cells, Treg, Th17, and Tfh17 cells were specifically reduced in the PAD+NIC group. $CD21^{lo}$ B cells and Tfh cells were increased in frequencies, but not in absolute numbers in PAD+NIC.

Conclusion: The previously reported increased frequencies of $CD21^{lo}$ B cells and Tfh cells are the indirect result of reduced naive B-cell and T-cell numbers. Hence, correct interpretation of immunophenotyping of immunodeficiencies is critically dependent on absolute cell counts. Finally, the defects in naive B- and T-cell numbers suggest a mild combined immunodeficiency in PAD patients with NIC. Together with the reductions in Th17, Treg, and Tfh17 numbers, these key differences could be utilized as biomarkers to support definitive diagnosis and to predict for disease progression.

Keywords: predominantly antibody deficiency, common variable immunodeficiency, autoimmunity, X-linked agammaglobulinemia, follicular helper T cells, CD21^{lo} B cells, naive T cells, EuroFlow

INTRODUCTION

Predominantly antibody deficiency (PAD) represents the largest group of primary immunodeficiencies (PIDs) and includes up to 70% of all patients (1–5). The hallmark of PAD is a history of severe and recurrent sinopulmonary infections and poor vaccination responses underpinned by impaired B-cell differentiation and antibody production. As such, these patients require lifelong immunoglobulin replacement therapy (IgRT) and prophylactic antibiotics (3, 4).

The archetypical PAD is agammaglobulinemia (6), with patients lacking all serum Ig isotypes as well as circulating B cells. The majority of patients are boys suffering from X-linked agammaglobulinemia (XLA) as a result of mutations in the gene encoding Bruton's tyrosine kinase (*BTK*) (7, 8), an enzyme pivotal in the development of B cells. Autosomal recessive agammaglobulinemia is typically the result of mutations in other components of the pre-B-cell receptor complex or in B-cell transcription factors (9–15).

In a minority of PAD patients with circulating B cells, monogenic defects underpinning clinical phenotype, and pathophysiology have been identified. Most involve B-cell receptor signaling components or molecules required for T: B cell interactions (2, 5, 15–27). With the advancements in genomics, genetic diagnosis is now feasible for 20–30% of patients (28–30). However, for the remainder, diagnosis is typically made by ways of exclusion of clinical and general immunological characteristics (5).

Common variable immunodeficiency (CVID) is the most well-defined PAD (2, 5) and is defined diagnostically by reduced total serum IgG and IgA and/or IgM levels in the presence of impaired vaccination responses and recurrent bacterial infections (31–35). Less well-defined PADs include unclassified hypogammaglobulinemia (HGG), defined by reduced IgG levels but normal IgM and IgA levels; specific polysaccharide antibody deficiency (SpAD), defined by normal serum Ig isotypes but the absence of specific antibody responses to vaccination; and IgG subclass deficiency (IGSCD), defined by normal total IgG levels but reduced levels of one or more IgG subclasses (2, 5, 36).

In addition to recurrent infections and resulting complications, up to 68% of PAD patients suffer from non-infectious complications (NICs), which typically include autoimmunity, autoinflammation, gastrointestinal disease, and lymphoid malignancies (3, 37–43). NICs are most frequent in, but not exclusive to, CVID patients (36, 38, 44). The dominant presentation of NIC can overshadow infectious problems and thereby complicate diagnosis of PAD. Furthermore, NICs are often hard to treat, rendering patients at risk of early morbidity, and high mortality (38, 44, 45).

From the early 2000s, immunophenotyping of the B-cell compartment has been utilized to improve PAD diagnosis and has formed the basis of two classification systems: Freiburg (46) and EUROclass (47). In both strategies, CD19^{+} B cells are delineated using normally low Ig switched memory B-cell (smB) frequencies (CD19^{+}CD27^{+}IgM^{-}IgD^{-}) and abnormally high proportions of B cells with reduced CD21 expression (CD21^{lo} B cells) to distinguish subsets. In addition, to these two cell subsets, the EUROclass classification also uses abnormally high frequencies of transitional B cells (CD19^{+}CD27^{-}CD38^{+}) for further subgrouping. Subsequently, more detailed studies have been applied to define immunophenotypes for subgroups in patients with CVID or PAD (36, 48, 49). Despite the identification of clearly distinct phenotypes, these have thus far provided limited prognostic value to predict clinical progression or disease complications. The strongest association found to date is the expansion of CD21^{lo} B cells in patients with splenomegaly (47, 50). In addition, marked reductions in total, Ig switched memory, and marginal zone B cells were found to be associated with splenomegaly (47). Furthermore, the presence of any form of autoimmune disease in CVID patients was associated with expansion of CD21^{lo} B cells (46) and significant reductions in plasmablasts (47) and Ig smBs (37). A proportional expansion of transitional B cells was found to be associated with lymphadenopathy, whereas CVID patients with granulomatous disease presented with significant reductions in Ig class-switched memory and marginal zone B cells (47).

Although PAD is by definition a disease resulting from defective antibody production, multiple studies have demonstrated that disturbances in T and natural killer (NK) cell homeostasis likely contribute to the disease etiology and pathophysiology. Specifically, decreased circulating NK-cell numbers in CVID and XLA patients were found to be associated with severe bacterial infections and granulomas (51, 52). Pronounced CD4 T-cell lymphopenia occurs in some CVID patients (44, 53), and reductions in naive CD4 T cells were associated with splenomegaly (53), autoimmunity, and polyclonal lymphoproliferation. Reductions in naive CD8 T-cell numbers have also been associated with autoimmunity in CVID patients (54). In addition, follicular T helper cells

Abbreviations: CT, cortisone; CVID, common variable immunodeficiency; HGG, hypogammaglobulinemia; IGSCD, IgG subclass deficiency; IgRT, immunoglobulin replacement therapy; MS, multiple sclerosis; PBS, phosphate-buffered saline; RA, rheumatoid arthritis; SLE, systemic lupus erythematosus; SpAD, specific polysaccharide antibody deficiency; XLA, X-linked agammaglobulinemia.

(Tfh), regulatory T cells (Treg), and Th17 cell disturbances have been identified in PAD patients. In particular, XLA patients who lack B-cell follicles have reduced numbers of circulating Tfh cells (54), whereas in CVID patients with autoimmunity and/or splenomegaly, increased proportions of circulating Tfh have been observed (37, 55–57). Furthermore, reduced absolute numbers (54) and frequencies of Treg (58, 59) have been described in CVID patients with autoimmunity and/or splenomegaly, and these reductions are associated with the expansion of $CD21^{lo}$ B cells (59). Th17 cells were also decreased in number and frequency in CVID, paralleled by expansions of $CD21^{lo}$ B cells and activated CD4 T cells with no link to clinical manifestations (60). Finally, interleukin (IL)-2 and interferon gamma (IFN-γ) production by CD4 T cells was higher in patients with hepatomegaly, and chemokine receptor CCR5 known to be expressed on Th1 cells was shown to be higher on CD4 T cells in patients with granulomas (61), implying Th1 bias in these patients.

The many published abnormalities in circulating B and T cells, with several potentially correlating with specific clinical phenotypes, stress the need for high-quality and reproducible immunophenotyping of circulating lymphocytes in PAD patients. The EuroFlow consortium has developed standards for instrument setup and sample preparation (62) and multicolor panels to examine PAD patients (63, 64). We here utilized this expertise to develop a compact 11-color flow cytometry panel that was applied to our cohort of 62 adult PAD patients to identify abnormalities in the B- and T-cell compartments, specifically aiming to discriminate between patients with and without NICs.

MATERIALS AND METHODS

Patients

From November 2015 to June 2019, 62 adult patients with a clinical diagnosis of PAD were enrolled in a low-risk research study to examine their blood leukocyte subsets (projects Alfred Health 109/15 and Monash University CF15/771-2015-0344). All patients consented to the collection of their medical information and a donation of 40 ml of blood. In parallel, 59 adult healthy controls were enrolled in a low-risk reference value study (Monash University project 2016-0289) and consented to collection of basic demographics (age, sex, and history of immunological and hematological diseases) and donation of 40 ml of blood. The study was conducted according to the principles of the Declaration of Helsinki and was approved by local human research ethics committees.

Assessment of Absolute Numbers of Leukocyte and Lymphocyte Subsets

Absolute numbers of leukocytes were determined using a lyse-no-wash method within 24 h of blood sampling in Vacutainers containing EDTA (BD Biosciences). Fifty microliters of whole blood was added to a TruCount tube (BD Biosciences) together with an antibody cocktail of 20 µl to stain CD3, CD4, CD8, CD16, CD45, and CD56 (**Supplementary Figure 1** and **Supplementary Tables 1, 2, 5**). Following incubation for 15 min at room temperature, 500 µl of 0.155 M NH_4Cl was added to lyse red blood cells for 15 min. Subsequently, the mixture was stored in the dark at 4°C prior to acquisition on a flow cytometer within 2 h.

Design of Three Multicolor Tubes for Staining B- and T-Cell Subsets

The design of the tubes was based on the EuroFlow PID antibody panels (64), which had undergone stringent testing and optimization in a multi-laboratory setting. In contrast to the EuroFlow PID initiative, we undertook a research study of adult patients with the intent to examine all cell subsets in all enrolled individuals. Hence, the PID orientation tube (PIDOT) (63, 65) was not included, as the data obtained would be redundant with subsequent lineage-specific analysis. In addition, we had access to 11 fluorescent parameters. This enabled us to merge the EuroFlow pre-GC and post-GC tubes, which share six of the eight markers into one B-cell tube with 12 markers in 10 fluorescent channels (**Supplementary Figure 2** and **Supplementary Tables 1–3**). For eight of the 12 markers, the same reagents were used as in the eight-color EuroFlow panel (64). The same antibody clones were used for CD5, CD21, and CD38, with a different fluorescent label; and for CD19, different clone (SJ25C1) and fluorochrome were used.

Similarly, the EuroFlow SCID/RTE and T-cell tubes were combined into one 11-parameter T-effector tube. Of the 11 markers, seven were identical to those of the EuroFlow protocol (64). For CD3 and HLA-DR, the same clones were used on different fluorochromes, and for CCR7 (CD197), a different clone (G043H7) and another fluorochrome were used. CD45RA was newly inserted in this tube, as this is present in the EuroFlow PIDOT, whereas CD62L was not included owing to redundancy with the CCR7 marker (**Supplementary Figure 3** and **Supplementary Tables 1–3**).

Finally, an 11-color Th-subset tube was designed based on our previous work (66) with the objective to use membrane markers to distinguish Treg (67, 68), helper T-cell subsets (Th) (69, 70), and Tfh (71, 72), and their subsets (73) (**Supplementary Figure 4** and **Supplementary Tables 1–3**). This resulted in a panel of three tubes (B cell, T effector, and T helper) in addition to the TruCount analysis (**Supplementary Table 1**), and these were run for all patients and controls enrolled in the study.

Sample Preparation for B-Cell and T-Cell Subset Tubes

To gain detailed insight into the composition of the lymphocyte compartment, including robust identification of small cell populations such as plasma cell subsets, standard operating procedures (SOPs) from the EuroFlow consortium were adopted for acquisition of high cell numbers (1–5 × 10^6 total nucleated cells) (74–76). The bulk-lysis-stain technique was performed (62, 74). Briefly, samples (up to 2 ml) were diluted in a total volume of 50 ml of an NH_4Cl hypotonic solution, gently mixed, and incubated for 15 min at room temperature on a roller. Then, nucleated cells were centrifuged and washed twice in phosphate-buffered saline (PBS) containing 0.5% bovine

TABLE 1 | Demographics, clinical details, and diagnostic results of the patients in this study.

	Healthy controls ($n = 59$)	All patients ($n = 62$)	PAD–NIC ($n = 23$)	PAD+NIC ($n = 30$)	XLA ($n = 9$)
DEMOGRAPHICS					
Median age (years; range)					
At inclusion	30 (20–71)	43 (18–82)	46 (19–73)	44 (23–82)	24 (18–59)
At diagnosis	N/A	35 (2 months to 74 years)	45 (18–73)	36 (12–74)	9 (2 months to 13 years)
Female sex (%)	33 (58%)	34 (55%)	14 (61%)	20 (67%)	0
Clinical diagnosis					
Agammaglobulinemia (%)	0	10 (16%)	1 (4%)	0	9 (100%)
CVID (%)	0	32 (52%)	9 (39%)	23 (77%)	0
HGG (%)	0	13 (21%)	7 (30%)	6 (20%)	0
IGSCD (%)	0	1 (2%)	1 (4%)	0	0
SpAD (%)	0	6 (9%)	5 (22%)	1 (3%)	0
IMMUNOLOGICAL PRESENTATION					
Decreased serum immunoglobulin levels					
IgG (%)	N/A	40/54 (74%)	14/23 (61%)	26/30 (87%)	0/1#
IgA (%)	N/A	46/61 (75%)	15/23 (65%)	24/30 (80%)	8/8 (100%)
IgM (%)	N/A	34/61 (56%)	11/23 (48%)	15/30 (50%)	8/8 (100%)
Impaired vaccination responses (%)	N/A	25/30 (83%)	12/16 (75%)	12/14 (86%)	N/A#
Reduced cell numbers					
B cells (%)	N/A	24 (39%)	3 (13%)	12 (40%)	9 (100%)
T cells (%)	N/A	17 (27%)	5 (22%)	11 (37%)	2 (22%)
TREATMENT					
IgRT at sampling (%)	N/A	46 (74%)	11 (48%)	25 (83%)	9 (100%)
IgRT started after inclusion (%)	N/A	12 (19%)	7 (30%)	5 (17%)	N/A
Immunomodulators* (%)	N/A	8 (13%)	3 (13%)	4 (13%)	1 (11%)

Reference ranges: IgG, 6.1–16.2 g/L; IgA, 0.85–4.99 g/L; IgM, 0.35–2.42 g/L; B cells, 97–614 cells/μl; T cells, 830–2,430 cells/μl.
(B- and T-cell reference ranges were derived from the 5th and 95th percentiles of our healthy controls).
#Serum IgG levels and vaccination responses not assessed owing to historic nature of disease.
**On immunomodulators within 6 months prior to blood sampling.*
PAD, predominantly antibody deficiency; NIC, non-infectious complications; XLA, X-linked agammaglobulinemia; CVID, common variable immunodeficiency; HGG, hypogammaglobulinemia; IGSCD, IgG subclass deficiency; SpAD, specific polysaccharide antibody deficiency; IgRT, immunoglobulin replacement therapy; IGSCD, IgG subclass deficiency. A subset of patients has been reported in a recent publication (77).

serum albumin (BSA). Subsequently, the surface membrane markers on nucleated cells were stained with the corresponding antibody mixtures.

Flow Cytometer Setup

All flow cytometry was performed across three instruments in our flow core facility that contained either four lasers (BD LSRII and BD LSRFortessa) or five lasers (BD LSRFortessa X-20) with a nearly identical setup for the shared four lasers (**Supplementary Table 4**). Instrument setup and calibration were performed using EuroFlow SOPs as previously described in detail (**Supplementary Table 5**) (62), with in-house optimization for the additional three fluorescent channels (V610, V710, and YG610).

Data Analysis and Statistics

All data were analyzed with FACS DIVA v8.0.1 (BD Biosciences) and FlowJo v10 software packages (FlowJo, LLC). Reference ranges were defined as being within the 5th and 95th percentiles of absolute cell numbers from our 59 adult controls. Statistical analysis for multiple-group comparison was performed with the non-parametric Kruskal-Wallis test. If significant, pairwise comparisons were made with the non-parametric Mann-Whitney *U* test. Statistical analysis of sampling distributions was assessed with the chi-square test. For all tests, $p < 0.05$ was considered significant.

RESULTS

Clinical and Immunological Features of Predominantly Antibody Deficiency Patients

Sixty-two PAD patients were recruited in a prospective research study from a teaching hospital in Melbourne, Australia. Median age of the patients was 43 years (range, 18–82 years), and 34 were female (**Table 1**). CVID was the most common clinical diagnosis in 52% of all patients, followed by 21% with HGG, 16% with agammaglobulinemia, 9% with SpAD, and 2% with IGSCD. Of the 10 patients diagnosed with agammaglobulinemia,

TABLE 2 | Complications in patients with predominantly antibody deficiency.

	All patients ($n = 62$)	PAD–NIC ($n = 23$)	PAD+NIC ($n = 30$)	XLA ($n = 9$)
INFECTIOUS COMPLICATIONS				
URTI (%)	49 (79%)	17 (74%)	24 (80%)	8 (89%)
Sinusitis (%)	48 (77%)	16 (70%)	24 (80%)	8 (89%)
Otitis (%)	20 (32%)	7 (30%)	7 (23%)	6 (67%)
LRTI (%)	49 (79%)	17 (74%)	25 (83%)	8 (89%)
Bronchitis (%)	8 (13%)	4 (17%)	4 (13%)	0
Pneumonia (%)	38 (61%)	12 (52%)	20 (67%)	7 (78%)
Bronchiectasis (%)	17 (27%)	4 (17%)	8 (27%)	5 (56%)
Gastrointestinal (%)	4 (6%)	0	4 (13%)	0
Giardia (%)	4 (6%)	0	4 (13%)	0
Other sites*	8 (13%)	1 (4%)	6 (20%)	1 (11%)
NON-INFECTIOUS COMPLICATIONS				
GLILD (%)	1 (2%)	0	1 (3%)	0
Autoimmunity (total) (%)	18 (29%)	0	18 (60%)	0
Musculoskeletal (%)	5 (8%)	0	5 (17%)	0
Cytopenia (%)	6 (10%)	0	6 (20%)	0
Endocrine (%)	3 (5%)	0	3 (10%)	0
Splenomegaly (%)	4 (6%)	0	4 (13%)	0
Lymphadenopathy (%)	1 (2%)	0	1 (3%)	0
Gastrointestinal disease total) (%)	11 (18%)	0	11 (37%)	0
Enteropathy (%)	10 (16%)	0	10 (33%)	0
Colitis (%)	2 (3%)	0	2 (7%)	0
Granulomatous disease (%)	3 (5%)	0	3 (10%)	0
Malignancy (%)	2 (3%)	0	2 (7%)	0
Solid Organ (%)	2 (3%)	0	2 (7%)	0
Hematological (%)	0	0	0	0#

PAD, predominantly antibody deficiency; PAD–NIC, PAD without non-infectious complications; PAD+NIC, PAD with non-infectious complications; XLA, X-linked agammaglobulinemia; GLILD, granulomatous-lymphocytic interstitial lung disease.
**Other includes osteomyelitis, pertussis, prostatitis, and systemic viral infection.*
#One XLA patient developed an acute precursor-B-cell leukemia 6 months after inclusion in this study (78).

nine were male and genetically confirmed to have XLA (**Table 1** and **Supplementary Tables 6, 7**). The other 53 patients did not undergo any genetic testing.

All patients presented with infectious manifestations (**Table 2** and **Supplementary Table 6**), and these were generally confined to the respiratory tract: sinusitis (77%), pneumonia (61%), and otitis (32%) with frequent complications of bronchiectasis (27%). Infections of the gastrointestinal tract and other sites, such as the prostate and bone, were less frequently involved (19%). Of all 62 patients, 30 (48%) presented with at least one NIC, with autoimmunity being the most frequent (29%), followed by gastrointestinal (18%), and granulomatous diseases (5%; **Table 2**). At the time of inclusion in the study, 46 (74%) patients were treated with IgRT. A further 12 (19%) newly diagnosed patients commenced IgRT directly after inclusion. Eight patients (13%) had been prescribed immunomodulators within 6 months prior to inclusion (**Table 1**). Three patients were treated with immunomodulators for asthma or for IgRT tolerability, which were deemed unrelated to their PAD, and thus, these patients were defined as PAD–NIC.

Serum IgG levels prior to commencement of IgRT were obtained from medical records of 47 patients (**Table 1**), and in 40/47 (85%), these were below the normal range. Serum IgA and IgM concentrations were available for 61 patients, and of these, 46 (75%) had reduced IgA and 34 (56%) had reduced IgM. The results of vaccination responses in most cases to polysaccharide pneumococcal vaccine were documented for 30 patients and impaired in 25 (83%). B- and T-cell numbers were below the normal range (<5th percentile of our healthy control cohort) for 39 and 27% of all patients, respectively. A total of 11% of patients had a reduction of both B- and T-cell numbers (**Table 1**). B-cell numbers were below the normal range for all nine XLA patients, with two patients (22%) also having reduced T-cell numbers.

For further immunological analysis, the PAD patient cohort was divided into three groups: 9 patients with genetically diagnosed XLA, 23 PAD patients without NICs (PAD–NIC), and 30 with NICs (PAD+NIC). The nine XLA patients presented with infectious complications only, and these included respiratory infections (89%). Five XLA patients (56%) had evidence of bronchiectasis; this incidence was 2-fold higher than in other PAD groups (17% in PAD–NIC; 27% in PAD+NIC). Of the 32 CVID patients, 23 (72%) presented with one or more NICs (**Table 2**), whereas only a minority of patients diagnosed with HGG or SpAD presented with NIC. By definition, PAD+NIC patients displayed a more severe and complex clinical phenotype (**Table 2**) and were diagnosed at a younger age than were PAD–NIC patients (median age at diagnosis: 3 vs. 45 years).

All classifications of patients were undertaken alongside those of 59 healthy controls (median age 30 years and 55% females). The healthy controls and the non-XLA PAD patients were classified according to the Freiburg and EUROclass definitions (47, 79) on the basis of their B-cell phenotypes (**Table 3**). According to the Freiburg classification, 95% of controls had normal frequencies of smBs and no increases in $CD21^{lo}$ B cells (group II), with the remaining 5% having low smB (Ib). The majority of all PAD patients (29; 55%) had reduced smB frequencies (Ia/Ib; $p < 0.0001$ vs. controls). Seven PAD patients had increased frequencies of $CD21^{lo}$ B cells (Ia), and the majority of these patients ($n = 5$) were in the PAD+NIC group. According to the EUROclass scheme, all controls had normal smB and $CD21^{lo}$ B-cell frequencies (**Table 3**). Of all PAD patients, 12 (22%) had reduced smB frequencies and 13 (25%) had increased $CD21^{lo}$ B-cell frequencies. Slightly more PAD+NIC patients had reduced smB and increased $CD21^{lo}$ B cells than had PAD–NIC, but these differences were not significant ($CD21^{lo}$ expansion, $p = 0.06$).

Overall, our patient cohort is diverse in clinical and immunological presentations, in line with previously reported cohorts of adult PAD (38, 44). Importantly, PAD–NIC and PAD+NIC groups are seemingly different in their immunological profiles. With almost equally large PAD–NIC and PAD+NIC groups and a substantial group of genetically diagnosed XLA patients, this cohort is well-suited to examine immunological differences that associate with the presence of NICs.

TABLE 3 | Classification of PAD patients according to the Freiburg and EUROclass definitions.

	Healthy controls ($n = 59$)	All PAD[a] ($n = 53$)	PAD–NIC ($n = 23$)	PAD+NIC ($n = 30$)
FREIBURG				
Ia (smB−21lo)	0	7 (13%)	2 (9%)	5 (16%)
Ib (smB−21norm)	3 (5%)	22 (42%)	8 (36%)	14 (47%)
II (smB+21lo or norm)	56 (95%)	24 (45%)	13 (55%)	11 (37%)
EUROCLASS				
B−	0	3 (6%)	2 (9%)	1 (3%)
B+smB−21normTrnorm	0	5 (9%)	3 (13%)	2 (7%)
B+smB−21normTrhi	0	1 (2%)	0	1 (3%)
B+smB−21loTrnorm	0	5 (9%)	0	5 (17%)
B+smB−21loTrhi	0	1 (2%)	0	1 (3%)
B+smB+21norm	59 (100%)	31 (58%)	15 (65%)	16 (53%)
B+smB+21lo	0	7 (14%)	3 (13%)	4 (14%)

PAD, predominantly antibody deficiency; NIC, non-infectious complications; smBs, switched memory B cells, 21, CD21; Tr, transitional B cells.

Freiburg classification undertaken on patients with ≥1% B cells in lymphocyte gate; definitions (79): smB−, <0.4% $CD28^{+}IgD^{-}$ B cells within lymphocytes; 21lo, ≥20% B cells are $CD21^{lo}$.

EUROclass definitions (47): B−, <1% of lymphocytes; smB−, <2% of B cells; 21^{lo}, ≥10% B cells are $CD21^{lo}$; Trhi, >9% of B cells are transitional ($CD38^{hi}CD27^{-}$).

[a]Excluding patients with a clinical diagnosis of X-linked agammaglobulinemia (XLA), as these were all B cell negative.

Reduced Numbers of Lymphocytes in Predominantly Antibody Deficiency Patients

As a large fraction of the non-XLA PAD patients had B- and/or T-cell numbers below the normal range of controls (**Table 1**), we first examined the numbers of leukocyte and lymphocyte subsets in our patient groups (**Supplementary Figures 1, 5** and **Supplementary Table 3**). Circulating numbers of granulocytes and monocytes in both PAD–NIC and PAD+NIC were similar to those of controls, whereas these were significantly increased in XLA patients (**Supplementary Figures 5A,B**). In contrast, total lymphocytes, and NK cells were significantly reduced in both PAD groups as compared with controls, whereas these were normal in the XLA group (**Supplementary Figures 5C,D**).

Reduced Total, Naive, and IgM Memory B Cells in Predominantly Antibody Deficiency Patients With Non-infectious Complications

Further detailed analysis of the B-cell compartment was restricted to the 59 controls and the 53 non-XLA PAD patients, as B cells were completely absent in the XLA patients (**Figure 1A**). Numbers of circulating B cells were significantly reduced in the PAD+NIC, but not in the PAD–NIC group (**Figure 1B**). Within the peripheral B-cell compartment, frequencies of IgM memory, Ig switched memory, and plasmablasts were significantly lower in both PAD–NIC and PAD+NIC compared with controls (**Figure 1C**). Frequencies of naive B cells were increased in both patient groups. However, when expressed as absolute numbers, these were actually normal in PAD–NIC and significantly reduced in PAD+NIC (**Figures 1C,D** and **Supplementary Figure 6A**). IgG and IgA smBs remained reduced in terms of absolute numbers in both PAD groups. In contrast, absolute numbers of IgM memory B cells were normal in PAD–NIC whereas reduced in PAD+NIC (**Figures 1C,D** and **Supplementary Figures 6A,B**). Finally, $CD21^{lo}$ B-cell frequencies were increased in the PAD+NIC group, but the absolute numbers of circulating $CD21^{lo}$ B cells were normal (**Figure 1C**).

Taken together, both PAD–NIC and PAD+NIC have severely reduced numbers of Ig smBs. In addition, as a group, PAD+NIC patients have reduced numbers of circulating total, naive, and IgM memory B cells.

Reduced Naive CD4 and CD8 T Cells in Predominantly Antibody Deficiency Patients

In addition to the lymphocyte, NK-cell, and B-cell abnormalities, the PAD–NIC and PAD+NIC groups had significantly lower numbers of circulating T cells than had controls. These concerned all three major lineages: TCRγδ T cells in PAD–NIC and both CD4 and CD8 T cells in both PAD groups. In contrast, only two XLA patients had reduced total T-cell numbers (**Figure 2A**).

To examine the nature of the T-cell abnormalities, we delineated the CD4 and CD8 lineages into $CCR7^{+}CD45RO^{-}$ naive (Tn), $CCR7^{+}CD45RO^{+}$ central memory (Tcm), $CCR7^{-}CD45RO^{+}$ effector memory (TemRO), and $CCR7^{-}CD45RO^{-}$ effector memory (TemRA) T cells (**Supplementary Figure 3** and **Supplementary Table 3**). Frequencies and absolute numbers of naive CD4 and CD8 T cells were reduced in both PAD–NIC and PAD+NIC, but not in XLA patients (**Figures 2B,C**). To examine the association between naive CD4 and naive CD8 T-cell counts, we performed correlation analysis of these in both the healthy control and the patient cohorts. This revealed a reasonable positive correlation for controls ($r = 0.32$; $p < 0.05$) and strong correlation for total group of 53 non-XLA PAD patients ($r = 0.63$; $p < 0.0001$; **Figure 3A**). As PAD+NIC patients also had reduced naive B cells, we examined their association with naive CD4 and CD8 T cells. No correlations were found in the control group, but naive B-cell numbers were positively correlated with naive CD4 T cells ($r = 0.53$; $p < 0.0001$) and naive CD8 cells ($r = 0.48$; $p < 0.0001$; **Figures 3B,C**).

PAD+NIC had increased frequencies of CD4 Tcm and TemRO, but as a result of the reduced total CD4 T cells, these were normal in terms of numbers (**Figure 2B**). Early-, intermediate-, and late-differentiated TemRO and TemRA cells were distinguished by the progressive loss of CD27 and/or CD28 (80) (**Supplementary Figure 3**). Within the CD4 TemRO compartment, numbers of early-differentiated cells were increased in PAD–NIC and XLA whereas reduced in PAD+NIC. Intermediate-TemRO cell numbers were reduced in PAD–NIC, and late-TemRO numbers were increased in XLA (**Supplementary Figure 7A**). Intermediate-TemRA

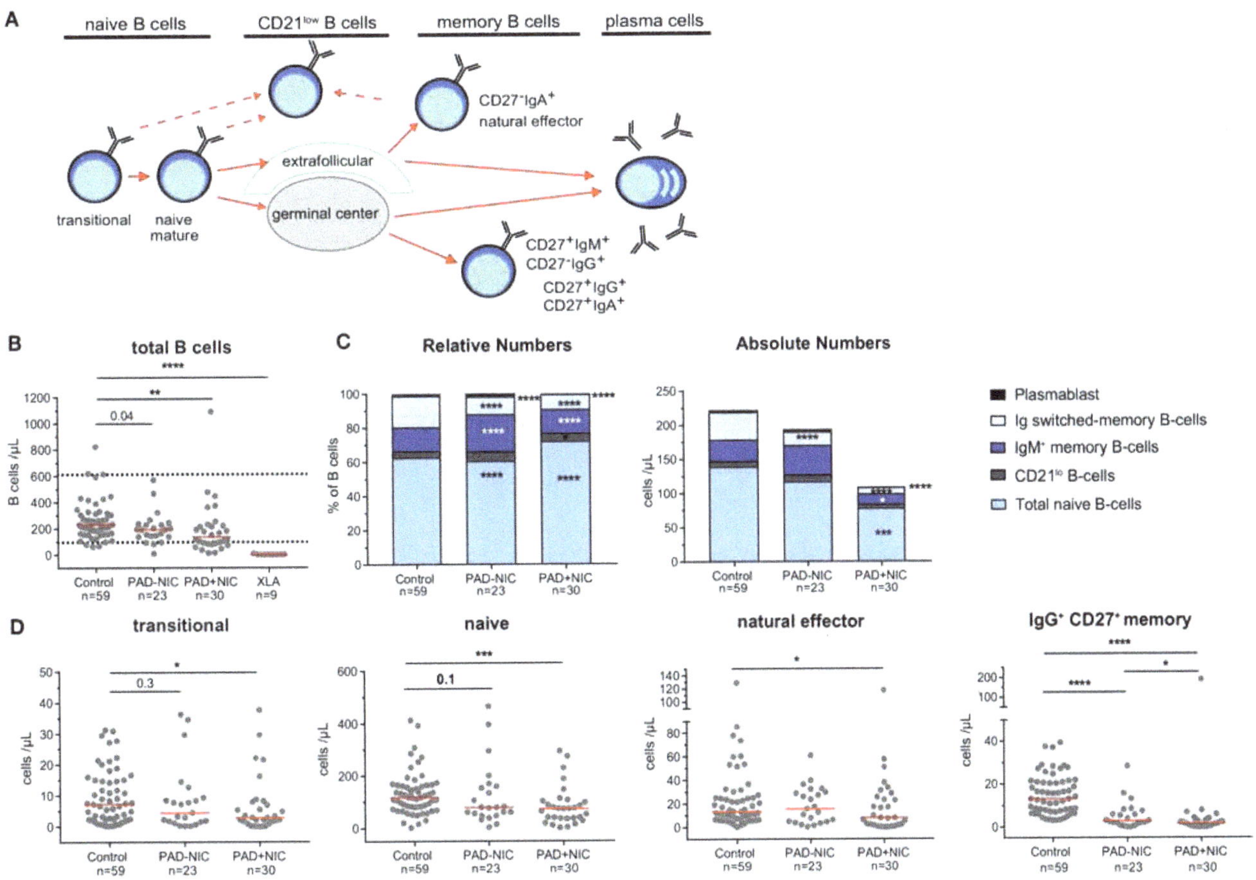

FIGURE 1 | B-cell abnormalities in PAD patients. **(A)** Schematic overview of naive and memory B-cell subsets. **(B)** Absolute numbers of total B cells. Horizontal dotted lines represent the 5th and 95th percentiles of the healthy control group and were used as reference ranges. **(C)** Relative numbers and absolute numbers of B-cell subsets. **(D)** Absolute numbers of transitional, naive, natural effector, and IgG$^+$ CD27$^+$ memory B cells. For gating strategy and population definitions, see **Supplementary Figure 2** and **Supplementary Table 3**. PAD, predominantly antibody deficiency; NIC, noninfectious complications. Statistics were performed with the Kruskal–Wallis test, followed by Mann–Whitney tests for pairwise comparisons. $^*p < 0.5$, $^{**}p < 0.01$, $^{***}p < 0.001$, and $^{****}p < 0.0001$.

numbers were reduced in PAD+NIC, but proportions were unchanged (**Supplementary Figure 7B**). CD8 TemRO numbers were not different between patients and controls (**Supplementary Figure 7C**), whereas CD8 TemRA early and intermediate cell subsets were significantly reduced in all three patient groups (**Supplementary Figure 7D**).

Overall, both PAD–NIC and PAD+NIC patients exhibit a marked reduction in circulating T cells, mainly as a result of reductions in the naive CD4 and CD8 T-cell subsets.

Altered Treg and Th Cell Composition in Predominantly Antibody Deficiency Patients With Non-infectious Complications

To analyze whether Th numbers were altered in PAD patients with and without NIC, we delineated Treg, Th, Tfh, and their subsets (**Supplementary Table 3** and **Supplementary Figure 4**). Total Treg numbers and their respective naive and memory subsets were significantly lower in PAD+NIC than in controls, whereas these were not changed in PAD–NIC and XLA patients (**Figure 4A**). The subset of follicular regulatory T(fr) cells was also specifically decreased in PAD+NIC patients (**Figure 4A**). Within the Th cells, four subsets were defined (i.e., Th1, Th2, Th17, and Th17.1), which are each associated with responses to distinct types of pathogens. No alterations were observed for Th1 (bacterial and viral pathogens) or Th2 cells (extracellular pathogens; data not shown). In contrast, Th17-cell numbers (bacterial and fungal pathogens) were specifically reduced only in PAD+NIC as compared with controls ($p = 0.005$). Finally, numbers of Th17.1 cells (IL-17 and IFN-γ double producers) were reduced in both PAD–NIC and PAD+NIC, but not in XLA patients (**Figure 4B**).

Finally, we enumerated Tfh numbers, as these are critical for providing help to B cells in germinal center responses. Absolute numbers of Tfh cells were not different between controls, PAD–NIC, and PAD+NIC, whereas these were significantly reduced in XLA patients ($p \leq 0.0001$). Within the total Tfh population, a similar distinction of four subsets was made as for the Th

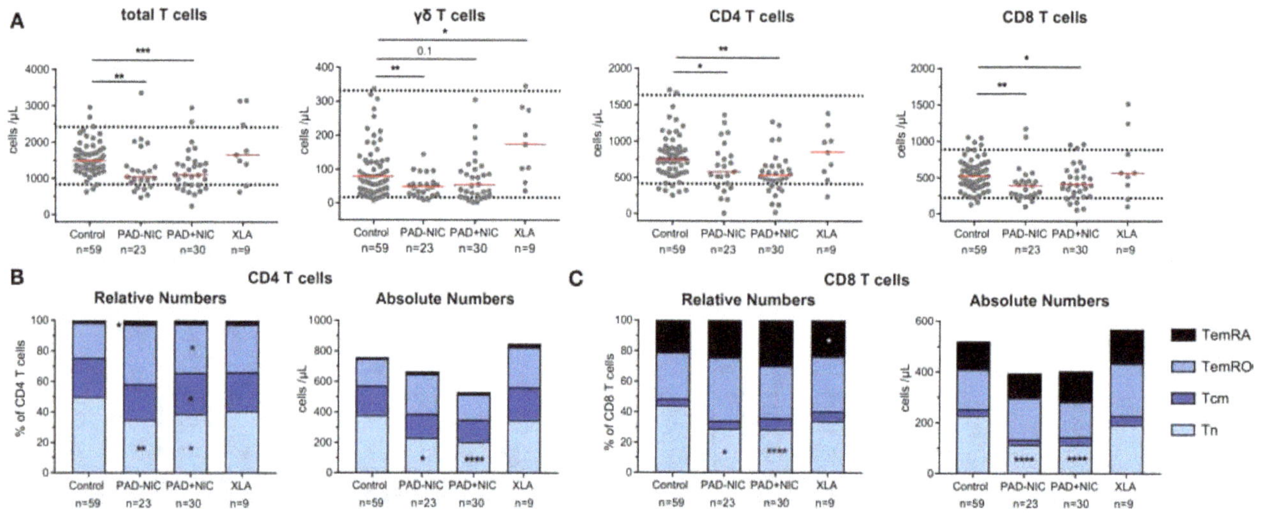

FIGURE 2 | Reduced naive T-cell numbers in PAD patients. **(A)** Absolute numbers of total T cells, γδ T cells, CD4 T cells, and CD8 T cells. Horizontal dotted lines represent the 5th and 95th percentiles as calculated in healthy controls. Relative and absolute numbers of **(B)** CD4 T-cell subsets and **(C)** CD8 T-cell subsets. Naive (Tn; $CCR7^{+}CD45RO^{-}$), central memory (Tcm; $CCR7^{+}CD45RO^{+}$), effector memory (TemRO; $CCR7^{-}CD45RO^{-}$), and effector memory CD45RA revertant (TemRA; $CCR7^{-}CD45RO^{-}$). For gating strategy and population definitions, see **Supplementary Figure 3** and **Supplementary Table 3**. PAD, predominantly antibody deficiency; NIC, non-infectious complications. Statistics were performed with the Kruskal–Wallis test, followed by Mann–Whitney tests for pairwise comparisons. $^{*}p < 0.5$, $^{**}p < 0.01$, $^{***}p < 0.001$, and $^{****}p < 0.0001$.

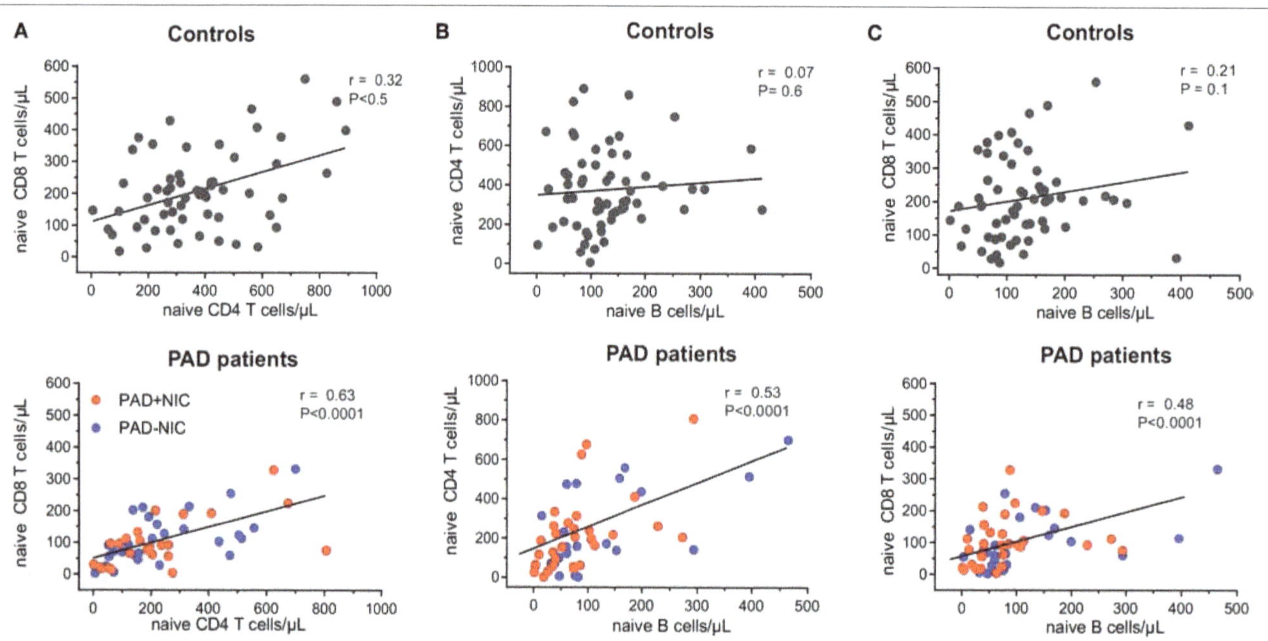

FIGURE 3 | Correlation between naive B- and T-cell numbers in healthy controls and PAD patients. Correlation between absolute numbers of **(A)** naive CD4 and naive CD8 T cells, **(B)** naive B and naive CD4 T cells, and **(C)** naive B and naive CD8 T cells were assessed in healthy controls and PAD patients. Trend lines depict linear correlations for controls (top row; $n = 59$) and total group of non-XLA PAD patients (bottom row = 53). PAD, predominantly antibody deficiency; NIC, non-infectious complications; XLA, X-linked agammaglobulinemia. Statistics were performed using Spearman's rank correlation.

subsets: Tfh1, Tfh2, Tfh17.1, and Tfh17 (73). Of these, only Tfh17 was significantly reduced in the PAD+NIC and XLA groups as compared with controls (**Figure 4C**).

Taken together, the CD4 T-cell compartment was most severely affected in PAD+NIC patients with significantly reduced Treg, Th17, Th17.1, and Tfh17 numbers.

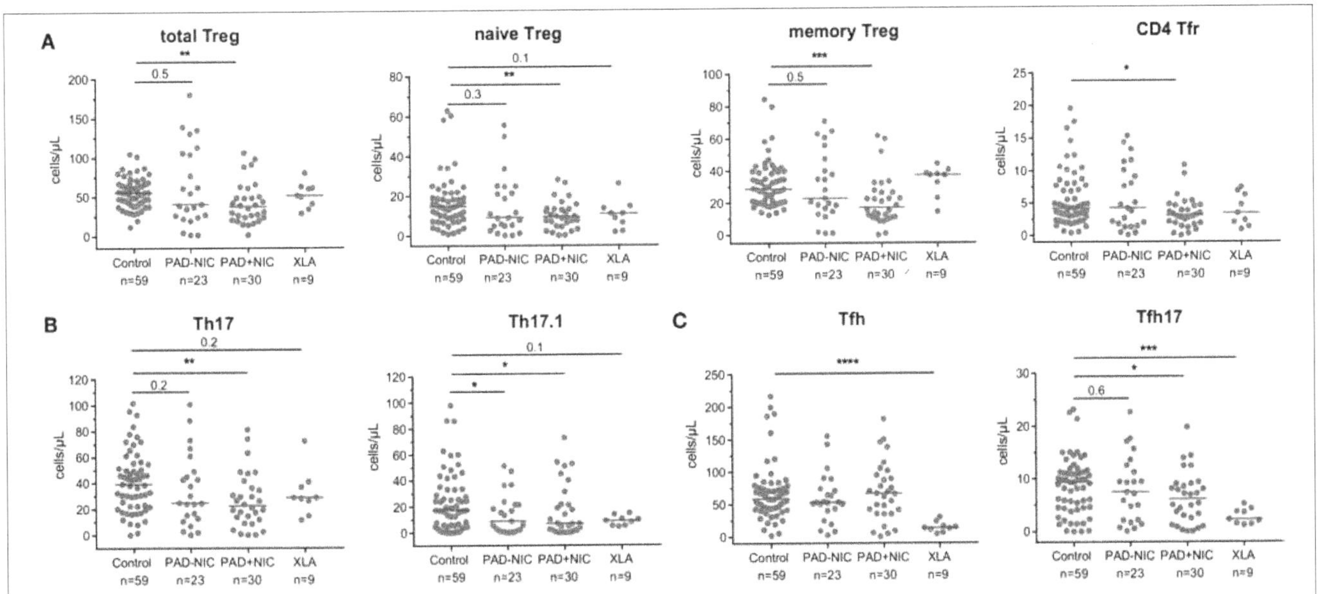

FIGURE 4 | Reduced Treg and helper T-cell numbers in PAD patients with non-infectious complications. **(A)** Total Treg, naive Treg, memory Treg, and CD4 Tfr cells. **(B)** Th17 and Th17.1 cells. **(C)** Total Tfh and Tfh17 cells. All numbers represent cells per microliter of blood. For gating strategy and population definitions, see **Supplementary Figure 4** and **Supplementary Table 3**. PAD, predominantly antibody deficiency; NIC, non-infectious complications. Statistics were performed with the Kruskal–Wallis test, followed by Mann–Whitney tests for pairwise comparisons. $^{*}p < 0.5$, $^{**}p < 0.01$, $^{***}p < 0.001$, and $^{****}p < 0.0001$.

Misinterpretation of Relative Numbers in the Context of Reduced Absolute Cell Numbers

Similar to previous reports, we observed in our cohort that PAD+NIC patients had a significantly increased proportion of CD21^{lo} B cells (**Figures 1B, 5**). However, when expressed as absolute numbers of cells per microliter blood, CD21^{lo} B cells were normal in our cohort (**Figure 5B**). In fact, the increased proportion of CD21^{lo} B cells was the result of a reduction in total B-cell numbers in the PAD+NIC group. Thus, the increased proportion of CD21^{lo} B cells did not reflect an increase in this subset but rather a decrease of other, mainly naive B cells. In parallel, we confirmed previous reports (37, 55, 56, 81) of increased proportions of Tfh in the PAD+NIC group (**Figure 5**). However, absolute numbers of Tfh were normal in the context of reduced total CD4 T cells (**Figures 5C,D**). Thus, the relative expansion does not reflect an abnormality in Tfh but rather is the result of abnormally low total T cells, mainly due to the reduction in the naive subset.

DISCUSSION

Here we present the results of a standardized approach for extensive immunophenotyping of the B- and T-cell compartments in patients with PAD. Irrespective of the presence of NIC, PAD patients show reduced Ig smBs, Th17.1 cells, and naive CD4 and CD8 T cells. In addition, the group of patients with NICs has severe reductions in total B-cell, Th17, Treg, and Tfh17 numbers. Finally, expansions of CD21^{lo} B-cell and Tfh-cell frequencies are the product of reduced total B-cell and T-cell numbers, and not of absolute increases. Thus, our results demonstrate the importance of structured immunophenotypic analysis with the inclusion of absolute cell numbers to delineate affected cell types in PAD patients with NICs.

We here examined a cohort of 62 PAD patients. These included nine genetically diagnosed XLA patients, who were all diagnosed in early childhood and, prior to inclusion into our study, suffered from infectious complications only. Although the XLA group was by far the smallest, it does represent a homogenous group of patients with a B-cell intrinsic defect to be used as patient controls for our PAD–NIC and PAD+NIC immunophenotying. The vast majority of the other PAD patients were diagnosed with CVID (32; 52%) or HGG (13; 21%). This is in line with previous reports from teaching hospitals and is most likely reflective of the skewed population seen in tertiary care (36, 38, 44, 49). In our cohort, the most frequent infections were of the respiratory tract (13%, upper respiratory tract infection [URTI] only; 21% lower respiratory tract infection [LRTI] only; 66% URTI plus LRTI), with the most prevalent NIC being autoimmunity (60%) (38, 44, 82–85), which is reflective of other clinical studies. Furthermore, the significantly higher incidence of NIC in patients with a CVID diagnosis (72%) vs. all other non-XLA PAD (35%; $p = 0.01$) is similar to that of previous reports (36, 38, 44, 83). In terms of patient numbers, it falls short of multi-institute cohort analyses of clinical and basic immunological features (38, 44, 83, 86). However, our cohort of 62 patients relates well to other immunophenotyping studies (37, 46, 48, 51–53, 79, 87) and is larger than most studies (37, 46, 55, 58–61, 79). Moreover, the division into almost equally sized groups of PAD–NIC ($n = 23$) and PAD+NIC ($n = 30$) and a genetically defined XLA patient control group ($n = 9$)

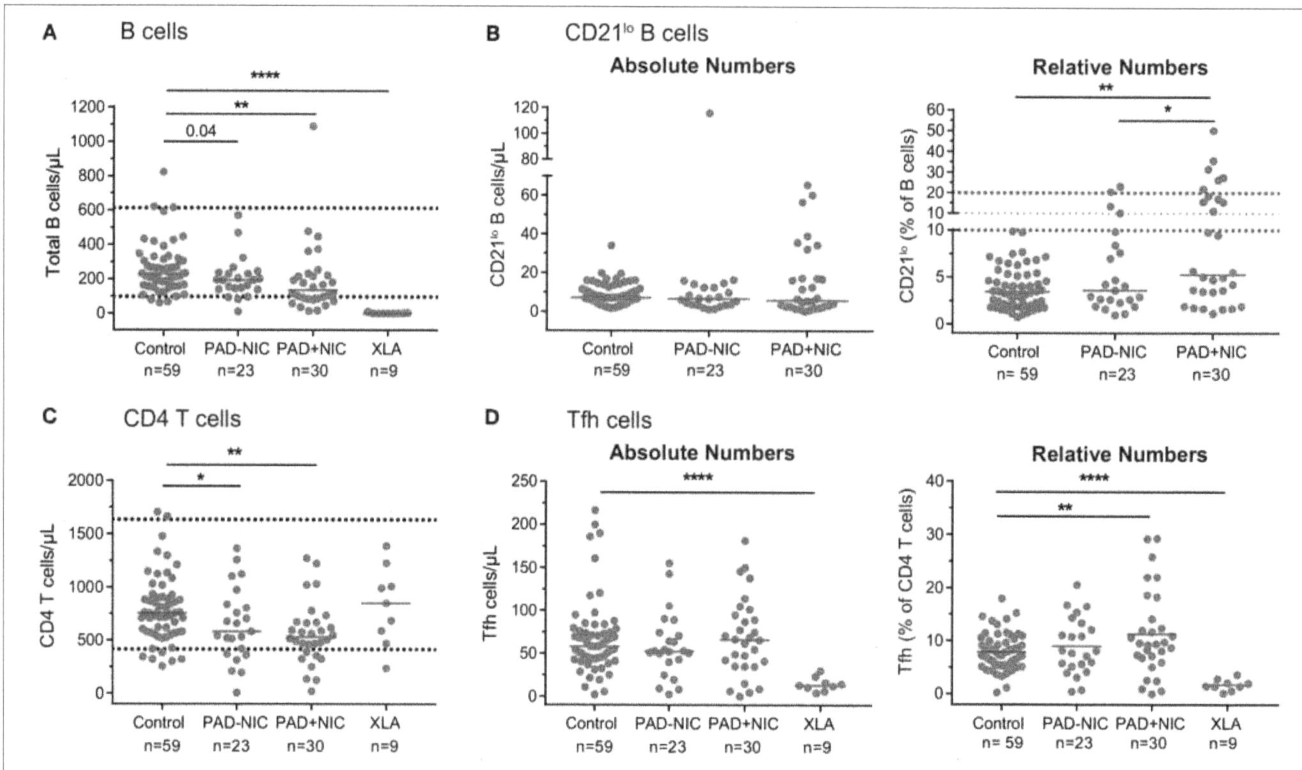

FIGURE 5 | Pitfalls in interpretation of relative expansions of cell subsets in the context of reduced absolute total cell numbers. **(A)** Absolute numbers of total B cells. Horizontal dotted lines represent the 5th and 95th percentiles from the healthy controls. **(B)** Absolute numbers and relative frequencies of CD21^{lo} B cells. Horizontal dotted lines denote the upper thresholds for CD21^{lo} expansions in the Freiburg (red) and EUROclass (blue) classification schemes. **(C)** Absolute numbers of total CD4 T cells. **(D)** Absolute numbers and relative frequencies of Tfh cells. For gating strategies, see **Supplementary Figure 2** (CD21^{lo} B cells) and **Supplementary Figure 4** (Tfh cells). PAD, predominantly antibody deficiency; NIC, non-infectious complications. Statistics were performed with the Kruskal–Wallis test, followed by Mann–Whitney tests for pairwise comparisons. $^{*}p < 0.5$, $^{**}p < 0.01$, and $^{****}p < 0.0001$.

is well-suited for examination of common and NIC-associated abnormalities. The high prevalence of NICs in adult PAD patients in our study likely associates with later onset of symptoms (86) and delayed diagnosis in these patients (38, 44). The clinical and immunological presentations of our patient cohort are diverse, in line with previously published studies. Thus, this cohort is highly representative for the in-depth analysis of immunological differences that segregate with the presence of NICs.

In our study, reduced B-cell numbers segregated with the presence of NICs. Further in-depth examination of the B-cell compartment revealed significant reductions in Ig smBs and plasmablasts in both PAD groups, which was in line with a recent PAD study (48). However, unlike previous reports (37, 47), in our cohort, these abnormalities did not segregate with NICs such as splenomegaly, granulomatous disease, and autoimmunity. In contrast, we observed specific reductions in serum IgM levels and IgM memory B-cell numbers in PAD+NIC patients. As IgM has a role in preventing autoimmunity by promoting phagocytic clearance of cell debris including autoantigen (88, 89), it is possible that this defect contributes to the autoimmune pathophysiology in patients with PAD+NIC.

In addition to the reduced memory B cells, naive B cells were significantly reduced in the PAD+NIC group. As naive B cells form the largest proportion of total B cells, this reduction is mostly responsible for the reduced total B-cell numbers. The cause of reduced B-cell numbers is unclear and could be related to either reduced production from bone marrow precursors or reduced survival in the periphery. Gene defects underlying either of these processes have been reported in patients with an antibody deficiency syndrome (2). Importantly, the reductions in naive B cells correlated with reduced naive CD4 and CD8 T cells (see *Discussion* below) and could be part of a more general lymphocyte production and/or survival defect that contributes to disease pathology. Finally, the reduction in naive B-cell numbers highlights the importance of measuring absolute cell numbers, as this will affect proportions of other cell subsets (e.g., CD21^{lo} B cells; see below) and lead to misinterpretation of indirect findings.

We here show that the expansion of CD21^{lo} B cells, which is reportedly associated with autoimmunity and splenomegaly in CVID patients (46, 47), was only observed in PAD+NIC patients when presented as frequency of total B cells, but not in terms of absolute cell numbers. Expansion of this B-cell subset has also been identified in numerous chronic infections and autoimmune and granulomatous diseases. Specifically, increased frequencies and numbers of CD21^{lo} B cells have been observed in Crohn's disease (90), Sjögren's syndrome (91), and poor HIV controllers (92). In addition, increased CD21^{lo} B-cell frequencies have also been identified in rheumatoid arthritis (RA) (93, 94), scleroderma (94), systemic lupus erythematosus (SLE) (95), and multiple sclerosis (MS) (96). Similar to PAD+NIC, absolute numbers of CD21^{lo} B cells are normal in RA (93), and the increased frequencies of CD21^{lo} B cells were the result of reduced naive and memory B-cell numbers (93). This segregates PAD+NIC and RA from Crohn's disease, Sjögren's syndrome, and HIV in which the absolute numbers of CD21^{lo} B cell are increased and might be indicative of distinct pathophysiologies.

Total CD4 and CD8 T-cell numbers were significantly lower in both PAD–NIC and PAD+NIC groups as a result of a reduction in the naive subsets. In contrast to other studies where naive T-cell deficiencies associated with NICs such as splenomegaly (53, 54), this link was not observed in our study. In addition, as memory T-cell numbers were unaffected, we postulate that decreased total CD4 and CD8 T-cell numbers are as a result of smaller numbers of naive T cells. Although PAD has long been considered to result from disturbances in B-cell homeostasis, it is becoming more evident that defective T-cell responses also play a role in disease pathogenesis. In particular, reductions in naive CD4 and CD8 T cells will likely impair immunity in primary infection and vaccination, thus rendering patients more prone to severe and often lethal infections, as shown in studies of aging and HIV infection (97–100).

Further dissection of the CD4 T-cell compartment in our cohort revealed abnormalities in Treg, Th, and Tfh cells. Treg-cell numbers were specifically low in PAD+NIC patients, in line with previous reports (54, 58, 59). This concerned both thymus-derived, naive Treg, and peripherally induced memory Treg. It is very tempting to speculate that the Treg deficiency contributes to the autoimmune pathology, similar to what has been proposed for patients with type 1 diabetes, MS, and SLE (101–106). Still, it remains unclear what causes the reduction and how this contributes to NIC. Potentially, the reduction is related to the reduced total naive T cells and might be reflective of either impaired production from the thymus, or increased maturation into effector memory cells as a result of the high infectious pressure in PAD patients.

Although the precise role of Th17.1 cells in immunity has not yet been fully elucidated, decreased Th17.1 counts have been linked to increased susceptibility to bacterial infection in other immunocompromised patients, including those with hyper-IgE syndrome and HIV/AIDS (107–112). In addition to the function of Th17 cells in controlling infections, these cells have been shown to promote antibody production by B cells (60). Thus, reductions in these cell numbers might contribute to the impaired antibody responses in PAD patients.

In line with previous reports, we observed increased frequencies of Tfh cells in patients with NIC (37, 55, 57). However, we also determined the absolute Tfh numbers and found that these were similar to those of controls. Thus, rather than a role of increased Tfh cells in CVID and autoimmunity (37, 55, 57, 113–115), it might be an altered distribution of Tfh subsets that contributes to disease pathology. Importantly, in PAD+NIC patients, the most potent B-cell helpers, Tfh17 cells, are significantly reduced. This could potentially link the inefficient antibody responses to pathological B cell responses, driven by, for example, the other Tfh cell subsets.

In our study, we utilized membrane markers only for the delineation of Th, Tfh, and Treg cells. In literature, multiple phenotypic definitions have been used to assess Th cells (cytoplasmic IFN-γ, IL-4, IL-10, and IL-17), Tfh cells (CD4$^+$CXCR5$^+$, CD4$^+$CXCR5$^+$PD-1$^+$, or CD4$^+$CXCR5$^+$ICOS$^+$), and Treg cells (CD4$^+$CD25$^+$CD127$^{lo/-}$ or CD4$^+$CD25$^+$FoxP3$^+$) (71, 72, 116, 117). Although intracellular FoxP3 and cytokine expression represents the gold standard protocols for the delineation of Treg and Th subsets, respectively, these protocols are laborious and not easily amenable to high-throughput analyses. The surface markers utilized to define Treg and Th subsets in our panel have previously been demonstrated to correlate well with intracellular FoxP3 (116) and cytokine expression (117, 118). Therefore, we are convinced that the gating strategies we applied were highly specific. Without the need for *in vitro* activation and/or cytoplasmic staining, our protocol is more straightforward, making it quicker and more easily scalable for adoption in diagnostic laboratories.

Here, we have identified B- and T-cell biomarkers associated with NICs in patients with PAD. Humoral and cellular deficiencies have previously been associated with aging contributing to susceptibility to infection and NIC development including autoimmunity and cancer. This is particularly the case for declining numbers of naive B and T cells (74, 119–121). Thus, it could be suggested that PAD–NIC represent a precursor group whom with aging will develop NICs. However, the lower median age at diagnosis of the PAD+NIC group (25 vs. 45 years in PAD–NIC) suggests that it is more likely that the PAD–NIC and PAD+NIC patients suffer from distinct pathophysiologies.

CVID demonstrates intrinsic clinical, immunological, and genomic heterogeneity complicating diagnosis resulting in decreased overall survival rates (82, 122, 123). Over the past 5 years, criteria utilized to define CVID have been expanded to include total and naive CD4 T-cell quantification, in addition to the assessment of B-cell subsets and clinical parameters of disease. These updated criteria enable the exclusion of patients with combined immunodeficiency (CID) on the basis of demonstration of severe reductions in naive CD4 T cells. It was suggested that reduced proportions of naive CD4 T cells (<10% CD4 T cells) rather than decreased CD4 counts (<200 cells/μl) are more sensitive in the definition of CID, further highlighting the validity of simultaneously quantifying absolute and relative numbers in patient diagnostics and prognostication protocols. Utilizing the updated criteria, the authors redefined previously published patients on the basis of the updated criteria. Here, 2% patients previously defined as CVID were redefined as CID (122–124). Application of these updated criteria to our CVID group would redefine five (16%) patients as CID. The distinction between CVID and CID is extremely important, as a higher incidence of pneumonia, lymphoma, granulomas, autoimmunity, and enteropathy (2, 5, 123), in addition to lower B-cell and naive CD4 T-cell numbers, accounts for the lower 5-year survival rate in CID patients (123). Thus, unlike PAD patients where IgRT is sufficient for disease management, some patients with CID will require life-saving stem cell transplantation. Hence, the utilization of our panel would aid in the identification and correct classification of patients who progress to CID, as well as PAD patients at risk of developing NICs. We do realize that the differences in cellular immunophenotypes observed in PAD patients with and without NIC will need to be verified in independent international PAD cohorts. Ideally, these markers should be analyzed longitudinally in early-diagnosed patients without NIC to validate if abnormalities will predict disease progression and development of NIC. Therefore, the immunophenotypic defects outlined here could guide genomic analysis of patients, to enable precise diagnosis and predictive prognostic information, as well as guide targeted patient treatment with the potential to limit diagnostic delay, as well as reduce the incidence of early mortality and high morbidity associated with NICs in these patients.

AUTHOR CONTRIBUTIONS

MZ, RO'H, and JB conceptualized the study and designed the experiments. EE, JB, PA, RS, PC, JC, FH-L, and MZ collected and interpreted the data. EE and PA performed the experiments. EE and MZ wrote the manuscript. All authors critically read, commented on, and approved the final version of the manuscript.

FUNDING

This work was supported by the Australian National Health and Medical Research Council (NHMRC; Senior Research Fellowship 1117687 for MZ) and the Jeffrey Modell Foundation.

ACKNOWLEDGMENTS

We gratefully acknowledge the technical support of Mr. Samuel De Jong and Dr. Malgorzata Gorniak, sample collection by the Alfred pathology collection service and Medical Day unit, advice on panel design by Mrs. Christina Grosserichter-Wagener and Dr. Tomas Kalina, collation of clinical data by Dr. Marsus Pumar, and maintenance of the flow cytometers by the AMREP flow core facility.

REFERENCES

1. Gathmann B, Grimbacher B, Beaute J, Dudoit Y, Mahlaoui N, Fischer A, et al. The European internet-based patient and research database for primary immunodeficiencies: results 2006-2008. *Clin Exp Immunol.* (2009) 157 (Suppl 1):3–11. doi: 10.1111/j.1365-2249.2009.03954.x
2. Picard C, Bobby Gaspar H, Al-Herz W, Bousfiha A, Casanova JL, Chatila T, et al. International union of immunological societies: 2017 primary immunodeficiency diseases committee report on inborn errors of immunity. *J Clin Immunol.* (2018) 38:96–128. doi: 10.1007/s10875-017-0464-9
3. Durandy A, Kracker S, Fischer A. Primary antibody deficiencies. *Nat Rev Immunol.* (2013) 13:519–33. doi: 10.1038/nri3466
4. Lucas M, Lee M, Lortan J, Lopez-Granados E, Misbah S, Chapel H. Infection outcomes in patients with common variable immunodeficiency disorders: relationship to immunoglobulin therapy over 22 years. *J Allergy Clin Immunol.* (2010) 125:1354–60.e1354. doi: 10.1016/j.jaci.2010.02.040
5. Bousfiha A, Jeddane L, Picard C, Ailal F, Bobby Gaspar H, Al-Herz W, et al. The 2017 IUIS phenotypic classification for primary immunodeficiencies. *J Clin Immunol.* (2018) 38:129–43. doi: 10.1007/s10875-017-0465-8
6. Bruton OC. Agammaglobulinemia. *Pediatrics.* (1952) 9:722–8.
7. Tsukada S, Saffran DC, Rawlings DJ, Parolini O, Allen RC, Klisak I, et al. Deficient expression of a B cell cytoplasmic tyrosine kinase in human X-linked agammaglobulinemia. *Cell.* (1993) 72:279–90. doi: 10.1016/0092-8674(93)90667-F
8. Vetrie D, Vorechovsky I, Sideras P, Holland J, Davies A, Flinter F, et al. The gene involved in X-linked agammaglobulinaemia is a member of the src family of protein-tyrosine kinases. *Nature.* (1993) 361:226–33. doi: 10.1038/361226a0
9. Dobbs AK, Yang T, Farmer D, Kager L, Parolini O, Conley ME. Cutting edge: a hypomorphic mutation in Igβ (CD79b) in a patient with immunodeficiency and a leaky defect in B cell development. *J Immunol.* (2007) 179:2055–9. doi: 10.4049/jimmunol.179.4.2055
10. Ferrari S, Lougaris V, Caraffi S, Zuntini R, Yang J, Soresina A, et al. Mutations of the Igβ gene cause agammaglobulinemia in man. *J Exp Med.* (2007) 204:2047–51. doi: 10.1084/jem.20070264
11. Minegishi Y, Coustan-Smith E, Rapalus L, Ersoy F, Campana D, Conley ME. Mutations in Igα (CD79a) result in a complete block in B-cell development. *J Clin Invest.* (1999) 104:1115–21. doi: 10.1172/JCI7696
12. Minegishi Y, Coustan-Smith E, Wang YH, Cooper MD, Campana D, Conley ME. Mutations in the human lambda5/14.1 gene result in B cell deficiency and agammaglobulinemia. *J Exp Med.* (1998) 187:71–7. doi: 10.1084/jem.187.1.71
13. Minegishi Y, Rohrer J, Coustan-Smith E, Lederman HM, Pappu R, Campana D, et al. An essential role for BLNK in human B cell development. *Science.* (1999) 286:1954–7.
14. Yel L, Minegishi Y, Coustan-Smith E, Buckley RH, Trubel H, Pachman LM, et al. Mutations in the mu heavy-chain gene in patients with agammaglobulinemia. *N Engl J Med.* (1996) 335:1486–93. doi: 10.1056/NEJM199611143352003
15. van Zelm MC, Geertsema C, Nieuwenhuis N, de Ridder D, Conley ME, Schiff C, et al. Gross deletions involving IGHM, BTK, or Artemis: a model for genomic lesions mediated by transposable elements. *Am J Hum Genet.* (2008) 82:320–32. doi: 10.1016/j.ajhg.2007.10.011
16. van Zelm MC, Reisli I, van der Burg M, Castano D, van Noesel CJ, van Tol MJ, et al. An antibody-deficiency syndrome due to mutations in the CD19 gene. *N Engl J Med.* (2006) 354:1901–12. doi: 10.1056/NEJMoa051568
17. van Zelm MC, Smet J, Adams B, Mascart F, Schandene L, Janssen F, et al. CD81 gene defect in humans disrupts CD19 complex formation and leads to antibody deficiency. *J Clin Invest.* (2010) 120:1265–74. doi: 10.1172/JCI39748
18. Thiel J, Kimmig L, Salzer U, Grudzien M, Lebrecht D, Hagena T, et al. Genetic CD21 deficiency is associated with hypogammaglobulinemia. *J Allergy Clin Immunol.* (2012) 129:801–10.e806. doi: 10.1016/j.jaci.2011.09.027

19. Angulo I, Vadas O, Garcon F, Banham-Hall E, Plagnol V, Leahy TR, et al. Phosphoinositide 3-kinase delta gene mutation predisposes to respiratory infection and airway damage. *Science.* (2013) 342:866–71. doi: 10.1126/science.1243292
20. Lucas CL, Kuehn HS, Zhao F, Niemela JE, Deenick EK, Palendira U, et al. Dominant-activating germline mutations in the gene encoding the PI(3)K catalytic subunit p110delta result in T cell senescence and human immunodeficiency. *Nat Immunol.* (2014) 15:88–97. doi: 10.1038/ni.2771
21. Kuijpers TW, Bende RJ, Baars PA, Grummels A, Derks IA, Dolman KM, et al. CD20 deficiency in humans results in impaired T cell-independent antibody responses. *J Clin Invest.* (2010) 120:214–22. doi: 10.1172/JCI40231
22. Tuijnenburg P, Lango Allen H, Burns SO, Greene D, Jansen MH, Staples E, et al. Loss-of-function nuclear factor kappaB subunit 1 (NFKB1) variants are the most common monogenic cause of common variable immunodeficiency in Europeans. *J Allergy Clin Immunol.* (2018) 142:1285–96. doi: 10.1016/j.jaci.2018.01.039
23. Warnatz K, Bossaller L, Salzer U, Skrabl-Baumgartner A, Schwinger W, van der Burg M, et al. Human ICOS deficiency abrogates the germinal center reaction and provides a monogenic model for common variable immunodeficiency. *Blood.* (2006) 107:3045–52. doi: 10.1182/blood-2005-07-2955
24. Lee CE, Fulcher DA, Whittle B, Chand R, Fewings N, Field M, et al. Autosomal-dominant B-cell deficiency with alopecia due to a mutation in NFKB2 that results in nonprocessable p100. *Blood.* (2014) 124:2964–72. doi: 10.1182/blood-2014-06-578542
25. Shi C, Wang F, Tong A, Zhang XQ, Song HM, Liu ZY, et al. NFKB2 mutation in common variable immunodeficiency and isolated adrenocorticotropic hormone deficiency: a case report and review of literature. *Medicine.* (2016) 95:e5081. doi: 10.1097/MD.0000000000005081
26. Lucas CL, Zhang Y, Venida A, Wang Y, Hughes J, McElwee J, et al. Heterozygous splice mutation in PIK3R1 causes human immunodeficiency with lymphoproliferation due to dominant activation of PI3K. *J Exp Med.* (2014) 211:2537–47. doi: 10.1084/jem.20141759
27. van Zelm MC, Bartol SJ, Driessen GJ, Mascart F, Reisli I, Franco JL, et al. Human CD19 and CD40L deficiencies impair antibody selection and differentially affect somatic hypermutation. *J Allergy Clin Immunol.* (2014) 134:135–44. doi: 10.1016/j.jaci.2013.11.015
28. Maffucci P, Filion CA, Boisson B, Itan Y, Shang L, Casanova JL, et al. Genetic diagnosis using whole exome sequencing in common variable immunodeficiency. *Front Immunol.* (2016) 7:220. doi: 10.3389/fimmu.2016.00220
29. Bogaert DJ, Dullaers M, Lambrecht BN, Vermaelen KY, De Baere E, Haerynck F. Genes associated with common variable immunodeficiency: one diagnosis to rule them all? *J Med Genet.* (2016) 53:575–90. doi: 10.1136/jmedgenet-2015-103690
30. de Valles-Ibanez G, Esteve-Sole A, Piquer M, Gonzalez-Navarro EA, Hernandez-Rodriguez J, Laayouni H, et al. Evaluating the genetics of common variable immunodeficiency: monogenetic model and beyond. *Front Immunol.* (2018) 9:636. doi: 10.3389/fimmu.2018.00636
31. Ameratunga R, Brewerton M, Slade C, Jordan A, Gillis D, Steele R, et al. Comparison of diagnostic criteria for common variable immunodeficiency disorder. *Front Immunol.* (2014) 5:415. doi: 10.3389/fimmu.2014.00415
32. Boileau J, Mouillot G, Gerard L, Carmagnat M, Rabian C, Oksenhendler E, et al. Autoimmunity in common variable immunodeficiency: correlation with lymphocyte phenotype in the French DEFI study. *J Autoimmun.* (2011) 36:25–32. doi: 10.1016/j.jaut.2010.10.002
33. ImmunodeficienciesESF. (2017). *New Clinical Diagnosis Criteria for the ESID Registry.* Geneva. Available online at: https://esid.org/Working-Parties/Registry/Diagnosis-criteria
34. Conley ME, Notarangelo LD, Etzioni A. Diagnostic criteria for primary immunodeficiencies. *Representing PAGID (Pan-American Group for Immunodeficiency) and ESID (European Society for Immunodeficiencies). Clin Immunol.* (1999) 93:190–7.
35. Bonilla FA, Barlan I, Chapel H, Costa-Carvalho BT, Cunningham-Rundles C, de la Morena MT, et al. International Consensus Document (ICON): common variable immunodeficiency disorders. *J Allergy Clin Immunol Pract.* (2016) 4:38–59. doi: 10.1016/j.jaip.2015.07.025
36. Driessen GJ, Dalm VA, van Hagen PM, Grashoff HA, Hartwig NG, van Rossum AM, et al. Common variable immunodeficiency and idiopathic primary hypogammaglobulinemia: two different conditions within the same disease spectrum. *Haematologica.* (2013) 98:1617–23. doi: 10.3324/haematol.2013.085076
37. Romberg N, Le Coz C, Glauzy S, Schickel JN, Trofa M, Nolan BE, et al. Patients with common variable immunodeficiency with autoimmune cytopenias exhibit hyperplastic yet inefficient germinal center responses. *J Allergy Clin Immunol.* (2019) 143:258–65. doi: 10.1016/j.jaci.2018.06.012
38. Slade CA, Bosco JJ, Binh Giang T, Kruse E, Stirling RG, Cameron PU, et al. Delayed diagnosis and complications of predominantly antibody deficiencies in a cohort of australian adults. *Front Immunol.* (2018) 9:694. doi: 10.3389/fimmu.2018.00694
39. Wang N, Hammarstrom L. IgA deficiency: what is new? *Curr Opin Allergy Clin Immunol.* (2012) 12:602–8. doi: 10.1097/ACI.0b013e3283594219
40. Jolles S. The variable in common variable immunodeficiency: a disease of complex phenotypes. *J Allergy Clin Immunol Pract.* (2013) *1*:545–6. doi: 10.1016/j.jaip.2013.09.015
41. Yazdani R, Azizi G, Abolhassani H, Aghamohammadi A. Selective IgA deficiency: epidemiology, pathogenesis, clinical phenotype, diagnosis, prognosis and management. *Scand J Immunol.* (2017) 85:3–12. doi: 10.1111/sji.12499
42. Chapel H, Lucas M, Patel S, Lee M, Cunningham-Rundles C, Resnick E, et al. Confirmation and improvement of criteria for clinical phenotyping in common variable immunodeficiency disorders in replicate cohorts. *J Allergy Clin Immunol.* (2012) 130:1197–8.e1199. doi: 10.1016/j.jaci.2012.05.046
43. Cunningham-Rundles C. The many faces of common variable immunodeficiency. *Hematology Am Soc Hematol Educ Program.* (2012) 2012:301–5. doi: 10.1182/asheducation.V2012.1.301.3798316
44. Resnick ES, Moshier EL, Godbold JH, Cunningham-Rundles C. Morbidity and mortality in common variable immune deficiency over 4 decades. *Blood.* (2012) 119:1650–7. doi: 10.1182/blood-2011-09-377945
45. Odnoletkova I, Kindle G, Quinti I, Grimbacher B, Knerr V, Gathmann B, et al. The burden of common variable immunodeficiency disorders: a retrospective analysis of the European Society for Immunodeficiency (ESID) registry data. *Orphanet J Rare Dis.* (2018) 13:201. doi: 10.1186/s13023-018-0941-0
46. Warnatz K, Wehr C, Drager R, Schmidt S, Eibel H, Schlesier M, et al. Expansion of CD19(hi)CD21(lo/neg) B cells in common variable immunodeficiency (CVID) patients with autoimmune cytopenia. *Immunobiology.* (2002) 206:502–13. doi: 10.1078/0171-2985-00198
47. Wehr C, Kivioja T, Schmitt C, Ferry B, Witte T, Eren E, et al. The EUROclass trial: defining subgroups in common variable immunodeficiency. *Blood.* (2008) 111:77–85. doi: 10.1182/blood-2007-06-091744
48. Blanco E, Perez-Andres M, Arriba-Mendez S, Serrano C, Criado, I., Del Pino-Molina, L, et al. *Defects in memory B-cell and plasma cell subsets expressing different immunoglobulin-subclasses in patients with CVID and immunoglobulin subclass deficiencies. J Allergy Clin Immunol.* (2019) 144:809–24. doi: 10.1016/j.jaci.2019.02.017
49. Driessen GJ, van Zelm MC, van Hagen PM, Hartwig NG, Trip M, Warris A, et al. B-cell replication history and somatic hypermutation status identify distinct pathophysiologic backgrounds in common variable immunodeficiency. *Blood.* (2011) 118:6814–23. doi: 10.1182/blood-2011-06-361881
50. Warnatz K, Schlesier M. Flowcytometric phenotyping of common variable immunodeficiency. *Cytometry B Clin Cytom.* (2008) 74:261–71. doi: 10.1002/cyto.b.20432
51. Ebbo M, Gerard L, Carpentier S, Vely F, Cypowyj S, Farnarier C, et al. Low Circulating natural killer cell counts are associated with severe disease in patients with common variable immunodeficiency. *EBioMed.* (2016) 6:222–30. doi: 10.1016/j.ebiom.2016.02.025
52. Aspalter RM, Sewell WA, Dolman K, Farrant J, Webster AD. Deficiency in circulating natural killer (NK) cell subsets in common variable immunodeficiency and X-linked agammaglobulinaemia. *Clin Exp Immunol.* (2000) 121:506–14. doi: 10.1046/j.1365-2249.2000.01317.x
53. Giovannetti A, Pierdominici M, Mazzetta F, Marziali M, Renzi C, Mileo AM, et al. Unravelling the complexity of T cell abnormalities in common variable immunodeficiency. *J Immunol.* (2007) 178:3932–43. doi: 10.4049/jimmunol.178.6.3932
54. Bateman EA, Ayers L, Sadler R, Lucas M, Roberts C, Woods A, et al. T cell phenotypes in patients with common variable immunodeficiency disorders: associations with clinical phenotypes in comparison with other

groups with recurrent infections. *Clin Exp Immunol.* (2012) 170:202–11. doi: 10.1111/j.1365-2249.2012.04643.x

55. Coraglia A, Galassi N, Fernandez Romero DS, Juri MC, Felippo M, Malbran A, et al. Common variable immunodeficiency and circulating TFH. *J Immunol Res.* (2016) 2016:4951587. doi: 10.1155/2016/4951587
56. Unger S, Seidl M, van Schouwenburg P, Rakhmanov M, Bulashevska A, Frede N, et al. The TH1 phenotype of follicular helper T cells indicates an IFN-γ-associated immune dysregulation in patients with CD21low common variable immunodeficiency. *J Allergy Clin Immunol.* (2018) 141:730–40. doi: 10.1016/j.jaci.2017.04.041
57. Romberg ND, Hsu I, Price CC, Cunningham-Rundles C, Meffre E. Expansion of circulating t follicular helper cells in CVID patients with autoimmune cytopenias. *J Allergy Clin Immunol.* (2014) 133:AB162. doi: 10.1016/j.jaci.2013.12.586
58. Melo KM, Carvalho KI, Bruno FR, Ndhlovu LC, Ballan WM, Nixon DF, et al. A decreased frequency of regulatory T cells in patients with common variable immunodeficiency. *PLoS ONE.* (2009) 4:e6269. doi: 10.1371/journal.pone.0006269
59. Arumugakani G, Wood PM, Carter CR. Frequency of Treg cells is reduced in CVID patients with autoimmunity and splenomegaly and is associated with expanded CD21lo B lymphocytes. *J Clin Immunol.* (2010) 30:292–300.
60. Barbosa RR, Silva SP, Silva SL, Melo AC, Pedro E, Barbosa MP, et al. Primary B-cell deficiencies reveal a link between human IL-17-producing CD4 T-cell homeostasis and B-cell differentiation. *PLoS ONE.* (2011) 6:e22848. doi: 10.1371/journal.pone.0022848
61. Kutukculer N, Azarsiz E, Aksu G, Karaca NE. CD4+CD25+Foxp3+ T regulatory cells, Th1 (CCR5, IL-2, IFN-γ) and Th2 (CCR4, IL-4, Il-13) type chemokine receptors and intracellular cytokines in children with common variable immunodeficiency. *Int J Immunopathol Pharmacol.* (2016) 29:241–51. doi: 10.1177/0394632015617064
62. Kalina T, Flores-Montero J, van der Velden VH, Martin-Ayuso M, Bottcher S, Ritgen M, et al. EuroFlow standardization of flow cytometer instrument settings and immunophenotyping protocols. *Leukemia.* (2012) 26:1986–2010. doi: 10.1038/leu.2012.122
63. van der Burg M, Kalina T, Perez-Andres M, Vlkova M, Lopez-Granados E, Blanco E, et al. The euroFlow PID orientation tube for flow cytometric diagnostic screening of primary immunodeficiencies of the lymphoid system. *Front Immunol.* (2019) 10:246. doi: 10.3389/fimmu.2019.00246
64. van Dongen JJM, van der Burg M, Kalina T, Perez-Andres M, Mejstrikova E, Vlkova M, et al. EuroFlow-based flowcytometric diagnostic screening and classification of primary immunodeficiencies of the lymphoid system. *Front Immunol.* 10:1271. doi: 10.3389/fimmu.2019.01271
65. van der Velden VH, Flores-Montero J, Perez-Andres M, Martin-Ayuso M, Crespo O, Blanco E, et al. *Optimization and testing of dried antibody* tube: the EuroFlow LST and PIDOT tubes as examples. *J Immunol Methods.* (2017) S0022-1759(17)30095-9. doi: 10.1016/j.jim.2017.03.011
66. Heeringa JJ, Rijvers L, Arends NJ, Driessen GJ, Pasmans SG, van Dongen JJM, et al. IgE-expressing memory B cells and plasmablasts are increased in blood of children with asthma, food allergy, and atopic dermatitis. *Allergy.* (2018) 73:1331–6. doi: 10.1111/all.13421
67. Liu W, Putnam AL, Xu-Yu Z, Szot GL, Lee MR, Zhu S, et al. CD127 expression inversely correlates with FoxP3 and suppressive function of human CD4+ T reg cells. *J Exp Med.* (2006) 203:1701–11. doi: 10.1084/jem.20060772
68. Seddiki N, Santner-Nanan B, Martinson J, Zaunders J, Sasson S, Landay A, et al. Expression of interleukin (IL)-2 and IL-7 receptors discriminates between human regulatory and activated T cells. *J Exp Med.* (2006) 203:1693–700. doi: 10.1084/jem.20060468
69. Annunziato F, Cosmi L, Liotta F, Maggi E, Romagnani S. The phenotype of human Th17 cells and their precursors, the cytokines that mediate their differentiation and the role of Th17 cells in inflammation. *Int Immunol.* (2008) 20:1361–8. doi: 10.1093/intimm/dxn106
70. Bonecchi R, Bianchi G, Bordignon PP, D'Ambrosio D, Lang R, Borsatti A, et al. Differential expression of chemokine receptors and chemotactic responsiveness of type 1 T helper cells (Th1s) and Th2s. *J Exp Med.* (1998) 187:129–34. doi: 10.1084/jem.187.1.129
71. Breitfeld D, Ohl L, Kremmer E, Ellwart J, Sallusto F, Lipp M, et al. Follicular B helper T cells express CXC chemokine receptor 5, localize to B cell follicles, and support immunoglobulin production. *J Exp Med.* (2000) 192:1545–52. doi: 10.1084/jem.192.11.1545
72. Schaerli P, Willimann K, Lang AB, Lipp M, Loetscher P, Moser B. CXC chemokine receptor 5 expression defines follicular homing T cells with B cell helper function. *J Exp Med.* (2000) 192:1553–62. doi: 10.1084/jem.192.11.1553
73. Ma CS, Wong N, Rao G, Avery DT, Torpy J, Hambridge T, et al. Monogenic mutations differentially affect the quantity and quality of T follicular helper cells in patients with human primary immunodeficiencies. *J Allergy Clin Immunol.* (2015) 136.e1001. doi: 10.1016/j.jaci.2015.05.036
74. Blanco, E., Perez-Andres, M., Arriba-Mendez, S., Contreras-Sanfeliciano, T., Criado, I., Pelak, O., et al. Age-associated distribution of normal B-cell and plasma cell subsets in peripheral blood. *J Allergy Clin Immunol.* (2018) 141:2208–19.e2216.
75. Flores-Montero J, Sanoja-Flores L, Paiva B, Puig N, Garcia-Sanchez O, Bottcher S, et al. Next generation flow for highly sensitive and standardized detection of minimal residual disease in multiple myeloma. *Leukemia.* (2017) 31:2094–103. doi: 10.1038/leu.2017.29
76. Theunissen P, Mejstrikova E, Sedek L, van der Sluijs-Gelling AJ, Gaipa G, Bartels M, et al. Standardized flow cytometry for highly sensitive MRD measurements in B-cell acute lymphoblastic leukemia. *Blood.* (2017) 129:347–57. doi: 10.1182/blood-2016-07-726307
77. Verstegen RHJ, Aui PM, Watson E, De Jong S, Bartol SJW, Bosco JJ, et al. Quantification of T-cell and B-cell replication history in aging, immunodeficiency, and newborn screening. *Front Immunol.* (2019) 10:2084. doi: 10.3389/fimmu.2019.02084
78. van Zelm MC, Pumar M, Shuttleworth P, Aui PM, Smart JM, Grigg A, et al. Functional antibody responses following allogeneic stem cell transplantation for TP53 mutant pre-B-ALL in a patient with X-linked agammaglobulinemia. *Front Immunol.* (2019) 10:895. doi: 10.3389/fimmu.2019.00895
79. Warnatz K, Denz A, Drager R, Braun M, Groth C, Wolff-Vorbeck G, et al. Severe deficiency of switched memory B cells (CD27(+)IgM(-)IgD(-)) in subgroups of patients with common variable immunodeficiency: a new approach to classify a heterogeneous disease. *Blood.* (2002) 99:1544–51. doi: 10.1182/blood.V99.5.1544
80. van den Heuvel D, Jansen MA, Dik WA, Bouallouch-Charif H, Zhao D, van Kester KA, et al. Cytomegalovirus- and epstein-barr virus-induced T-cell expansions in young children do not impair naive T-cell populations or vaccination responses: the generation R study. *J Infect Dis.* (2016) 213:233–42. doi: 10.1093/infdis/jiv369
81. Romberg N, Chamberlain N, Saadoun D, Gentile M, Kinnunen T, Ng YS, et al. CVID-associated TACI mutations affect autoreactive B cell selection and activation. *J Clin Invest.* (2013) 123:4283–93. doi: 10.1172/JCI69854
82. Cunningham-Rundles C. Common variable immune deficiency: dissection of the variable. *Immunol Rev.* (2019) 287:145–61. doi: 10.1111/imr.12728
83. Chapel H, Lucas M, Lee M, Bjorkander J, Webster D, Grimbacher B, et al. Common variable immunodeficiency disorders: division into distinct clinical phenotypes. *Blood.* (2008) 112:277–86. doi: 10.1182/blood-2007-11-124545
84. Agarwal S, Cunningham-Rundles C. Autoimmunity in common variable immunodeficiency. *Curr Allergy Asthma Rep.* (2009) 9:347–52. doi: 10.1007/s11882-009-0051-0
85. Warnatz K, Voll RE. Pathogenesis of autoimmunity in common variable immunodeficiency. *Front Immunol.* (2012) 3:210. doi: 10.3389/fimmu.2012.00210
86. Gathmann B, Mahlaoui N, Ceredih GL, Oksenhendler E, Warnatz K, European Society for Immunodeficiencies Registry Working P. Clinical picture and treatment of 2212 patients with common variable immunodeficiency. *J Allergy Clin Immunol.* (2014) 134:116–26. doi: 10.1016/j.jaci.2013.12.1077
87. Stuchly J, Kanderova V, Vlkova M, Hermanova I, Slamova L, Pelak O, et al. Common variable immunodeficiency patients with a phenotypic profile of immunosenescence present with thrombocytopenia. *Sci Rep.* (2017) 7:39710. doi: 10.1038/srep39710
88. Boes M. Role of natural and immune IgM antibodies in immune responses. *Mol Immunol.* (2000) 37:1141–9. doi: 10.1016/s0161-5890(01)00025-6
89. Chen Y, Park YB, Patel E, Silverman GJ. IgM antibodies to apoptosis-associated determinants recruit C1q and enhance dendritic cell phagocytosis of apoptotic cells. *J Immunol.* (2009) 182:6031–43. doi: 10.4049/jimmunol.0804191
90. Timmermans WM, van Laar JA, van der Houwen TB, Kamphuis LS, Bartol SJ, Lam KH, et al. B-cell dysregulation

in crohn's disease is partially restored with infliximab therapy. *PLoS ONE.* (2016) 11:e0160103. doi: 10.1371/journal.pone.0160103
91. Saadoun D, Terrier B, Bannock J, Vazquez T, Massad C, Kang I, et al. Expansion of autoreactive unresponsive CD21-/low B cells in Sjogren's syndrome-associated lymphoproliferation. *Arthritis Rheum.* (2013) 65:1085–96. doi: 10.1002/art.37828
92. van den Heuvel D, Driessen GJ, Berkowska MA, van der Burg M, Langerak AW, Zhao D, et al. Persistent subclinical immune defects in HIV-1-infected children treated with antiretroviral therapy. *AIDS.* (2015) 29:1745–56. doi: 10.1097/QAD.0000000000000765
93. McComish J, Mundy J, Sullivan T, Proudman SM, Hissaria P. Changes in peripheral blood B cell subsets at diagnosis and after treatment with disease-modifying anti-rheumatic drugs in patients with rheumatoid arthritis: correlation with clinical and laboratory parameters. *Int J Rheum Dis.* (2015) 18:421–32. doi: 10.1111/1756-185X.12325
94. Rubtsov AV, Rubtsova K, Fischer A, Meehan RT, Gillis JZ, Kappler JW, et al. Toll-like receptor 7 (TLR7)-driven accumulation of a novel CD11c(+) B-cell population is important for the development of autoimmunity. *Blood.* (2011) 118:1305–15. doi: 10.1182/blood-2011-01-331462
95. Wehr C, Eibel H, Masilamani M, Illges H, Schlesier M, Peter HH, et al. A new CD21low B cell population in the peripheral blood of patients with SLE. *Clin Immunol.* (2004) 113:161–71. doi: 10.1016/j.clim.2004.05.010
96. Claes N, Fraussen J, Vanheusden M, Hellings N, Stinissen P, Van Wijmeersch B, et al. Age-associated B cells with proinflammatory characteristics are expanded in a proportion of multiple sclerosis patients. *J Immunol.* (2016) 197:4576–83. doi: 10.4049/jimmunol.1502448
97. Fagnoni FF, Vescovini R, Passeri G, Bologna G, Pedrazzoni M, Lavagetto G, et al. Shortage of circulating naive CD8(+) T cells provides new insights on immunodeficiency in aging. *Blood.* (2000) 95:2860–8. doi: 10.1182/blood.V95.9.2860.009k35_2860_2868
98. Rabin RL, Roederer M, Maldonado Y, Petru A, Herzenberg LA, Herzenberg LA. Altered representation of naive and memory CD8 T cell subsets in HIV-infected children. *J Clin Invest.* (1995) 95:2054–60. doi: 10.1172/JCI117891
99. Roederer M, Dubs JG, Anderson MT, Raju PA, Herzenberg LA, Herzenberg LA. CD8 naive T cell counts decrease progressively in HIV-infected adults. *J Clin Invest.* (1995) 95:2061–6. doi: 10.1172/JCI117892
100. Anyimadu H, Pingili C, Sivapalan V, Hirsch-Moverman Y, Mannheimer S. The impact of absolute CD4 count and percentage discordance on pneumocystis jirovecii pneumonia prophylaxis in HIV-infected patients. *J Int Assoc Provid AIDS Care.* (2018) 17:2325958218759199. doi: 10.1177/2325958218759199
101. Long SA, Buckner JH. CD4+FOXP3+ T regulatory cells in human autoimmunity: more than a numbers game. *J Immunol.* (2011) 187:2061–6. doi: 10.4049/jimmunol.1003224
102. Brusko TM, Wasserfall CH, Clare-Salzler MJ, Schatz DA, Atkinson MA. Functional defects and the influence of age on the frequency of CD4+ CD25+ T-cells in type 1 diabetes. *Diabetes.* (2005) 54:1407–14. doi: 10.2337/diabetes.54.5.1407
103. Putnam AL, Vendrame F, Dotta F, Gottlieb PA. CD4+CD25high regulatory T cells in human autoimmune diabetes. *J Autoimmun.* (2005) 24:55–62. doi: 10.1016/j.jaut.2004.11.004
104. Astier AL, Meiffren G, Freeman S, Hafler DA. Alterations in CD46-mediated Tr1 regulatory T cells in patients with multiple sclerosis. *J Clin Invest.* (2006) 116:3252–7. doi: 10.1172/JCI29251
105. Huan J, Culbertson N, Spencer L, Bartholomew R, Burrows GG, Chou YK, et al. Decreased FOXP3 levels in multiple sclerosis patients. *J Neurosci Res.* (2005) 81:45–52. doi: 10.1002/jnr.20522
106. Zhang B, Zhang X, Tang F, Zhu L, Liu Y. Reduction of forkhead box P3 levels in CD4+CD25high T cells in patients with new-onset systemic lupus erythematosus. *Clin Exp Immunol.* (2008) 153:182–7. doi: 10.1111/j.1365-2249.2008.03686.x
107. Peck A, Mellins ED. Precarious balance: Th17 cells in host defense. *Infect Immun.* (2010) 78:32–8. doi: 10.1128/IAI.00929-09
108. Crum-Cianflone N, Weekes J, Bavaro M. Recurrent community-associated methicillin-resistant Staphylococcus aureus infections among HIV-infected persons: incidence and risk factors. *AIDS Patient Care STDS.* (2009) 23:499–502. doi: 10.1089/apc.2008.0240
109. Hirschtick RE, Glassroth J, Jordan MC, Wilcosky TC, Wallace JM, Kvale PA, et al. Bacterial pneumonia in persons infected with the human immunodeficiency virus. *Pulmonary complications of HIV* infection study group. *N Engl J Med.* (1995) 333:845–51.
110. Minegishi Y, Saito M, Nagasawa M, Takada H, Hara T, Tsuchiya S, et al. Molecular explanation for the contradiction between systemic Th17 defect and localized bacterial infection in hyper-IgE syndrome. *J Exp Med.* (2009) 206:1291–301. doi: 10.1084/jem.20082767
111. Milner JD, Brenchley JM, Laurence A, Freeman AF, Hill BJ, Elias KM, et al. Impaired T(H)17 cell differentiation in subjects with autosomal dominant hyper-IgE syndrome. *Nature.* (2008) 452:773–6. doi: 10.1038/nature06764
112. Paulson ML, Freeman AF, Holland SM. Hyper IgE syndrome: an update on clinical aspects and the role of signal transducer and activator of transcription 3. *Curr Opin Allergy Clin Immunol.* (2008) 8:527–33. doi: 10.1097/ACI.0b013e3283184210
113. Xie J, Cui D, Liu Y, Jin J, Tong H, Wang L, et al. Changes in follicular helper T cells in idiopathic thrombocytopenic purpura patients. *Int J Biol Sci.* (2015) 11:220–9. doi: 10.7150%2Fijbs.10178
114. Gensous N, Charrier M, Duluc D, Contin-Bordes C, Truchetet ME, Lazaro E, et al. T follicular helper cells in autoimmune disorders. *Front Immunol.* (2018) 9:1637. doi: 10.3389/fimmu.2018.01637
115. Romme Christensen J, Bornsen L, Ratzer R, Piehl F, Khademi M, Olsson T, et al. Systemic inflammation in progressive multiple sclerosis involves follicular T-helper, Th17- and activated B-cells and correlates with progression. *PLoS ONE.* (2013) 8:e57820. doi: 10.1371/journal.pone.0057820
116. Rodriguez-Perea AL, Arcia ED, Rueda CM, Velilla PA. Phenotypical characterization of regulatory T cells in humans and rodents. *Clin Exp Immunol.* (2016) 185:281–91. doi: 10.1111/cei.12804
117. Annunziato F, Cosmi L, Santarlasci V, Maggi L, Liotta F, Mazzinghi B, et al. Phenotypic and functional features of human Th17 cells. *J Exp Med.* (2007) 204:1849–61. doi: 10.1084/jem.20070663
118. Sallusto F, Lanzavecchia A. Heterogeneity of CD4+ memory T cells: functional modules for tailored immunity. *Eur J Immunol.* (2009) 39:2076–82. doi: 10.1002/eji.200939722
119. Kilpatrick RD, Rickabaugh T, Hultin LE, Hultin P, Hausner MA, Detels R, et al. Homeostasis of the naive CD4+ T cell compartment during aging. *J Immunol.* (2008) 180:1499–507. doi: 10.4049/jimmunol.180.3.1499
120. Czesnikiewicz-Guzik M, Lee WW, Cui D, Hiruma Y, Lamar DL, Yang ZZ, et al. T cell subset-specific susceptibility to aging. *Clin Immunol.* (2008) 127:107–18. doi: 10.1016/j.clim.2007.12.002
121. Wertheimer AM, Bennett MS, Park B, Uhrlaub JL, Martinez C, Pulko V, et al. Aging and cytomegalovirus infection differentially and jointly affect distinct circulating T cell subsets in humans. *J Immunol.* (2014) 192:2143–55. doi: 10.4049/jimmunol.1301721
122. von Spee-Mayer C, Koemm V, Wehr C, Goldacker S, Kindle G, Bulashevska A, et al. Evaluating laboratory criteria for combined immunodeficiency in adult patients diagnosed with common variable immunodeficiency. *Clin Immunol.* (2019) 203:59–62. doi: 10.1016/j.clim.2019.04.001
123. Bertinchamp R, Gerard L, Boutboul D, Malphettes M, Fieschi C, Oksenhendler E, et al. Exclusion of Patients with a Severe T-cell defect improves the definition of common variable immunodeficiency. *J Allergy Clin Immunol Pract.* (2016) 4:1147–57. doi: 10.1016/j.jaip.2016.07.002
124. Chapel H. Common variable immunodeficiency disorders (CVID) - diagnoses of exclusion, especially combined immune defects. *J Allergy Clin Immunol Pract.* (2016) 4:1158–9. doi: 10.1016/j.jaip.2016.09.006

19

Delineating Human B Cell Precursor Development with Genetically Identified PID Cases as a Model

*Marjolein W. J. Wentink[1], Tomas Kalina[2], Martin Perez-Andres[3], Lucia del Pino Molina[4], Hanna IJspeert[1], François G. Kavelaars[5], Arjan C. Lankester[6], Quentin Lecrevisse[3], Jacques J. M. van Dongen[6], Alberto Orfao[3], and Mirjam van der Burg[1,7]** **on behalf of the EuroFlow PID consortium***

[1] Department of Immunology, Erasmus MC, University Medical Center Rotterdam, Rotterdam, Netherlands, [2] Department of Paediatric Haematology and Oncology, Second Faculty of Medicine, Charles University and University Hospital Motol, Prague, Czechia, [3] Department of Medicine-Service Cytometry, Cancer Research Center (IBMCC-CSIC/USAL) and University of Salamanca, Salamanca, Spain, [4] Department of Clinical Immunology, La Paz University Hospital, Lymphocyte Pathophysiology in Immunodeficiencies Group La Paz Institute for Health Research (IdiPAZ), Madrid, Spain, [5] Department of Hematology, Erasmus MC, University Medical Center Rotterdam, Rotterdam, Netherlands, [6] Department of Immunohematology and Blood Transfusion, Leiden University Medical Center, Leiden, Netherlands, [7] Department of Pediatrics, Leiden University Medical Center, Leiden, Netherlands

***Correspondence:**
Mirjam van der Burg
M.van_der_Burg@lumc.nl

B-cell precursors (BCP) arise from hematopoietic stem cells in bone marrow (BM). Identification and characterization of the different BCP subsets has contributed to the understanding of normal B-cell development. BCP first rearrange their immunoglobulin (Ig) heavy chain (IGH) genes to form the pre-B-cell receptor (pre-BCR) complex together with surrogate light chains. Appropriate signaling via this pre-BCR complex is followed by rearrangement of the Ig light chain genes, resulting in the formation, and selection of functional BCR molecules. Consecutive production, expression, and functional selection of the pre-BCR and BCR complexes guide the BCP differentiation process that coincides with corresponding immunophenotypic changes. We studied BCP differentiation in human BM samples from healthy controls and patients with a known genetic defect in V(D)J recombination or pre-BCR signaling to unravel normal immunophenotypic changes and to determine the effect of differentiation blocks caused by the specific genetic defects. Accordingly, we designed a 10-color antibody panel to study human BCP development in BM by flow cytometry, which allows identification of classical preB-I, preB-II, and mature B-cells as defined via BCR-related markers with further characterization by additional markers. We observed heterogeneous phenotypes associated with more than one B-cell maturation pathway, particularly for the preB-I and preB-II stages in which V(D)J recombination takes place, with asynchronous marker expression patterns. Next Generation Sequencing of complete IGH gene rearrangements in sorted BCP subsets unraveled their rearrangement status, indicating that BCP differentiation does not follow a single linear pathway. In conclusion, B-cell development in human BM is not a linear process, but a rather complex network of parallel pathways dictated by V(D)J-recombination-driven checkpoints and pre-BCR/BCR mediated-signaling occurring during B-cell production and selection. It can also be described as asynchronous, because precursor B-cells do not differentiate as full population between the different stages, but rather transit as a continuum, which seems influenced (in part) by V-D-J recombination-driven checkpoints.

Keywords: next generation sequence (NGS), immunoglobulin repertoire, bone marrow, flow cytometry, precursor B-cell

INTRODUCTION

B cells arise from hematopoietic stem cells in bone marrow (BM) and develop in a stepwise manner (1, 2). Identification and characterization of the different B-cell precursor (BCP) subsets contributes to the understanding of normal B-cell development (3, 4). Currently, it is accepted that expression of the PAX5 transcription factor triggers commitment to the B-cell lineage through the expression of B-cell specific genes such as CD79a (or Igα) and CD19, while suppressing B-lineage inappropriate genes. Since cytoplasmic expression of CD79a (cyCD79a) is one of the first signs of B-cell lineage commitment, human cyCD79a+ CD19- cells are defined as pro-B cells, followed by CD19 expression in pre-B-I cells. During this stage, V-D-J recombination of the immunoglobulin (Ig) heavy chain (IGH) locus is initiated by the recombination activating genes (RAG1 and RAG2) (5–11). If this rearrangement process results in a functional protein, Igμ heavy chain is expressed in the cytoplasm (cyIgμ), which defines the pre-BII-stage. Whenever rearrangement of the first allele does not result in a productive Igμ molecule, the second allele will be rearranged. Igμ is expressed on the cell membrane together with the surrogate light chains λ14.1 and VpreB as pre-B-cell receptor (pre-BCR) (12, 13). Pre-BCR signaling triggers a cascade of events including downregulation of the recombination machinery to ensure allelic exclusion and subsequent proliferation, followed by opening of the Ig light chain (IGL) locus, which is being rearranged under the influence of a second expression wave of RAG1 and RAG2 (10, 14). After successful IGL rearrangement, a functional BCR in the form of a complete IgM molecule is expressed on the cell surface membrane, defining progression to the immature B-lymphocyte stage. Subsequent IgD expression on the plasma membrane of IgM^+ immature B-cell leads to the differentiation into mature naive B-lymphocytes, which are released from BM to peripheral blood (PB). In addition to the above described changes in rearrangement status and expression of Ig molecules, BCP undergo also other maturation-associated immunophenotypic changes. Whereas, Pro-B cells express stem cell markers such as CD34 and CD10, later stages start to express B-cell specific markers such as CD19 and CD20. Additionally, cells that are in their rearrangement process express TdT in two waves, one during the IGH gene rearrangements and another during the IGL gene rearrangement which ensures junctional diversity by random addition of non-templated nucleotides at the joining sites of the V, D, and J genes. Expression of these markers and the different variants of the immunoglobulin (BCR) complex-molecules can be studied with flow-cytometry (15).

Most knowledge about B cell development in BM came from mouse studies; however, detailed insight into normal human BCP development is important to identify and unravel pathophysiological processes in hematological malignancies and primary immunodeficiencies (PID), caused by genetic defects (16). In turn, BCP analysis in genetically-defined PID can help elucidating the role of specific genes in BCP development (13, 17), because absence (or dysfunction) of essential proteins cause a full or incomplete block of maturation at specific developmental stages (18–20).

Here, we studied BCP differentiation in BM from both healthy controls and patients with a well-defined genetic defect in V(D)J recombination or pre-BCR signaling, to further unravel the normal immunophenotypic profiles of BM BCP at distinct stages of maturation and to determine the type of differentiation blockades caused by specific genetic defects. In multiple cycles of design, testing, evaluation, and redesign, we developed a 10-color antibody combination and applied novel data analysis strategies based on multivariate (principal component and viSNE) analysis (21) that allowed more detailed characterization of previously described BCP populations. This 10-color antibody combination was first validated against a conventional 4-color panel (7, 15, 18, 22). Secondly, we analyzed Ig gene rearrangement status and the gating strategy based on BCR-associated markers (cyCD79a, cyIgμ, IgM, IgD, CD19) was compared with gating based on membrane markers such as CD10 and CD20, as also done in the literature (7, 23–25). Gating based on BCR-associated markers allowed us to define the crucial steps of B cell development better than gating based on other non-BCR-associated surface markers alone, while intracellular markers emerged as essential to adequately delineate BCP development.

MATERIALS AND METHODS

Bone Marrow Samples

BM samples from healthy controls were left over samples from healthy children who donated BM for transplantation into a diseased sibling or were collected from patients that had a BM biopsy to rule out other diseases than lymphoid PID. The latter BM samples were considered to be normal when no malignant cells were detected in combination with a normal BCP differentiation pattern upon standard diagnostic testing. Patient BM samples were collected for PID-diagnostics. Both normal BM samples and patient BM samples in this study were obtained with informed consent according to the guidelines of the local medical ethics committee of the Erasmus MC (MEC-2013-026) and the LUMC (P08.001).

Flow Cytometric Immunophenotyping and Repertoire Analysis of Bone Marrow

Flow cytometric immunophenotyping of BM samples was performed on a LSR Fortessa (BD Biosciences, San Jose, CA) with instrument setting according to EuroFlow SOP (26). Following the EuroFlow bulk-lysis SOP (26, 27), cells were stained for surface membrane (sm) and intracellular markers in two consecutive steps. The following surface stainings -fluorochrome conjugate (clone)- were used: IgM-BV510 (MHM-88) CD38-BV605 (HIT2) and CD20-PB (2H7) were all from Biolegend (San Diego, CA); CD34-APC (8G12) and IgD-PeCF594 (IA6) were both from BD Biosciences); CD19-PC7 (J3-119) was purchased from Beckman Coulter (Fullerton, CA); and CD10-APC-C750 (HI10a) was obtained from Cytognos (Salamanca, Spain). Sustained cells were fixed and permeabilized using the Fix&Perm reagent kit (An der Grub, Vienna, Austria) according to manufacturer's instructions, and further stained for intracellular markers: IgM-PerCPcy5.5 (MHM-88) from Biolegend; TdT-FITC (HT6) purchased from (Supertechs, Rockville, MD); and CD79a-PE (HM47) purchased from Beckman Coulter) (see **Table 1** for complete panel).

Patient BM samples were analyzed in parallel with a diagnostic 4-color panel as previously described (7, 18), for comparison of the new 10-color panel to the 4-color diagnostic panel (gold standard). Based on the 4-color protocol the main precursor B-cell populations were defined as follows: pro-B-cells as $CD22^+CD19^-$; pre-B-I cells as $CD19^+cyIg\mu^-$, pre-B-II cells as $CD19^+cyIg\mu^+IgM^-$; immature cells as $CD19^+IgM^+IgD^-$ and $CD19^+IgM^+IgD^+$. For calculation the composition of the precursor B-cell compartment mature B-cells are excluded, because mature B-cells can also arise from peripheral contamination. An overview of the antibodies used in all panels can be found in **Table 1**.

For data was analysis with Infinicyt (Version 1.8, Cytognos) and Cytobank (Cytobank, Inc, Santa Clara, CA, USA) software programs were used. Principle component analysis was performed with the Infinicyt software. This method calculates the most discriminating projections based on selected parameters, into a single Automated Population Separator (APS) bi-dimensional graph. Multiple APS graphs (APS1, APS2 etc.) can be generated, depending on which parameters contribute more or less to the principle components on the X-axis and Y-axis. ViSNE projection (21) was calculated using Cytobank (Cytobank, Inc, Santa Clara, CA, USA) (28). This method generates a 2D dotplot in which the X- and Y-axis are defined by virtual parameters called tSNE1 and tSNE2, in which all events are projected integrating information on all selected parameters. In a viSNE plot the distance of one event to other events represents how similar events are, with the most similar events plotting closest to each other (21).

For repertoire analysis, two BM samples without malignant cells and with normal BCP differentiation (determined with standard diagnostic testing) were enriched for B cells using a RosetteSepp human B-cell enrichment cocktail (Stem cell Technologies, Vancouver, Canada) according to the manufacturer's instructions, as described elsewhere (29). Subsequently, the B-cell enriched samples were frozen in liquid nitrogen and thawed prior to sorting. Sorting was done with the same 10-color antibody combinations as described above on an FACS Aria-III flow cytometer (BD Biosciences). After sorting, cells were washed and DNA was isolated using a direct lysis procedure as described elsewhere (30). From this DNA, *IGH* rearrangements were amplified in a 2-step PCR and sequenced by NGS. *IGH* rearrangements were amplified (35 cycles) using the forward VH1-6 FR2 and reverse JH consensus EuroClonality/BIOMED-2 primers, extended with Illumina P5 and P7 adapter sequence (31). Subsequently, PCR products were purified by gel extraction (Qiagen, Valencia, CA), followed by a nested PCR reaction (12 cycles) to include the sample-specific indices and Illumina sequencing adapters using primers from the Illumina TruSeq Custom Amplicon Index Kit (Illumina, San Diego, CA). The final PCR product concentration was measured using the Quant-it Picogreen dsDNA assay (Invitrogen, Carlsbad, CA). The libraries were analyzed by NGS (221 bp paired-end) on the MiSeq platform (Illumina, San Diego, CA, USA) with use of an Illumina MiSeq Reagent Kit V3, according to the manufacturer's protocol (Illumina, San Diego, CA, USA). Paired sequences were aligned using paired-end read merger (PEAR) (32), and the fastq files were converted to fasta files (33). Subsequently, the sequences were trimmed to remove the primer sequence and uploaded in IMGT/High-V-Quest (34); subsequently, the IMGT output files were analyzed using the ARGalaxy tool (https://bioinf-galaxian.erasmusmc.nl/argalaxy) (35). For analysis only a single sequence per clone (defined as same V gene, same J gene and the nucleotide sequence of the CDR3 region) were included. In-frame IGH rearrangements were defined to have an in-frame rearrangement without a stop codon. Unproductive IGH rearrangements were either out-of-frame rearrangements or in-frame rearrangements with a stop codon.

TABLE 1 | Composition and technical information on reagents of the 10-color EuroFlow BCP tube.

Fluorochrome	PB	BV510	BV605	FITC	PE	PE-CF594	PerCP-Cy5,5	PE-Cy7	APC	Alexa750
Target	CD20	IgM	CD38	TdT	CD79a	IgD	cyIgM	CD19	CD34	CD10
clone	2H7	MHM-88	HIT2	HT6	HM47	IA6	MHM-88	J3-119	8G12	HI10a
Volsume (undiluted)	1 µl	1.3 µl	1 µl	10 µl	5 µl	3 µl	2.5 µl	5 µl	2.5 µl	5 µl

Shaded fields indicate intracellular markers.

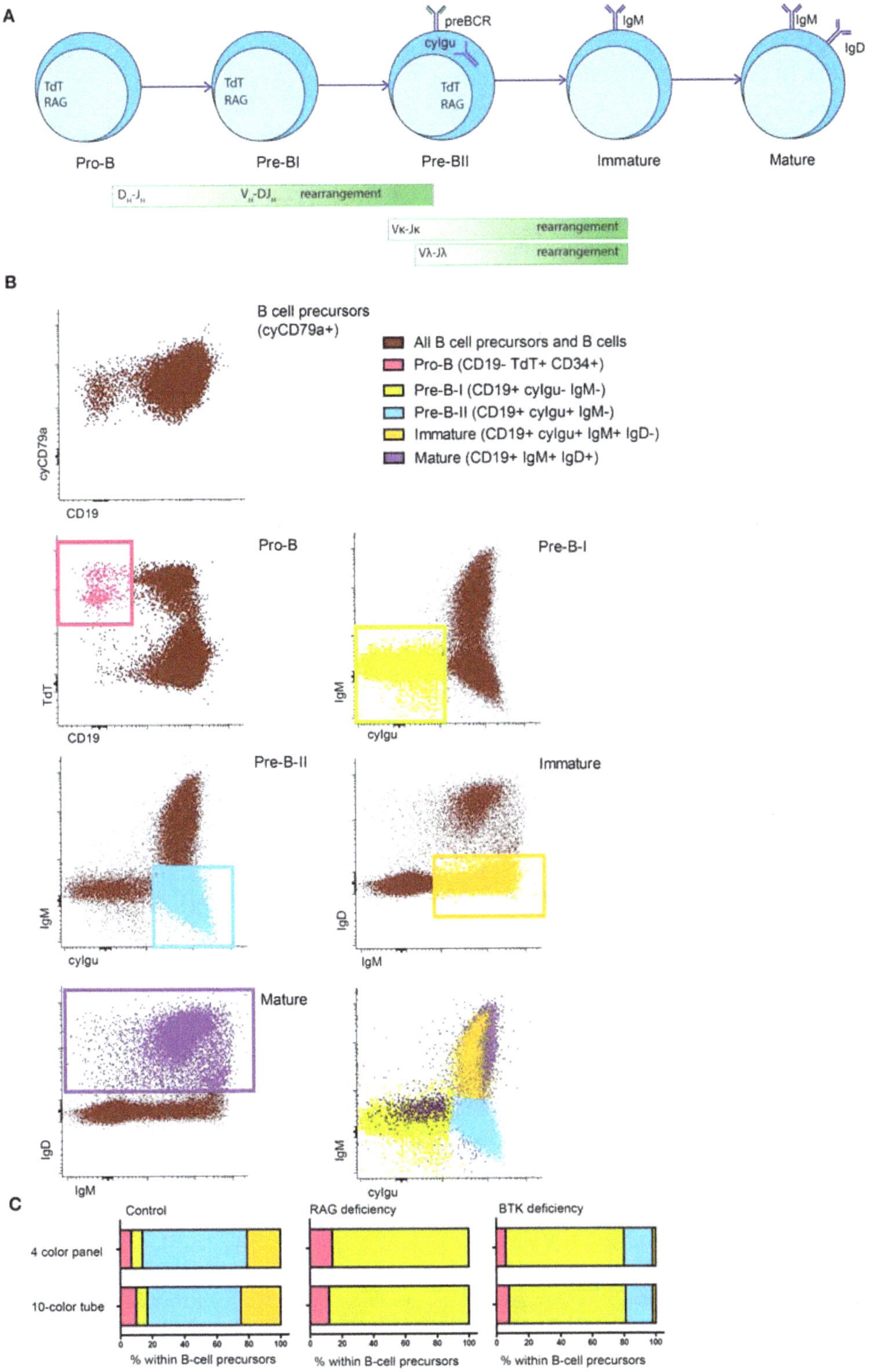

FIGURE 1 | Major BCP subsets in human bone marrow. **(A)** Schematic representation of the BCP subsets in human bone marrow, the green bars indicate when recombination processes take place. **(B)** Population definition based on BCR-related markers. All cyCD79a expressing cells are considered BCP or B cells. Pro-B cells are defined as CD19- TdT+, pre-BI cells are defined as CD19+ cyIgμ- IgM-, pre-BII cells are defined as CD19+ cyIgμ+ IgM-, immature B cells are defined as CD19+ IgM+ IgD- and mature B cells are defined as CD19+ IgM+ IgD+. **(C)** BCP subset distribution in the same sample that was acquired in parallel with two different panels. Population definition was in both cases done as indicated above.

RESULTS

Subset Definition Based on BCR-Associated Markers Is Consistent Between Different Panels

To study human BM, we designed and validated a 10-color flowcytometry antibody combination to be stained in a single tube (**Table 1**), to make optimal use of available material and integrate information about both intracellular and extracellular markers on each individual cell. This 10-color tube was tested against a previously validated 4-color diagnostic panel (7, 18) using BM samples from healthy controls and PID patients. B cells and BCP were defined as cyCD79a+. The five major B-cell populations (pro-B, pre-BI, preB-II, immature and mature B cells) (**Figure 1A**) were gated based on the staining profiles for the BCR-associated markers CD19, nTdT, cyIgμ, IgM, and IgD (**Figure 1B** and **Supplementary Material**), as defined by the previously observed subset distribution with the 4-color panel used as gold standard. Since IgMD^{+} cells (mature B cells) can also be detected in peripheral blood (PB), they were not considered as a formal BCP stage. In ten independent (n = 4 controls and 6 patients) samples both panels revealed the same precursor B-cell subset distribution, as illustrated by three representative cases in **Figure 1C**: one of normal BCP development, a RAG deficient patient and a BTK deficient patient. This indicates that gating based on BCR-associated markers is consistent between both panels and gives comparable results in both healthy controls and PID patients with defects in BCR signaling or V(D)J recombination (**Figure 1C**).

B-Cell Populations Defined Based on BCR-Associated Markers Only Show Heterogeneous Intra-Population Phenotypes

Based on BCR-associated markers only (cyCD79a, CD19, cyIgμ, IgM, and IgD), 4 distinct subsets of BCP were identified/defined as described above. Further analysis of the expression profiles for other markers (i.e. TdT, CD34, CD10, CD20, and CD38) within these four B-cell populations showed highly heterogeneous patterns, particularly within pre-BI and pre-BII BCP (**Figure 2A**). Thus, pre-BI BCP were mainly TdT+ and CD34+, but some cells had lost one or both markers, while, at the same time, they were CD10+ and CD20- ruling out they could be unswitched memory B-cells. Similarly heterogeneous patterns of expression were observed for CD10 and CD38 (most cells being positive but a minority negative) and CD20 (most cells CD20- but some were CD20+), pointing out the existence of multiple subsets of pre-BI cells (**Figure 2A**). In turn, pre-BII cells, were cyIgμ-positive while mostly negative for CD34 and TdT, but with some CD34+ and TdT+ pre-B-II cells. CD20 expression was highly heterogeneous within this population with progressively more CD20 molecules per cell (**Figure 2A**). Multivariate (e.g., viSNE) analysis confirmed the presence of minor subsets of TdT− CD34− pre-BI B-cells and CD34+ TdT+ pre-BII cells, both populations showing progressively higher expression levels of CD20, similarly to immature B-lymphocytes (**Figure 2B**).

Asynchronous Expression of Non-BCR-Associated Markers in BCP Stages Defined by BCR-Associated Patterns

In order to gain further insight into the relationship between the pattern of expression of non-Ig related markers and cyIgμ, we compared BM pre-BI and pre-BII cells from controls to patients with RAG-deficiency and BTK-deficiency. As described above a fraction of all pre-BI cells in controls, loses CD34 and/or TdT expression, and some upregulate CD20 (**Figure 3**). In RAG-deficient patient, TdT expression remains intact, but loss of CD34 together with some upregulation of CD20 was observed. Thus, it appears that BCP can lose CD34 and upregulate CD20 in the absence of a functionally rearranged heavy chain while they do not loose TdT. In BTK-deficiency a similar profile was observed. In addition, within the pre-BII BCP of controls and BTK-deficient patients, some cells retained CD34 and/or TdT expression, although they already expressed cyIgμ. Since RAG deficient patients do not have pre-BII cells, we could not compare this subset for these patients. Altogether, there results point out the existence of different kinetics of expression of BCR-associated and other non-BCR-related markers during normal B-cell maturation. Additionally, RAG or BTK deficient cells can lose CD34 expression, without downregulating TdT.

Dissection of Multiple BCP Maturation Pathways in BM

Multivariate analysis of normal BM BCP based on all markers evaluated simultaneously revealed the existence of up to three (parallel) distinct maturation pathways, where the BCR-associated cyIgM and CD20 represent the major discriminating markers (**Supplemental Figure 1**). Based on a data set of 5 healthy control BM samples, a reference BM profile was built using the APS1 view –Principal Component (PC) 1 *vs.* PC2- of the in Infinicyt software (36) (**Figure 4A**), after plotting the 2SD lines corresponding to each reference population of normal BCP. Once this reference profile has been built, BCP events from a sixth, independent healthy donor was plotted against it (**Figure 4B**), the events neatly falling within the ranges of the other 5 healthy controls BM samples. In contrast, when BM BCP from a patient with RAG-deficiency and another child with BTK-deficiency were plotted against the reference profile, profiles with a clear blockade appeared with most cells exclusively present within the first maturation pathway. In the BTK deficient patient, a small fraction of the BCP cells reached the pre-B-II stage (**Figure 4C**). Furthermore, in this representation, some patient cells fell outside the 2SD lines of both pre-BI and pre-BII suggesting the existence of aberrant phenotypic profiles.

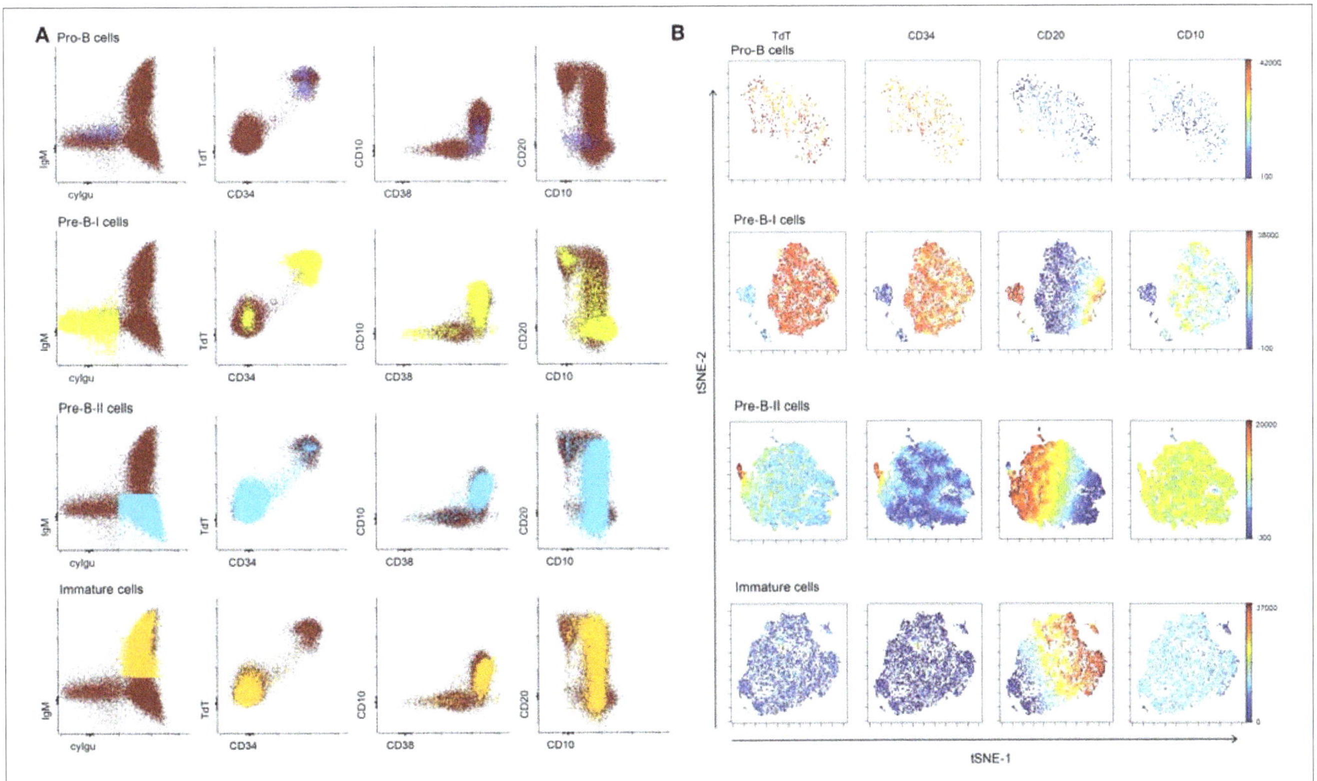

FIGURE 2 | Heterogeneity within BCP subsets. **(A)** Dotplots of a representative normal bone marrow sample, showing all cyCD79a+ B cells in bone marrow. Populations of interest are highlighted in a different color: pro-B cells in pink, pre-B-I cells in green, pre-B-II cells in blue, immature cells in orange. **(B)** Results of a viSNE analysis of individual B-cell precursor subsets, represented by tSNE-1 vs. tSNE-2 plots. The color scale represents the intensity of the stain for individual markers: TdT, CD34, CD20, CD10, and CD38.

IGH Gene Rearrangement Profile of BCP at the pre-BI and pre-BII Stage Showing Distinct Patterns of Expression of CD34 and TdT

When we focused on the cells that were neither within the 2SD interval of the pre-BI cells nor in the 2SD interval of pre-BII cells, we found that they are present in normal BCP differentiation (between 1 and 3% of all BCP cells), although not as many as in the patient samples (**Figure 5A**). These cells are defined as pre-BI or pre-BII based on the absence or presence of cyIgμ, but the expression of TdT, CD34, CD10, and CD20 is asynchronous with their cyIgμ status (**Figure 5B**). We can divide the pre-BI cells in true pre-BI cells that are CD19+ cyIgμ- CD34+ TdT+ (pre-BI+/+) and another, more heterogeneous group that is CD19+ cyIgμ- but where CD34 and or TdT expression is negative (pre-BI-/-). These cells are not switched memory B cells coming from peripheral blood, because they all express both CD10 and CD38. The same split can be made within the pre-BII cells, dividing them in pre-BII cells that are CD19+ cyIgμ+ CD34− TdT− (pre-BII-/-) and a heterogeneous group that is CD19+, cyIgμ+ but that still have CD34, TdT or both these markers (pre-BII+/+). In the APS views that are based on all BCPs, these cells end up between pre-BI and pre-BII. If we create an APS view of only the pre-BI and pre-BII stages, we can examine how heterogeneous these populations are (**Figures 5C,D**).

Rearrangement Status Classifies the Intermediate Stages

To further dissect this, we sorted the pre-B populations into four populations: pre-BI +/+ (CD19+ cyIgμ- CD34+ TdT+), pre-BI-/- (CD19+ cyIgμ− CD34- TdT−), pre-BII-/- (CD19+ cyIgμ+ CD34− TdT−) and pre-BII+/+ (CD19+ cyIgμ+ CD34+ TdT+). We isolated DNA from these subsets and sequenced complete IGH rearrangements using next-generation sequencing. We found that in the pre-BI+/+ cells, the majority of complete rearrangements is non-productive with an in-frame: non-productive ratio of 1:9, which is in line with the observation that these cells do not express cyIgu, yet (**Figure 5E**). In the pre-BII-/- cells, the in-frame: non-productive ratio is 4:1, with ~80% of rearrangements in frame, which is in line with the observation that these cells all express cyIgu. In the pre-BI-/- population, the in-frame: non-productive ratio is 3:1, and in the pre-BII +/+ population, this ratio is also 3:1. In these populations, the relative amount of in-frame complete rearrangements is approximately the same, however, in one population the cells do not express cyIgu, whereas they do in the other populations. This indicates that in the pre-BI-/- cells in-frame rearrangements are present,

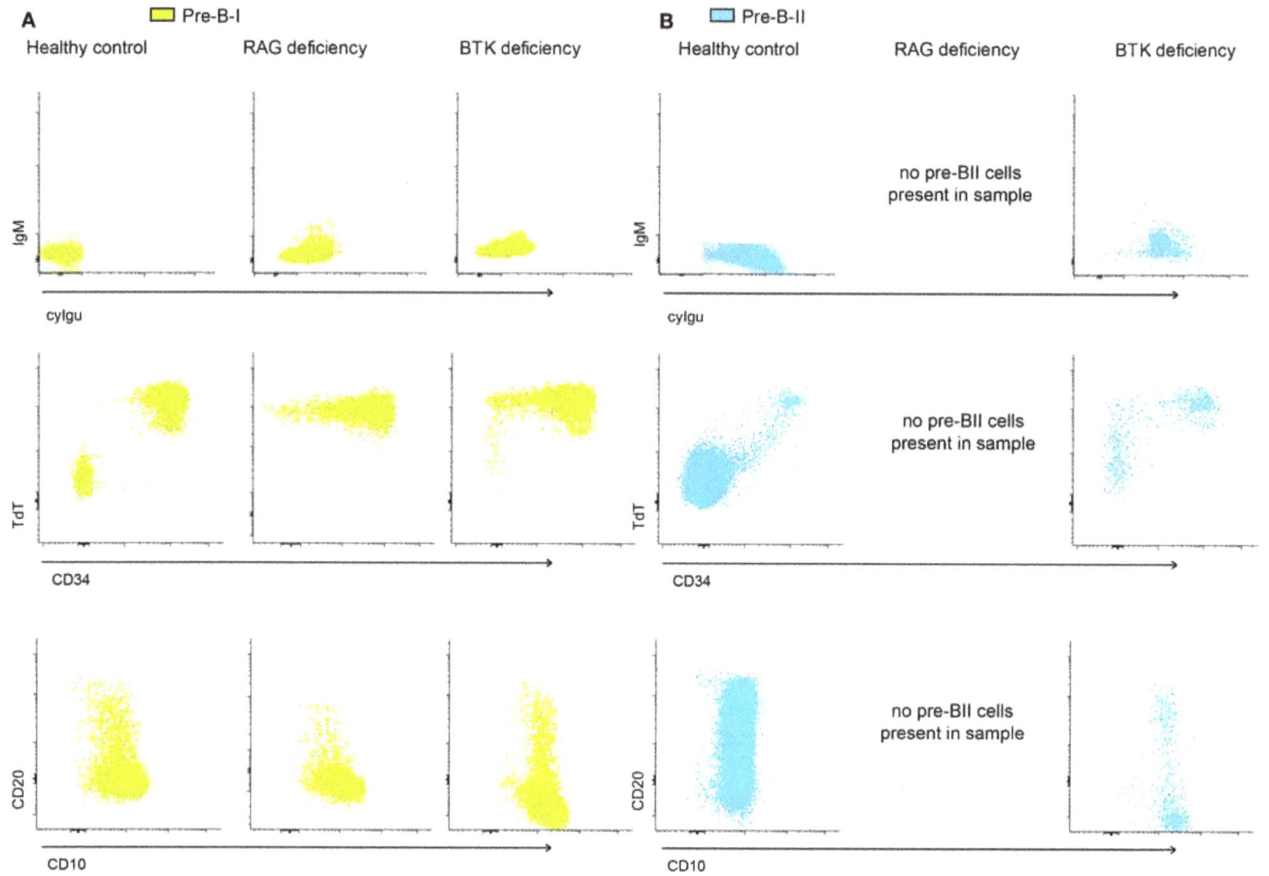

FIGURE 3 | pre-BI and pre-BII marker expression in control and patient samples. **(A)** Dot plots representing pre-BI cells from a control sample, and two patient samples, indicating the uncoupling of expression of cyIgμ and surface markers like CD34, CD20, and CD10. In both the control and the patients, cells without cyIgμ can lose CD34 expression and gain CD20 expression. **(B)** Dot plots representing pre-BII cells from a control sample, and two patient samples. In both the control and the patients, cells with cyIgμ expression can still express CD34 and TdT, and CD20 expression is heterogeneous.

but they are either not productive (i.e., not leading to a functional protein) or they are not (yet) expressed. The pre-BII +/+ already express cyIgu, but did not yet downregulate CD34 and TdT. In addition, we analyzed the CDR3 lengths of the productive rearrangements as well as proportion of IGH CDR3s with $\geq$3, 2, 1, or 0 positive charges (**Figures 5F,G**). The CDR3 lengths of productive rearrangements of pre-B-I-/- cells were longer than the productive rearrangements of pre-B-I +/+ and pre-B-II cells, which could be explained by a lower number of nucleotide deletions. The proportions of IGH CDR3 charges did not differ between the four subpopulations.

DISCUSSION

In this study, we designed and validated a 10-color flow cytometry panel, to study human BCP development in BM of immune deficient patients at crucial developmental thresholds in more detail than was done previously. In our standardized measurements, we could reliably gate populations according to BCR-related markers. This allowed us to superimpose PID samples over healthy controls and describe the deviations from normal development as found in patients. Unexpectedly, when we included information from additional (non-BCR) markers, we found heterogeneity, especially within the preB-I and preB-II populations, during which V(D)J recombination takes place with expression of surface markers that seem asynchronous to the expression of cyIgμ. NGS analysis of complete IGH rearrangements in sorted populations was used to determine the rearrangement status at the DNA level.

We showed that BCR-related marker based population definition is consistent over samples and different panels, but this results in heterogeneous populations when other markers, like CD34, TdT, and CD20 are considered. Upon more in-depth study of expression patterns of these markers, we found that in some specific populations, expression of these markers is asynchronous to the process of BCR-formation. This effect is more visible in patients with defects in V(D)J-recombination. Specifically, we found that CD20 can be upregulated in the absence of cyIgμ expression and that cells can lose TdT expression and CD34 expression without having expression of heavy chain protein in the cytoplasm.

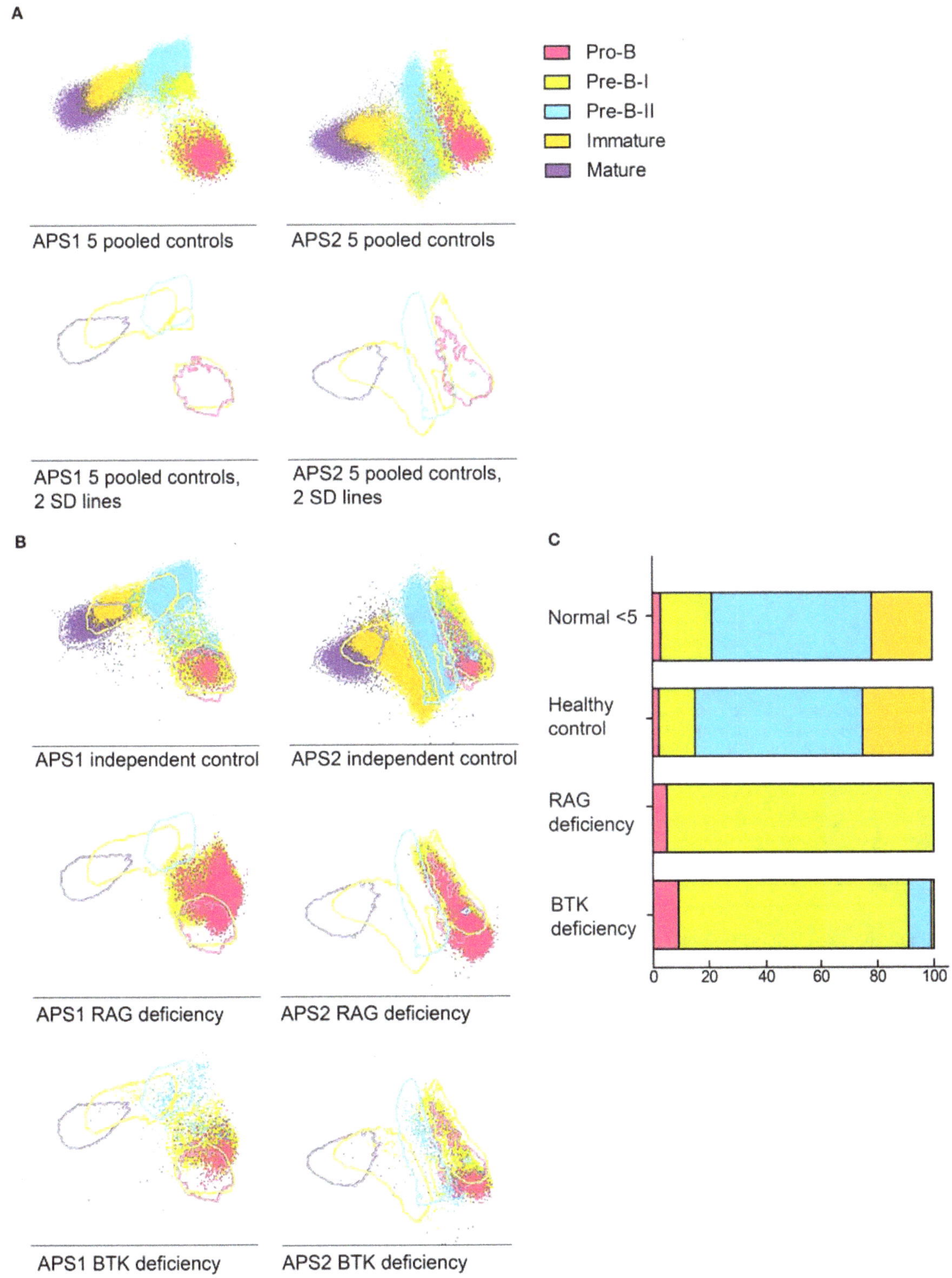

FIGURE 4 | Supervised APS view of BCP populations in healthy bone marrow ($n = 5$) indicated by lines at 2SD intervals. **(A)** BCP populations in a pool of 5 healthy bone marrow samples that were used to create the APS view. Lines indicate the 2 SD range of each population, dot indicate individual cells. The different populations are indicated by the different colors. **(B)** 2 SD lines of BCP populations derived from a pool of 5 healthy donors, dots indicate total BCP from a sixth healthy donor, a RAG deficient patient and a BTK deficient patient, plotted against the reference pool. **(C)** Bars indicate the BCP subset distribution of each sample, compared to age matched controls (<5 years).

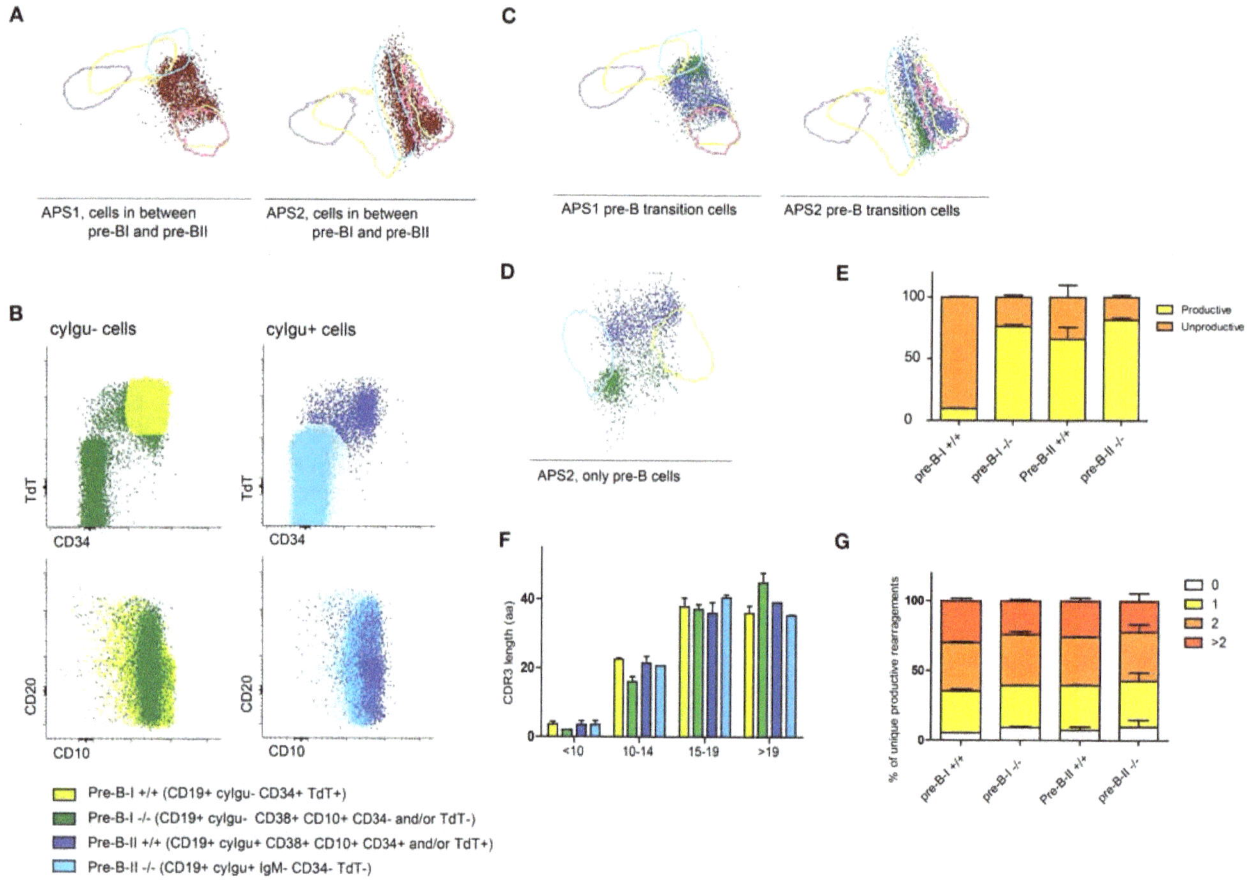

FIGURE 5 | Further dissection of the BCP compartment. **(A)** APS views indicating the cells that are outside the 2SD lines of the pre-B-I and pre-B-II populations of healthy controls. **(B)** Expression of CD34, TdT, CD10, and CD20 within cyIgμ- (in green) and cyIgμ+ cells. All cells here are CD19+ CD10+ CD38+ indicating that they are bone marrow derived B cells. **(C)** APS views indicating the cells that are outside the 2SD lines of the pre-BI and pre-BII populations of healthy controls, color coded as in B. **(D)** APS view supervised on pre-BI and pre-BII cells, separating the transitioning pre-B cells further. **(E)** Distribution of in-frame and out-of-frame DNA-rearrangements in sorted pre-B subpopulations. **(F)** CDR3 length of productive rearrangements of the four sorted pre-B-I and pre-B-II populations. **(G)** The proportion of CDR3 regions with ≥3, 2, 1, or 0 positive charges.

We combined the population-gating based strategy that is often used in flow cytometry with principle component analysis. We showed that the BCP populations seem to overlap, indicating a continuous process rather that a step-wise differentiation. This is in line with asynchronous marker expression that we see between surface markers e.g. each cell seems to up-and-down regulate its phenotype markers at its own pace. Even more, some phenotype markers that were previously thought to be V(D)J-recombination dependent, seem to progress even in the absence of cyIgμ expression, as indicated by loss of CD34 and gain of CD20 in patients with genetic defects in V(D)J-recombination. Some of the cellular phenotypes that we found in controls are more common in genetically defined patient samples. This indicates that, even though cells cannot successfully rearrange their IgH-locus, as is the case in RAG deficiency (10, 37), they will still lose CD34 expression as if they are progressing to the next stage. In addition to that, we found that CD20 expression is gradually increasing over the course of several stages. However, CD20 expression is heterogeneous in many populations. Especially in patient samples, we often detected high CD20 expression in populations that were assumed to be early in B-cell differentiation. Even though the exact role of CD20 on B cells is not found yet, it is still a useful marker indicating B-cell development and if highly expressed in combination with loss of CD10 and CD38, indicating maturity of the B cells. CD20 expression does not seem to be related with BCR-rearrangement.

Both in PID patients and in control samples, we identified cells outside the reference borders of the defined populations (e.g., pre-BI and pre-BII) in the APS plots, although the cell numbers were much lower in control samples. Especially in the RAG deficient patient this is striking, because it seems as if some cells can progress in surface marker expression by expressing CD20 and loosing CD34, without having a functionally rearranged heavy chain. This further supports the idea that expression of CD20 and CD34 is not in all cells strictly linked to IGH gene rearrangement status.

To further dissect this, we sorted preB-I and preB-II cells and further divided these populations based on their CD34 and TdT expression. DNA extracted from these cell populations was used to study complete IGH-rearrangements using NGS. In preB-I+/+ cells we showed that close to 90% of detectable IGH gene rearrangements are non-productive. Since these cells do not express cyIgu yet, we hypothesize that these cells have not yet obtained an in-frame IGH rearrangement, and thus they still express CD34 and TdT. In preB-II cells that are CD34- TdT-, around 75% of detectable IGH rearrangements were in-frame. These cells all express cyIgu, and some have an non-productive rearrangement on one allele combined with an in-frame rearrangement on the second allele, which explains the 25% of non-productive rearrangements in this population. The preB-II +/+ cells also contain ~75% of in-frame rearrangements. Possibly, these cells have only just completed their in-frame rearrangement, starting already expressing cyIgu but still need to downregulate CD34 and TdT. However, our data is not sufficient to conclude this. Also, we detected around 75% in-frame rearrangements in preB-I-/- cells. These cells have an in frame IGH rearrangement at the DNA level, but they do not (yet?) express cyIgu protein. To further investigate this, single-cell analysis on DNA, RNA and protein level might give further insight in how and why V(D)J recombination status and phenotypic marker expression are linked.

In conclusion, we have designed and validated a standardized 10-color staining and analytical tools for the analysis of BCP compartment in human BM. Our data indicate that BCP differentiation is not a single linear differentiation pathway, but rather a complex process of V(D)J recombination-driven checkpoints, divergence, parallel pathways and convergence to form a unique and functional BCR. The data also support the notion that B cell maturation is asynchronous, implying that precursor B-cells do not differentiate as full population between the different stages, but rather transit as a continuum, which can be influenced in part by V(D)J recombination-driven checkpoints. Due to this continuum, small populations of cells are captured as they transit between stages and, thus, have intermediate patterns of marker expression. Understanding the process of BCP differentiation requires an integrated approach of single-cell DNA, RNA and protein analysis, which can be applied for studying blockades in BCP differentiation pathways of genetically defined immunodeficient patients. We propose that our immunophenotyping panel can be used in multi-center studies with the standardization stringency developed by the EuroFlow consortium (26), thus allowing to mutually compare the data-files generated on patients with primary immunodeficiency with those of individuals with undisturbed B cell development.

AUTHOR CONTRIBUTIONS

MB, TK, AO, and JD: contributed conception and design of the study. MW, TK, MP-A, LM, HI, FK, AL, and QL: performed the data acquisition and data analysis. MW and MB wrote the manuscript. All authors contributed to manuscript, read, and approved the submitted version.

FUNDING

TK were supported by Ministry of Education, Youth and Sports NPU I no. LO1604 and CZ.2.16/3.1.00/21540. The EuroFlow meetings and development of the 10-color BCP-BM tube was supported by the EuroFlow Consortium. The IGH repertoire studies were supported by the Dutch Organization for Scientific Research (NWO/ZonMW VIDI grant 91712323 to MB).

ACKNOWLEDGMENTS

The authors would like to thank Ingrid Pico-Knijnenburg and Peter J. M. Valk for help with the NGS runs.

REFERENCES

1. Ghia P, ten Boekel E, Rolink AG, Melchers F. B-cell development: a comparison between mouse and man. *Immunol Today.* (1998) 19:480–5. doi: 10.1016/S0167-5699(98)01330-9
2. LeBien TW. Fates of human B-cell precursors. *Blood.* (2000) 96:9–23. doi: 10.1182/blood.V96.1.9
3. Loken MR, Shah VO, Dattilio KL, Civin CI. Flow cytometric analysis of human bone marrow. II. Normal B lymphocyte development. *Blood.* (1987) 70:1316–24. doi: 10.1182/blood.V70.5.1316.1316
4. Loken MR, Shah VO, Hollander Z, Civin CI. Flow cytometric analysis of normal B lymphoid development. *Pathol Immunopathol Res.* (1988) 7:357–70. doi: 10.1159/000157129

5. Busslinger M. Transcriptional control of early B cell development. *Annu Rev Immunol.* (2004) 22:55–79. doi: 10.1146/annurev.immunol.22.012703.104807
6. Ghia P, ten Boekel E, Sanz E, de la Hera A, Rolink A, Melchers F. Ordering of human bone marrow B lymphocyte precursors by single-cell polymerase chain reaction analyses of the rearrangement status of the immunoglobulin H and L chain gene loci. *J Exp Med.* (1996) 184:2217–29. doi: 10.1084/jem.184.6.2217
7. van Zelm MC, van der Burg M, de Ridder D, Barendregt BH, de Haas EF, Reinders MJ, et al. Ig gene rearrangement steps are initiated in early human precursor B cell subsets and correlate with specific transcription factor expression. *J Immunol.* (2005) 175:5912–22. doi: 10.4049/jimmunol.175.9.5912
8. Meffre E, Milili M, Blanco-Betancourt C, Antunes H, Nussenzweig MC, Schiff C. Immunoglobulin heavy chain expression shapes the B cell receptor repertoire in human B cell development. *J Clin Invest.* (2001) 108:879–86. doi: 10.1172/JCI13051
9. Geier JK, Schlissel MS. Pre-BCR signals and the control of Ig gene rearrangements. *Semin Immunol.* (2006) 18:31–9. doi: 10.1016/j.smim.2005.11.001
10. Oettinger MA, Schatz DG, Gorka C, Baltimore D. RAG-1 and RAG-2, adjacent genes that synergistically activate V(D)J recombination. *Science.* (1990) 248:1517–23. doi: 10.1126/science.2360047
11. van Gent DC, McBlane JF, Ramsden DA, Sadofsky MJ, Hesse JE, Gellert M. Initiation of V(D)J recombinations in a cell-free system by RAG1 and RAG2 proteins. *Curr Top Microbiol Immunol.* (1996) 217:1–10. doi: 10.1007/978-3-642-50140-1_1
12. Herzog S, Reth M, Jumaa H. Regulation of B-cell proliferation and differentiation by pre-B-cell receptor signalling. *Nat Rev Immunol.* (2009) 9:195–205. doi: 10.1038/nri2491
13. Espeli M, Rossi B, Mancini SJ, Roche P, Gauthier L, Schiff C. Initiation of pre-B cell receptor signaling: common and distinctive features in human and mouse. *Semin Immunol.* (2006) 18:56–66. doi: 10.1016/j.smim.2005.11.002
14. Stadhouders R, de Bruijn MJ, Rother MB, Yuvaraj S, Ribeiro de Almeida C, Kolovos P, et al. Pre-B cell receptor signaling induces immunoglobulin kappa locus accessibility by functional redistribution of enhancer-mediated chromatin interactions. *PLoS Biol.* (2014) 12:e1001791. doi: 10.1371/journal.pbio.1001791
15. van Lochem EG, van der Velden VH, Wind HK, te Marvelde JG, Westerdaal NA, van Dongen JJ. Immunophenotypic differentiation patterns of normal hematopoiesis in human bone marrow: reference patterns for age-related changes and disease-induced shifts. *Cytometry B Clin Cytom.* (2004) 60:1–13. doi: 10.1002/cyto.b.20008
16. Gathmann B, Grimbacher B, Beauté J, Dudoit Y, Mahlaoui N, Fischer A, et al. The European internet-based patient and research database for primary immunodeficiencies: results 2006-2008. *Clin Exp Immunol.* (2009) 157(Suppl. 1):3–11. doi: 10.1111/j.1365-2249.2009.03954.x
17. Schiff C, Lemmers B, Deville A, Fougereau M, Meffre E. Autosomal primary immunodeficiencies affecting human bone marrow B-cell differentiation. *Immunol Rev.* (2000) 178:91–8. doi: 10.1034/j.1600-065X.2000.17804.x
18. Noordzij JG, de Bruin-Versteeg S, Comans-Bitter WM, Hartwig NG, Hendriks RW, de Groot R, et al. Composition of precursor B-cell compartment in bone marrow from patients with X-linked agammaglobulinemia compared with healthy children. *Pediatr Res.* (2002) 51:159–68. doi: 10.1203/00006450-200202000-00007
19. Noordzij JG, Verkaik NS, van der Burg M, van Veelen LR, de Bruin-Versteeg S, Wiegant W, et al. Radiosensitive SCID patients with Artemis gene mutations show a complete B-cell differentiation arrest at the pre-B-cell receptor checkpoint in bone marrow. *Blood.* (2003) 101:1446–52. doi: 10.1182/blood-2002-01-0187
20. Pearl ER, Vogler LB, Okos AJ, Crist WM, Lawton AR, Cooper MD. B lymphocyte precursors in human bone marrow: an analysis of normal individuals and patients with antibody-deficiency states. *J Immunol.* (1978) 120:1169–75.
21. Amir el-AD, Davis KL, Tadmor MD, Simonds EF, Levine JH, Bendall SC, et al. viSNE enables visualization of high dimensional single-cell data and reveals phenotypic heterogeneity of leukemia. *Nat Biotechnol.* (2013) 31:545–52. doi: 10.1038/nbt.2594
22. Anzilotti C, Kienzler AK, Lopez-Granados E, Gooding S, Davies B, Pandit H, et al. Key stages of bone marrow B-cell maturation are defective in patients with common variable immunodeficiency disorders. *J Allergy Clin Immunol.* (2015) 136:487–90 e2. doi: 10.1016/j.jaci.2014.12.1943
23. Dulau Florea AE, Braylan RC, Schafernak KT, Williams KW, Daub J, Goyal RK, et al. Abnormal B-Cell Maturation in the Bone Marrow of Patients with Germline Mutations in PIK3CD. *J Allergy Clin Immunol.* (2016) 139:1032–5.e6. doi: 10.1016/j.jaci.2016.08.028
24. Lougaris V, Baronio M, Masneri S, Lorenzini T, Cattivelli K, Tampella G, et al. Correlation of bone marrow abnormalities, peripheral lymphocyte subsets and clinical features in uncomplicated common variable immunodeficiency (CVID) patients. *Clin Immunol.* (2016) 163:10–3. doi: 10.1016/j.clim.2015.12.006
25. Kohn LA, Seet CS, Scholes J, Codrea F, Chan R, Zaidi-Merchant S, et al. Human lymphoid development in the absence of common gamma-chain receptor signaling. *J Immunol.* (2014) 192:5050–8. doi: 10.4049/jimmunol.1303496
26. Kalina T, Flores-Montero J, van der Velden VH, Martin-Ayuso M, Böttcher S, Ritgen M, et al. EuroFlow standardization of flow cytometer instrument settings and immunophenotyping protocols. *Leukemia.* (2012) 26:1986–2010. doi: 10.1038/leu.2012.122
27. Flores-Montero J, Sanoja-Flores L, Paiva B, Puig N, Garcia-Sanchez O, Böttcher S, et al. Next Generation Flow for highly sensitive and standardized detection of minimal residual disease in multiple myeloma. *Leukemia.* (2017) 31:2094–2103. doi: 10.1038/leu.2017.29
28. Kotecha N, Krutzik PO, Irish JM. Web-based analysis and publication of flow cytometry experiments. *Curr Protoc Cytom.* (2010) Chapter:Unit10.17. doi: 10.1002/0471142956.cy1017s53
29. Pelák O, KuŽílková D, Thürner D, Kiene ML, Stanar K, Stuchlý J, et al. Lymphocyte enrichment using CD81-targeted immunoaffinity matrix. *Cytometry A.* (2017) 91:62–72. doi: 10.1002/cyto.a.22918
30. van der Burg M, Kreyenberg H, Willasch A, Barendregt BH, Preuner S, Wątzinger F, et al. Standardization of DNA isolation from low cell numbers for chimerism analysis by PCR of short tandem repeats. *Leukemia.* (2011) 25:1467–70. doi: 10.1038/leu.2011.118
31. van Dongen JJ, Langerak AW, Brüggemann M, Evans PA, Hummel M, Lavender FL, et al. Design and standardization of PCR primers and protocols for detection of clonal immunoglobulin and T-cell receptor gene recombinations in suspect lymphoproliferations: report of the BIOMED-2 Concerted Action BMH4-CT98-3936. *Leukemia.* (2003) 17:2257–317. doi: 10.1038/sj.leu.2403202
32. Zhang J, Kobert K, Flouri T, Stamatakis A. *PEAR:* a fast and accurate Illumina Paired-End reAd mergeR. *Bioinformatics.* (2014) 30:614–20. doi: 10.1093/bioinformatics/btt593
33. Blankenberg D, Gordon A, Von Kuster G, Coraor N, Taylor J, Nekrutenko A, et al. Manipulation of FASTQ data with Galaxy. *Bioinformatics.* (2010) 26:1783–5. doi: 10.1093/bioinformatics/btq281
34. Alamyar E, Duroux P, Lefranc MP, Giudicelli V, Alamyar E. IMGT((R)) tools for the nucleotide analysis of immunoglobulin (IG) and T cell receptor (TR) V-(D)-J repertoires, polymorphisms, and IG mutations: IMGT/V-QUEST and IMGT/HighV-QUEST for NGS. *Methods Mol Biol.* (2012) 882:569–604. doi: 10.1007/978-1-61779-842-9_32

35. IJspeert H, van Schouwenburg PA, van Zessen D, Pico-Knijnenburg I, Stubbs AP, van der Burg M, et al. antigen receptor galaxy: a user-friendly, web-based tool for analysis and visualization of T and B Cell receptor repertoire data. *J Immunol.* (2017) 198:4156–65. doi: 10.4049/jimmunol.1601921
36. Costa ES, Pedreira CE, Barrena S, Lecrevisse Q, Flores J, Quijano S, et al. Automated pattern-guided principal component analysis vs expert-based immunophenotypic classification of B-cell chronic lymphoproliferative disorders: a step forward in the standardization of clinical immunophenotyping. *Leukemia.* (2010) 24:1927–33. doi: 10.1038/leu.2010.160
37. Notarangelo LD, Villa A, Schwarz K. RAG and RAG defects. *Curr Opin Immunol.* (1999) 11:435–42. doi: 10.1016/S0952-7915(99)80073-9

Permissions

All chapters in this book were first published by Frontiers; hereby published with permission under the Creative Commons Attribution License or equivalent. Every chapter published in this book has been scrutinized by our experts. Their significance has been extensively debated. The topics covered herein carry significant findings which will fuel the growth of the discipline. They may even be implemented as practical applications or may be referred to as a beginning point for another development.

The contributors of this book come from diverse backgrounds, making this book a truly international effort. This book will bring forth new frontiers with its revolutionizing research information and detailed analysis of the nascent developments around the world.

We would like to thank all the contributing authors for lending their expertise to make the book truly unique. They have played a crucial role in the development of this book. Without their invaluable contributions this book wouldn't have been possible. They have made vital efforts to compile up to date information on the varied aspects of this subject to make this book a valuable addition to the collection of many professionals and students.

This book was conceptualized with the vision of imparting up-to-date information and advanced data in this field. To ensure the same, a matchless editorial board was set up. Every individual on the board went through rigorous rounds of assessment to prove their worth. After which they invested a large part of their time researching and compiling the most relevant data for our readers.

The editorial board has been involved in producing this book since its inception. They have spent rigorous hours researching and exploring the diverse topics which have resulted in the successful publishing of this book. They have passed on their knowledge of decades through this book. To expedite this challenging task, the publisher supported the team at every step. A small team of assistant editors was also appointed to further simplify the editing procedure and attain best results for the readers.

Apart from the editorial board, the designing team has also invested a significant amount of their time in understanding the subject and creating the most relevant covers. They scrutinized every image to scout for the most suitable representation of the subject and create an appropriate cover for the book.

The publishing team has been an ardent support to the editorial, designing and production team. Their endless efforts to recruit the best for this project, has resulted in the accomplishment of this book. They are a veteran in the field of academics and their pool of knowledge is as vast as their experience in printing. Their expertise and guidance has proved useful at every step. Their uncompromising quality standards have made this book an exceptional effort. Their encouragement from time to time has been an inspiration for everyone.

The publisher and the editorial board hope that this book will prove to be a valuable piece of knowledge for researchers, students, practitioners and scholars across the globe.

List of Contributors

Michael Bitar, Andreas Boldt, Marie-Theres Freitag and Ulrich Sack
Medical Faculty, Institute of Clinical Immunology, University of Leipzig, Leipzig, Germany

Bernd Gruhn
Department of Pediatrics, Jena University Hospital, Jena, Germany

Ulrike Köhl
Medical Faculty, Institute of Clinical Immunology, University of Leipzig, Leipzig, Germany
Hannover Medical School, Institute of Cellular Therapeutics, Hannover, Germany
Fraunhofer Institute for Immunology and Cell Therapy (IZI), Leipzig, Germany

Patricia A. Merkel and Vijaya Knight
Section of Allergy and Immunology, Department of Pediatrics, University of Colorado School of Medicine, Denver, CO, United States

Terri Lebo
Advanced Diagnostic Laboratories, National Jewish Health, Denver, CO, United States

Manisha Rajan Madkaikar, Snehal Shabrish, Manasi Kulkarni, Jahnavi Aluri, Aparna Dalvi, Madhura Kelkar and Maya Gupta
Department of Paediatric Immunology and Leukocyte Biology, National Institute of Immunohematology (ICMR), Mumbai, India

Samuel Cern Cher Chiang, Jack J. Bleesing and Rebecca A. Marsh
Division of Bone Marrow Transplantation and Immune Deficiency, Cincinnati Children's Hospital Medical Center, Cincinnati, OH, United States
Department of Pediatrics, University of Cincinnati, Cincinnati, OH, United States

Jacques J. M. van Dongen
Department of Immunohematology and Blood Transfusion, Leiden University Medical Center, Leiden, Netherlands

Marjolein Wentink
Department of Immunology, Erasmus MC, Rotterdam, Netherlands

Melissa Dullaers
Ablynx, A Sanofi Company, Zwijnaarde, Belgium

Tomas Kalina and Ester Mejstrikova
Department of Pediatric Hematology and Oncology, University Hospital Motol, Charles University, Prague, Czechia

Elena Blanco, Alberto Orfao and Martin Perez-Andres
Department of Medicine, Cancer Research Centre (IBMCC, USAL-CSIC), Cytometry Service (NUCLEUS), University of Salamanca (USAL), Institute of Biomedical Research of Salamanca (IBSAL), Salamanca, Spain
Biomedical Research Networking Centre Consortium of Oncology (CIBERONC), CB/16/12/00233, Instituto Carlos III, Madrid, Spain

Marcela Vlkova
Institute of Clinical Immunology and Allergology, St. Anne's University Hospital Brno, Masaryk University, Brno, Czechia

Eduardo Lopez-Granados
Department of Immunology, Hospital Universitario La Paz, Madrid, Spain

Anne-Kathrin Kienzler
Experimental Medicine Division, Nuffield Department of Medicine, University of Oxford, Oxford, United Kingdom

Jan Philippé
Department of Laboratory Medicine, University Hospital Ghent, Ghent, Belgium

Ana E. Sousa
Faculdade de Medicina, Instituto de Medicina Molecular, Universidade de Lisboa, Lisbon, Portugal

Menno C. van Zelm
Department of Immunology, Erasmus MC, Rotterdam, Netherlands
Department of Immunology and Pathology, Central Clinical School, Alfred Hospital, Monash University, Melbourne, VIC, Australia

Mirjam van der Burg
Department of Immunology, Erasmus MC, Rotterdam, Netherlands
Department of Pediatrics, Leiden University Medical Center, Leiden, Netherlands

Edgar Borges de Oliveira Jr.
Immunogenic Inc., São Paulo, Brazil

Ester Mejstríková, Vendula Šinkorova, Jan Stuchly and Tomas Kalina
Department of Paediatric Haematology and Oncology, Second Faculty of Medicine, Charles University and University Hospital Motol, Prague, Czechia

Alberto Orfao, Martin Perez-Andres and Elena Blanco
Department of Medicine, Cancer Research Centre (IBMCC, USAL-CSIC), Cytometry Service (NUCLEUS), University of Salamanca (USAL), Institute of Biomedical Research of Salamanca (IBSAL), Salamanca, Spain
Biomedical Research Networking Centre Consortium of Oncology (CIBERONC), Instituto de Salud Carlos III, Madrid, Spain

Eduardo Lopez-Granados
Immunology, Universitario La Paz, Madrid, Spain

Carolien Bonroy
Laboratory for Clinical Biology and Hematology, University Hospital Ghent, Ghent, Belgium

Ana E. Sousa
Faculdade de Medicina, Instituto de Medicina Molecular, Universidade de Lisboa, Lisbon, Portugal

Anne-Kathrin Kienzler
BRC-Translational Immunology Lab, University of Oxford, Oxford, United Kingdom

Menno C. van Zelm
Department of Immunology and Pathology, Central Clinical School, Monash University, Melbourne, VIC, Australia

Jacques J. M. van Dongen
Department of Immunology, Erasmus MC, Rotterdam, Netherlands
Department of Immunohematology and Blood Transfusion, Leiden University Medical Center Leiden, Netherlands

Amit Rawat, Kanika Arora, Jitendra Shandilya, Pandiarajan Vignesh, Deepti Suri, Gurjit Kaur, Rashmi Rikhi, Vibhu Joshi, Jhumki Das, Babu Mathew and Surjit Singh
Allergy Immunology Unit, Department of Pediatrics, Advanced Pediatrics Center, Post Graduate Institute of Medical Education and Research, Chandigarh, India

Andreja N. Kopitar and Alojz Ihan
Faculty of Medicine, Institute of Microbiology and Immunology, University of Ljubljana, Ljubljana, Slovenia

Tadej Avčin
Department of Allergology, Rheumatology and Clinical Immunology, University Children's Hospital, University Medical Center Ljubljana, Ljubljana, Slovenia
Department of Pediatrics, Faculty of Medicine, University of Ljubljana, Ljubljana, Slovenia

Gašper Markelj and Štefan Blazina
Department of Allergology, Rheumatology and Clinical Immunology, University Children's Hospital, University Medical Center Ljubljana, Ljubljana, Slovenia

Miha Oražem
Department of Radiation Oncology, Institute of Oncology Ljubljana, Ljubljana, Slovenia

Maruša Debeljak
Unit for Special Laboratory Diagnostics, University Children's Hospital, University Medical Center Ljubljana, Ljubljana, Slovenia

Annelies Emmaneel, Sofie Van Gassen and Yvan Saeys
Department of Applied Mathematics, Computer Science and Statistics, Ghent University, Ghent, Belgium
Data Mining and Modeling for Biomedicine, VIB Center for Inflammation Research, Ghent, Belgium

Delfien J. Bogaert and Filomeen Haerynck
Primary Immunodeficiency Research Lab, Center for Primary Immunodeficiency Ghent, Jeffrey Modell Diagnosis and Research Center, Ghent University Hospital, Ghent, Belgium
Department of Internal Medicine and Pediatrics, Ghent University, Ghent, Belgium

Simon J. Tavernier
Primary Immunodeficiency Research Lab, Center for Primary Immunodeficiency Ghent, Jeffrey Modell Diagnosis and Research Center, Ghent University Hospital, Ghent, Belgium
Department of Biomedical Molecular Biology, Ghent University, Ghent, Belgium
Unit of Molecular Signal Transduction in Inflammation, VIB Center for Inflammation Research, Ghent, Belgium

Otavio Cabral-Marques and Antonio Condino-Neto
Department of Immunology, Institute of Biomedical Sciences, University of São Paulo, São Paulo, Brazil

Lena F. Schimke
Department of Rheumatology and Clinical Immunology, Faculty of Medicine, Center for Chronic Immunodeficiency (CCI), Medical Center-University of Freiburg, University of Freiburg, Freiburg im Breisgau, Germany

Nadia El Khawanky
Department of Hematology, Oncology and Stem Cell Transplantation, Freiburg University Medical Center, Freiburg im Breisgau, Germany
Precision Medicine Theme, The South Australian Health and Medical Research Institute (SAHMRI), Adelaide, SA, Australia

Rodrigo Nalio Ramos
INSERM U932, SiRIC Translational Immunotherapy Team, Institut Curie, Paris Sciences et Lettres Research University, Paris, France

Basel K. Al-Ramadi
Department of Medical Microbiology and Immunology, College of Medicine and Health Sciences, UAE University, Al Ain, United Arab Emirates

Gesmar Rodrigues Silva Segundo
Department of Pediatrics, Federal University of Uberlandia Medical School, Uberlândia, Brazil

Hans D. Ochs
Department of Pediatrics, University of Washington School of Medicine, and Seattle Children's Research Institute, Seattle, WA, United States

Menno C. van Zelm
Department of Immunology and Pathology, Central Clinical School, Monash University, Melbourne, VIC, Australia
Allergy, Asthma and Clinical Immunology Service, Department of Respiratory, Allergy and Clinical Immunology (Research), Central Clinical School, Monash University, The Alfred Hospital, Melbourne, VIC, Australia
The Jeffrey Modell Diagnostic and Research Centre for Primary Immunodeficiencies in Melbourne, Melbourne, VIC, Australia

Pei M. Aui and Samuel De Jong
Department of Immunology and Pathology, Central Clinical School, Monash University, Melbourne, VIC, Australia
The Jeffrey Modell Diagnostic and Research Centre for Primary Immunodeficiencies in Melbourne, Melbourne, VIC, Australia

Paul U. Cameron
The Jeffrey Modell Diagnostic and Research Centre for Primary Immunodeficiencies in Melbourne, Melbourne, VIC, Australia
Department of Infectious Diseases, Alfred Hospital and Monash University, Melbourne, VIC, Australia
The Peter Doherty Institute for Infection and Immunity, University of Melbourne and Royal Melbourne Hospital, Melbourne, VIC, Australia

Fiona Hore-Lacy, Robyn E. O'Hehir, Robert G. Stirling and Julian J. Bosco
Allergy, Asthma and Clinical Immunology Service, Department of Respiratory, Allergy and Clinical Immunology (Research), Central Clinical School, Monash University, The Alfred Hospital, Melbourne, VIC, Australia
The Jeffrey Modell Diagnostic and Research Centre for Primary Immunodeficiencies in Melbourne, Melbourne, VIC, Australia

Rita Polito and Aurora Daniele
Dipartimento di Scienze e Tecnologie Ambientali Biologiche Farmaceutiche, Università degli Studi della Campania "Luigi Vanvitelli," Caserta, Italy
CEINGE-Biotecnologie Avanzate Scarl, Naples, Italy

Ersilia Nigro
CEINGE-Biotecnologie Avanzate Scarl, Naples, Italy
Dipartimento di Scienze Mediche Traslazionali, Allergologia e Immunologia Clinica, Università degli Studi di Napoli Federico II, Naples, Italy

Antonio Pecoraro, Arturo Genovese and Giuseppe Spadaro
Dipartimento di Scienze Mediche Traslazionali, Allergologia e Immunologia Clinica, Università degli Studi di Napoli Federico II, Naples, Italy

Franco Perna and Alessandro Sanduzzi
Dipartimento di Medicina Clinica e Chirurgia, Università degli Studi di Napoli "Federico II," Naples, Italy

Julia I. Ellyard, Robert Tunningley, Ayla May Lorenzo, Amelia Cook, David A. Fulcher and Carola G. Vinuesa
Department of Immunology and Infectious Diseases, Australian National University, Canberra, ACT, Australia
Centre for Personalised Immunology, John Curtin School of Medical Research, Australian National University, Canberra, ACT, Australia

Simon H. Jiang
Department of Immunology and Infectious Diseases, Australian National University, Canberra, ACT, Australia
Centre for Personalised Immunology, John Curtin School of Medical Research, Australian National University, Canberra, ACT, Australia
Department of Nephrology, The Canberra Hospital, Canberra, ACT, Australia

Ann-Maree Hatch and Anastasia Wilson
Centre for Personalised Immunology, John Curtin School of Medical Research, Australian National University, Canberra, ACT, Australia

Maria Ludovica Monaco
CEINGE-Biotecnologie Avanzate Scarl, Naples, Italy

Rochna Chand and Matthew C. Cook
Department of Immunology and Infectious Diseases, Australian National University, Canberra, ACT, Australia
Centre for Personalised Immunology, John Curtin School of Medical Research, Australian National University, Canberra, ACT, Australia
Department of Immunology, The Canberra Hospital, Canberra, ACT, Australia

Dipti Talaulikar
Department of Hematology, The Canberra Hospital, Canberra, ACT, Australia

Rosa Anita Fernandes and Emilia Faria
Allergy and Clinical Immunology Department, Centro Hospitalar e Universitário de Coimbra, Coimbra, Portugal

Martin Perez-Andres, Elena Blanco, Ignacio Criado, Julia Almeida, Vitor Botafogo and Alberto Orfao
Department of Medicine, Cancer Research Centre (IBMCC, USAL-CSIC), Cytometry Service (NUCLEUS), University of Salamanca (USAL), Salamanca, Spain
Institute of Biomedical Research of Salamanca (IBSAL), Salamanca, Spain
Biomedical Research Networking Centre on Cancer-CIBER-CIBERONC (CB16/12/00400), Institute of Health Carlos III, Madrid, Spain

Maria Jara-Acevedo
Institute of Biomedical Research of Salamanca (IBSAL), Salamanca, Spain
Biomedical Research Networking Centre on Cancer-CIBER-CIBERONC (CB16/12/00400), Institute of Health Carlos III, Madrid, Spain
Sequencing DNA Service, NUCLEUS, University of Salamanca, Salamanca, Spain

Rita R. Barbosa
Faculdade de Medicina, Instituto de Medicina Molecular João Lobo Antunes, Universidade de Lisboa, Lisbon, Portugal

Artur Paiva
Flow Cytometry Unit—Clinical Pathology Department, Centro Hospitalar e Universitário de Coimbra, Coimbra, Portugal
Ciências Biomédicas Laboratoriais, ESTESC-Coimbra Health School, Instituto Politécnico de Coimbra, Coimbra, Portugal
Faculty of Medicine, Coimbra Institute for Clinical and Biomedical Research (iCBR), University of Coimbra, Coimbra, Portugal

Ines Coutinho
Dermatology Department, Centro Hospitalar e Universitário de Coimbra, Coimbra, Portugal

Jacques J. M. van Dongen
Department of Immunohematology and Blood Transfusion, Leiden University Medical Center, Leiden, Netherlands

Carmela Giancotta, Cristina Cifaldi and Maria Chiriaco
Unit of Immunology and Infectious Diseases, Academic Department of Pediatrics, Bambino Gesù Children's Hospital, Rome, Italy

Enrico Attardi
Unit of Immunology and Infectious Diseases, Academic Department of Pediatrics, Bambino Gesù Children's Hospital, Rome, Italy
Department of Experimental and Clinical Medicine, University of Florence, Florence, Italy

Nicola Cotugno
Department of Systems Medicine, University of Rome Tor Vergata, Rome, Italy
Research Unit of Congenital and Perinatal Infection, Academic Department of Pediatrics, Children's Hospital Bambino Gesù, Rome, Italy

Silvia Di Cesare, Donato Amodio, Andrea Finocchi, Gigliola Di Matteo, Paolo Rossi and Caterina Cancrini
Unit of Immunology and Infectious Diseases, Academic Department of Pediatrics, Bambino Gesù Children's Hospital, Rome, Italy,
Department of Systems Medicine, University of Rome Tor Vergata, Rome, Italy

Paolo Palma
Research Unit of Congenital and Perinatal Infection, Academic Department of Pediatrics, Children's Hospital Bambino Gesù, Rome, Italy

Ana Serra-Caetano, Pedro Rosmaninho, Alexandre A. S. F. Raposo, Mariana Fonseca and Ana E. Sousa
Faculdade de Medicina, Instituto de Medicina Molecular João Lobo Antunes, Universidade de Lisboa, Lisbon, Portugal
Centro de Imunodeficiências Primárias, Centro Académico de Medicina de Lisboa, Centro Hospitalar Universitário Lisboa Norte and Faculdade de Medicina da Universidade de Lisboa and Instituto de Medicina Molecular, Lisbon, Portugal

Margarida Gama-Carvalho and Marcelo L. M. Pereira
Faculty of Sciences, BioISI-Biosystems & Integrative Sciences Institute, University of Lisboa, Lisbon, Portugal

Susana L. Silva, Sara P. Silva, Ana Berta Sousa and Rui M. M. Victorino
Faculdade de Medicina, Instituto de Medicina Molecular João Lobo Antunes, Universidade de Lisboa, Lisbon, Portugal
Centro de Imunodeficiências Primárias, Centro Académico de Medicina de Lisboa, Centro Hospitalar Universitário Lisboa Norte and Faculdade de Medicina da Universidade de Lisboa and Instituto de Medicina Molecular, Lisbon, Portugal
Centro Hospitalar Universitário Lisboa Norte, Hospital de Santa Maria, Lisbon, Portugal

Martin Pérez-Andrés and Elena Blanco
Department of Medicine, Cancer Research Centre (IBMCC, USAL-CSIC), Cytometry Service (NUCLEUS), Institute of Biomedical Research of Salamanca (IBSAL), University of Salamanca (USAL), Salamanca, Spain
Biomedical Research Networking Centre on Cancer-CIBER-CIBERONC, Number CB16/12/00400, Institute of Health Carlos III, Madrid, Spain

Lennart Hammarstrom
Department of Laboratory Medicine, Karolinska Institutet, Stockholm, Sweden

Cindy S. Ma and Stuart G. Tangye
Immunology Division, Garvan Institute of Medical Research, Sydney, NSW, Australia
Faculty of Medicine, St. Vincent's Clinical School, UNSW Sydney, Sydney, NSW, Australia
Clincial Immunogenomics Research Consortium Australia, Darlinghurst, NSW, Australia

Emily S. J. Edwards and Pei M. Aui
Department of Immunology and Pathology, Central Clinical School, Monash University and The Alfred Hospital, Melbourne, VIC, Australia
The Jeffrey Modell Diagnostic and Research Centre for Primary Immunodeficiencies in Melbourne, Melbourne, VIC, Australia

Robert G. Stirling, Paul U. Cameron, Josh Chatelier, Fiona Hore-Lacy and Julian J. Bosco
The Jeffrey Modell Diagnostic and Research Centre for Primary Immunodeficiencies in Melbourne, Melbourne, VIC, Australia
Allergy, Asthma and Clinical Immunology Service, Department of Respiratory, Allergy and Clinical Immunology (Research), Central Clinical School, The Alfred Hospital, Melbourne, VIC, Australia

Robyn E. O'Hehir and Menno C. van Zelm
Department of Immunology and Pathology, Central Clinical School, Monash University and The Alfred Hospital, Melbourne, VIC, Australia
The Jeffrey Modell Diagnostic and Research Centre for Primary Immunodeficiencies in Melbourne, Melbourne, VIC, Australia
Allergy, Asthma and Clinical Immunology Service, Department of Respiratory, Allergy and Clinical Immunology (Research), Central Clinical School, The Alfred Hospital, Melbourne, VIC, Australia

Marjolein W. J. Wentink and Hanna IJspeert
Department of Immunology, Erasmus MC, University Medical Center Rotterdam, Rotterdam, Netherlands

Tomas Kalina
Department of Paediatric Haematology and Oncology, Second Faculty of Medicine, Charles University and University Hospital Motol, Prague, Czechia

Martin Perez-Andres, Quentin Lecrevisse and Alberto Orfao
Department of Medicine-Service Cytometry, Cancer Research Center (IBMCC-CSIC/USAL) and University of Salamanca, Salamanca, Spain

Lucia del Pino Molina
Department of Clinical Immunology, La Paz University Hospital, Lymphocyte Pathophysiology in Immunodeficiencies Group La Paz Institute for Health Research (IdiPAZ), Madrid, Spain

François G. Kavelaars
Department of Hematology, Erasmus MC, University Medical Center Rotterdam, Rotterdam, Netherlands

Arjan C. Lankester and Jacques J. M. van Dongen
Department of Immunohematology and Blood Transfusion, Leiden University Medical Center, Leiden, Netherlands

Mirjam van der Burg
Department of Immunology, Erasmus MC, University Medical Center Rotterdam, Rotterdam, Netherlands
Department of Pediatrics, Leiden University Medical Center, Leiden, Netherlands

Index

www.ingramcontent.com/pod-product-compliance
Lightning Source LLC
LaVergne TN
LVHW080951210926
848485LV00004B/815
* 9 7 8 1 6 4 6 4 7 5 7 3 5 *